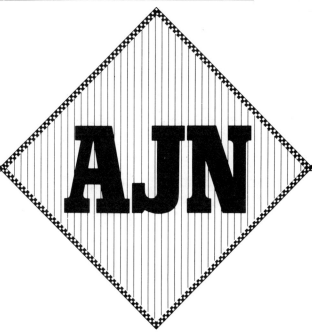

THE QUESTION AND ANSWER BOOK

FOR THE NCLEX-RN EXAMINATION

Coordinators for this Edition

Mariann C. Lovell, RN, MS. *Assistant Professor of Nursing, Wright State University, Dayton, OH*
B. Patricia Nix, RN, MSN. *Instructor of Nursing, Henry Ford Community College, Dearborn, MI*
Mary Paquette, MN, RN. *Assistant Professor, California State University, LA, Los Angeles, CA*
Paulette D. Rollant, MSN, RN, CCRN. *Assistant Professor, Emory University; President, Multi-Resources, Inc., Atlanta, GA*

Contributing Authors for this Edition

Paula J. Albertson, BSN, RN. *Clinical Nurse, National Institutes of Health, Bethesda, MD*
M. Regina Asaro, BSN, RN. *Psychiatric Nurse, National Institutes of Health, Bethesda, MD*
Diane J. Baker, BSN, RN. *Psychiatric Nurse, National Institutes of Health, Bethesda, MD*
Deborah DiGiaro, MS, RN. *Psychotherapist, Northridge, CA*
Silva Foxpuglisi, MS, RN. *Associate Professor, California State University, Long Beach, CA*
Elizabeth C. Kaiser, MSN, RN. *Coordinator, Psychiatric Consultation Liaison Nursing Service, Hospital of the University of Pennsylvania, Philadelphia, PA*
Susan L. W. Krupnick, MSN, CCRN, CEN, CS, RN. *Psychiatric Consultation Liaison Nurse, Hospital of the University of Pennsylvania Medical Center, Philadelphia, PA*
Elizabeth J. Lipp, MS, RN. *Instructor, Wright State University School of Nursing, Dayton, OH*
Mary-Charles Santopietro, EdD, MS, EdM, RN. *Clinical Director, Mental-Health Nursing, Suburban Hospital, Bethesda, MD*
Jean H. Woods, PhD, RNCS. *Assistant Professor, Temple University College of Allied Health Professions, Department of Nursing, Philadelphia, PA*
Marybeth Young, RN, MSN. *Assistant Professor, Maternal-Child Health Nursing, Niehoff School of Nursing, Loyola University, Chicago, IL*

Contributing Authors for Previous Edition

Janis P. Bellack, MN, RN
Kay Bensing, MA, RN
Louise Bradford, RN, MSN
Nancy Jo Bush, MN, RN
Geraldine C. Colombraro, MA, RN
Olivian DeSouza, MSN, RN

Gita L. Dhillon, MEd, RN
Cynthia Dunsmore, MS, RN
Janice M. Dyehouse, MSN, RN
Doris S. Edwards, MS, RN
Lou Ann T. Emerson, MSN, RN
Linda Finke, MSN, RN
Julia B. George, PhD, RN
Jo Ann Gragnani, MS, MA, RN
Cynthia Smith Greenberg, MS, RN, CPNP
Carol Seal Hildebrand, MSN, RN
Wendy B. Hollis, MN, RN
Carolyn Kay Jass, MS, RN
Ann L. Jessop, MSN, RN
Phyllis Walls Juett, MSN, RN
Michele M. Kamradt, EdD, RN
Shari Wazney Keba, MSN, RN
Retha Vornholt Keenan, MSN, RN
Marie Trava King, MAN, RN
Deborah Koniak, EdD, RN
Beverly Kopala, MS, RN
Judith K. Leavitt, MEd, RN
Mariann C. Lovell, MS, RN
Esther Matassarin-Jacobs, PhD, MSN, MEd, RN
Edwina A. McConnell, PhD, MS, RN
Michele Michael, MSN, RN
Mary Ann Niehaus, MSN, RN
B. Patricia Nix, MSN, RN
Joan Webster Reighley, MN, RN
Constance Ritzman, MSN, RN
Mary-Charles Santopietro, EdD, MS, EdM, RN
Victoria Schoolcraft, MSN, RN
Virginia Madden Shea, MS, RN
Brenda Hanson Smith, MSN, RNC
Janet Trigg, MSN, RN
Quilla D.B. Turner, PhD, MN, RN
Deborah L. Ulrich, MA, RN
Esther Coto Walloch, MN, RN
Gail D. Wegner, MS, RN
Elizabeth Elder Weiner, PhD, RN
Donna J. Woodside, EdD, RN
Nancy K. Worley, MSN, RN
Marybeth Young, MSN, RN

THE AMERICAN JOURNAL OF NURSING COMPANY

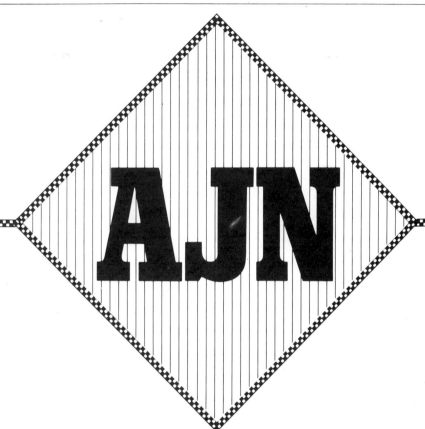

THE QUESTION AND ANSWER BOOK

FOR THE NCLEX-RN EXAMINATION

 WILLIAMS & WILKINS

Baltimore • Hong Kong • London • Sydney

Editor: Rose Mary Carroll-Johnson
Associate Editor: Linda Napora
Design: Catherine Chambers
Production: Anne Seitz

Accurate indications, adverse reactions, and dosage schedules for drugs are provided in this book, but it is possible that they may change. The reader is urged to review the package information data of the manufacturers of the medications mentioned.

First Edition 1984

Printed in the United States of America

Library of Congress Cataloging in Publication Data

AJN, the question and answer book.
    p.   cm.
  At head of title: The American Journal of Nursing Company.
  Companion v. to: AJN . . . nursing boards review for the NCLEX-RN examination.
  Includes bibliographies and index.
  ISBN 0-683-09539-0
  1. Nursing—Examinations, questions, etc. I. American Journal of Nursing Company.
II. AJN . . . nursing boards review for the NCLEX-RN examination.
  [DNLM: 1. Nursing—examination questions. WY 18 A3125]
RT55.A37 1988   610.73'076—dc19   87-31811
DNLM/DLC for Library of Congress   CIP

| | | | | | 88 | 89 | 90 | 91 | 91 |
| 1 | 2 | 3 | 4 | 5 | 6 | 7 | 8 | 9 | 10 |

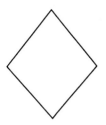

Foreword

One of the final steps before full admission to the nursing profession is to document achievement of basic knowledge for safe and effective nursing practice. The *AJN Question and Answer Book* provides guidance to assist you in preparation for the test-taking experience. It is not a substitute for your educational program, but it is an excellent supplemental resource prior to the NCLEX-RN exam and to entry into practice.

Nursing is confronted with many new challenges in addressing health care now and in preparation for the future. Changes in health care delivery and in health care practices are evident throughout the country, and the proposed resolutions for the future can only be described as transitional. Perhaps the challenges are best summarized by the statement "the prospects never looked brighter and the problems never looked tougher."

Nursing has a history of commitment and compassion in working with others to plan and to deliver health care. As new graduates in nursing, you can build upon the achievements of nursing to address the current and future challenges of the health field. John Gardner, in *No Easy Victories*, speaks to the need for a commitment of mind and heart in times of change. As you enter the practice of nursing, may each of you continue to learn and to provide nursing care that reflects thoughtful and compassionate commitment to health care for all people.

Lorene Fisher, MA, RN, FAAN
Professor and Dean
Wayne State University
College of Nursing
Detroit, Michigan

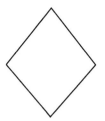

Editor's Note

There are events that occur in our lives that we remember more vividly than others. For a registered nurse, taking the "state board exam" seems to be one of those events. Also memorable is the pre-exam study period.

There used to be only one review book available (that made selection easy). Now there are many texts available, and all show agreement on one point—at least part of your study time should be devoted to answering practice questions.

On the pages of this book you will find over 1900 practice questions. They were written and edited by registered nurses. The questions reflect client situations across the lifespan, and every effort has been made to ensure that the information offered is not only accurate, but clear.

Part of the book has been organized in such a way that it corresponds to the *AJN Nursing Boards Review*. In this edition, we have extrapolated enough questions to devise two complete sample NCLEX-type exams. The index will help you locate questions on a particular topic.

Also included in this edition are expanded rationales for the correct answer. We have included more information about why the wrong answers are wrong. If you still desire more information about a given answer, each rationale refers you to a section of the *AJN Nursing Boards Review* where you can find out more about the topic.

The appendices categorize the questions according to the steps of the nursing process and client needs. Decisions regarding the categories were made after consultation with the contributing authors and the National Council of State Boards of Nursing. You will be tested on your abilities to *apply the steps of the nursing process*, not on your ability to assign a category to an individual question.

We believe that this book of questions, in conjunction with the *AJN Nursing Boards Review*, offers you excellent preparation to pass the NCLEX-RN. YOU CAN DO IT! Best of luck in your nursing career.

Rose Mary Carroll-Johnson, MN, RN

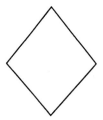

Preface

All of us who have ever been involved—as the AJN Company has for many years—in review courses, appreciate the stress under which you are operating right now. Regardless of how well you did in nursing school, you are in the midst of a special cram time, sorting your knowledge in preparation for the NCLEX-RN.

You have made a good beginning in choosing this book, which will help you to organize your studying and make the most of this period. The *AJN Question and Answer Book* has been developed by expert curriculum committees made up of top clinical faculty who are very experienced in teaching our highly successful nursing review courses. They are knowledgeable not only in their own areas of expertise but in knowing how to help you focus on the NCLEX-RN format. The book contains two full sample tests and many, many additional questions to help you get comfortable in answering multiple-choice questions.

If you want a still greater sense of security about your exam, please do call us for information about an AJN Nursing Boards Review course. Our toll-free number is (800) 223–2282; in New York State, call (212) 582–8820 collect.

One more thing—our very best wishes to you for success in the exam and throughout your nursing career. You have chosen a wonderful career. Welcome to it.

Thelma M. Schorr, RN
President and Publisher
American Journal of Nursing Company

◇ Introduction

Each year, students attending our AJN Nursing Boards Review courses have always asked for more practice questions to study on their own. To meet this need, the American Journal of Nursing Company publishes the *AJN Question and Answer Book*. A companion to the *AJN Nursing Boards Review* book, this new revised edition is organized for you to practice testing your knowledge.

Section 1 explains in detail the NCLEX testing format and scoring methodology. Strategies to help you read questions more carefully and select the correct answer are included to increase your test-wiseness. Techniques to help you reduce your stress on the day of the examination are also presented. Read this section first and refer to it as often as necessary for reinforcement whenever you encounter any difficulties understanding any questions or the rationales for the answers.

Sections 2 through 5 contain over 1100 questions and rationales that have been organized according to the following content areas:

— Nursing Care of the Client with Psychosocial, Psychiatric/Mental Health Problems
— Nursing Care of the Adult
— Nursing Care of the Childbearing Family
— Nursing Care of the Child

Develop a system for review by first doing those questions in the content area where you feel least secure. The contents for each section will help you locate questions which test specific health problems within that section. Based on your answers and your understanding of the correct rationales, you may decide you need to review content in a specific area using your textbooks or the *AJN Nursing Boards Review* book. Appropriate reprints of articles from *The American Journal of Nursing* and *MCN: The American Journal of Maternal/Child Nursing* have been included to further enhance your knowledge.

In the appendices at the back of the book you will find that each question has been categorized according to the nursing process (assessment, analysis, planning, implementation, and evaluation) and client needs (environmental safety, physiologic integrity, psychosocial integrity, and health promotion). These appendices will help you to assess your knowledge and ability in each of these areas.

Section 6 includes two complete NCLEX-RN-type examinations for practice. The test items have been carefully mixed for content. When you feel ready, set aside time for each examination. The goal is to answer each book (95 questions) within 90 minutes.

Give yourself a break between each section of the examination. To determine your score, divide the number of your correct answers by the total number of questions on the examination. A score of less than 75% indicates you need to spend more time reviewing in those areas indicated by the questions you answered incorrectly. It may also be helpful to review again the test-taking strategies outlined in Section 1.

The test items in this book have been prepared by our national faculty who teach in the AJN Nursing Boards Review course. All are instructors, clinical specialists, and/or authors in their clinical speciality. They, as well as all of us involved in the production of this book at the American Journal of Nursing Company and at Williams & Wilkins, wish you every success on your NCLEX-RN examination and in your career as a registered professional nurse.

Remember—you are a graduate of a professional nursing school and you DO know this material!

Patricia Jones, MEd, RN
Director
Professional Seminars Division

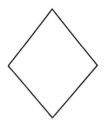

Contents

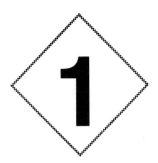

Preparing for the NCLEX-RN

Marybeth Young, MSN, RN

Section 1: Preparing for the NCLEX-RN

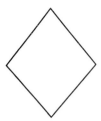

Preparing for the NCLEX-RN

Keys to Success on the State Boards

Know the Test Format
- An integrated exam
- Single response, multiple-choice items
- Based on measurement of safe nursing behaviors for common health problems

Review Concepts
- Growth and development pharmacology
- Effects of culture and nutrition on health
- The nursing process
- Systems of health care decision making

Where Should You Begin?
- What is the area of least confidence?

How Should You Prepare?
- Consider your strengths and how you review or learn effectively.

Available Resources
- Review course notes and texts.
- Consider a review program.
- Use human resources and support services.

Strategies to Promote Success
- Begin with self-evaluation.
- Sharpen test-taking skills.
- Learn methods to reduce stress.
- Be self-confident.

Just Before the Exam
- Get a night's sleep.
- Avoid late cramming.
- Eat breakfast.

During the NCLEX
- Be precise in marking answer spaces.
- Use time wisely.
- Be "test-wise."
- Keep emotions in control.

Used with permission.   © 1982 M.Young, B.Kopala

Pretest

Please respond to the following questions by darkening the circle next to the *best* option.
1. Test items on the NCLEX-RN are multiple choice with
   - ○ 1. one single correct response.
   - ○ 2. multiple-multiple options.
2. The average time available to answer each item in the four test sections is about

- ○ 1. 20 seconds.
- ○ 2. 30 seconds.
- ○ 3. 45 seconds.
- ○ 4. 60 seconds.
3. There are approximately the same number of test items measuring
   - ○ 1. knowledge of pediatric and medical/surgical nursing.
   - ○ 2. understanding of each nursing process phase.
   - ○ 3. nursing judgment in acute and community settings.
   - ○ 4. applied knowledge and recall of information.
4. Scoring of the licensure exam depends on the
   - ○ 1. total of right minus wrong answers.
   - ○ 2. percentage of test items completed.
   - ○ 3. difficulty level of the questions.
   - ○ 4. actual number of correct responses.

Reading the following section may make the difference between passing and failing the licensing exam.

Preparing for the Licensure Exam

Planning for Review

You made a career choice that has required long-range planning and an investment of time, energy, and money. Now, your preparation for the NCLEX-RN examination (State Boards) requires the same thoughtful planning. *Passing* will be confirmation of your professional competence. This section of the book is designed to help you achieve that goal.

A summary of the exam format, suggested cognitive strategies, and approaches to reduce tension should help you develop a personal plan for preparation and review. You will then be able to use the nursing review that follows to organize specialty knowledge for a broader understanding of safe practice.

While the content is basic, there are many unique features in this text; take a few moments to become familiar with the layout. Notice that the *nursing process* is the basis for patient care. Each assessment and implementation is in priority sequence; goals and evaluations are patient centered. Space is available in the margin to indicate, with a symbol or check, those areas needing further attention.

The content is supplemented with tables, summaries, and illustrations to clarify and reinforce knowledge of specific health problems. Additionally, at the end of each section there are reprints of articles for fuller reference.

Featured after the review materials are four separate practice tests, simulating the actual NCLEX exam, which may be used in several ways. You may select one test and complete it under time control similar to the 1 minute per one item exam. Or you may select several case studies and answer the questions that follow as you review the specific content, then referring to the correct answer and rationale, compare your problem-solving skills with those of testing experts. Return to the content outline or a nursing text as needed to clarify doubts or improve understanding. Look for patterns of test-taking difficulty as you review the test responses. Evaluation of your own test-taking skills is a major step toward improving that ability, and gives more meaningful feedback than a tally of errors.

When you are familiar with the book, map out a personal plan for preparation and review. If independent study is anticipated, set realistic goals within the time available. Begin with the content areas that seem less familiar or about which you feel insecure—your results on national standardized tests could serve as a guide. By beginning with the greatest challenge and reinforcing that knowledge, your confidence is renewed.

Know the Test Format

Just as the novice driver needs to know what to expect on the state driving test, each graduate nurse needs a clear idea of the licensure exam format. Knowing that you have some questions about the NCLEX format, the following brief summary will provide answers.

Success on a national examination is required for entry to professional practice. The same multiple-choice test is administered simultaneously throughout the United States each February and July. Although the future may bring individualized computer testing, the current process assembles masses in large, impersonal settings in each state.

There are approximately 93 test items on each of four separate, integrated sections. (A few of the questions are "pilot items" and do not count.) Situations and questions represent a variety of patient health problems. One case study describing the needs of an elderly diabetic cared for at home may be followed by another case study focusing on the problems of a hospitalized adolescent amputee. Test items focus on critical requirements for safe nursing practice rather than separately testing knowledge of specialties such as adult medical-surgical or pediatric nursing.

How the Test is Scored

The grading method differs significantly from the standardized achievement or aptitude tests used in college placement. Instructions given prior to the SAT or ACT urge the high school student to avoid guessing. Directions given to you in the nursing licensure exam stress that guessing is not penalized. The **pass/fail** score is based on the number of correct responses, which are equally weighted. Success on the exam reflects demonstration of minimal competence. Completing all the questions becomes a critical goal because of this grading process. An educated guess may contribute to a passing score, if you can narrow the four options to two possibilities. The probability then is 50% for making a correct choice by guess.

Applied knowledge, rather than mere recall of facts, is measured in most test questions. Case studies present a specific situation, followed by six or more questions. In order to answer those questions, you will need to transfer knowledge from clinical experience and classroom learning to meet the patient's needs. Expect to find the test questions challenging and of varied levels of difficulty. Application of knowledge may be subtle, such as asking for a toy appropriate for a hospitalized toddler in a body cast; or an emergency situation such as a roadside birth may be described. Remember that care standards are based on general principles; problems implied in the setting often do not affect priorities for care.

The National Council of State Boards of Nursing organizes the licensure examination around a specific framework: the *Nursing Process, and Categories of Human Needs.* Each is summarized briefly, and implications for testing are suggested.

The nursing process provides organization for the test as it does for actual care planning in every clinical setting. Each nursing process phase is equally important in resolving health problems. This consistency is immediately evident to test takers who perceive this equal emphasis. These same graduates are quick to point out that the number of items testing maternity or psychiatric nursing are not equal. Table 1.1 suggests possible test item focus for each phase of the nursing process.

Health Needs are four categories of client needs. Based on the ANA Nursing Social Policy Statement and research on the role of the beginning practitioner, these Needs are detailed in tables 1.2 and 1.3. Emphasis is on physiologic integrity, safe care, and health promotion/maintenance.

Concepts basic to understanding human needs are another exam focus. Among these are Maslow's hierarchy of needs, the teaching-learning process, therapeutic communication, crisis intervention, and developmental theory. Anatomy, physiology, pathophysiology, asepsis, pharmacology, nutrition, management principles, accountability, and mental health concepts are also basic to the practice of nursing, and are incorporated into many test items.

Note that meeting the physiologic and emotional needs of patients suggests that priority setting is critical. If a patient has a severe alteration in fluid/gas exchange related to dehydration, the psychosocial problems are not attended to until after the immediate physiologic needs are met. Life-threatening conditions must be resolved initially.

Test features include several aids of importance to you as a test taker. As there is no separate answer sheet, responses are marked by filling in circles to the left of each option. All stray pencil marks and underlining must be erased before turning in the test booklet so that the scanner does not pick them up during the grading process. Mathematical calculations for drugs and IV flow rates may be written on the blank page provided for that purpose. This is also an ideal "scratch sheet" to note items you wish to skip initially and then re-examine after completing most of the exam.

In summary, the NCLEX test plan has been developed to measure critical thinking and nursing competence. Knowing the framework of the exam should dispel some of your fears, and help you to anticipate and prepare for the testing reality. When the actual date arrives, do not think about the "test

---

Table 1.1 Test Item Focus Suggested by the Nursing Process

Phase	Possible Item Focus
Assessment	• Identifying data base • Selecting appropriate means to gather data • Gathering patient/family history • Preparing for/understanding diagnostic tests • Understanding need for further assessment
Analysis	• Identifying potential/actual problems • Listing problems in priority sequence • Interpreting diagnostic test results
Planning	• Setting measurable long-/short-term goals • Identifying priorities for goals • Involving patient/family in process • Examining a suggested plan • Modifying an existing plan • Sharing plan with patient/family/staff
Implementation	• Carrying out nursing actions • Understanding rationale for care • Identifying priorities for care • Calculating dosage accurately • Administering medications/IVs safely • Suggesting diet modifications • Supporting coping styles • Communicating appropriately to patient/family • Teaching to developmental/knowledge level • Ensuring safety/comfort • Preventing infection/injury • Responding to emergencies • Recording/sharing information • Teaching/supervising staff
Evaluation	• Comparing outcomes to goals set • Examining response to therapy, medications • Asking patient pertinent questions • Interpreting patient's feedback • Identifying learning outcomes • Understanding effects of surgery • Recognizing complications of treatment • Communicating feedback on outcomes to staff • Reassessing as needed • Revising plan when indicated

---

Table 1.2 Human Needs

Categories	Nursing Focus
Safe, effective care environment	Coordinating care Ensuring quality Setting goals Promoting Safety Preparing client for treatments/procedures Implementing care
Physiologic integrity	Promoting adaptation Identifying/reducing risks Fostering mobility Ensuring comfort Providing care
Psychosocial Integrity	Promoting adaptation Facilitating coping
Health promotion/maintenance	Promoting growth and development Directing self-care Fostering support systems Preventing/early treatment of disease

Table 1.3 Test Item Focus suggested by Categories of Human Needs

Human Needs Category	Possible Test Item Focus
Safe, effective environment	Understanding basic principles Using management skills Implementing protective measures Promoting safety Ensuring client/family rights Preventing spread of infection
Physiologic integrity	Managing emergencies Using body mechanics Providing comfort measures Using equipment safely Understanding effects of immobility Recognizing untoward responses to therapy/procedures
Psychosocial integrity	Identifying mental health concepts Recognizing behavior change Referring to resources Implementing appropriate care
Health promotion/maintenance	Understanding family systems Teaching nutrition Promoting wellness Recognizing adaptive changes to health alterations Teaching for childbearing Supporting the dying/family Fostering immune responses

Table 1.4 Cognitive Strategies for Success

• Prepare	for safe practice
• Plan a review	to broaden knowledge
• Read carefully	for understanding
• Identify key words	to focus attention
• Narrow options	by critical thinking
• Use educated guess	not random choice
• Set priorities	based on health risk
• Trust decisions	avoid many erasures

plan'' but concentrate on the challenge of each case study and its questions. Just as the driver attends to the road test without wondering ''what is being tested now?'', you need only to address the problem-solving task.

Cognitive and Affective Keys to Success

There are three factors that are important in your achievement of success: *reading,* which affects both reviewing and test taking; *test wiseness,* which has been defined as the ability to use a test and situation to demonstrate learning; and the ability to *control tension* in a major examination, freeing the mind to concentrate on the written questions. While each of these factors is interrelated, each is discussed separately. Suggestions and strategies are offered for use during your licensure exam experience.

Cognitive Strategies to Promote Success

(see table 1.4)
Reading with concentration is a learned skill that is critical for study, review, and examination performance. During advance preparation for the

NCLEX, select an environment that is well lighted and that suits your learning style. Avoid reading on a bed: its comfort may induce sleep rather than reinforce knowledge. Gather all materials in advance for the planned study session, including appropriate texts, notes, and marker pens to highlight critical content or material needing subsequent review.

Skim the content outline, then read for understanding. Look up any unfamiliar terms. Note all further questions that come to mind as you review information. Use your knowledge of anatomy and physiology to visualize the impact of a specific health alteration. Review the disease process and its impact on prevention, restoration, and rehabilitation.

When reading test items as practice or in a real situation, be especially observant for key words. Select the critical ideas from the case study. Notice cues such as age, health habits, and coping mechanisms used. Clearly identify the focus of the question (e.g., the concerned parent, the ill child). Use your knowledge of nursing to think through the question and consider possible responses, even before reading all possible options.

As you consider each situation and question, be sure to control the time spent. During each 90-minute test section you will not have the luxury of time to thoughtfully reread and reflect. For this reason, it is wise to omit the very complex situations that may take several minutes to resolve. Return to those challenges after completing the less difficult items.

While you must read carefully to understand the questions, avoid reading into the words more than is actually stated. Assume that the health care agency described is ideal and well staffed. If you feel that the patient's needs would be met by a midnight snack of milk and fruit, do not qualify this with, ''. . . but it may not be available at night.''

During the exam, you have no resource for defining vocabulary. Use the sentence context to deduce the meaning of unfamiliar words. Refer back to the case study for insight and clarification.

One word of caution about rereading prior questions during the test. Occasionally, a series of items covers several days of care for one patient. Do not alter care priorities for the day of admission, based on results of later diagnostic tests. This is not possible in clinical practice and is a destructive testing strategy.

Test wiseness implies that you have skills available to call upon during an examination, that you know what these are, and are ready to use them. These are not tricks but cognitive approaches to the multiple choice format. Forget the ways you have "psyched out" a professor's tests. Do not anticipate patterns of responses, or frequent use of "2" (the second option) as the BEST response. Realize that the testing service has constructed an excellent examination from the many items submitted by faculty and practitioners across the country. Grammar and length of options are consistent. Past graduates have described the NCLEX as a well-constructed test.

During both the review and the actual exam, consider carefully each option as it resolves the problem suggested. Try to eliminate one or two responses that do not clearly answer the question. Refer back to the test item to clarify the focus. Then, just as you would in a clinical situation, make a decision based on your knowledge of nursing. Or use the "educated guess" approach to select the better option of two possibilities. Trust your decisions! Unless a flash of inspiration strikes later, do not randomly change answers. Self-doubt leads to reduced confidence and often to increased errors.

One approach to the complexity of priority setting for items is to treat the question as a series of true-false statements. This is particularly helpful if all nursing implementations suggested are appropriate, but you are asked to select a *BEST* or *FIRST* action. When reading the stem and each option, ask yourself, "Is the life or well-being of the client at risk if this action is *not* performed initially?" If oxygenation is altered, that physiologic need clearly dictates priority assessments, an emergency plan, and immediate intervention. Other problems may not suggest such a clear solution, and require applied knowledge.

Consider an example of a priority test item:

5. Mrs. Lee is admitted through the emergency room following a bicycle accident in which she suffered a simple fracture of her left foot. During the initial assessment, it is obvious that she is in severe pain. The foot appears swollen and bruised, and is wrapped in an elastic bandage. Which goal is appropriate to meet her needs initially? The patient will
   - ○ 1. accept limited mobility.
   - ○ 2. comply with teaching.
   - ○ 3. experience pain relief.
   - ○ 4. adapt to body-image change.

Using the "true-false" approach, ask yourself, "Does the short-term goal 'accepting mobility limitations' meet her immediate needs?" That option, as well as the others, is an appropriate goal; however her priority need at this time is comfort. Thus the selection of option "3" is the best initial goal.

Communications test items present a special challenge. As in actual practice, nonverbal cues and the specific setting affect the communication process. When reading such questions, consider all factors. Realize that the presence of quotation marks does not automatically signal therapeutic use of self. Identify the type of interaction suggested in the case study (see table 1.5). Apply basic principles, and avoid blocks to effective communications. Base your choice on sound rationale, rather than selecting a response that sounds like you.

Consider the following situation and test items.

6. The nurse employed in a student health center has a varied practice. Maintaining health records for all students is one responsibility. Pre-entrance health requirements include documentation of immunity to measles, polio, and rubella. While taking a health history, a freshman asks why the male students need protection from rubella.

Table 1.5	Focus of Communications Test Items
Type of Interaction	**Approach**
Interview	Asking purposeful questions Using appropriate vocabulary Listening to responses Maintaining confidentiality
Information giving	Describing test/procedure Clarifying data Explaining treatment
Teaching/ learning	Assessing learning needs Using developmentally appropriate terms Giving instructions Demonstrating care Reinforcing knowledge Seeking return demonstration Involving family Evaluating learning
Therapeutic use of self	Establishing trust Developing goal direction Listening actively Clarifying, reflecting Sharing observations Anticipating needs Exploring coping styles Reinforcing positive behavior Supporting Referring for help

Suggest an appropriate response to his question.

○ 1. "University policy dictates equal requirements."
○ 2. "This recommendation follows national guidelines."
○ 3. "These rules ensure minimal exposure on campus."
○ 4. "Elimination of rubella depends on mass immunity."

7. A young woman student asks the nurse about the administration of the tuberculin test during a routine physical assessment. In addition to explaining the purpose of the test, teaching includes which of the following?

○ 1. "Keep the arm dry today; check back in 48 hours if redness develops."
○ 2. "Do not scratch the area; stop in to have it read in 48-72 hours."
○ 3. "Place a Band-Aid on the site; call if there is itching or swelling."
○ 4. "Avoid the sun today; let me know if there is bruising or inflammation."

8. After a seminar on substance abuse, a student asks to speak privately to the nurse. "I am very upset about a close friend who is drinking heavily, is abusive and needs help. I care about him; I am confused and don't know where to turn." Select an appropriate response to the student.

○ 1. "Send your friend over here for help."
○ 2. "Let's talk about what you're feeling."
○ 3. "There are many resources for alcoholism."
○ 4. "Why are you so upset about his problem?"

9. A student treated for a strep infection misses a follow-up appointment. When telephone contact is made, the student apologizes for the missed appointment, but tearfully explains that a brother was assaulted and the family is under great stress. The following day, when she reports for a throat culture, she appears tense and distracted. Which of the following would be an appropriate approach?

○ 1. Allow her to talk if she mentions the attack.
○ 2. Avoid asking questions about the incident.
○ 3. Suggest she discuss matters with a therapist.
○ 4. Ask how she is handling her feelings.

Each of these questions explores nurse-client interactions. Question #6 focuses on giving information based on sound rationale. While each option may be true, "4" best answers the "why" of the student, and is factual. For question #7, a teaching interaction, the correct choice is "2". Notice that each option has a partially correct statement.

The student in question #8 needs a chance to share feelings ("2"). Asking "why" about feelings or behavior is a block to therapeutic communication. Similarly, the woman in question #9 should be asked about her feelings, with a goal of crisis support ("4"). Notice that the last two items focus on the same need, but one is interactive while the second asks about an approach.

If you responded with confidence to these sample items, acknowledge the success. More important, continue to learn from the review of communications techniques, and apply that knowledge in test taking.

In summary, refer to suggested testing strategies periodically, use those that are helpful, and discover that test wiseness can make a difference in demonstrating your nursing knowledge.

Affective Strategies for Success

It is difficult to separate cognitive from emotional factors in test performance. There are, however, distinctly separate ways to prepare for the mental and the affective tasks facing you as you take the licensure examination.

Long-range goals must include realistic life plans. Anticipate the time that study and review demand; avoid a major life change that increases pressure. While a wedding date may be difficult to reschedule, consider delaying other emotionally charged events. Even a three-week vacation prior to the NCLEX may create tension over travel plans, finances, and limited study time.

Realistically evaluate your usual response to challenges such as the NCLEX. Look at past successes and ways you maintain energy and confidence. How have you reacted to other major exams? What physiologic or emotional responses to stress are common for you? Many graduates report gastrointestinal distress during the test, or lapses in concentration during a long day of problem solving. Thoughts may drift. Occasional "failure fantasies" are reported. Anger about a specific test item is common, with feedback such as, "I could have written better answers to that question!"

In order to use your mind to the fullest and to demonstrate that you are a competent nurse, you need to control the effects of anxiety. Several effective ways exist, including relaxation methods

- progressive muscle relaxation and tension (face to neck to shoulders and down)
- slow deep breathing and deliberate calming
- guided imagery and a restful setting
- meditation
- prayer

- positive thoughts
- focus on a confident self

Select the methods of stress reduction that have worked for you in the past, learn new approaches and practice them occasionally during times of tension. For example, to use imagery, think of a place and time that are most peaceful for you. Close your eyes for a moment and visualize the surroundings, the scents, the quiet sounds. Feel the warmth and the energy. Enjoy the calm. Revisit the imaged scene each time you are fatigued from studying. Change the picture as you need to, until it is a perfect relaxing pause. Recall the image during moments in the examination when you need a recharging break. You will feel your spirits lift.

Close to the test date, plan your travel to the exam site. If distances are reasonable, visit the building in advance to familiarize yourself with the route and alternatives. Consider seasonal problems that may affect travel time.

Anticipate that the massive test setting will be overwhelming. Plan ways that you can block out the environmental stimuli, the noisy lobby, the last-minute review recitations and the test item post-mortems. Plan to replace those distractions with other activities: a walk outside at lunch, a brief nap on the steps, or a discussion of a television comedy. This is one time in your professional life that *your* needs are a priority. Do what you must to remain calm and confident.

On the exam days, meet your needs for comfort and nutrition. Dress in nonconstricting and attractive clothing that makes you feel good about yourself. It is wise to carry a jacket in anticipation of temperature change in the large hall. Eat breakfast, but avoid excessive caffeine and fluids so that distracting trips to the rest room are avoided during the test. Carry fruit, a container of juice, and other quick-energy sources for the break.

If you know that you always have a tension headache during a long day of concentration, carry a remedy with you. Prepare for other usual problems with antacids and cough drops. Then you can remain attentive to the paper-and-pencil task.

Expect at least one unfamiliar health problem among the exam situations. Remain confident that you can transfer knowledge from related concepts. Do not let an emotional response destroy your concentration with an angry comment such as, ''Why would they ask about *that* condition.'' Rather, say to yourself, ''Maybe that item doesn't count. I can try to answer it.'' Or just omit that set of questions initially and return to it later.

The keys to success lie within you. Discover your strengths and potential by preparing mentally and emotionally for the exam experience. Study, review, practice test-taking strategies, and learn how to reduce personal tension. The rewards begin with your license to practice as a professional nurse. You are needed, and welcomed as a colleague.

References

Jacobs, A., Fivars, G., & Fitzpatrick, R. (1982). What the new test will test. *American Journal of Nursing, 82*(4), 625–626.

Jacobs, A., et al. (1978). *Critical requirements for safe effective nursing practice*. Kansas City, MO: American Nurses' Association.

National Council of State Boards of Nursing. (1983). Developing, constructing and scoring the national council licensure examination. *Issues 4*(1,2), 1–8.

———*Test plan for the registered nurse state board test pool examination*. (1980). Chicago: Author.

Test wiseness—Test taking skills for the adult. (1978). New York: McGraw-Hill.

Young, M., & Kopala, B. (1981). Plan for success: Preparing for the 1982 state boards. *Imprint, 28*(6), 50–51, 70–71, 85.

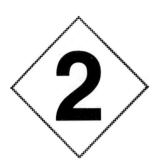

Nursing Care of the Client with Psychosocial, Psychiatric/Mental Health Problems

Coordinator

Mary Paquette, MN, RN

Contributors to this Edition

Paula J. Albertson, BSN, RN
M. Regina Asaro, BSN, RN
Diane J. Baker, BSN, RN
Deborah DiGiaro, MS, RN
Silva Foxpuglisi, MS, RN
Elizabeth C. Kaiser, MSN, RN
Susan L. W. Krupnick, MSN, CCRN, CEN, CS, RN
Mary-Charles Santopietro, EdD, MS, EdM, RN
Jean H. Woods, PhD, RNCS

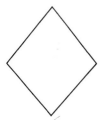

Questions

Joan Washington, RN, has been assigned as co-facilitator for a group of elderly residents in a local nursing home. The group of residents is composed of 8 men aged 70 to 85; the purpose of the group is to promote social interaction.

1. During the first meeting, Miss Washington introduces herself and asks each member to do the same. What additional information will be most useful to the nurse at this time?
   ○ 1. The reasons for each resident's admission to the nursing home
   ○ 2. A sociocultural history of each resident
   ○ 3. The usual activity patterns of each resident
   ○ 4. The interaction patterns in the group

2. When Miss Washington asks the group what kinds of things they would like to do together, the only responses she receives are comments such as, "You tell us, you're the leader," or, "Why do we need to come to this group anyway?" This behavior probably means
   ○ 1. Miss Washington has not explained the purpose of the group clearly enough.
   ○ 2. the residents are anxious (a typical response).
   ○ 3. the residents are angry about being in the group.
   ○ 4. an interpretation of these comments is not possible after only 1 meeting.

3. During 1 group meeting, Mr. Pankowski tells everyone of his apprehension about going to his daughter's for a weekend visit. What would your best response be?
   ○ 1. "We wouldn't let you go if you weren't able."
   ○ 2. "Maybe others in the group have had similar feelings."
   ○ 3. "Have you ever had those feelings before?"
   ○ 4. "Mr. Abraham, tell Mr. Pankowski how you handled similar feelings."

4. Over a period of several weeks, Mr. Abels has monopolized most of the conversation in the group. How might the group facilitator best handle this?
   ○ 1. Take him aside and kindly tell him that others deserve a chance to talk too.
   ○ 2. Ignore Mr. Abels's comments, and they will occur less often.
   ○ 3. Share your perception with the group.
   ○ 4. Transfer Mr. Abels to another group.

Jane Thomas is a 57-year-old woman who was admitted to the psychiatric unit over the weekend. She says she is quite angry and thoroughly disgusted, even though she is smiling.

5. Which of the following best describes Mrs. Thomas's behavior?
   ○ 1. Suspicious
   ○ 2. Demanding
   ○ 3. Incongruent
   ○ 4. Resistant

6. What is the best response to this behavior?
   ○ 1. "Your smile does not match what you are saying, Mrs. Thomas."
   ○ 2. "I wonder what you're really thinking, Mrs. Thomas."
   ○ 3. "Tell me more about your anger."
   ○ 4. "What were you thinking just now?"

7. Mrs. Thomas reflects on what the nurse has said and begins to think silently. After 1 minute, what would be an appropriate response for the nurse to make?
   ○ 1. Continue to allow her time to think.
   ○ 2. Ask her, "Did I say something wrong?"
   ○ 3. Tell her, "I'm concerned about your silence, Mrs. Thomas."
   ○ 4. Tell her, "Just say the first thing that comes to mind Mrs. Thomas."

8. Which of the following information would be most useful to discuss at today's client-care meeting?
   ○ 1. Diagnosis
   ○ 2. Case history
   ○ 3. Psychologic testing
   ○ 4. Approaches for present behavior

9. Mrs. Thomas begins to become more reclusive and refuses to leave her room. What is the best nursing response when initiating contact with her?
   - ○ 1. "Come, let's go play some cards."
   - ○ 2. "Have I done something to frighten you?"
   - ○ 3. "I would like to stay with you for awhile."
   - ○ 4. "You seem concerned about something. What's on your mind?"

Ruby Sanchez comes to the mental health clinic and relates that since the death of her husband she feels "really miserable." She states in a loud voice, "How could he do this to me. I just won't have it."

10. Which of the following stages of the grief reaction is Mrs. Sanchez most likely displaying at this time?
    - ○ 1. Denial
    - ○ 2. Anger
    - ○ 3. Depression
    - ○ 4. Resolution

11. Which of the following statements made by Mrs. Sanchez would be the most important in determining whether her response is normal or pathologic?
    - ○ 1. "My husband died 1 week ago."
    - ○ 2. "Most everything makes me cry."
    - ○ 3. "We were married for 42 years."
    - ○ 4. "We didn't have much in common in later years."

12. Based upon the data given by Mrs. Sanchez, which of the following would be the most appropriate statement of the nursing problem?
    - ○ 1. Prolonged grief reaction related to death of husband
    - ○ 2. Anger related to loss of husband
    - ○ 3. Denial related to feelings of guilt
    - ○ 4. Feelings of depression related to interference in marital bond

13. What is the most therapeutic initial nursing approach to use in assisting Mrs. Sanchez to deal with her feelings?
    - ○ 1. Assist her to see the positive aspects of the relationship with her husband.
    - ○ 2. Describe the stages of the grieving process to her.
    - ○ 3. Assist her to express the feelings she is experiencing.
    - ○ 4. Tell her that in time she will feel better.

Della Quale is a 36-year-old married woman. She has 2 daughters, ages 7 and 9. She lives with her children and her husband, Dan, a 38-year-old construction foreman. Mrs. Quale has a history of cancer of the breast and had a radical mastectomy 6 years ago. Until 2 months ago, she was in excellent health. At that time, she began to complain of severe back pain and to lose weight rapidly. Examination and surgery have revealed inoperable cancerous tumors on her spine, and she has been admitted to the oncology unit for palliative chemotherapy and radiation treatment. On admission, she is quiet and withdrawn, a thin, frail woman. She speaks only when spoken to and eats and drinks only when someone feeds her.

14. What is the nurse's highest priority in caring for the client at this time?
    - ○ 1. Help the client deal with her family's feelings of their impending loss.
    - ○ 2. Encourage verbal expression of the client's anger.
    - ○ 3. Ensure the client receives adequate nutrition and hydration.
    - ○ 4. Allow the client to use any form of denial that she chooses.

15. Mrs. Quale continues to lose weight and refuses to move from her bed or to turn herself. This behavior may result in 3 of the following consequences. Which is *not* likely to occur?
    - ○ 1. Formation of decubitus ulcers
    - ○ 2. More energy to express her feelings to the nursing staff
    - ○ 3. Anger and hostility from the nursing staff toward the client
    - ○ 4. Contractures of the extremities

16. Mrs. Quale refuses to see her children or to talk with them on the telephone. Such behavior may lead to
    - ○ 1. an understanding by the client of the family's need for empathy.
    - ○ 2. moving through the grief process more quickly.
    - ○ 3. rejection by the client's children.
    - ○ 4. client understanding of the changes in her body image and self-esteem.

17. One evening the physician meets with Mrs. Quale and her husband to discuss her discharge with hospice care. Mrs. Quale is visibly distressed and later that night suffers an episode of respiratory arrest. Her medical condition is treated and stabilized, but she is visibly weakened and remains withdrawn. Which of the following nursing actions will *not* be therapeutic at this time?
○ **1.** Turning and positioning the client as needed
○ **2.** Having the nurse consider her own feelings and beliefs about dying
○ **3.** Sitting with the client quietly
○ **4.** Encouraging her to feed and bathe herself to regain some autonomy

18. When working with the dying client and the family, the nurse understands that 3 of the following are very likely to occur. Which one is *not*?
○ **1.** The family will respond to the dying member much as they have handled other major crisis situations.
○ **2.** The client will proceed through each of the stages of dying, regardless of outside help.
○ **3.** The family's greatest needs may be for competent physical care for the ill member and empathy for their situation.
○ **4.** The young child may see death as something others experience.

Mr. and Mrs. Carlson have recently learned that their 3-year-old daughter Jeannie has an untreatable malignant tumor.

19. Because Jeannie is 3 years old, the nurse can expect her to have which of the following views of death?
○ **1.** Someone bad will carry her away.
○ **2.** Death occurs but it is not permanent.
○ **3.** Death and absence are the same.
○ **4.** Everyone must die.

20. Which of the following would probably *not* be effective in helping Jeannie express her reactions and feelings about her situation?
○ **1.** Provide her with dolls and puppets to play with and pretend one is an ill girl.
○ **2.** Provide paper and colors for her to draw with and have her tell you about her drawings.
○ **3.** Set up a regular time each day for her to talk about her feelings and concerns.
○ **4.** Read stories and talk about how the children in the stories feel.

Gail Miller is a 27-year-old woman admitted to the surgical unit of a general hospital following an accident in a small airplane. In the accident, her husband, the pilot, was killed. Mrs. Miller has a fractured left femur and some minor abrasions and contusions, but is physiologically in stable condition. She has a 2-year-old son.

21. The day after admission, the nurse enters Mrs. Miller's room to find the shades drawn and Mrs. Miller in bed sobbing quietly. The most therapeutic response by the nurse would be
○ **1.** "It's a beautiful day outside. Let's get some sunshine in here."
○ **2.** "I heard about the accident. Would you like to talk about it?"
○ **3.** "I'll come back when you are feeling better."
○ **4.** "It's not good for you to sit in here in the dark."

22. Mrs. Miller is exhibiting a normal response to grief. Which of the following would most likely be considered an *abnormal* grief response?
○ **1.** A period of preoccupation with the deceased person
○ **2.** A period of emotional numbness
○ **3.** Hoarding sleep medications
○ **4.** Expressing angry feelings

23. Which of the following would be most helpful to Mrs. Miller as she progresses through the grief process?
○ **1.** Give antidepressant medication.
○ **2.** Schedule numerous activities for her in order to keep her mind occupied.
○ **3.** Arrange for a surprise visit from her son.
○ **4.** Allow her to work through the grief process at her own pace.

24. A week following Mrs. Miller's admission, her physician informs her that her admission tests reveal that she is pregnant. The nurse enters her room to find her crying hysterically. Which of the following would be most effective?
○ **1.** Tell her that you will return later when she has had a chance to gain control.
○ **2.** Tell her that you will sit with her until she is ready to talk.
○ **3.** Administer a sedative.
○ **4.** Ask her if she would like you to sit with her.

25. Two days after learning of her pregnancy, Mrs. Miller tells the nurse, "I'm going to have an abortion. I can't bear the thought of raising another child by myself." What is the best response?
    ○ 1. "Well, it sounds as though you have already made a decision."
    ○ 2. "You may be acting too hastily."
    ○ 3. "It's your decision, but I'd be happy to talk with you about it."
    ○ 4. "You might be sorry in a year or 2."

Ashley Carlisle, a newlywed, comes to the mental-health clinic because of "nervousness." She relates to the nurse that "my stomach has butterflies a lot of the time. I haven't missed any work, but it's getting harder because I can't concentrate on anything very long."

26. What level of anxiety is Mrs. Carlisle most likely experiencing?
    ○ 1. Mild
    ○ 2. Moderate
    ○ 3. Severe
    ○ 4. Panic

27. Which of the following would be the best way to begin taking Mrs. Carlisle's nursing history?
    ○ 1. "Tell me about your husband."
    ○ 2. "What are you feeling now?"
    ○ 3. "Have you ever felt this way before?"
    ○ 4. "Does anyone else in your family ever get these feelings?"

Joan Taber calls out to the nurse's station every 10 minutes asking for something. She is a 67-year-old client who is 2 days post-op after a hip pinning.

28. Which of the following is the most important action for the nurse to take in regard to Miss Taber's behavior?
    ○ 1. Observe her behavior at regular intervals to obtain a baseline.
    ○ 2. Observe her ability to carry out her activities of daily living.
    ○ 3. Assess her need for pain medicine.
    ○ 4. Assess her reaction to the anesthetic.

29. Select the best plan of nursing care for Miss Taber.
    ○ 1. Respond only when called on by her.
    ○ 2. Administer pain medicine to her.
    ○ 3. Respond to her at consistent intervals when she is not requesting something.
    ○ 4. Explain to her that the nurse has other clients to care for.

30. This nursing action expressed above is important because the nurse needs to
    ○ 1. allay anxiety.
    ○ 2. present reality.
    ○ 3. respond to the client's need for safety.
    ○ 4. avoid reinforcing demanding behavior.

31. Which of the following explains the major difference between normal anxiety and the syndrome associated with anxiety reactions?
    ○ 1. Normal anxiety is constant; an anxiety reaction is intermittent and rather short-lived.
    ○ 2. Normal anxiety is free-floating; in an anxiety reaction, there is an impending sense within the person that something bad will happen.
    ○ 3. An anxiety reaction is seldom controllable and usually must run its course.
    ○ 4. Normal anxiety is a fact of life and seldom becomes an anxiety reaction.

32. Miss Taber says to the nurse, "Dr. Wells has surely botched my case. I can't believe they'd let him continue to practice." The appropriate response of the nurse is
    ○ 1. "Dr. Wells is a fine doctor and one worthy of respect."
    ○ 2. "Dr. Wells has been sued before, and his practice is questionable."
    ○ 3. "You seem to have some concerns about Dr. Wells."
    ○ 4. "Dr. Wells usually provides good care."

Martin Oren is experiencing anxiety. He is married, has three children, and just lost his job as a coal miner. He comes into the hospital with severe indigestion and fears that he has a serious stomach disorder.

33. Signs and symptoms associated with anxiety are
    ○ 1. complaints of apprehension, narrowed perception, stomach pains, restlessness.
    ○ 2. inability to get to sleep, early morning awakening, 10 lb weight loss, lack of energy.
    ○ 3. ideas of reference, grandiose delusions, hallucinations, delusions.
    ○ 4. indifference, elated behavior, feeling better in the morning, overeating.

34. If Mr. Oren goes into panic the nurse would most likely note which of the following symptoms?
- ○ **1.** Persecutory delusions, ideas of reference, rhyming
- ○ **2.** Greatly reduced perception, extreme discomfort, extreme agitation
- ○ **3.** Fugue state, amnesia, multiple personalities
- ○ **4.** Extreme agitation, mood depression, stream of thought

35. Nursing care during panic reaction would most likely include
- ○ **1.** allowing the client to express thoughts and feelings.
- ○ **2.** reality orientation.
- ○ **3.** problem solving.
- ○ **4.** helping the client to express and deal with anger.

36. Which of the following criteria should the nurse best use to evaluate Mr. Oren's care?
- ○ **1.** Coherence of thought processes and reality orientation
- ○ **2.** Absence of behavioral signs of nervousness and effective use of coping mechanisms
- ○ **3.** Cycle of mood swings
- ○ **4.** Self reports of experiencing less fear

John Luzinski, a 40-year-old, married man, has demonstrated increasing reluctance to leave his home over the past 3 months. He has been absent from his job frequently, and 1 month ago the job was terminated. Since that time, he has not been outside his home. His wife informed their family physician, who arranged for him to be brought to the psychiatric hospital for evaluation.

37. From the information provided, Mr. Luzinski most likely displays symptoms of
- ○ **1.** acrophobia.
- ○ **2.** agoraphobia.
- ○ **3.** astraphobia.
- ○ **4.** claustrophobia.

38. The ego-defense mechanism being used by Mr. Luzinski is which of the following?
- ○ **1.** Denial
- ○ **2.** Displacement
- ○ **3.** Substitution
- ○ **4.** Symbolization

39. What is the most effective technique in the treatment of Mr. Luzinski's condition?
- ○ **1.** Confrontation to determine if the fear is real
- ○ **2.** Immediate exposure to the situation he fears
- ○ **3.** Distraction each time he mentions the subject
- ○ **4.** Gradual desensitization by controlled exposure to the situation he fears

40. To decrease the anxiety experienced when exposed to his situational phobia, Mr. Luzinski is started on a medication regimen. Which of the following would most likely be prescribed for him?
- ○ **1.** The antipsychotic fluphenazine (Prolixin) 2 mg TID, PO
- ○ **2.** The antipsychotic chlorpromazine (Thorazine) 25 mg BID, PO
- ○ **3.** The antidepressant amitriptyline (Elavil) 25 mg BID, PO
- ○ **4.** The anxiolytic diazepam (Valium) 2 mg TID, PO

41. Which of the following activities attended by Mr. Luzinski would probably indicate he is progressing satisfactorily?
- ○ **1.** Milieu group in the dayroom
- ○ **2.** Occupational therapy in the adjunctive-therapy room
- ○ **3.** Recreational therapy on the outside volleyball court
- ○ **4.** Sunday dinner in the hospital cafeteria

Maria Morgan is a 16-year-old high school student brought to the psychiatric hospital by her mother. Since she was a small child, she has been preoccupied with excessive cleanliness, refusing to play in areas where she might soil her clothing, and bathing several times a day. Recently she has begun to scrub her underarm areas so frequently that the skin is excoriated and bleeding. She states that she does not wish to offend anyone by her body odor. She is admitted with a diagnosis of obsessive-compulsive disorder.

42. Maria's symptoms most likely represent which of the following?
- ○ **1.** A method of receiving attention
- ○ **2.** A method of reducing anxiety
- ○ **3.** A delusional method of reducing anxiety
- ○ **4.** A manipulative method of avoiding socialization

43. Which ego-defense mechanisms are most prominently utilized in this disorder?
- ○ **1.** Introjection and projection
- ○ **2.** Compensation and isolation
- ○ **3.** Displacement and undoing
- ○ **4.** Rationalization and repression

44. What is the best rationale to explain Maria's type of disorder?
○ **1.** Anger is internalized and turned against the self.
○ **2.** Intellectualization fails as a defense mechanism.
○ **3.** Trust was never established in early significant relationships.
○ **4.** A distressing thought is cancelled out by some type of action.

45. Select the factors that are most important for the nurse to assess about Maria.
○ **1.** Actions, life events, unresolved conflicts, activities of daily living
○ **2.** Silly behavior, thought patterns, associations, delusions
○ **3.** Nervousness, vital signs, body language, impending sense of doom
○ **4.** Involvement of involuntary muscles, fears, attention level, sleeping disorders

46. When you formulate the initial nursing care plan for Maria, which of the following should receive the highest priority?
○ **1.** Client will maintain her role in the family.
○ **2.** Client will eliminate her washing behavior.
○ **3.** Client will verbalize the underlying cause of her behavior.
○ **4.** Client will reestablish skin integrity.

47. Initially the nurse will most likely consider which of the following in planning care for Maria?
○ **1.** She will require strict limit setting in order to conform to the unit schedules.
○ **2.** She will need extra time to perform her rituals, so her anxiety will be manageable.
○ **3.** She will need to be isolated in order to feel less anxious about proximity to other clients.
○ **4.** She will need to be confronted about the senselessness of her behavior.

48. Which of the following is most important in planning nursing care for Maria?
○ **1.** Use reality orientation.
○ **2.** Set limits on washing behavior.
○ **3.** Administer diazepam (Valium) 5 mg as ordered.
○ **4.** Use assertiveness training.

49. Maria relates that she likes to watch TV but is fearful of sitting on the chairs in the dayroom. What would be the most therapeutic intervention?
○ **1.** Sterilize one of the chairs in the dayroom and reserve it for Maria.
○ **2.** Move the TV into Maria's room.
○ **3.** Permit Maria to stand while watching TV.
○ **4.** Insist that she sit in the chair.

50. Three of the following interventions are appropriate. Which one is not?
○ **1.** Allow her to complete her ritual, once she has begun.
○ **2.** Allow her to make choices in her schedule.
○ **3.** Prevent her ritualistic behavior, once she has begun adjunctive therapy.
○ **4.** Provide protection from physical discomfort caused by her ritualistic behavior.

51. Which statement would be the most appropriate guideline when considering possible outcomes of Maria's care?
○ **1.** If given an antipsychotic medication, she has a good chance of completely eliminating her symptoms.
○ **2.** If psychotherapy is used intensively, she will be able to deal with her repressed feelings and completely eliminate her symptoms.
○ **3.** If Maria is given sufficient opportunities to succeed in activities, her self-esteem will improve and her symptoms will be eliminated.
○ **4.** It is appropriate to develop methods to limit and confine symptoms, since these behaviors are very resistant to treatment.

52. Which of the following criteria would be used to evaluate Maria?
○ **1.** A reduction of washing behavior and resumption of daily activities
○ **2.** Intact thought processes grounded in reality
○ **3.** Able to go to school without fear
○ **4.** Self-reports of decreased anxiety

53. Which statement best demonstrates Maria's understanding of her problem?
○ **1.** "I suppose you think washing under my arms all the time is a crazy thing to do."
○ **2.** "I feel so clean when I get done washing, but it just doesn't last very long."
○ **3.** "I know I'm getting better, because I don't have as much body odor as I did in the beginning."
○ **4.** "I really don't think I have a problem. It's important to be clean if you want to have dates."

Tina Otis, 18 years old, is admitted to an inpatient psychiatric unit. She is 5 ft, 7 in tall and weighs 95 lb. She attends a local university, where she is an excellent student. She appears weak and yet exercises heavily, especially after meals. Her condition is diagnosed as anorexia nervosa. She has been dieting to lose weight and sees herself as needing to lose at least 25 more pounds to "get rid of my fat hips."

54. Three of the following conditions are characteristic of the anorexic client. Which one is *not*?
- ○ **1.** Amenorrhea
- ○ **2.** Delayed psychosexual development
- ○ **3.** A familial pattern
- ○ **4.** Tachycardia

55. Miss Otis exhibits much of the behavior considered typical of clients suffering from anorexia nervosa. Which of the following behaviors could be considered *atypical*?
- ○ **1.** Hoarding food
- ○ **2.** Eating only low-calorie foods
- ○ **3.** Napping frequently to conserve energy
- ○ **4.** Strenuous exercising

56. Which of the following has the highest priority in the treatment of this client?
- ○ **1.** Negotiate a behavioral contract with the client.
- ○ **2.** Teach her the basics of good nutrition.
- ○ **3.** Institute measures to restore electrolyte and nutritional balance.
- ○ **4.** Observe her closely for 2 hours after each meal.

57. In setting up Miss Otis's treatment plan, 3 of the following would be appropriate. Which one would be *inappropriate*?
- ○ **1.** Provide opportunities for her to pick her menu and observe that nutritious and high-calorie foods are included.
- ○ **2.** Provide positive reinforcement for each pound gained.
- ○ **3.** Encourage Miss Otis to be more independent.
- ○ **4.** Allow her quiet time in her room after each meal.

58. When monitoring Miss Otis's eating patterns, it is essential for the nurse to recognize that she
- ○ **1.** has an alteration in the functioning of the hypothalamus, which affects the appetite center.
- ○ **2.** is unable to eat properly because of a physiologic lack of appetite.
- ○ **3.** represses normal stomach hunger.
- ○ **4.** is aware of the sensation of hunger.

59. Miss Otis is started on a behavior modification program. She is encouraged to eat 3 well-balanced meals each day and to attempt to gain at least one-half pound each day. Each time she accomplishes this, she is allowed an additional privilege on the unit. This is an example of which of the following behavior modification techniques?
- ○ **1.** Avoidance of punishment
- ○ **2.** Positive reinforcement
- ○ **3.** Negative reinforcement
- ○ **4.** Generalization

60. Miss Otis continues to deny her problems and remains aloof from the staff and peers on the unit. Which of the following approaches would be the most effective?
- ○ **1.** Point out that she will be force fed if she does not improve her eating habits.
- ○ **2.** Let her eat as little as she wishes, as she will not continue to lose weight after a plateau is reached.
- ○ **3.** Involve her in the preparation of her treatment plan, assisting in decisions concerning food, exercise, and hygiene.
- ○ **4.** Assign her a roommate who has good eating habits, so she will become more interested in good nutrition.

61. Which of the following is the most appropriate nursing response when Miss Otis describes her hips as fat?
- ○ **1.** "Actually you're too skinny; you don't look good that way."
- ○ **2.** "Look here in the mirror. You can see your hips are not fat."
- ○ **3.** "Your hips seem fat to you, but actually you are very thin."
- ○ **4.** "It's difficult for me to understand how you can do this to yourself."

Horace Babcock is admitted to the mental health unit for evaluation. He has a 5-year history of numerous medical admissions for severe, intermittent headaches. Despite extensive diagnostic workups and tests that have revealed no organic basis for his symptoms, he continues to believe he is ill. He holds a responsible job as an accountant, is married, and is the father of 2 young children.

62. Mr. Babcock's symptoms are most characteristic of which of the following diagnostic categories?
- ○ **1.** Hypochondriasis
- ○ **2.** Psychosomatic illness
- ○ **3.** Conversion disorder
- ○ **4.** Dissociative reaction

63. The day after admission, Mr. Babcock tells the nurse that he will be unable to participate in group therapy because his headaches have increased. What is the most therapeutic response from the nurse?
   ○ 1. "Describe the pain to me."
   ○ 2. "Go to your room and lie down. I'll call your doctor."
   ○ 3. "You must go to group therapy. It's part of your treatment."
   ○ 4. "Let's sit down and talk a bit about what group therapy involves."

64. Diazepam (Valium) 5 mg TID is ordered for Mr. Babcock. This drug is primarily effective in the treatment of which of the following?
   ○ 1. Hallucinations
   ○ 2. Delusions
   ○ 3. Anxiety
   ○ 4. Mania

65. Mr. Babcock is discharged with a prescription for diazepam (Valium) 5 mg TID. When teaching him how to use the medication at home, the nurse would *exclude* which of the following instructions?
   ○ 1. "Do not combine medication with alcohol."
   ○ 2. "If you need to take any other medication while taking this drug, consult with your physician first."
   ○ 3. "Valium decreases muscular coordination and mental alertness, so use caution when driving."
   ○ 4. "Drink at least 8 glasses of water daily, as Valium will dehydrate you."

Tina Manchester, a 33-year-old widow and mother of 4 children, was visiting a neighbor when her house burned down. Her children were at home alone when the fire occurred. The 2 oldest children, aged 10 and 8, were killed. The baby, Chrissie, 2 months old, and Danny, 4 years old, survived, but were badly burned. Four months later, Tina was still waking at night with nightmares about the incident. She kept remembering the sight of the fireman carrying her children out of the burning home. She could not turn on a stove and see flames without becoming very anxious and scared. She visits a local mental health clinic and receives a diagnosis of post-traumatic stress disorder.

66. When describing the fire to the nurse at the clinic, Mrs. Manchester clearly leaves out part of the story. The best nursing response would be to
   ○ 1. ask several questions to help her remember what happened.
   ○ 2. allow her to tell as much of the story as she is comfortable relating.
   ○ 3. realize that she probably does not remember those parts of the story that are not painful.
   ○ 4. tell her that she must not hold back information if she wants to improve.

67. Mrs. Manchester says she feels very guilty about the children's deaths. She says, "I wish it had been me that died in the fire." Which of these responses is most appropriate for the nurse to make?
   ○ 1. "Your feelings are normal for this type of accident, and we can talk more about them."
   ○ 2. "Your feelings are different than most parents in this type of situation, so let's explore them further."
   ○ 3. "Then who would take care of Chrissie and Danny?"
   ○ 4. "Do you have a plan to kill yourself?"

68. One of the goals the nurse and Mrs. Manchester have agreed upon is that she will increase her involvement in out-of-the-home activities. Which of the following actions will probably be most effective in helping her achieve that goal?
   ○ 1. Join a Parents Without Partners group
   ○ 2. Take a 1-week trip out of town
   ○ 3. Plan on taking the children to a film once a week
   ○ 4. Join a group of parents whose children died from accidental causes

69. The mental health clinic has an emergency crisis intervention team to provide immediate care to prevent post-traumatic stress disorder. According to the Public Health Model, this is an example of
   ○ 1. primary prevention.
   ○ 2. secondary prevention.
   ○ 3. tertiary prevention.
   ○ 4. early diagnostic care.

Ada Cohen, aged 60, is admitted to the hospital with symptoms of increasing forgetfulness, irritability, decreasing concentration, and feelings that others are out to get her. The medical diagnosis is Alzheimer's disease.

70. In view of the medical diagnosis, which of the following pieces of information would be most useful to obtain in planning nursing care?
○ **1.** Family history concerning other members with similar disorders
○ **2.** Her previous occupation, hobbies, diversional activities
○ **3.** Her past medical history
○ **4.** Major stressors in her life

71. Three of the following statements are true about this disease. Which one is *incorrect*?
○ **1.** There is degeneration of the cortex and atrophy of the cerebrum.
○ **2.** Death usually occurs 1 to 10 years following onset.
○ **3.** There is progressive deterioration of intellectual function and changes in personality and behavior.
○ **4.** The etiology of this disease is well known and fairly uniform.

72. Memory loss for recent events is the most common symptom during the early stages of Alzheimer's disease. Of the following actions, which one will probably *not* help?
○ **1.** Answer questions repeatedly as needed using short, simple sentences.
○ **2.** Place a large calendar next to the client's bed.
○ **3.** Place the client's name in large letters outside of the door to her room.
○ **4.** Tell the client she is getting increasingly forgetful.

73. Mrs. Cohen has difficulty remembering where her room is on the unit. Which of the following would best help her to alleviate this problem?
○ **1.** Paint the door to her room light blue.
○ **2.** Assign her a buddy who will help her when she gets lost.
○ **3.** Put her picture and her name in large letters on the door to her room.
○ **4.** Assign her a room next to the nurses' station so the staff can assist her as necessary.

74. Mrs. Cohen's food intake is only marginally adequate, due, in part, to her inability to sit at the table and concentrate for the length of time necessary to eat the meal. Which approach would be most likely to ensure a nutritionally adequate intake?
○ **1.** Order a full liquid diet that will take her less time to eat.
○ **2.** Feed Mrs. Cohen.
○ **3.** Order 6 small, nutritionally balanced meals.
○ **4.** Offer small amounts of food whenever she appears ready to eat.

75. During a visit, Mr. Cohen asks to speak to the nurse. He tearfully tells her that his son and daughter are urging him to place Mrs. Cohen in a nursing home. Which of the following is the best response?
○ **1.** "Your wife will recover soon. Just give her time."
○ **2.** "Our social service department has a list of the best nursing homes in the area that you may want to consider."
○ **3.** "When you are finished visiting your wife, come up to the nursing station. I'll find a quiet place where we can talk."
○ **4.** "I'm sure you will be able to take care of your wife at home without that much difficulty."

Glenn Jones is a 33-year-old client admitted to the psychiatric unit with a diagnosis of major depression. He has been hospitalized twice before with this diagnosis. He speaks negatively of himself and states that he has a history of recurrent depression. He has demonstrated no suicidal ideation and is not on "suicide" status at present, although he has been suicidal during previous hospitalizations. He is quiet and withdrawn and responds slowly to all stimuli.

76. Mr. Jones seems less lethargic today and agrees to participate in the occupational therapy program. To help make the session most successful for Mr. Jones, the nurse would do which one of the following?
○ **1.** Set up a large number of projects for Mr. Jones to choose from.
○ **2.** Introduce Mr. Jones to the other clients in occupational therapy.
○ **3.** Help to structure Mr. Jones's participation in occupational therapy to facilitate successful completion of one specific small task.
○ **4.** Stay away from the client while he is in occupational therapy, so that he is free to express himself.

77. Mr. Jones is to receive nortriptyline (Aventyl) 100 mg daily. Of the following side effects, which one is *not* expected with this medication?
○ **1.** Blurred vision
○ **2.** Ataxia
○ **3.** Urinary retention and delayed micturition
○ **4.** Potentiation of the action of other medications

78. Which of the following behaviors or symptoms is Mr. Jones most likely to demonstrate?
    ○ 1. Lack of cooperation with staff
    ○ 2. Flight of ideas
    ○ 3. Increased motor activity
    ○ 4. Decreased short-term memory

79. Which of the following nursing actions is considered nontherapeutic?
    ○ 1. Identifying the aspects of cognitive changes that are important to the client
    ○ 2. Taking responsibility for the client's physical safety
    ○ 3. Refusing to acknowledge or discuss irrational demands
    ○ 4. Evaluating the effect of the antidepressant medication on the client

Barney Chung, a 60-year-old widower, was brought by his son to the hospital after exhibiting increasingly withdrawn behavior over a period of 3 months. He had been living alone since coming to this country 12 years ago. He has been widowed 15 years, and he worked as a tailor until his retirement 3 years ago. He is now refusing to eat or bathe, must be escorted to the bathroom, and does not respond verbally when addressed.

80. When orienting Mr. Chung to the unit, which of the following guidelines would be most appropriate?
    ○ 1. Ensure he meets everyone on the unit as soon as possible.
    ○ 2. Accompany him to his room and stay with him, only giving a minimum of information.
    ○ 3. Accompany him to all activities, so he will be encouraged to participate.
    ○ 4. Assign him to a room with a talkative roommate, so he will not feel isolated.

81. In severe depression, which of the following defense mechanisms is commonly found?
    ○ 1. Introjection
    ○ 2. Projection
    ○ 3. Suppression
    ○ 4. Repression

82. What is the most common cause of symptoms of depression that Mr. Chung exhibits?
    ○ 1. A hormonal imbalance
    ○ 2. A problem with sexual identity
    ○ 3. An unresolved parental conflict
    ○ 4. A sense of real or imagined loss

83. In planning activities for Mr. Chung during the initial stages of hospitalization, which of the following is most appropriate?
    ○ 1. Give him only 1 activity a day, so he will not become fatigued.
    ○ 2. Prepare a schedule of activities for him to follow each day.
    ○ 3. Let him choose what he wants to do each day.
    ○ 4. Wait until he indicates a willingness to participate before providing any activities.

84. During the first few days of his hospitalization, Mr. Chung comes to the dayroom when escorted but does not yet respond verbally. Which of the following statements would be most therapeutic?
    ○ 1. "I will sit with you, Mr. Chung. You may wish to talk later."
    ○ 2. "I will sit with you, Mr. Chung, so that you won't hurt yourself."
    ○ 3. "You won't get better if you don't talk to others, Mr. Chung."
    ○ 4. "I will sit with you, Mr. Chung. It's important for you to be comfortable in the dayroom."

85. Mr. Chung will be started on therapy with an antidepressant drug. The most appropriate choice would be which of the following?
    ○ 1. The tricyclic imipramine (Tofranil) 50 mg TID, PO
    ○ 2. The tricyclic amitryptyline (Elavil) 150 mg TID, PO
    ○ 3. The MAO inhibitor isocarboxazid (Marplan) 30 mg TID, PO
    ○ 4. The MAO inhibitor phenelzine sulfate (Nardil) 50 mg TID, PO

86. The possibility of suicide is a most important concern in the care of depressed clients. During which period is Mr. Chung most likely to attempt suicide?
    ○ 1. When he is mute and unlikely to tell anyone about it
    ○ 2. When he is ready to go home
    ○ 3. When his family goes on vacation
    ○ 4. When he begins to demonstrate improvement

87. The most important priority in caring for a client who is a high suicide risk is to
   - ○ 1. administer tranquilizers, so the client will be less suicidal.
   - ○ 2. monitor location and behavior constantly.
   - ○ 3. change the subject whenever suicide is mentioned, so ideation is less.
   - ○ 4. keep the client in isolation to prevent other clients from witnessing a possible attempt.

88. Mr. Chung has improved slowly. He consents to a series of electroconvulsive therapy treatments (ECT). Prior to the first treatment, he becomes anxious and states he does not wish to go to the treatment room. Which of the following is the most appropriate response?
   - ○ 1. "You'll be asleep, Mr. Chung, and won't remember anything."
   - ○ 2. "I'll call your doctor, Mr. Chung, and let him know you have changed your mind about the treatment."
   - ○ 3. "You don't have to go, Mr. Chung. You have the right to refuse a treatment like this."
   - ○ 4. "I'll go with you, Mr. Chung, and I'll be there throughout the treatment."

89. What are the most common side effects of ECT?
   - ○ 1. Headache and dizziness
   - ○ 2. Nausea and vomiting
   - ○ 3. Confusion and memory loss
   - ○ 4. Diarrhea and urinary incontinence

90. Which of the following medications is used in conjunction with ECT?
   - ○ 1. Succinylcholine (Anectine) as a muscle relaxant
   - ○ 2. Methohexital (Brevital) as an anesthetic
   - ○ 3. Atropine sulfate as an anticholinergic
   - ○ 4. All of the above medications are used in conjunction with ECT.

91. Mr. Chung continues to improve and now attends group therapy daily. The most important benefit he would derive from this is
   - ○ 1. improved socialization skills.
   - ○ 2. improved reality orientation.
   - ○ 3. greater insight into his problems through the concept of universality.
   - ○ 4. greater insight and knowledge of self through feedback provided by group members.

Phyllis Rafferty's history reveals that she has had 8 depressive episodes during the last 5 years and has been treated with a number of antidepressants, antipsychotic medications, and psychotherapy during this time. During her current hospitalizaion, several consults are held with psychiatrists who specialize in the treatment of depression. The decision is made, with the approval of the client and her daughter, to try electroconvulsive therapy (ECT).

92. One of the chief benefits of ECT is that it
   - ○ 1. shortens the hospitalization period.
   - ○ 2. often enables a client to be more accessible to psychotherapy.
   - ○ 3. decreases the need for medication.
   - ○ 4. enables the client to terminate psychiatric treatment.

93. Which of the following is *not* a nursing responsibility for ECT?
   - ○ 1. Remove dentures, hairpins, etc.
   - ○ 2. Administer medications, such as muscle relaxant, as ordered.
   - ○ 3. Prep the client as if she were going to OR.
   - ○ 4. Carry out the ECT treatment.

94. In order to deal effectively with the side effects that follow ECT, the first nursing action would be to do which of the following?
   - ○ 1. Reintegrate client into the therapeutic milieu.
   - ○ 2. Orient the client to place, time, and person.
   - ○ 3. Provide environmental stimulation as soon as treatment is completed for the day.
   - ○ 4. Place client on bedrest for remainder of the day.

Esther Bell has been admitted to a locked unit; her diagnosis is severe depression with history of suicidal ideation and insomnia. She is a 52-year-old, divorced woman and is unemployed. She expresses feelings of hopelessness, anger at hospitalization, and self-deprecation. She reports having repeated thoughts of suicide and has a plan to "crash my car and die."

95. Upon completing the initial assessment, the nurse most accurately determines that Mrs. Bell's suicidal risk is at which level?
   - ○ 1. Low
   - ○ 2. Medium
   - ○ 3. High
   - ○ 4. In remission

96. Which of the following is *not* a high-risk group for suicidal behavior?
   - ○ 1. The elderly
   - ○ 2. Adolescents
   - ○ 3. Alcohol/drug abusers
   - ○ 4. People in their 30s

97. Mrs. Bell has treatment orders that include suicide precautions. Which of the following is *not* considered a suicide precaution?
    ○ 1. Searching personal effects for toxic agents (drugs or alcohol)
    ○ 2. Removing sharp instruments (razor blades, sewing equipment, glass bottles, knives)
    ○ 3. Removing clothes that could be made into straps (belts, stockings, pantyhose)
    ○ 4. Asking the client to focus on positive feelings

98. The nurse knows that severe depression may also be classified as a
    ○ 1. somatoform disorder.
    ○ 2. affective disorder.
    ○ 3. anxiety disorder.
    ○ 4. personality disorder.

99. On what basis is the distinction made between severe and mild depression?
    ○ 1. Somatic and motor activity
    ○ 2. Suicidal ideation
    ○ 3. Duration of symptoms
    ○ 4. Client's age at onset

100. Mrs. Bell continues to be concerned about insomnia and wants to nap in the daytime. Which of the following short-term goals is *not* appropriate for this client?
    ○ 1. Client will discuss feelings and concerns about sleep.
    ○ 2. Client will state that she was able to get some sleep during the night.
    ○ 3. Client will take several naps during the day.
    ○ 4. Client will participate in exercise and activity in the daytime.

101. Nursing actions for the insomnia problem should include which of the following?
    ○ 1. Ignore sleep patterns and complaints about insomnia.
    ○ 2. Reassure the client that insomnia is not a serious problem.
    ○ 3. Encourage short naps during the day.
    ○ 4. Assist the client to establish a bedtime routine to promote rest and sleep.

102. Mrs. Bell has been transferred to an open unit from the locked unit. Her physician has ordered imipramine (Tofranil). Tofranil is a(n)
    ○ 1. tricyclic drug.
    ○ 2. phenothiazine.
    ○ 3. MAO inhibitor.
    ○ 4. antianxiety agent.

103. The nurse teaches Mrs. Bell about Tofranil. Which statement is correct about this drug?
    ○ 1. Takes 2 to 4 weeks to take effect
    ○ 2. May cause urinary frequency
    ○ 3. May cause increased salivation
    ○ 4. Should only be taken when the client is severely depressed

104. Which of the following would *not* be appropriate questions for the nurse to ask when assessing the depressed client?
    ○ 1. "What are your expectations of yourself?"
    ○ 2. "How do you cope with anger?"
    ○ 3. "What kinds of things are pleasurable for you?"
    ○ 4. "Don't you know that it is morally wrong to think of suicide?"

105. Which of the following would be the most appropriate goal for a nursing diagnosis of "ineffective individual coping related to feelings of hopelessness and anger"?
    ○ 1. The client will deny feelings of hopelessness and anger.
    ○ 2. The client will demonstrate cheerful affect.
    ○ 3. The client will voice no complaints.
    ○ 4. The client will share feelings with nurse and others.

106. Which of the following actions would be *least* effective in assisting the client cope with painful feelings?
    ○ 1. Focus on the positive aspects of life.
    ○ 2. Encourage the client to share feelings.
    ○ 3. Assist the client to identify feelings.
    ○ 4. Provide reality orientation and encourage realistic expectations of self.

107. Mrs. Bell refuses to discuss discharge plans. She states she "can't go home alone, and no one wants to come live with me." Which of the following is the most appropriate action?
    ○ 1. Accept her appraisal of the situation and encourage exploration of alternatives.
    ○ 2. Call her family and work with them on plans for discharge.
    ○ 3. Allow Mrs. Bell to discuss other topics of interest.
    ○ 4. Insist that Mrs. Bell discuss discharge to her family home.

108. Mrs. Bell ruminates about her failures in relationships and work. Which of the following would be an *ineffective* intervention for rumination?
   - ○ **1.** Introduce communication that expands her narrow frame of reference.
   - ○ **2.** Tell her to stop ruminating about failure and to speak of positive goals.
   - ○ **3.** Provide opportunities for activity and exercise.
   - ○ **4.** Assist the client to reevaluate her strengths and weaknesses.

109. Mrs. Bell is angry with the nursing staff and her physician for continuing to discuss discharge planning. Three of the following nursing actions are appropriate to this situation. Which one is *not* appropriate?
   - ○ **1.** Encourage client to verbalize feelings and concerns.
   - ○ **2.** Utilize simple, direct explanations and open-ended questions.
   - ○ **3.** Make plans with the client for physical activity and exercise.
   - ○ **4.** Ignore angry outbursts; tell the client to remain calm.

Eunice King, a 42-year-old woman, is admitted to the intensive care unit. She is accompanied by her husband, who tells the nurse that he recently asked his wife for a divorce. He left the house yesterday to go on a 3-day business trip. Some of his meetings were cancelled, and he returned home today to find his wife unconscious. An empty bottle that had contained sleeping pills was on the bedside table.

110. In assessing the seriousness of Mrs. King's suicide attempt, which of the following facts is the most important?
   - ○ **1.** She is unconscious.
   - ○ **2.** She used a potentially lethal method.
   - ○ **3.** She planned the attempt for a time when she thought no rescue was possible.
   - ○ **4.** She did not leave a suicide note.

111. The following day, Mrs. King regains consciousness. She is in tears and tells the nurse, "I'm a failure at everything, as a woman, as a wife; and I've even failed at killing myself." When interpreting this statement, which of the following is *least* likely to be correct?
   - ○ **1.** Mrs. King is depressed.
   - ○ **2.** Mrs. King is remorseful about her suicide attempt, and therefore, it is unlikely that she will make a second attempt.
   - ○ **3.** Mrs. King is feeling hopeless, and the potential for another suicide attempt is great.
   - ○ **4.** Mrs. King is ambivalent about whether she wants to live or die.

112. A few days later, Mrs. King is transferred from the intensive care unit to the psychiatric unit. Which of the following nursing interventions has the highest priority?
   - ○ **1.** Remove all potentially harmful items from the client's room.
   - ○ **2.** Allow the client to express feelings of hopelessness and helplessness.
   - ○ **3.** Stress the client's capabilities and strengths in order to increase self-esteem.
   - ○ **4.** Observe the client closely for suicidal ideation or gestures.

113. A week after admission, Mrs. King comes to breakfast in a new dress; her hair and makeup are immaculate; and she is quite cheerful. She tells the nurse that she is going to ask her physician for a weekend pass. What does the nurse need to know regarding this change in behavior and affect?
   - ○ **1.** Realize that the client is improving and discontinue suicide precautions.
   - ○ **2.** Realize that her first weekend at home will be difficult and offer anticipatory guidance.
   - ○ **3.** Realize that a decrease in depression may be indicative of renewed suicide potential and monitor the client carefully.
   - ○ **4.** Realize that depressed clients often have mood swings and no intervention is probably necessary.

114. The treatment team decides that one of the goals in treating Mrs. King is to increase her self-esteem. Which of the following is the most appropriate way of doing this in the early stages of treatment?
    ○ 1. Suggest that she make her bed and keep her room in order.
    ○ 2. Introduce her to another client who is an excellent chess player and suggest that he teach her to play.
    ○ 3. Suggest that she lead the evening sing-along.
    ○ 4. Since she is an excellent cook, suggest that she start a cooking class for the other clients.

115. Another treatment goal for Mrs. King is reduction of dependency. Which of the following is an *inappropriate* way to reduce dependency needs in a client?
    ○ 1. Provide only the help needed.
    ○ 2. Encourage the client to solve her own problems.
    ○ 3. Rotate the staff caring for the client frequently.
    ○ 4. Encourage participation in unit activities.

Dorothy Pinsky, a 49-year-old homemaker, was recently admitted to the psychiatric unit because of anxiety and suicidal behavior. Her adult life has always been centered on her family and home. Her 2 oldest children are married and live in nearby towns; her 2 youngest children are away at college. She had expressed feelings of hopelessness and somatic complaints prior to hospitalization.

116. Mrs. Pinsky presents the typical symptoms of which of the following?
    ○ 1. Paranoid schizophrenia
    ○ 2. Manic-depressive reaction, manic phase
    ○ 3. Psychotic depression
    ○ 4. Substance abuse

117. Which of the following is the most important nursing action at this time?
    ○ 1. Monitor her food intake.
    ○ 2. Institute suicide precautions.
    ○ 3. Encourage her interest in her family.
    ○ 4. Reassure her that her physical complaints are unwarranted.

118. Mrs. Pinsky is indeed a potential suicide victim. She is most likely to commit suicide
    ○ 1. immediately after admission.
    ○ 2. at the point of her deepest depression.
    ○ 3. when the depression begins to lift.
    ○ 4. just prior to discharge.

119. Mrs. Pinsky's psychiatrist is thinking of changing her medicine to a monamine oxidase (MAO) inhibitor. Of the following characteristics, which one should the nurse be most aware of?
    ○ 1. They are short acting.
    ○ 2. They cause tachycardia.
    ○ 3. They cause an increase in appetite.
    ○ 4. They potentiate the effects of other drugs.

120. Mrs. Pinsky will begin electroconvulsive therapy (ECT) today. She tells the nurse that she is very afraid. The best response is
    ○ 1. "Don't be afraid, your doctor has had 18 years experience in giving ECT."
    ○ 2. "It's not good for you to worry so much."
    ○ 3. "You do seem frightened; I will stay with you."
    ○ 4. "Most people say the same thing; so you are not alone."

Sixty-two-year-old Rose Magrone is admitted to the psychiatric unit with a diagnosis of agitated depression.

121. Which of the following behaviors would you *not* expect to observe with this diagnosis?
    ○ 1. Extreme restlessness
    ○ 2. Pacing
    ○ 3. Handwringing
    ○ 4. Sleeping 10 to 12 hours per day

122. The physician orders amitriptyline HCl (Elavil) 25 mg TID for Mrs. Magrone. Which classification of psychotropic drugs includes amitriptyline HCl (Elavil)?
    ○ 1. Tricyclic antidepressants
    ○ 2. Monamine oxidase inhibitors
    ○ 3. Phenothiazines
    ○ 4. Antihistamines

123. A few days after starting the medication, Mrs. Magrone complains of a dry mouth, constipation, and blurred vision. These symptoms are characteristic of the action of this drug on which of the following body systems?
    ○ 1. Cardiovascular
    ○ 2. Endocrine
    ○ 3. Autonomic nervous
    ○ 4. Respiratory

124. Mrs. Magrone takes her medication as ordered. Three days later, she still exhibits signs of agitation, anxiety, and restlessness. What is the most likely explanation for this?
    ○ 1. She is not actually taking the medication.
    ○ 2. She is not responding to the medication.
    ○ 3. Symptomatic relief is not usually achieved until 2 to 4 weeks after therapy is started.
    ○ 4. The dosage is too small to be effective.

125. Mrs. Magrone refuses to take the next scheduled dose of her medication, because she finds the side effects too annoying. Which of the following is the most effective nursing action?
- ○ **1.** Tell Mrs. Magrone that skipping 1 dose is not important.
- ○ **2.** Explain to her that the side effects will diminish in a few days.
- ○ **3.** Ask her to discuss the side effects with her physician.
- ○ **4.** Advise her that she will probably have to get electroconvulsive therapy if she fails to take her medication.

Sarah Perkins, aged 35, is admitted to the hospital because of increasing feelings of extreme worthlessness and sinfulness, uninterest in eating and personal hygiene, weight loss, and problems with sleep. These problems began shortly after Mrs. Perkins learned that her husband was having an affair with her best friend. A diagnosis of major depression with psychotic features is made.

126. During the initial interview, Mrs. Perkins states, "I really can't blame him. He's such a fine person, and I'm such a terrible wife." How might the nurse best respond?
- ○ **1.** "Everyone has good qualities, Mrs. Perkins. I'm sure you do too."
- ○ **2.** "Tell me why you think you're so terrible?"
- ○ **3.** "You're not feeling very good about yourself right now."
- ○ **4.** "You'll feel better about yourself after a few days in the hospital."

127. Mrs. Perkins's response to this situation may be most likely viewed as
- ○ **1.** normal, because of the severity of the precipitating stress.
- ○ **2.** a reaction to what she perceives as a severe blow to her security.
- ○ **3.** the result of a maturational crisis.
- ○ **4.** transitory and likely to be self-limiting.

128. The nurse notes that Mrs. Perkins is having difficulty making decisions. Which approach would be most therapeutic?
- ○ **1.** Firmly, but kindly, indicate that she is expected to make decisions.
- ○ **2.** Explain how important decision making is to her recovery.
- ○ **3.** Provide an opportunity for her to make small decisions when she appears ready to do so.
- ○ **4.** Do not ask her to make decisions.

129. Mrs. Perkins stays in her room most of the time and is not interested in any activities or persons on the unit. Which action by the nurse would be most therapeutic?
- ○ **1.** Allow her the time alone that she requires.
- ○ **2.** Require her to attend at least 1 activity per day.
- ○ **3.** Spend short, frequent periods of time with her.
- ○ **4.** Explain that becoming more active will help her feel better.

130. Mrs. Perkins is to receive a series of electroconvulsive therapy (ECT) treatments. Which of the following understandings about this procedure is most important when providing care to the client?
- ○ **1.** The preparation for this is basically the same as for any procedure where general anesthesia is used.
- ○ **2.** ECT is not very effective in the treatment of endogenous or melancholic depressions, so Mrs. Perkins should not get her hopes up.
- ○ **3.** ECT is highly controversial and is used only as a last resort.
- ○ **4.** ECT has no short-term side effects.

131. Before her first treatment, Mrs. Perkins is quite anxious. Which action by the nurse would be most therapeutic?
- ○ **1.** Adminster diazepam (Valium) 10 mg IM.
- ○ **2.** Encourage her to sit quietly in her room and breathe deeply.
- ○ **3.** Take her to the dayroom for a cup of coffee.
- ○ **4.** Remain with her and discuss topics she introduces.

132. What nursing action would be most appropriate for Mrs. Perkins following ECT?
- ○ **1.** Remain quietly with her until the confusion subsides.
- ○ **2.** Ask her to remain in bed until the physician arrives.
- ○ **3.** Assess her orientation to time, place, and person by frequent assessment.
- ○ **4.** Call her by name and reorient her to the unit as soon as possible.

133. One day while talking with the nurse, Mrs. Perkins states, "I guess I haven't been thinking very clearly. I'm beginning to think that there may be other ways of dealing with the things that have been happening in my life." This statement best indicates which phase of the nurse-client relationship?
   ○ 1. Initiating
   ○ 2. Working
   ○ 3. Terminating
   ○ 4. Orienting

Muriel Moskovitz, a 42-year-old homemaker, is admitted to the psychiatric unit with a diagnosis of psychotic depression.

134. The nurse's first priority is to
   ○ 1. establish reality orientation.
   ○ 2. ensure client safety.
   ○ 3. promote self-esteem.
   ○ 4. improve cognitive perceptions.

135. While interviewing Mrs. Moskovitz, the nurse asked what led to her coming to the hospital. She said, "I'm wicked and it's God's wrath." The most appropriate therapeutic response by the nurse would be which of the following?
   ○ 1. "You are not wicked, Mrs. Moskovitz."
   ○ 2. "What do you mean by that?"
   ○ 3. "Why is God punishing you?"
   ○ 4. "We'll talk about this later."

136. Mrs. Moskovitz's physician prescribes a course of electroconvulsive treatments for the client. She asks you what is going to happen to her. Which of the following is the most appropriate explanation to give her?
   ○ 1. "You will have a small seizure that will help you to forget what is bothering you."
   ○ 2. "Electrodes will be placed on your temples, and a light electrical shock will be delivered to your brain."
   ○ 3. "The anesthesiologist will put you to sleep, and you will not even be aware of what is happening."
   ○ 4. "You will be given something to help you relax, and you will not feel the actual shock."

137. After Mrs. Moskovitz's first electroconvulsive treatment, the nurse stays with her and the physician leaves. After initially regaining consciousness, Mrs. Moskovitz seems to go to sleep. What would the nurse do?
   ○ 1. Try to awaken her.
   ○ 2. Let her sleep.
   ○ 3. Summon the physician.
   ○ 4. Administer a prescribed stimulant.

138. Mrs. Moskovitz is slow about getting herself dressed and ready for breakfast. What should the nurse do?
   ○ 1. Permit her to take as much time as she wishes.
   ○ 2. Tell her she will not get breakfast if she arrives late.
   ○ 3. Serve her breakfast in her room.
   ○ 4. Help her to get dressed and get to breakfast.

139. Mrs. Moskovitz says to the nurse, "I'm really not worth all the time it takes for you to help me." What is the best response for the nurse to make?
   ○ 1. "Even though you feel that way, I am here to help you."
   ○ 2. "You should not think of yourself that way."
   ○ 3. "I don't have anything else I have to do right now."
   ○ 4. "Soon you will be able to start doing more for yourself, so it won't take so much of my time."

140. After 3 weeks of treatment, Mrs. Moskovitz begins to take more responsibility for herself and expresses an interest in getting ready for discharge. What should the nurse do?
   ○ 1. Assess Mrs. Moskovitz's current level of self-esteem.
   ○ 2. Institute suicide precautions.
   ○ 3. Encourage her to become more involved with the activities on the ward.
   ○ 4. Discuss with her her denial of the long-term effects of her depression.

141. Mrs. Moscovitz tells the nurse, "I feel guilty, now that my children are grown, because I didn't do more for them when they were little." Which is the most therapeutic response for the nurse to make?
   ○ 1. "What have your children done to make you feel that way?"
   ○ 2. "Parents often feel guilty about things that have to do with their children."
   ○ 3. "You probably did the best you could for them."
   ○ 4. "What other feelings do you have toward your children besides guilt?"

142. The day before her discharge, Mrs. Moscovitz is late for her last interview with the nurse. When the nurse mentions the late arrival, Mrs. Moscovitz blurts out, "Don't nag me! I'm an adult." What is the best response for the nurse to make?
    ○ 1. "You feel angry when it seems as though someone's nagging you."
    ○ 2. "You're not acting as we would expect an adult to act."
    ○ 3. "It must be hard for you to think of leaving the hospital."
    ○ 4. "Being on time is part of being responsible for yourself."

Marilyn Brooks has been brought to the hospital by her husband, who states she has become increasingly agitated and overactive during the past 2 weeks. She did not sleep last night. Upon admission, Mrs. Brooks refuses to sit down and continues to move about rapidly, speaking in a loud, tense voice.

143. The medical-biologic model of psychiatric illness is based on 3 of the following assumptions. Which assumption is *not* a tenet of this model?
    ○ 1. A client suffering from emotional disturbances has an illness or defect.
    ○ 2. The illness has characteristic symptoms or syndromes.
    ○ 3. Mental illnesses are properly within the charge of the physician.
    ○ 4. Psychiatric illness stems from social and environmental conditions.

144. The manic behavior displayed by Mrs. Brooks is best explained by which of the following statements?
    ○ 1. Repression is used to avoid inner feelings of loneliness and poor self-esteem.
    ○ 2. Suppression is used to avoid inner feelings of dependency and inadequacy.
    ○ 3. Displacement is used to shift inner feelings to the environment.
    ○ 4. Denial is used to avoid inner feelings of depression.

145. Which of the following would be the best initial response to Mrs. Brooks?
    ○ 1. "I'm glad to see you have so much energy today, Mrs. Brooks."
    ○ 2. "I need you to help me pass the breakfast trays, Mrs. Brooks."
    ○ 3. "Let me introduce you to another new client, Mrs. Brooks."
    ○ 4. "I will go with you to your room, Mrs. Brooks."

146. When managing Mrs. Brooks's behavior on the unit, which of the following actions would *not* be helpful?
    ○ 1. Suggest activities that require her attention for long periods of time.
    ○ 2. Attempt to minimize environmental stimuli.
    ○ 3. Encourage her to use the craft hammer for making a leather belt in occupational therapy.
    ○ 4. Use distracting techniques when necessary to channel her attention appropriately.

147. The physician orders lithium therapy. The therapeutic blood level is maintained between which of the following?
    ○ 1. 0.5 to 1.5 mEq/liter
    ○ 2. 1.0 to 1.5 mEq/liter
    ○ 3. 0.5 to 1.5 mg/ml
    ○ 4. 1.0 to 1.5 mg/ml

148. As a part of a teaching plan on lithium carbonate, clients are instructed to have lithium levels determined every 1 to 3 months. Which statement best describes the reason for this?
    ○ 1. Lithium carbonate can produce potassium depletion.
    ○ 2. Triglyceride levels can increase as the lithium level increases.
    ○ 3. Lithium carbonate in large quantities produces sedation.
    ○ 4. There is a very narrow margin of safety between the therapeutic level and toxic level of lithium carbonate.

149. Which of the following symptoms would Mrs. Brooks most likely exhibit if she developed mild lithium toxicity?
    ○ 1. Urinary retention, increased appetite, abdominal distension
    ○ 2. Dry mouth, decreased appetite, constipation
    ○ 3. Macular rash, fever, hematuria
    ○ 4. Nausea, muscle weakness, polydipsia

150. As his wife begins to improve, Mr. Brooks states he wishes her to return home and asks what he can do to help his wife after discharge. Which of the following would be the most appropriate information to give Mr. Brooks?
    ○ 1. Get someone to stay with her, since she probably will not be stable enough to be left alone.
    ○ 2. While his wife remains on lithium therapy, it is necessary to have her blood lithium levels monitored regularly.
    ○ 3. Manic-depressive illness is hereditary, so they should never have any children.
    ○ 4. Ensure she has a prescription for tranquilizers, so that she can start taking them if her symptoms of mania recur.

151. Mrs. Brooks receives instructions about lithium before discharge. Learning has most probably occurred when she notifies the outpatient clinic that she has experienced which of the following?
    ○ 1. Vomiting and diarrhea for 48 hours
    ○ 2. Swollen lymph nodes
    ○ 3. Dry mouth
    ○ 4. Symptoms of an upper respiratory tract infection

John Peters, a 60-year-old investment analyst, was admitted to the psychiatric unit with an admission diagnosis of manic-depressive disorder, manic phase, and alcohol abuse. His wife left him a week ago. Two days ago, he was counseled by his work supervisor for telling several clients to sell all their stocks immediately and not to ask questions.

152. In obtaining a family history, which of the following would the nurse most expect to find?
    ○ 1. A high incidence of childhood illnesses
    ○ 2. Alcohol or drug abuse as a young adult
    ○ 3. Parents were divorced when he was a child
    ○ 4. One parent was described as being "very happy" or "very down"

153. The diagnostic category, affective disorders, includes extremes in mood and affect. Of the following, which is *not* characteristic of a manic-depressive disorder?
    ○ 1. Vegetative behavior
    ○ 2. Hypomanic behavior
    ○ 3. Thought disorder
    ○ 4. Clang associations

154. Which of the following is *not* characteristic of manic-depressive clients in a manic phase?
    ○ 1. Potential for violence
    ○ 2. Attempt to boss the staff around
    ○ 3. Denial of feelings of depression and sadness
    ○ 4. Hypersomnolence

155. Upon Mr. Peters's admission, his son said to the nursing staff, "You had better do your job right and calm him down." Which of the following responses would be most helpful at this time?
    ○ 1. "You must really be fed up. I've never seen anyone this maniacal."
    ○ 2. "You must be very worn out dealing with your father's behavior. It will be very helpful to both of you that you brought him to the hospital."
    ○ 3. "I can appreicate your embarrassment. He is really high, isn't he?"
    ○ 4. "Your father is acting aggressively in order to avoid feeling depressed."

156. Despite evidence to the contrary, Mr. Peters tells the nurse to, "Go get your money. The banks have failed. Only I know this." In assessing Mr. Peters's behavior, what do his remarks most likely indicate?
    ○ 1. Short attention span
    ○ 2. Irritability
    ○ 3. Thought disorder
    ○ 4. Overtalkativeness

157. The psychiatrist orders lithium carbonate, 300 mg, QID, PO, for Mr. Peters. The laboratory results indicate a serum lithium level of 1.5 mEq/liter. Which nursing action is most appropriate?
    ○ 1. Suggest that the psychiatrist repeat the test.
    ○ 2. Withhold the next dose of lithium and notify the psychiatrist.
    ○ 3. Administer the next dose of lithium.
    ○ 4. Observe Mr. Peters's degree of pressured speech.

158. For clients taking lithium, it is critical that the nurse observe the client's food intake. Lithium toxicity is most likely to occur if the client has insufficient intake of which of the following?
    ○ 1. Fat and carbohydrates
    ○ 2. Potassium and iron
    ○ 3. Sodium and fluids
    ○ 4. Protein

159. The nursing history is a vital component of the nursing process. Which of the following, obtained through the history, is most likely to contraindicate treatment of a client with lithium?
    ○ **1.** Kidney damage
    ○ **2.** High suicide risk
    ○ **3.** High level of physical activity
    ○ **4.** Hyperthyroidism

160. In order to provide Mr. Peters with the most therapeutic environment during his hospitalization, which of the following would be most important for the nurse to keep in mind?
    ○ **1.** Assign him to a semiprivate room with another client who has a similar problem.
    ○ **2.** Assign him to a private room.
    ○ **3.** Realize that the presence or absence of a roommate is not particularly important for him.
    ○ **4.** Place him in the seclusion-quiet room and in restraints as soon as possible after admission.

161. In order to intervene effectively when Mr. Peters is talking rapidly and indicating a flight of ideas, the nursing staff would consistently remind him to do which of the following?
    ○ **1.** Verbalize how he feels about his work as an investment analyst and his behavior.
    ○ **2.** Tell himself that his verbalizations are a flight of ideas, which is indicative of his depression.
    ○ **3.** Speak more slowly, so that he can be understood better.
    ○ **4.** Describe as many details of his problems as possible.

162. To help reduce the overt aggression demonstrated by Mr. Peters, the nursing staff would utilize 3 of the following measures. Which measure would *not* be indicated?
    ○ **1.** Participation in competitive games
    ○ **2.** Physical exercise
    ○ **3.** Reduction in environmental stimuli
    ○ **4.** Encouraging the client to discuss feelings associated with angry behavior

163. In planning for Mr. Peters's discharge and future functioning, it is important for his son to be aware of his father's need for education about health. Client education would most likely include which of the following aspects?
    ○ **1.** Recognize behaviors that indicate increased excitement such as irritability, agitation, and verbal and motor hyperactivity.
    ○ **2.** Teach the son to make most major decisions for his father.
    ○ **3.** Encourage the father to handle business matters quickly and aggressively.
    ○ **4.** Teach father and son all possible drug toxicities.

164. In evaluating Mr. Peters's readiness for discharge, the client should demonstrate 3 of the following. Which would *not* be indicative of readiness for discharge?
    ○ **1.** Self-care
    ○ **2.** Stating requests appropriately and negotiating power with staff and other clients
    ○ **3.** Frequent expressions of anger and hostility
    ○ **4.** A decrease in manipulative or acting-out behaviors

165. The psychiatric-mental health nurse who assesses psychiatric clients in the emergency room encounters Mr. Peters 6 months postdischarge. He is hyperverbal, rude, hostile, and insulting to the emergency room staff. When conducting the initial nursing assessment, the most important question to ask early in the interview is
    ○ **1.** "Were you embarrassed when you returned to work?"
    ○ **2.** "Are you and your wife still separated?"
    ○ **3.** "Have you stopped taking your lithium?"
    ○ **4.** "Is it difficult for you to talk about your problem?"

William White is a 42-year-old salesman of boats and outdoor equipment for water recreation. He has a history of mood swings. His wife finally persuaded him to admit himself to the hospital following his latest episode of extremely unusual behavior. She reported that he's excited because he is the top salesperson in the company, but added that many of the sales were initiated by her husband's having put his own money down as deposits. When the final contracts are due, she said, he will become very depressed because he won't be able to get his money back in order to pay his own bills.

166. When assessing Mr. White's behavior, the nurse will most likely note which one of the following behaviors?
    ○ 1. Withdrawal from reality
    ○ 2. Overactivity
    ○ 3. Associative looseness
    ○ 4. Inappropriate affect

167. During the first few days on the unit, Mr. White comes up to the nurse several times and says, "You're an asshole." How would the nurse best deal with this inappropriate language?
    ○ 1. Ignore the language.
    ○ 2. Interpret the meaning to Mr. White.
    ○ 3. Tell him that kind of language will not be tolerated.
    ○ 4. Seclude him until his speech is less offensive.

168. Mr. White may fail to eat because he
    ○ 1. feels he does not deserve to eat.
    ○ 2. feels the food is poisoned.
    ○ 3. is too busy.
    ○ 4. does not like hospital food.

169. After 1 week on the unit, Mr. White has lost 10 lb. Which of the following will be most likely to prevent further weight loss?
    ○ 1. Increase the size of his portions at each meal.
    ○ 2. Remain with him at meals to ensure he eats everything.
    ○ 3. Restrict between-meals snacks, so that he will be more hungry at mealtime.
    ○ 4. Provide between-meal, nutritious foods that Mr. White can eat in brief time periods.

170. Mr. White refuses to eat, stating that he has too much to do. Which of the following is the best nursing response?
    ○ 1. "Come and eat at the table."
    ○ 2. "Here is a sandwich for you to eat."
    ○ 3. "You will be able to work later."
    ○ 4. "What are you doing that takes so much of your time?"

171. Mr. White is scheduled for occupational therapy (OT). The chief aim of OT for Mr. White is
    ○ 1. to teach social skills for group living.
    ○ 2. to stimulate interest in the environment.
    ○ 3. to provide a constructive outlet for excessive energy.
    ○ 4. to provide an environment where confrontation and reality testing are maximized.

Monica Wendall is a 17-year-old mother of an 8-month-old son. The nurse is discussing the baby's progress with Mrs. Wendall during a regularly scheduled visit to the well-baby clinic. Mrs. Wendall expresses her frustration over her baby's recent illness and reveals her fear of harming the baby and her feelings of wanting to throw the baby to the floor.

172. When assessing the mother's potential for child abuse, which factor from the mother's past history would be most important to know?
    ○ 1. Whether the mother has completed high school
    ○ 2. The mother's age at menarche
    ○ 3. Whether the mother, as a child, was physically abused by her parents
    ○ 4. The socioeconomic status of the mother's family of origin

173. When assessing the mother's current potential for child abuse, which factor is the most important to determine?
    ○ 1. Is the mother currently pregnant?
    ○ 2. Has the mother actually harmed the baby?
    ○ 3. Did the mother want the baby at the time of birth?
    ○ 4. Has the mother cared for small children before, such as baby-sitting or caring for younger siblings?

174. In planning for this family's care, the nurse would do best to consider which of the following facts about teenage mothers?
    ○ 1. They often have unrealistic expectations about the love and caring they will receive from the baby.
    ○ 2. They often have realistic expectations of the baby's patterns of growth and development.
    ○ 3. They often have adequate knowledge about the child care, nutrition, and health needs of the baby.
    ○ 4. They usually have excellent role models for parenting from their own parents.

175. Based on the current information and client needs, which of the following clinic-sponsored programs would be the most appropriate initial referral for Mrs. Wendall?
    ○ 1. The birth control clinic
    ○ 2. The nutritional counseling program
    ○ 3. Early childhood development and parenting classes
    ○ 4. Classes in first aid and cardiopulmonary resuscitation

Roberta Lane is a 42-year-old, married mother of 4 children ages 23, 21, 17, and 9. Mrs. Lane appears at the medical clinic this morning with a bandaged nose and a black eye. As you enter the examining room, Mrs. Lane laughs, points to her face and says, "See this! My husband did this. I was in the emergency room 4 hours the other night getting patched up. He really did a good job on me this time." With that comment, Mrs. Lane becomes sad and stares at the floor.

176. Which of the following approaches is most appropriate when responding to Mrs. Lane's comment?
    ○ 1. Respect Mrs. Lane's need to deny the problem and do not probe further into the issue.
    ○ 2. Comment that if Mrs. Lane is not going to put a stop to this situation there is not much the nurse can do to help.
    ○ 3. Acknowledge Mrs. Lane's sadness and ask directly about the circumstances surrounding this current battering incident.
    ○ 4. Refer Mrs. Lane for psychotherapy.

177. The nurse's attitudes toward women who remain in a relationship in which multiple battering incidents have occurred often influence his/her ability to be helpful to these women. Which of the following feelings are most commonly experienced by the nurse?
    ○ 1. Apathy and ignoring behavior
    ○ 2. Frustration and disappointment
    ○ 3. Guilt and shame
    ○ 4. Denial and repression

178. Which of the following attitudes, if conveyed by health care professionals, inhibits self-disclosure by the battered women?
    ○ 1. Indifference to the seriousness of the situation
    ○ 2. Concern over the detail of the situation
    ○ 3. Interest in previous medical records to determine the history of the battering incidences
    ○ 4. Feeling that the victim brought the battering on herself

179. When planning her care, which of the following is most important for Mrs. Lane?
    ○ 1. The phone numbers of the local crisis hot line and the local battered-women's shelter
    ○ 2. Referral to a psychotherapist
    ○ 3. Referral to assertiveness training classes for women
    ○ 4. No referral will be needed unless the battering occurs again or is witnessed by an adult.

Thomas Benson, a 14-year-old boy, is admitted to an inpatient psychiatric unit with the diagnosis of conduct disorder. He has been running away from home, taking illegal drugs, skipping classes, and now he has been arrested for shoplifting. His family is very discouraged and do not feel they can control him at home.

180. The nurse assigned to Tom can expect him to behave in which of the following ways the first few days on the unit?
    ○ 1. Exhibit depressed and withdrawn behavior
    ○ 2. Express a desire to spend most of the time alone
    ○ 3. Tease and bait the staff
    ○ 4. Display good interpersonal skills

181. This behavior is primarily Tom's way of
    ○ 1. avoiding or expressing feelings of anger or depression.
    ○ 2. attempting to make friends.
    ○ 3. behaving like a normal teenager.
    ○ 4. denying his lack of social and intellectual abilities.

182. The most appropriate initial goal of nursing care will be which of the following?
    ○ 1. Client will sit and talk with a primary nurse for 30 minutes daily.
    ○ 2. Client will verbalize his understanding of why his family feels frustrated with him.
    ○ 3. Client will decrease acting-out behavior.
    ○ 4. Client will increase contact with other clients.

183. The most appropriate action for Tom's early treatment would be to
    ○ 1. have the client's friends visit daily.
    ○ 2. have the client discuss with the nurse why his family is upset with him.
    ○ 3. set firm and definite limits on his acting-out behavior.
    ○ 4. allow the client to use abusive language until he is able to regain some control.

Susan Porter has been hospitalized in an alcohol-rehabilitation unit for 3 weeks. She was given a pass, but has returned to the psychiatric unit in an agitated state. She spits on the primary nurse and then kicks her and tries to choke her. Despite efforts to encourage verbalization, Miss Porter continues to try to be physically abusive. Using a team approach, the staff members place Miss Porter in 4-point (all extremities) leather restraints and reassure her that they will help her regain control of herself.

184. Miss Porter's history indicates that during her drinking bouts, she has periods of amnesia and blackouts; when she withdraws from drinking she has delirium tremens. Given this history, the multidisciplinary health team assigned to this client would best conclude that her alcoholism is in which stage?
○ **1.** Early
○ **2.** Middle
○ **3.** Late or chronic
○ **4.** Recovered

185. When dealing with a potentially violent client, staff would use 3 of the following alternatives to restraints and seclusion. Which one would be *inappropriate*?
○ **1.** Identify the anxiety, e.g., say, "It seems as though you feel very bad. Tell me what is going on."
○ **2.** Encourage the client to verbalize instead of act out, e.g., "What happened while you were out on pass that made you so angry?"
○ **3.** Sit close to client and provide reassurance, e.g., say "Let me give you some kind words."
○ **4.** Tell the client she is getting out of control and will have to be restrained if she refuses to take the prescribed medication.

186. If staff have sufficient time to prepare themselves to restrain a client, they should do all of the following. If it is vital to restrain the client quickly, which component can be done following the restraint procedure?
○ **1.** Obtain a physician's order for restraints.
○ **2.** Remove their own glasses, ties, earrings, pens, and any other articles that the client can seize to hurt them with.
○ **3.** Distract the client with a blanket or sheet.
○ **4.** Have 4 staff members available to avoid client and staff injury.

187. During the time that Miss Porter is in restraints, she experiences vivid hallucinations and persecutory delusions. She continues to be agitated and combative for several hours. Blood is drawn for drug screening. The most likely substance used by Miss Porter while on pass is
○ **1.** barbiturates.
○ **2.** opiates.
○ **3.** diazepam (Valium).
○ **4.** phencyclidine (PCP).

188. Three of the following behaviors indicate that the goals regarding the use of physical restraints have been met. Which one does *not*?
○ **1.** The client tolerates physical restraints.
○ **2.** The client verbalizes angry feelings and calms down considerably.
○ **3.** The client does not demonstrate aggressive behavior such as abusive language.
○ **4.** The client promises to quiet herself.

Lydia Smith, a 26-year-old nurse, was leaving the hospital at midnight at the end of her shift when she was sexually assaulted in the parking lot of the hospital. After the assault, Mrs. Smith went to the emergency room for treatment.

189. The initial treatment of a rape victim can significantly affect the psychologic impact the assault will have on the victim. The first information elicited from Mrs. Smith should be which of the following?
○ **1.** The marital state of the victim
○ **2.** The victim's perception of what occurred
○ **3.** Whether or not the rapist was known to her
○ **4.** How she feels about having an abortion if she becomes pregnant

190. Rape is generally considered to be an act of
○ **1.** aggression.
○ **2.** bestiality.
○ **3.** exposure.
○ **4.** sexual passion.

191. Mrs. Smith called her husband to come to the hospital. Which of the following statements is most often true about the reactions of significant others?
○ **1.** They are usually very supportive and helpful to the victim.
○ **2.** They are usually apathetic, because they do not empathize with the victim.
○ **3.** They may require time and professional assistance for resolution of this crisis.
○ **4.** They may derive positive experiences by providing emotional support for the victim.

192. Mrs. Smith may not have a true emotional crisis as a result of the assault. Which factor will contribute most to decreasing the severity of the trauma?
○ **1.** Support from counseling
○ **2.** Support from her nursing colleagues
○ **3.** Support from the hospital administration
○ **4.** Support from her husband and the effectiveness of her coping mechanisms

Sarah Long, a 35-year-old electrician, is brought by the police to the emergency room. The officer tells the triage nurse that Miss Long called the police to report a man had broken into her apartment and raped her. The nurse notes Miss Long has several bruises and lacerations on her face and is very quiet; she gives only her name.

193. What is the first action that the nurse should implement with Miss Long?
○ **1.** Obtain a specimen of semen for documentation for the future court case.
○ **2.** Suture lacerations and clean all wounds.
○ **3.** Call Miss Long's family.
○ **4.** Reassure Miss Long that she is safe and will not be harmed further.

194. In planning care for Miss Long, the nurse's first actions should be oriented towards
○ **1.** controlling symptoms.
○ **2.** the diagnosis.
○ **3.** the behavior.
○ **4.** her intellectual capacity.

195. The nurse has established a rapport with Miss Long. Which of the following would *not* be helpful during the early stages of crisis intervention?
○ **1.** Encourage her to identify the frightening events.
○ **2.** Help her to understand the crisis.
○ **3.** Assess her thoughts of suicide.
○ **4.** Identify her resources and support systems.

196. The use of crisis intervention is based on several important assumptions. Which of the following is *not* characteristic of the crisis model?
○ **1.** Interventions focus on immediate concrete problems rather than on many aspects of the client's life.
○ **2.** Interventions are consistent with the client's culture and life-style.
○ **3.** Interventions include the client's significant others.
○ **4.** Interventions will be initiated by the nurse and not by the client.

Nicholas Bonono is a 43-year-old, married man who is chronically suspicious and lacks trust in people. In the past few months, he has become convinced his brother is attempting to steal his property. Although he is still functioning in his position as an accountant, his family, marital, and social relationships have deteriorated. He is admitted to the hospital with a diagnosis of paranoid disorder.

197. Mr. Bonono demonstrates which of the following?
○ **1.** Persecutory hallucinations
○ **2.** Persecutory delusions
○ **3.** Persecutory illusions
○ **4.** Persecutory phobias

198. Which of the following ego-defense mechanisms are most prominently utilized by Mr. Bonono?
○ **1.** Denial and projection
○ **2.** Denial and repression
○ **3.** Displacement and projection
○ **4.** Displacement and repression

199. Since Mr. Bonono is mistrustful of others, which nursing action would be most appropriate?
○ **1.** Have him attend many activities, so he will meet as many clients and personnel as soon as possible.
○ **2.** Be very cheerful at all times, so he will sense positive feelings from the nursing staff.
○ **3.** Be consistent with personnel and schedules, so that structure is provided for his daily activities.
○ **4.** Utilize touch appropriately to reinforce reality.

200. Mr. Bonono is started on a regimen of chlorpromazine (Thorazine) 50 mg TID, PO. What is the primary reason for the use of psychotropic drugs?
○ **1.** To keep clients sedated and easier to manage
○ **2.** To alleviate symptoms, so that additional therapies may be more effective for clients
○ **3.** To assist clients in gaining insight into their problems
○ **4.** To improve the self-esteem of clients

201. The clients on the unit are going on a picnic in the park. What information should Mr. Bonono be given regarding the side effects of his medication before he leaves?
○ **1.** Wear a hat and a long-sleeved shirt.
○ **2.** Report constipation and fatigue.
○ **3.** Report dry mouth and a stuffy nose.
○ **4.** Watch for signs of jaundice.

202. Mr. Bonono says to the nurse, "I really have been intolerant of others all these years." Which response by the nurse is preferable?
- ○ **1.** "Why do you say that, Mr. Bonono?"
- ○ **2.** "With whom have you been intolerant, Mr. Bonono?"
- ○ **3.** "Tell me about it, Mr. Bonono."
- ○ **4.** "What will you do differently now, Mr. Bonono?"

Rodman Dooley is a 45-year-old man, whose wife has accompanied him to the hospital. Mrs. Dooley states that her husband has recently become very suspicious of their neighbors and has almost engaged in physical conflicts with 1 man on 2 occasions. He has accused other persons of trying to spy on him, when they are merely going about their own business. In the interview, Mrs. Dooley states that this behavior began a few weeks after Mr. Dooley was on an airplane that was hijacked to another country. The admissions officer decides to admit Mr. Dooley for observation.

203. What is the nurse's first priority in working with Mr. Dooley?
- ○ **1.** Help him to establish a trusting relationship.
- ○ **2.** Make him aware of the reality of the situation.
- ○ **3.** Improve his self-esteem.
- ○ **4.** Improve his social functioning.

204. Mr. Dooley states that he consented to being admitted only to please his wife and that there is really nothing wrong with him. What is the best nursing response?
- ○ **1.** "Why would she want you here if you didn't need help?"
- ○ **2.** "You have been creating some problems for her."
- ○ **3.** "The only way you will get help is if you admit you need it."
- ○ **4.** "What has been going on in your life lately?"

205. The nurse assigned to meet with Mr. Dooley is delayed 30 minutes by an emergency. Which of the following is the best action to take?
- ○ **1.** Acknowledge the lateness, but do not dwell on it.
- ○ **2.** Explain the reason for the delay.
- ○ **3.** Make another appointment with the client.
- ○ **4.** Apologize for being late.

206. Two nurses are discussing Mr. Dooley's progress, when the client unexpectedly walks around the corner and overhears his name. He says, "What were you saying about me?" Which is the best response for the nurse to make?
- ○ **1.** "We were discussing your progress."
- ○ **2.** "We often talk about clients."
- ○ **3.** "It would be better if we didn't talk about it."
- ○ **4.** "Does it bother you that we talk about you?"

207. Which of the following best indicates that Mr. Dooley is developing a trusting relationship with a nurse?
- ○ **1.** He recounts his delusions with the nurse.
- ○ **2.** The nurse can explain the reasons for his delusions.
- ○ **3.** He can describe his feelings to the nurse.
- ○ **4.** The nurse feels more at ease with him.

Sheila Dumas appears to be in her early twenties. She was found curled up in a corner of a bus station. When she was asked her name all she would say was, "good baby." The police brought her to the psychiatric unit. Miss Dumas's guardian is an aunt who has been responsible for her since her parents were killed when she was 10. The aunt reports that Miss Dumas has had similar episodes in the past. Her condition has been managed with medication, and she has not had a psychotic episode in over 2 years. The current episode occurred when Miss Dumas refused to continue taking her medication.

208. Which of the following areas should the nurse gather data about first?
- ○ **1.** The client's perception of reality
- ○ **2.** The client's physical condition
- ○ **3.** The observations of the client made by others in the bus station
- ○ **4.** The client's speech patterns

209. Whenever the nurse tries to talk with Miss Dumas, the client responds with baby talk or gibberish. How would the nurse react?
- ○ **1.** Correct her speech.
- ○ **2.** Discontinue efforts to communicate with her.
- ○ **3.** Give simple, explicit directions to her.
- ○ **4.** Request a consultation with a speech therapist for her.

210. The physician prescribes haloperidol (Haldol) 6 mg IM q30min for 3 doses. Which of the following would the nurse do prior to each dose?
○ **1.** Draw a blood specimen.
○ **2.** Do a neurologic check.
○ **3.** Offer her fluids.
○ **4.** Take her blood pressure.

211. After the third dose of the medication, Miss Dumas is still talking baby talk and appears to be hallucinating. What would the nurse do?
○ **1.** Call the physician for further orders.
○ **2.** Administer another dose of the medication.
○ **3.** Record the results of the medication.
○ **4.** Observe the client for an hour.

212. After the client is past the acute hallucinatory period, the physician orders 4 mg of haloperidol (Haldol) QID. Which of the following is the best explanation for the nurse to give the client about the side effects of the drug?
○ **1.** "This medication may make you feel a little light-headed, especially in the morning, but it will help your symptoms."
○ **2.** "You will probably experience considerable drowsiness with this drug, but it will help you function better."
○ **3.** "This medication has no major side effects, and it will help you to tell what is real from what you may be imagining."
○ **4.** "You will be able to stop using this drug before very long, because it will get rid of your disordered thinking."

213. Miss Dumas appears to be listening to something that must be an hallucination; the nurse does not hear it. What is the most appropriate nursing response?
○ **1.** Give her an additional dose of her antipsychotic medication.
○ **2.** Ignore the behavior.
○ **3.** Contact her physician and request a seclusion order.
○ **4.** Talk with her about what she is experiencing.

214. Miss Dumas says to the nurse, "My mama says I shouldn't talk to you." Which of the following is the most appropriate response?
○ **1.** "Your mother has been dead for over 10 years."
○ **2.** "When did she say that?"
○ **3.** "I think you don't want to talk to me."
○ **4.** "That's very real to you, but you need to talk to me."

215. Which of the following is the best way to get Miss Dumas to participate in recreational activity?
○ **1.** Ask her what sports she enjoys and find ways for her to join other clients in these activities.
○ **2.** Assign a staff member to play catch with her.
○ **3.** Give her a list of available choices and have her select her preference.
○ **4.** Give her time to develop an interest and initiate activity.

216. To what extent would the nurse encourage the involvement of Miss Dumas's aunt in her therapy?
○ **1.** Not at all, since Miss Dumas is an adult
○ **2.** Only as much as Miss Dumas requests
○ **3.** As much as the aunt can participate
○ **4.** The aunt should be encouraged to enter therapy herself.

Several weeks after her wedding, Jane O'Grady was brought to the hospital by her husband. He reported she had disrobed in the supermarket and had urinated on the floor while singing the "Battle Hymn of the Republic." Her husband emphasized that this was very unusual behavior, since she has always been reserved, rather shy, and religious. Mrs. O'Grady called the nurse "Holy Mary" and said she finally was in a place "where there are lots of saints." She also whispered that God talks to her through the television.

217. Mrs. O'Grady's present behavior and events which possibly led to her hospitalization are discussed at a team conference. Which of the following nursing actions should be given the highest priority?
○ **1.** Concentrate on helping her relate to her husband.
○ **2.** Concentrate on helping her relate to a few staff members.
○ **3.** Concentrate on having her improve her grooming and appearance.
○ **4.** Concentrate on getting her involved in social activities on the unit.

218. As you approach her, she says, "I don't want to talk." What is the best nursing response?
○ **1.** "You don't want to talk?"
○ **2.** "Why don't you want to talk to me?"
○ **3.** "There is no need to talk with me."
○ **4.** "I'll sit with you for awhile."

219. A nursing student and Mrs. O'Grady pass by a room where other nursing students and clients are involved in a grooming and makeup session. The nursing student explains, "These sessions are on Tuesday and Thursday afternoons. The women learn how to apply makeup." What is the rationale for this nursing student's response?
    ○ 1. Impress the other clients and the instructor
    ○ 2. Encourage the success of the nurse-client relationship
    ○ 3. Orient the client to reality
    ○ 4. Persuade the client to join the group

220. Mrs. O'Grady yells for the nurse. As the nurse arrives and enters her room, she says, "Do you see? There! God is appearing." Which of the following is the best nursing response?
    ○ 1. "No, I don't see Him, but I understand He is real to you."
    ○ 2. "He is not there. You must be imagining things."
    ○ 3. "Show me where God appears to you."
    ○ 4. "God is appearing?"

221. Your response when Mrs. O'Grady asks for confirmation of her hallucination is based on which one of the following?
    ○ 1. Agree that the client perceives the hallucination in order to avoid increasing the client's anxiety.
    ○ 2. Tell the client to reexamine her feelings.
    ○ 3. Give an honest reply with the focus on what the client believes to be real.
    ○ 4. Tell the client that she is imagining things.

222. Mrs. O'Grady's anxiety has increased since her admission 3 days ago. Which behavior is Mrs. O'Grady most likely to demonstrate?
    ○ 1. Receptive to psychotherapy
    ○ 2. Shows insight about the causes of her illness
    ○ 3. Less able to focus her attention on the reality of the situation
    ○ 4. Less inclined to talk with her husband

Chi Wu is admitted to the hospital because of increasing withdrawal. He moves very slowly and is largely uncommunicative. His medical diagnosis is schizophrenia, catatonic type.

223. The best initial goal is which of the following?
    ○ 1. Client will establish a trusting relationship with the nurse.
    ○ 2. Client will increase his social skills.
    ○ 3. Client will increase his level of communication.
    ○ 4. Client will be oriented to reality.

224. The nurse on the unit begins to establish a relationship with Mr. Wu. Which of the following would be most effective in establishing communication at this time?
    ○ 1. Sit quietly with Mr. Wu.
    ○ 2. Talk about current world problems.
    ○ 3. Ask about the problems Mr. Wu is experiencing now.
    ○ 4. Tell Mr. Wu about all of the activities on the unit.

225. Mr. Wu becomes more communicative. The nurse plans to include him in activities that will provide opportunities for socialization. Which of the following would be most appropriate?
    ○ 1. Square dancing in the gym
    ○ 2. Learning to play chess
    ○ 3. Picnicking on the hospital grounds
    ○ 4. Playing video games

226. After a week of therapy with chlorpromazine (Thorazine), the nurse notices that Mr. Wu walks with a shuffling gait. What action should be taken by the nurse?
    ○ 1. Take his blood pressure before the next dose.
    ○ 2. Withhold the drug until the symptom disappears.
    ○ 3. Suggest a neurologic consult.
    ○ 4. Obtain an order for an antiparkinsonian drug.

227. After the nurse has discussed an upcoming 3-week vacation, Mr. Wu stops coming to their scheduled meetings and begins spending more time alone in his room. What best explains his response?
    ○ 1. He feels threatened by the closeness of their relationship.
    ○ 2. He is having a cyclical exacerbation of his illness.
    ○ 3. He is responding to the impending loss.
    ○ 4. He does not feel the need for the relationship anymore.

Arthur Maling has been admitted to the substance-abuse unit. He is 51 years old and has a history of increasing alcohol ingestion over the last 35 years. He currently drinks 1½ quarts of whisky daily. He is married, but his wife has moved out of their home because of his drinking problem.

228. Which of these would most likely be included in Mr. Maling's admission orders?
   ○ **1.** High protein diet, vitamins C and B complex, chlordiazepoxide (Librium)
   ○ **2.** High fat diet, vitamins B complex and E, chlorpromazine (Thorazine)
   ○ **3.** Liquid diet, vitamins A and E, meperidine (Demerol)
   ○ **4.** Liquid diet, vitamins C and B complex, phenytoin (Dilantin)

229. Prolonged use of alcohol may result in damage to the central nervous system. This may present as Korsakoff's syndrome (severe memory loss and confabulation). What is the physiologic cause of this condition?
   ○ **1.** Encephalomalacia
   ○ **2.** Marked deficiency of vitamin B_1 (thiamine)
   ○ **3.** Convulsions during withdrawal
   ○ **4.** Dystonic reactions

230. That evening Mr. Maling begins to show signs of alcohol withdrawal. The first symptoms are
   ○ **1.** hypotension, bradycardia, and decreased salivation.
   ○ **2.** fever, dehydration, and convulsions.
   ○ **3.** tremors, nervousness, and diaphoresis.
   ○ **4.** vomiting, diarrhea, and incontinence.

231. If Mr. Maling experiences hallucinations during withdrawal, which would be the best nursing practice?
   ○ **1.** A quiet room, prn medication
   ○ **2.** Bed rest, soft music, fluids
   ○ **3.** Hot tea q2h, blood pressure check q30min, restraints
   ○ **4.** Ice cream q2h, blood pressure check q15min, restraints

232. Mrs. Maling comes to see her husband. After the visit, she asks the nurse about Al-Anon. Which is the best response?
   ○ **1.** "Al-Anon is a support group for families of alcoholics. How do you feel about joining?"
   ○ **2.** "Al-Anon is a support group for families of alcoholics. Do you feel you need this, since you haven't been living with your husband?"
   ○ **3.** "Al-Anon is a support group for families of alcoholics. I'm sure you'd get a lot of help from joining."
   ○ **4.** "Al-Anon is a support group for families of alcoholics. Everyone who has a spouse who abuses alcohol should join."

233. The chances of an alcoholic's becoming permanently sober are variable. Which factor is most necessary for Mr. Maling to be successful?
   ○ **1.** Willingness to atone for past behavior
   ○ **2.** Recognition of the problem and motivation to change
   ○ **3.** Support from his family and from his employer
   ○ **4.** Membership in Alcoholics Anonymous

234. Mr. Maling starts taking disulfiram (Antabuse). He will continue to take this after discharge. Which drugs should he be clearly instructed *not* to take?
   ○ **1.** Aspirin and acetaminophen (Tylenol)
   ○ **2.** Most cough medicines
   ○ **3.** Heart and blood pressure medications
   ○ **4.** Antacids and laxatives

235. Mr. Maling starts attending Alcoholics Anonymous (AA) meetings in the hospital prior to discharge. Which statement about Alcoholics Anonymous is most correct?
   ○ **1.** It is a therapy group in which membership is recommended after discharge from a substance-abuse program.
   ○ **2.** It is a self-help group where members acknowledge their illness and share experiences concerning abuse and control of alcohol intake.
   ○ **3.** It is a self-help group led by professionals who have achieved sobriety.
   ○ **4.** It is a therapy group that discourages relationships outside the organization.

236. Eight months after discharge, Mr. Maling returns to visit. He attends AA regularly, his wife has returned to him and attends Al-Anon regularly, and he remains on the disulfiram (Antabuse) regimen. Which is the best description of Mr. Maling?
   ○ **1.** A cured alcoholic
   ○ **2.** A former alcoholic
   ○ **3.** A recovering alcoholic
   ○ **4.** A recovered alcoholic

Bert Trysdale is a 19-year-old who was admitted at 4:35 A.M. to the orthopedic unit from surgery. He had fractured the shaft of his right femur in a motorcycle accident. The surgeon did an open reduction and inserted an intramedullary nail. Mr. Trysdale is in traction and a unit of whole blood is hanging. He has been sleeping, and his vital signs are stable.

237. When the nurse enters the room to hang the container with the IV fluid to follow the unit of blood, Mr. Trysdale is awake and alert. He says, "How about a pint of rye instead?" Which of the following is the most therapeutic response?
    ○ 1. "We don't have any of that in the hospital."
    ○ 2. "It's a little early in the day for that, isn't it?"
    ○ 3. "It sounds as though you feel you could use a drink."
    ○ 4. "Sorry, but liquor is not allowed in the hospital."

238. The nurse enters the room later to find Mr. Trysdale trying to undo his traction. How would the nurse respond?
    ○ 1. "The traction must be left in place, or more damage will be done to your leg. What is bothering you about it?"
    ○ 2. "You're in an awfully big hurry to get up. What made you try to undo your traction?"
    ○ 3. "If you aren't comfortable, maybe I can get you some sedation."
    ○ 4. "The traction is necessary to immobilize your leg, so that it can heal. You must leave it alone."

239. The nursing assessment notes on the evening shift say that Mr. Trysdale seems anxious, has tremors, is perspiring, and has requested something for nausea. When the nurse gives Mr. Trysdale his IM medication for nausea, he says, "Is that gonna put me out?" How would the nurse respond?
    ○ 1. "Do you want to be put out?"
    ○ 2. "This is only for your nausea."
    ○ 3. "Are you used to taking drugs?"
    ○ 4. "You seem to be having a difficult time."

240. Mr. Trysdale continues to complain of generalized discomfort. He is visibly more anxious by the end of the evening shift and has not been able to fall asleep. He has not taken anything by mouth all day, even though he received a general soft diet at dinner time. The nurse suspects Mr. Trysdale may be going through drug or alcohol withdrawal. What would the nurse do first?
    ○ 1. Call Mr. Trysdale's physician and discuss the symptoms.
    ○ 2. Observe Mr. Trysdale closely for further symptoms.
    ○ 3. Arrange to transfer Mr. Trysdale to the detoxification unit.
    ○ 4. Administer the sedative prescribed for Mr. Trysdale.

241. Mr. Trysdale begins screaming at 2:40 A.M. When the nurse enters the room, he is trying to get out of bed and is crying out, "They're all over the bed! Get me outta this bed!" How should the nurse respond?
    ○ 1. Gesture as if you were brushing off whatever Mr. Trysdale thinks he sees.
    ○ 2. Reassure Mr. Trysdale that there is nothing in his bed. Talk calmly and orient him to his surroundings.
    ○ 3. Speak in a calm voice until Mr. Trysdale has settled down; then get help to restrain him.
    ○ 4. Administer a dose of the tranquilizer that the physician ordered.

242. After initially calming down, Mr. Trysdale becomes agitated again. He says, "What's happening to me? Why are you keeping me here?" Which of the following is the best response?
    ○ 1. "We are trying to help you, but you must try to get control of yourself."
    ○ 2. "When was the last time you took drugs or had a drink? You seem to be going through substance withdrawal."
    ○ 3. "I think you are having withdrawal symptoms. We are going to take care of you and help you through this."
    ○ 4. "You must be quiet and not disturb the other patients. We are keeping you here because you are sick."

243. Which of the following supportive nursing measures is appropriate while Mr. Trysdale is acutely agitated?
○ **1.** Encourage ambulation for him every hour.
○ **2.** Offer fluids every 2 hours.
○ **3.** Provide distractions such as television.
○ **4.** Give mild, natural stimulants, such as coffee or tea.

244. After 3 days, Mr. Trysdale seems to be through the most dangerous stage of withdrawal. He has told the nurse that he has been a heavy drinker ever since he entered high school. He has never gone through withdrawal before, he says, and the experience has scared him enough that he wants to give up drinking. Which of the following goals has the highest priority for the client?
○ **1.** Client will admit to a drinking problem.
○ **2.** Client will give up the use of alcohol permanently.
○ **3.** Client will join Alcoholics Anonymous or similar self-help group and attend meetings.
○ **4.** Client will accept the support of others to give up drinking.

245. After being hospitalized for 2 weeks, Mr. Trysdale has learned crutch walking and is ready for discharge. The evening before he is to be discharged, the nurse enters his room and finds him drinking a can of beer. How should the nurse respond?
○ **1.** "It really is hard to give up drinking when you've been doing it for a long time."
○ **2.** "It is so disappointing to see that you are not willing to change your habits."
○ **3.** "After all the work you've done, how can you throw it away like this?"
○ **4.** "Are you testing me to see how I'll react?"

246. The day that Mr. Trysdale is discharged, he says to the nurse who has worked with him the most, "Even though I slipped up last night, I know I'm gonna be able to quit for good." How should the nurse respond?
○ **1.** "No matter how much you want to quit, it's going to be tough. Ask for help when you need it."
○ **2.** "I'm proud that you are getting back on track. We all slip sometimes."
○ **3.** "You haven't really committed yourself to giving up drinking. You're not going to get better until you do."
○ **4.** "Don't make promises you're not ready to keep. You're the only one you hurt when you act like you did last night."

Roy Clements, a 26-year-old man, is admitted to the hospital in an acute psychotic state. He crawls around the unit on his hands and knees, making barking sounds. He came in accompanied by several friends, who revealed that the client took an unknown amount of lysergic acid diethylamide (LSD).

247. LSD belongs to which of the following classifications of drugs?
○ **1.** Opiates
○ **2.** Barbiturates
○ **3.** Hallucinogenics
○ **4.** Stimulants

248. Which of the following is *not* characteristic of LSD?
○ **1.** Physical addiction
○ **2.** Psychologic dependence
○ **3.** Acute panic states
○ **4.** Heightened sensory perceptions

249. Drug-dependent clients respond best to
○ **1.** psychoanalysis.
○ **2.** behavior modification.
○ **3.** family therapy.
○ **4.** group therapy led by former drug abusers.

250. Immediately after admission to the unit, Mr. Clements's psychotic behavior worsens. He tears at his clothes and hair, attempts to smash the television set in the dayroom with a chair, and threatens to attack another client. The best immediate nursing action is to
○ **1.** turn off the TV to reduce stimulation.
○ **2.** place the client in seclusion.
○ **3.** ask the physician for a stat order for sedation.
○ **4.** restrain the client in a chair in the dayroom.

251. Of the following reasons for the use of seclusion, which one is *not* valid?
○ **1.** To reduce environmental stimulation
○ **2.** To prevent a client from hurting himself
○ **3.** To prevent a client from hurting others
○ **4.** To reduce the need for constant observation

252. Mr. Clements sees red spiders crawling on his bed. Which of the following is the appropriate nursing response?
○ **1.** "Come on, Mr. Clements, you're putting me on."
○ **2.** Swat at the red spiders as if to kill them in Mr. Clements's presence.
○ **3.** "I know you see the red spiders, Mr. Clements. I am not seeing any."
○ **4.** Logically explain that red spiders are not present in his bed.

253. Later, Mr. Clements states that he is the king of Siam, and as one of his subjects, the nurse should bow in his presence. Select the most appropriate nursing response.
○ **1.** Bow and pay respect to Mr. Clements.
○ **2.** "You must feel very powerful, Mr. Clements."
○ **3.** "If you're the king of Siam, I am Queen Jezebel."
○ **4.** Place him in seclusion until he is able to control himself.

254. Select the drug that best helps control hallucinations and delusions.
○ **1.** Haloperidol (Haldol)
○ **2.** Lithium carbonate
○ **3.** Diazepam (Valium)
○ **4.** Maprotiline (Ludiomil)

References

American Journal of Nursing Company. *AJN 1988 Nursing Boards Review*. Baltimore: Williams & Wilkins, 1987.

American Psychiatric Association. *Diagnostic and Statistical Manual of Mental Disorders*, 3rd Ed. Washington, DC: 1980.

Bergersen, B. and Goth, A. *Pharmacology in Nursing*, 14th Ed. St. Louis: Mosby, 1979.

Berner Howry, L., McGillis Bindler, R., and Tso, Y. *Pediatric Medications*. Philadelphia: Lippincott, 1981.

Burgess, A. and Lazare, A. *Psychiatric Nursing in the Hospital and the Community*, 3rd Ed. Englewood Cliffs, NJ: Prentice-Hall, 1981.

DeGennaro, M. et al. "Antidepressant Drug Therapy." *American Journal of Nursing*, July 1981:1304-10.

Dorland's Pocket Medical Dictionary, 21st Ed. Philadelphia: Saunders, 1968.

Figley, C. *Stress Disorders Among Vietnam Veterans: Theory Research and Treatment*. New York: Brunner/Mazel, 1978.

Gorton, J., and Partridge, R. (ed). *Practice and Management of Psychiatric Emergency Care*. St. Louis: Mosby, 1982.

Grace, H. and Camilleri, D. *Mental Health Nursing: A Sociopsychological Approach*. Dubuque, IA: Brown, 1981.

Haber, E. "Extrapyramidal Side Effects of Anti-Psychotic Medications." *American Journal of Nursing*, July 1981:1324-1328.

Haber, J. et al. *Comprehensive Psychiatric Nursing*, 2nd Ed. New York: McGraw-Hill, 1982.

Harris, E. "Lithium." *American Journal of Nursing*, July 1981:1310-15.

Hein, E. *Communication in Nursing Practice*, 2nd Ed. Boston: Little, Brown, 1980.

Huff, L. *People in Crisis: Understanding and Helping*, 2nd Ed. Menlo Park, CA: Addison Wesley, 1984.

Huppendavern, S. et al. "Post-traumatic Stress Disorders in Vietnam Veterans." *American Journal of Nursing*, 1982:1694-1704.

Lagerquist, S. et al. *Addison-Wesley's Nursing Examination Review*, 2nd Ed. Menlo Park, CA: Addison-Wesley, 1982.

Loebl, S. and Spratto, G. *Nurse's Drug Handbook*, 2nd Ed. New York: Wiley, 1980.

Pasquali, E. et al. *Mental Health Nursing: A Bio-psychocultural Approach*. St. Louis: Mosby, 1981.

Rodgers, J. et al. *Psychiatric Mental Health Nursing Review*, 2nd Ed. New York: Arco, 1980.

Stuart, G. and Sundeen, S. *Principles and Practices of Psychiatric Nursing*, 2nd Ed. St. Louis: Mosby, 1983.

Whaley, L. and Wong, D. *Nursing Care of Infants and Children*, 3rd Ed. St. Louis: Mosby, 1986.

Wilson, H. and Kneisl, C. *Psychiatric Nursing*, 2nd Ed. Menlo Park, CA: Addison-Wesley, 1983.

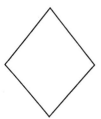

Section 2
Correct Answers

1. #4.	47. #2.	93. #4.	139. #1.
2. #2.	48. #2.	94. #2.	140. #1.
3. #2.	49. #3.	95. #3.	141. #4.
4. #3.	50. #3.	96. #4.	142. #1.
5. #3.	51. #4.	97. #4.	143. #4.
6. #1.	52. #1.	98. #2.	144. #4.
7. #1.	53. #1.	99. #1.	145. #4.
8. #4.	54. #4.	100. #3.	146. #1.
9. #3.	55. #3.	101. #4.	147. #1.
10. #2.	56. #3.	102. #1.	148. #4.
11. #1.	57. #4.	103. #1.	149. #4.
12. #2.	58. #3.	104. #4.	150. #2.
13. #3.	59. #2.	105. #4.	151. #1.
14. #3.	60. #3.	106. #1.	152. #4.
15. #2.	61. #3.	107. #1.	153. #4.
16. #3.	62. #1.	108. #2.	154. #4.
17. #4.	63. #4.	109. #4.	155. #2.
18. #2.	64. #3.	110. #3.	156. #3.
19. #3.	65. #4.	111. #2.	157. #3.
20. #3.	66. #2.	112. #1.	158. #3.
21. #2.	67. #1.	113. #3.	159. #1.
22. #3.	68. #4.	114. #1.	160. #2.
23. #4.	69. #2.	115. #3.	161. #3.
24. #4.	70. #2.	116. #3.	162. #1.
25. #3.	71. #4.	117. #2.	163. #1.
26. #2.	72. #4.	118. #3.	164. #3.
27. #2.	73. #3.	119. #4.	165. #3.
28. #1.	74. #3.	120. #3.	166. #2.
29. #3.	75. #3.	121. #4.	167. #1.
30. #4.	76. #3.	122. #1.	168. #3.
31. #2.	77. #4.	123. #3.	169. #4.
32. #3.	78. #1.	124. #3.	170. #2.
33. #1.	79. #3.	125. #2.	171. #3.
34. #2.	80. #2.	126. #3.	172. #3.
35. #1.	81. #1.	127. #2.	173. #2.
36. #2.	82. #4.	128. #3.	174. #1.
37. #2.	83. #2.	129. #3.	175. #3.
38. #2.	84. #1.	130. #1.	176. #3.
39. #4.	85. #1.	131. #4.	177. #2.
40. #4.	86. #4.	132. #4.	178. #4.
41. #3.	87. #2.	133. #2.	179. #1.
42. #2.	88. #4.	134. #2.	180. #3.
43. #3.	89. #3.	135. #2.	181. #1.
44. #4.	90. #4.	136. #4.	182. #3.
45. #1.	91. #4.	137. #2.	183. #3.
46. #4.	92. #2.	138. #4.	184. #3.

185. #3.	**203.** #1.	**221.** #3.	**239.** #4.
186. #1.	**204.** #4.	**222.** #3.	**240.** #1.
187. #4.	**205.** #2.	**223.** #1.	**241.** #2.
188. #4.	**206.** #1.	**224.** #1.	**242.** #3.
189. #2.	**207.** #3.	**225.** #3.	**243.** #2.
190. #1.	**208.** #2.	**226.** #4.	**244.** #4.
191. #3.	**209.** #3.	**227.** #3.	**245.** #1.
192. #4.	**210.** #4.	**228.** #1.	**246.** #1.
193. #4.	**211.** #1.	**229.** #2.	**247.** #3.
194. #3.	**212.** #1.	**230.** #3.	**248.** #1.
195. #2.	**213.** #4.	**231.** #1.	**249.** #4.
196. #4.	**214.** #4.	**232.** #1.	**250.** #2.
197. #2.	**215.** #2.	**233.** #2.	**251.** #4.
198. #1.	**216.** #3.	**234.** #2.	**252.** #3.
199. #3.	**217.** #2.	**235.** #2.	**253.** #2.
200. #2.	**218.** #4.	**236.** #3.	**254.** #1.
201. #1.	**219.** #3.	**237.** #3.	
202. #4.	**220.** #1.	**238.** #1.	

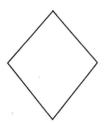

Correct Answers with Rationales

Editors note:

Two pieces of information are supplied at the end of each rationale. First, we tell you what part of the nursing process the question addresses. Second, in parentheses, you will find a reference to a section in the *AJN Nursing Boards Review* where a more complete discussion of the topic may be found should you desire more information.

1. **#4.** The present interaction pattern allows the nurse to work in the here and now and not proceed based on preconceived ideas. Present interaction includes not only verbal aspects (who talks to whom), but also nonverbal ones (e.g., facial expression, body movements, seating patterns). Options #1, #2, and #3 will be important later, once the group is established. IMPLEMENTATION (PSYCHOSOCIAL, MENTAL HEALTH, PSYCHIATRIC PROBLEMS/THERAPEUTIC USE OF SELF)

2. **#2.** The residents are anxious and their response is not unusual. This is the establishing phase of the group. While the nurse may not have clearly explained the purpose of the group, a characteristic of this stage is anxiety related to uncertainty over what will actually occur in the group. The members may express anger; however, it is usually a manifestation of anxiety at the beginning of a new experience. ANALYSIS (PSYCHOSOCIAL, MENTAL HEALTH, PSYCHIATRIC PROBLEMS/THERAPEUTIC USE OF SELF)

3. **#2.** The purpose of the group is interaction. Option #2 will permit discussion and possible problem solving by the entire group. #4 singles out 1 resident, in effect, closing the others out of the interaction. #1 is false reassurance and cuts off further exploration. Option #3 keeps the focus on an individual rather than encouraging group interaction. IMPLEMENTATION (PSYCHOSOCIAL, MENTAL HEALTH, PSYCHIATRIC PROBLEMS/THERAPEUTIC USE OF SELF)

4. **#3.** Commenting on your perceptions will allow the group to discuss their feelings and has the potential for serving as a learning situation. Monopolizing the conversation is a group issue and needs to be addressed in the group, not on an individual basis. Ignoring the behavior does not help Mr. Abels to learn how to be with other people appropriately. If transferred to another group, Mr. Abels will no doubt repeat the behavior, and it will give a message to other group members that exclusion is the penalty for not pleasing others. IMPLEMENTATION (PSYCHOSOCIAL, MENTAL HEALTH, PSYCHIATRIC PROBLEMS/THERAPEUTIC USE OF SELF)

5. **#3.** The client's verbal and nonverbal communication do not correspond. If she were angry and disgusted, she should not be smiling. Her words and behavior are incongruent. Mrs. Thomas is not demonstrating suspicious (fear of harm from others), demanding (unnecessary and insistent requests), or resistive (unwilling to cooperate) behavior. ANALYSIS (PSYCHOSOCIAL, MENTAL HEALTH, PSYCHIATRIC PROBLEMS/THERAPEUTIC USE OF SELF)

6. **#1.** The best way to deal with incongruence is to point out the inconsistency observed between verbal and nonverbal communication to the client. Options #2, #3, and #4 do not address the incongruent behavior and are not as helpful to the client. IMPLEMENTATION (PSYCHOSOCIAL, MENTAL HEALTH, PSYCHIATRIC PROBLEMS/THERAPEUTIC USE OF SELF)

7. **#1.** After the nurse has confronted her with the inconsistency, allow her some time to think about what was said before expecting her to respond. Option #3 is used with resistive, not thoughtful, silence. #2 reflects a lack of understanding of giving feedback and the need for the client to reflect upon the meaning of it before responding. #4 forces a response before the client is ready. IMPLEMENTATION (PSYCHOSOCIAL, MENTAL HEALTH, PSYCHIATRIC PROBLEMS/THERAPEUTIC USE OF SELF)

8. **#4.** The health care team can begin a plan of care based on initial assessment of behavior. Part of the plan of care will include approaches or possible interventions for specific behaviors displayed by the client. It is most likely that options #2 and #3 have not been completed or even initiated yet. #1 really does not pertain to nursing care. PLAN (PSYCHOSOCIAL, MENTAL HEALTH, PSYCHIATRIC PROBLEMS/THERAPEUTIC USE OF SELF)

9. **#3.** Clients who become more withdrawn are frequently regarded as needing human contact. This can best be done through a one-to-one relationship, beginning at the level the client is at. The nurse offers physical presence and avoids probing questions and does not demand options or participation that is premature. Options #2 and #4 reflect a lack of understanding of withdrawn behavior. IMPLEMENTATION (PSYCHOSOCIAL, MENTAL HEALTH, PSYCHIATRIC PROBLEMS/THERAPEUTIC USE OF SELF)

10. **#2.** From the data presented, both affect and words indicate anger. A statement such as ''It can't be true'' would indicate denial. Depression would show itself by crying, immobility, and inability to sleep and eat or sleeping and eating too much. Resolution would be shown by statements that acknowledge the death and view the deceased realistically. ANALYSIS (PSYCHOSOCIAL, MENTAL HEALTH, PSYCHIATRIC PROBLEMS/LOSS, DEATH AND DYING)

11. **#1.** This option provides information about the duration of the response. A normal grief reaction lasts for approximately 6 months and is usually resolved in 12 months. Options #2, #3, and #4 are normal grief reaction statements, but they do not help to discern between normal and dysfunctional grief. ASSESSMENT (PSYCHOSOCIAL, MENTAL HEALTH, PSYCHIATRIC PROBLEMS/LOSS, DEATH AND DYING)

12. **#2.** The problem being expressed at this time is anger. From the data provided, the anger seems to be associated with her husband's very recent death. She is not denying her feelings of guilt, nor is she experiencing depression at this time. ANALYSIS (PSYCHOSOCIAL, MENTAL HEALTH, PSYCHIATRIC PROBLEMS/LOSS, DEATH AND DYING)

13. **#3.** The abundance of feelings during the initial grieving process may leave the client anxious and confused. Talking about feelings (ventilation) aids in the reduction of anxiety and offers an opportunity to begin to work through the grief. Seeing the positive aspects of her husband occurs in the resolution stage. Educating the client to the grief process is important once the overwhelming feelings are explored. Option #4 is false reassurance and leaves the client feeling isolated and misunderstood. IMPLEMENTATION (PSYCHOSOCIAL, MENTAL HEALTH, PSYCHIATRIC PROBLEMS/LOSS, DEATH AND DYING)

14. **#3.** The client's basic physical needs must be met first. It would be more helpful if the nurse helped the family deal with their feelings at this point since the client is so very ill. Right now, the client does not have the energy to express anger and may not feel anger or be in touch with anger. The highest priority is physical care. PLAN (PSYCHOSOCIAL, MENTAL HEALTH, PSYCHIATRIC PROBLEMS/LOSS, DEATH AND DYING)

15. **#2.** Her behavior decreases her ability to express her feelings. Decubitus ulcers may result from immobility and associated stasis of blood flow. Nurses may feel anger toward client because Mrs. Quale is not demonstrating ''good patient'' behavior. Contractures in an already debilitated client are more likely with immobility. ANALYSIS (PSYCHOSOCIAL, MENTAL HEALTH, PSYCHIATRIC PROBLEMS/LOSS, DEATH AND DYING)

16. **#3.** The children may reject their mother as a defense against their perceived rejection by her. Since it may be too painful for Mrs. Quale to deal with her children, the separation keeps her from increasing her awareness of how they are actually feeling. Client may be afraid that her changed body image would repel her children and further decrease her self-esteem. She uses denial to protect herself from the changes and to fully experience her impending losses, thus prolonging the grief process. ANALYSIS (PSYCHOSOCIAL, MENTAL HEALTH, PSYCHIATRIC PROBLEMS/LOSS, DEATH AND DYING)

17. **#4.** The client may be unable to achieve this physically or mentally. Nursing care measures in option #1 are necessary. The nurse who explores her own feelings usually gains greater awareness and self-control; thus she is able to focus more on the client's need rather than her own needs. The presence of the nurse is usually comforting and connotes her acceptance of the client. IMPLEMENTATION (PSYCHOSOCIAL, MENTAL HEALTH, PSYCHIATRIC PROBLEMS/LOSS, DEATH AND DYING)

18. **#2.** A client may or may not experience each of the stages of dying, in order or not. People are usually consistent in their reactions to major crises. It is very important for the nurse to remember the needs of the family. A child's level of cognitive development will determine his/her response to death. ASSESSMENT (PSYCHOSOCIAL, MENTAL HEALTH, PSYCHIATRIC PROBLEMS/LOSS, DEATH AND DYING)

19. **#3.** To a 3-year-old, death is the same as going away for awhile. Six- to 9-year-olds personify death (someone bad carries them away). Five- to 6-year-olds believe death is reversible. Nine- to 10-year-olds recognize that everyone must die. ASSESSMENT (PSYCHOSOCIAL, MENTAL HEALTH, PSYCHIATRIC PROBLEMS/LOSS, DEATH AND DYING)

20. **#3.** Children generally do not express their emotions or concerns directly, especially to strangers such as hospital staff. They are able to express their concerns better through stories, drawings, or other forms of play as indicated in options #1, #2, and #4. Through these mediums, children may state directly how they feel or their emotions may be inferred through observation. IMPLEMENTATION (PSYCHOSOCIAL, MENTAL HEALTH, PSYCHIATRIC PROBLEMS/LOSS, DEATH AND DYING)

21. **#2.** This approach is direct. It allows the client to talk about her feelings but also allows her a choice. Options #1, #3, and #4 avoid dealing directly with Mrs. Miller's sorrow and grief. This may foster the client's repressing her grief and developing a delayed grief reaction. IMPLEMENTATION (PSYCHOSOCIAL, MENTAL HEALTH, PSYCHIATRIC PROBLEMS/LOSS, DEATH AND DYING)

22. **#3.** Suicidal thoughts are fairly common in reactive depression, but hoarding sleep medication indicates actual planning of a suicide attempt, which is an abnormal grief response. Options #1, #2, and #4 are common manifestations of a normal grief reaction. ASSESSMENT (PSYCHOSOCIAL, MENTAL HEALTH, PSYCHIATRIC PROBLEMS/LOSS, DEATH AND DYING)

23. **#4.** Although it is appropriate to offer support during the crisis period of a grief reaction, it is also important to allow the client to move through the process at her own pace. Mrs. Miller's depression is an expected stage of normal grief and she should be allowed to experience her sorrow rather than avoid it by medication or numerous activities. A surprise visit from her son could precipitate a flooding of overwhelming feelings which could be frightening to her and her 2-year-old son. Option #1 is an avoidance of the client's feelings and gives the message that crying is not acceptable. IMPLEMENTATION (PSYCHOSOCIAL, MENTAL HEALTH, PSYCHIATRIC PROBLEMS/LOSS, DEATH AND DYING)

24. **#4.** Although the nurse should offer emotional support at this time, allow Mrs. Miller the option of being alone since different persons cope with loss in different ways. IMPLEMENTATION (PSYCHOSOCIAL, MENTAL HEALTH, PSYCHIATRIC PROBLEMS/LOSS, DEATH AND DYING)

25. **#3.** This answer indicates the absence of a value judgment by the nurse, while allowing the client the option of discussing the decision. Option #1 is a premature closure of the subject. #2 and #4 are judgment statements that could provoke a defensive response. All 3 discourage further discussion of her feelings. IMPLEMENTATION (PSYCHOSOCIAL, MENTAL HEALTH, PSYCHIATRIC PROBLEMS/LOSS, DEATH AND DYING)

26. **#2.** In moderate anxiety, the person's ability to perceive and concentrate is decreased. Physical discomforts increase and overall level of functioning decreases. This client is still functioning and able to focus on work with effort, but her discomfort is increasing. At this point, the anxiety is moderate. Without intervention, it is likely to become severe, whereby the person's perceptual field is greatly reduced, time sense is distorted, and all behavior is aimed at getting relief. During mild anxiety, the person is alert and perceptual field is increased. When in a panic, the person's emotional tone is associated with awe, dread, and terror. ANALYSIS (PSYCHOSOCIAL, MENTAL HEALTH, PSYCHIATRIC PROBLEMS/ANXIOUS BEHAVIOR)

27. **#2.** This helps the client identify and express the feelings she is experiencing at the present time. It provides the nurse with more data to assist the client to recognize her anxiety and begin to relate her behavior to the feelings she is experiencing. It is best in the beginning of assessment to focus on the here-and-now and start with a general perspective rather than being directive or asking about past experiences. IMPLEMENTATION (PSYCHOSOCIAL, MENTAL HEALTH, PSYCHIATRIC PROBLEMS/ANXIOUS BEHAVIOR)

28. **#1.** In order to establish an effective behavior-modification program, baseline data must first be collected about the behavior (e.g., frequency, amount, time). Although options #2 and #3 are important because activities of daily living and pain contribute to the behavior, in themselves they do not provide a complete picture. Any reaction to the anesthetic would have already occurred. ASSESSMENT (PSYCHOSOCIAL, MENTAL HEALTH, PSYCHIATRIC PROBLEMS/ANXIOUS BEHAVIOR)

29. **#3.** The client is probably afraid that she will be left alone. Responding at consistent intervals when she is not calling for something will reduce the calling behavior and, one hopes, increase her confidence that she will be attended to. Her underlying fear can be dealt with by checking on her consistently and frequently. Option #1 promotes the client's frequent requests. Pain may not be the only reason she is uncomfortable. Option #4 only makes the client feel guilty and does not address the underlying problem of her fear of being alone. IMPLEMENTATION (PSYCHOSOCIAL, MENTAL HEALTH, PSYCHIATRIC PROBLEMS/ANXIOUS BEHAVIOR)

30. **#4.** If demanding behavior is reinforced, it will be repeated. To change undesired behavior, reinforce more appropriate behavior. Options #1 through #3 are also important, but are not as helpful for changing the behavior. PLAN (PSYCHOSOCIAL, MENTAL HEALTH, PSYCHIATRIC PROBLEMS/ANXIOUS BEHAVIOR)

31. **#2.** During an anxiety reaction, the client thinks that something bad will happen; with normal anxiety there is no such underlying feeling. Both have the same physiologic and psychologic manifestations. Normal anxiety is not constant; there can be a wide range of levels from mild to severe. An anxiety reaction can be controlled with proper interventions to reduce the level of panic. Normal anxiety can become an anxiety reaction when someone with inadequate coping mechanisms is under great stress. ASSESSMENT (PSYCHOSOCIAL, MENTAL HEALTH, PSYCHIATRIC PROBLEMS/ANXIOUS BEHAVIOR)

32. **#3.** The techniques used in option #3 are reflection and restatement. #1 defends the doctor; #2 agrees with the client, and #4 is reassurance; all of which are nontherapeutic statements because they do not allow further exploration of the client's concerns and feelings. IMPLEMENTATION (PSYCHOSOCIAL, MENTAL HEALTH, PSYCHIATRIC PROBLEMS/ANXIOUS BEHAVIOR)

33. **#1.** These are the physiologic and psychologic manifestations of anxiety. Characteristics of depression are listed in option #2; #3 describes thought disorders related to psychosis; and #4 is also characteristic of mania and depression. ASSESSMENT (PSYCHOSOCIAL, MENTAL HEALTH, PSYCHIATRIC PROBLEMS/ANXIOUS BEHAVIOR)

34. **#2.** The person in panic is severely agitated, which shows in verbal and nonverbal behavior. Option #1 lists symptoms of psychotic behaviors; option #3, neurotic anxiety states. Option #4 is only partially correct; mood depression is not usually characteristic of a panic reaction. ASSESSMENT (PSYCHOSOCIAL, MENTAL HEALTH, PSYCHIATRIC PROBLEMS/ANXIOUS BEHAVIOR)

35. #1. Stay calm and help the client mobilize thoughts and feelings. Option #3 is a cognitive skill that a person in panic may not be able to use until he has calmed down. Clients in a panic state are not out of touch with reality and are usually experiencing fear, dread, and terror, not anger. IMPLEMENTATION (PSYCHOSOCIAL, MENTAL HEALTH, PSYCHIATRIC PROBLEMS/ANXIOUS BEHAVIOR)

36. #2. The nurse must assess the psychologic and physiologic indicators of anxiety as well as the client's effective use of coping mechanisms. Incoherent thought processes, mood swings, or lack of reality orientation were never the problem. A more comprehensive evaluation than self-reporting is in order. EVALUATION (PSYCHOSOCIAL, MENTAL HEALTH, PSYCHIATRIC PROBLEMS/ANXIOUS BEHAVIOR)

37. #2. This is the most common phobia among those who seek treatment. Literally "fear of the marketplace" is displayed by those who specifically fear being in a public place from which they may not be able to escape. Acrophobia is the fear of heights; astraphobia is the fear or dread of thunder and lightning; claustrophobia is the fear of closed places. ANALYSIS (PSYCHOSOCIAL, MENTAL HEALTH, PSYCHIATRIC PROBLEMS/ANXIOUS BEHAVIOR)

38. #2. In a phobic disorder, the anxiety is displaced from the original source and then transferred, resulting in a phobia. Denial involves distorting reality so that the existence of threatening situations is negated. Substitution involves replacing the original unacceptable wish, drive, emotion, or goal with one that is more acceptable. Symbolization is an unconscious defense mechanism whereby one idea or object comes to stand for another because of some common aspect or quality in both. ASSESSMENT (PSYCHOSOCIAL, MENTAL HEALTH, PSYCHIATRIC PROBLEMS/ANXIOUS BEHAVIOR)

39. #4. The most common behavior modification technique used to treat phobic disorders is desensitization. Under controlled conditions, the client is gradually exposed to the object or situation feared. Confrontation is useful only when the client has the ability to hear the information and the readiness to work on the problem. Immediate exposure could create even greater anxiety. Distraction will not enable the client to overcome his fear and resume functioning. PLAN (PSYCHOSOCIAL, MENTAL HEALTH, PSYCHIATRIC PROBLEMS/ANXIOUS BEHAVIOR)

40. #4. Agoraphobia is classified as occurring with or without panic attacks. However, anxiety is experienced with exposure to the feared object or situation, and an anxiolytic may be prescribed at the beginning of desensitization. Fluphenazine and chlorpromazine are indicated for the treatment of psychosis. Amitriptyline is indicated for the treatment of depression. IMPLEMENTATION (PSYCHOSOCIAL, MENTAL HEALTH, PSYCHIATRIC PROBLEMS/ANXIOUS BEHAVIOR)

41. #3. Since agoraphobia is fear of the outside, his presence on the volleyball court would be indicative of his ability to leave the hospital building. Milieu group, occupational therapy, and Sunday dinner are held on the unit and, although they are important elements of the treatment program, the client is still in a closed environment. EVALUATION (PSYCHOSOCIAL, MENTAL HEALTH, PSYCHIATRIC PROBLEMS/ANXIOUS BEHAVIOR)

42. #2. The ritualistic behavior demonstrated by the client with an obsessive-compulsive disorder is considered a symbolic attempt to control anxiety. Obsessive-compulsive behaviors may result in attention but the behavior is an attempt to handle an anxiety-provoking situation. An obsessive-compulsive behavioral pattern is an uncontrollable impulse and may result in isolation, but it originates from a feeling of anxious dread and is persistently impelling, not manipulative. ANALYSIS (PSYCHOSOCIAL, MENTAL HEALTH, PSYCHIATRIC PROBLEMS/ANXIOUS BEHAVIOR)

43. **#3.** Displacement of the ego-dystonic idea into an unrelated and senseless activity temporarily lowers the anxiety of the individual. By carrying out the act, she attempts to undo the impulse she is unable to control. In introjection, a psychic representation of a loved or hated object is taken into one's ego system. In projection, a person attributes to another ideas, thoughts, feelings, and impulses that are a part of his/her inner perceptions but are unacceptable to him/her. Compensation is a conscious or unconscious defense mechanism by which a person tries to make up for an imagined or real deficiency, physical or psychologic or both. Isolation involves setting apart an idea from the feeling tone. Rationalization is an unconscious defense mechanism in which an irrational behavior, motive, or feeling is made to appear reasonable. Repression is an unconscious defense mechanism by which a person removes from consciousness those ideas, impulses, and affects that are unacceptable to him/her. ANAYLSIS (PSYCHOSOCIAL, MENTAL HEALTH, PSYCHIATRIC PROBLEMS/ANXIOUS BEHAVIOR)

44. **#4.** The obsessive-compulsive disorder is characterized by obsessive thoughts that are cancelled out by symbolic acts or rituals. Although the behavior is self-destructive, it is an attempt to control irrational thinking. This behavior does not involve an attempt to explain or justify it cognitively (intellectualization). Obsessive-compulsive behavior is described as being the result of fixation during the oral phase of development. ANALYSIS (PSYCHOSOCIAL, MENTAL HEALTH, PSYCHIATRIC PROBLEMS/ANXIOUS BEHAVIOR)

45. **#1.** Obsessive-compulsive clients are assessed for the ritualistic behavior, possible sources of conflict in life situations, the degree to which the ritual or repetitive behavior interferes with activities of daily living, and potential unresolved conflicts. Assessment of thought patterns, associations, and delusions would be important if the nurse believed the client to be psychotic. Options #3 and #4 must always be assessed; but in determining whether or not the client has an obsessive-compulsive disorder, the nurse must first determine the client's specific daily actions. ASSESSMENT (PSYCHOSOCIAL, MENTAL HEALTH, PSYCHIATRIC PROBLEMS/ANXIOUS BEHAVIOR)

46. **#4.** It is necessary to reestablish and maintain physiologic integrity while working on the long-range goal of decreasing the washing behavior. If this is not focused on initially, infection could result. Option #1 is a higher level of functioning. Once the client has stabilized physically (or concurrently), it is helpful to begin working on the problem behavior. Expression of feeling is important; understanding the "why" may or may not be a useful short-term goal. PLAN (PSYCHOSOCIAL, MENTAL HEALTH, PSYCHIATRIC PROBLEMS/ANXIOUS BEHAVIOR)

47. **#2.** Plan sufficient time for her to perform necessary rituals early in her treatment; to prohibit this behavior would induce extreme anxiety, as will strict limit-setting. The client's problem does not involve close proximity to others. The client already understands the behavior is irrational. PLAN (PSYCHOSOCIAL, MENTAL HEALTH, PSYCHIATRIC PROBLEMS/ANXIOUS BEHAVIOR)

48. **#2.** In dealing with ritualistic behavior, the nurse must help the client by setting limits on the destructive, repetitive behavior. Allow the client to carry out the behavior to some degree, but not to the point of injury. The client is in touch with reality and her primary problem does not involve assertive behavior. Medication may be ordered to help the client with uncontrollable anxiety. PLAN (PSYCHOSOCIAL, MENTAL HEALTH, PSYCHIATRIC PROBLEMS/ANXIOUS BEHAVIOR)

49. **#3.** This allows participation in a unit activity but does not call undue attention to or reinforce the obsessive-compulsive behavior. Option #1 would be an overreaction by the nurse and is inappropriate. Moving the TV does not address the problem and encourages isolation. #4 would likely result in the client becoming more anxious. IMPLEMENTATION (PSYCHOSOCIAL, MENTAL HEALTH, PSYCHIATRIC PROBLEMS/ANXIOUS BEHAVIOR)

50. **#3.** Providing Maria with a schedule will help limit her ritualistic behaviors but she should not be expected to prevent them altogether. The remaining actions would all be helpful. IMPLEMENTATION (PSYCHOSOCIAL, MENTAL HEALTH, PSYCHIATRIC PROBLEMS/ANXIOUS BEHAVIOR)

51. **#4.** There are no drugs to alleviate obsessive-compulsive symptoms, and these behaviors are very resistant to treatment. Nursing care plans can aim at modifying or limiting ritualistic behaviors rather than attempting to eliminate them altogether. Obsessive-compulsive clients are not psychotic. Options #2 and #3 may be true but initially the behavior must be controlled because of the physical threat. EVALUATION (PSYCHOSOCIAL, MENTAL HEALTH, PSYCHIATRIC PROBLEMS/ANXIOUS BEHAVIOR)

52. **#1.** To evaluate nursing care for the obsessive-compulsive client, look for a decrease in the ritualistic behavior and resumption of activities of daily living, such as personal care. Thought process regarding her obsessive beliefs and self-reports of reduced anxiety will need to be evaluated but are longer-term goals. EVALUATION (PSYCHOSOCIAL, MENTAL HEALTH, PSYCHIATRIC PROBLEMS/ANXIOUS BEHAVIOR)

53. **#1.** Obsessive-compulsive clients usually recognize the behavior is senseless and receive no pleasure from the activity. Anxiety and tension are only temporarily reduced. Options #2, #3, and #4 indicate no insight on the part of the client. ASSESSMENT (PSYCHOSOCIAL, MENTAL HEALTH, PSYCHIATRIC PROBLEMS/ANXIOUS BEHAVIOR)

54. **#4.** Bradycardia (not tachycardia) is characteristic with weight loss. Amenorrhea is a common finding. Delayed psychosexual development related to earlier unresolved issues of separation and individualization is frequently seen along with a familial pattern of a facade of happiness and harmony, which in reality covers underlying conflict and dysfunction among the family members. ASSESSMENT (PSYCHOSOCIAL, MENTAL HEALTH, PSYCHIATRIC PROBLEMS/ANXIOUS BEHAVIOR)

55. **#3.** These clients are not concerned with conserving energy; rather they typically exercise frequently in order to expend the number of calories equal to the amount they estimate they have consumed. Options #1, #2, and #4 are all commonly manifested behaviors in clients experiencing anorexia nervosa that demonstrate an intense interest in food and the relentless pursuit of thinness. ASSESSMENT (PSYCHOSOCIAL, MENTAL HEALTH, PSYCHIATRIC PROBLEMS/ANXIOUS BEHAVIOR)

56. **#3.** These clients are often in life-threatening electrolyte and nutritional imbalance. Death rates of up to 20% among diagnosed cases have been cited in the literature. Options #1, #2, and #4 are all important to implement after physiologic integrity is established. IMPLEMENTATION (PSYCHOSOCIAL, MENTAL HEALTH, PSYCHIATRIC PROBLEMS/ANXIOUS BEHAVIOR)

57. **#4.** It is important to keep an anorexic client within view of the staff for at least 1 hour after meals to discourage induction of vomiting. Options #1 and #3 promote some positive control and independence, which the client needs instead of starving herself to gain control. Providing support and reinforcement allays anxiety and increases compliance. IMPLEMENTATION (PSYCHOSOCIAL, MENTAL HEALTH, PSYCHIATRIC PROBLEMS/ANXIOUS BEHAVIOR)

58. **#3.** The anorexic denies and represses stomach hunger and, thus, is not aware of feeling hungry. Hypothalamic and physiologic functions are normal. ANALYSIS (PSYCHOSOCIAL, MENTAL HEALTH, PSYCHIATRIC PROBLEMS/ANXIOUS BEHAVIOR)

59. **#2.** A desired response is followed by a desired or positive consequence. Option #1 is the presentation of an aversive stimulus immediately following an undesired response. Option #3 occurs when the removal of a stimulus strengthens the tendency to behave in a certain way. Option #4 is the process of transferring learning from one situation to other similar situations. IMPLEMENTATION (PSYCHOSOCIAL, MENTAL HEALTH, PSYCHIATRIC PROBLEMS/ANXIOUS BEHAVIOR)

60. **#3.** Involvement in preparation and management of the treatment plan will help the client learn to be responsible. Threats create a power struggle that reenacts old familiar and pathologic family patterns. Option #2 can be life threatening since about 15% of anorexics die from starvation. #4 is not helpful because the core issue is control and self-image, not good eating habits. IMPLEMENTATION (PSYCHOSOCIAL, MENTAL HEALTH, PSYCHIATRIC PROBLEMS/ANXIOUS BEHAVIOR)

61. **#3.** Clients with anorexia nervosa see themselves as overweight regardless of how thin they are. Even when they look in the mirror, they see themselves as fat. The most appropriate nursing response is to tell them how the nurse sees their size, in a factual way without judgments or statements that may decrease their self-esteem. IMPLEMENTATION (PSYCHOSOCIAL, MENTAL HEALTH, PSYCHIATRIC PROBLEMS/ANXIOUS BEHAVIOR)

62. **#1.** Hypochondriasis is an exaggerated concern with one's physical health while having no organic pathologic condition (psychosomatic illness) and no loss of function (conversion disorder). Dissociation reaction is a mechanism for minimizing or avoiding anxiety by keeping parts of the individual's experience out of conscious awareness (e.g., amnesia, fugue state, multiple personality). ANALYSIS (PSYCHOSOCIAL, MENTAL HEALTH, PSYCHIATRIC PROBLEMS/ANXIOUS BEHAVIOR)

63. **#4.** These clients tend to react with increased anxiety to new and different situations. Clear and concise explanations of treatments and procedures help to allay the anxiety. The focus for intervention should not be the symptom (i.e., pain) but the precipitating event (i.e., group interaction). Option #2 fosters avoidance of the possible stressor(s) and encourages reliance on others to relieve the symptom (pain). #3 avoids any interaction by exerting authoritative control and sets up a possible power struggle. IMPLEMENTATION (PSYCHOSOCIAL, MENTAL HEALTH, PSYCHIATRIC PROBLEMS/ANXIOUS BEHAVIOR)

64. **#3.** Hallucinations, delusions, and mania would be treated with antipsychotic medication, not diazepam. IMPLEMENTATION (PSYCHOSOCIAL, MENTAL HEALTH, PSYCHIATRIC PROBLEMS/ANXIOUS BEHAVIOR)

65. **#4.** The first 3 options are true for diazepam (Valium). Valium and alcohol are both CNS depressants; the combination could severely depress the CNS. Valium can cause possible interactions/toxicity when taken with other medications. IMPLEMENTATION (PSYCHOSOCIAL, MENTAL HEALTH, PSYCHIATRIC PROBLEMS/ANXIOUS BEHAVIOR)

66. **#2.** As Mrs. Manchester deals with her feelings of guilt, anger, and fear, she will begin to remember the rest of the painful event. Allow her time to remember without probing. Asking questions might help the client to recall additional details of the story, but might also increase her anxiety and contribute to a sense of being overwhelmed by the situation. It is common for clients experiencing post-traumatic stress disorder to have lapses in memory regarding details that are too painful to remember. Telling the client that she is withholding information may only add to her sense of frustration, anxiety, and guilt. IMPLEMENTATION (PSYCHOSOCIAL, MENTAL HEALTH, PSYCHIATRIC PROBLEMS/ANXIOUS BEHAVIOR)

67. **#1.** For those with post-traumatic stress disorder, the pain of surviving and the accompanying guilt often lead to their wish that they too had died. For many survivors, the situation can compound their guilt if they feel they should have been at the scene of the trauma, or were there but survived when others did not. The client's feelings are those normally expressed in this type of situation. Option #3 does not convey a sense of acceptance of the feelings and only adds more guilt. It is important for the nurse to assess risk of suicide; however, option #4 is not sensitive to the client's feelings of guilt. IMPLEMENTATION (PSYCHOSOCIAL, MENTAL HEALTH, PSYCHIATRIC PROBLEMS/ANXIOUS BEHAVIOR)

68. **#4.** Support groups of people who have suffered similarly can be very helpful in teaching clients how to deal with the situation. They can also provide a forum where the client can express feelings in an accepting atmosphere. It might be helpful for the client to join Parents Without Partners after the crisis period in order to develop a support network for the future. An out-of-town trip might add to her sense of guilt about having left her children alone when the accident occurred. While planning weekly outings with her children might be helpful, the activities chosen should be more appropriate for their age group. IMPLEMENTATION (PSYCHOSOCIAL, MENTAL HEALTH, PSYCHIATRIC PROBLEMS/ANXIOUS BEHAVIOR)

69. **#2.** Crisis intervention, a form of secondary prevention, seeks to prevent psychiatric disorders through early intervention in order to allow the client to regain equilibrium. Primary prevention seeks to prevent psychiatric disorders through community education and special programs targeting high-risk groups. Tertiary prevention is aimed at reducing the long-term impact resulting from psychiatric disorders and includes rehabilitation programs. Early diagnostic care is ONLY one component of secondary prevention. PLAN (PSYCHOSOCIAL, MENTAL HEALTH, PSYCHIATRIC PROBLEMS/ANXIOUS BEHAVIOR)

70. **#2.** Knowledge of past occupations, hobbies, etc., will assist in keeping interactions reality based. Present medical conditions and past methods of coping with stress are more useful in planning nursing care than are prior medical history and stressors. Family history would not be helpful because the nurse is planning care for the individual client and not the family. S/he will not be able to help the family with similar disorders. ASSESSMENT (PSYCHOSOCIAL, MENTAL HEALTH, PSYCHIATRIC PROBLEMS/CONFUSED BEHAVIOR)

71. **#4.** The etiology of Alzheimer's disease is unknown. Options #1, #2, and #3 are true of Alzheimer's disease because the suspected virus attacks the tissue of the cerebral cortex causing progressive deterioration of intellectual functioning and behavior. ANALYSIS (PSYCHOSOCIAL, MENTAL HEALTH, PSYCHIATRIC PROBLEMS/CONFUSED BEHAVIOR)

72. **#4.** Realization that memory loss is occurring often causes anxiety and depression in these clients. The first 3 options will assist the client to remain oriented to time, person, and place for as long as possible. IMPLEMENTATION (PSYCHOSOCIAL, MENTAL HEALTH, PSYCHIATRIC PROBLEMS/CONFUSED BEHAVIOR)

73. **#3.** Her picture and name on the door draw upon long-term memory, which is more likely to remain intact. Mrs. Cohen would have a difficult time remembering the light blue door because of short-term memory loss. Assigning her a buddy or placing her close to the nurses' station will reinforce her feelings of dependency and loss of control. IMPLEMENTATION (PSYCHOSOCIAL, MENTAL HEALTH, PSYCHIATRIC PROBLEMS/CONFUSED BEHAVIOR)

74. **#3.** Serving smaller amounts of food at more frequent intervals will increase the probability of an adequate intake, as well as preserve the dignity of the client. A full liquid diet would not be palatable and would decrease her appetite. Feeding Mrs. Cohen would decrease her self-worth because of being forced to be in an unnecessarily dependent position. Serving food whenever Mrs. Cohen is ready could lead to an unbalanced diet; it is difficult to monitor the type of food and amount eaten. IMPLEMENTATION (PSYCHOSOCIAL, MENTAL HEALTH, PSYCHIATRIC PROBLEMS/CONFUSED BEHAVIOR)

75. **#3.** This response indicates a willingness to offer support and to allow Mr. Cohen to ventilate his feelings at a difficult time. Alzheimer's disease is a degenerating illness and she will progressively worsen. Option #2 is poorly timed. Mr. Cohen has not come to terms with this alternative solution. #4 reflects denial on the nurse's part. Alzheimer's disease clients require demanding care around the clock which may be too difficult for an elderly person. IMPLEMENTATION (PSYCHOSOCIAL, MENTAL HEALTH, PSYCHIATRIC PROBLEMS/CONFUSED BEHAVIOR)

76. **#3.** The client with major depression has low self-esteem, feelings of worthlessness, and very little physical energy. A structured, positive experience will help to increase self-esteem. Setting up too many tasks will overwhelm him. Introducing Mr. Jones to other people will make him feel more self-conscious. Staying away will reinforce the withdrawal and low self-esteem. Having him express himself freely is inappropriate in occupational therapy. IMPLEMENTATION (PSYCHOSOCIAL, MENTAL HEALTH, PSYCHIATRIC PROBLEMS/ELATED-DEPRESSIVE BEHAVIOR)

77. **#4.** Options #1, #2, and #3 are all side effects of nortriptyline, a tricyclic antidepressant. MAO inhibitors, not the tricyclics, potentiate the action of many other medications. ANALYSIS (PSYCHOSOCIAL, MENTAL HEALTH, PSYCHIATRIC PROBLEMS/ELATED-DEPRESSIVE BEHAVIOR)

78. **#1.** The depressed client is likely to demonstrate anger, withdrawal, or hostility at times. The other options are seen in mania. ASSESSMENT (PSYCHOSOCIAL, MENTAL HEALTH, PSYCHIATRIC PROBLEMS/ELATED-DEPRESSIVE BEHAVIOR)

79. **#3.** Refusal may be seen as rejection of the client. Focus on the client's needs. It is important to find out which changes the client wants to make. Depressed clients are more likely to make suicidal attempts. The nurse monitors the blood levels of the antidepressant because they have a critical therapeutic window effect, meaning that at a certain range in the blood they are most effective. IMPLEMENTATION (PSYCHOSOCIAL, MENTAL HEALTH, PSYCHIATRIC PROBLEMS/ELATED-DEPRESSIVE BEHAVIOR)

80. **#2.** The severely depressed client can best understand simple information, given slowly and directly. The presence of the nurse will be comforting to him in new surroundings. Introducing him to everyone and asking him to perform too many activities will be overwhelming. Placing him next to a talkative client would be a mismatch that would exaggerate Mr. Chung's quietness. IMPLEMENTATION (PSYCHOSOCIAL, MENTAL HEALTH, PSYCHIATRIC PROBLEMS/ ELATED-DEPRESSIVE BEHAVIOR)

81. **#1.** The depressed client introjects hostility and anger. Projection is a defense mechanism used in character disorders and by paranoid individuals. Suppression and repression are common defense mechanisms used in neurotic disorders. ASSESSMENT (PSYCHOSOCIAL, MENTAL HEALTH, PSYCHIATRIC PROBLEMS/ELATED-DEPRESSIVE BEHAVIOR)

82. **#4.** The perception that something or someone meaningful has been lost is the most important contributing factor in depression. Hormonal imbalance is related to postpartum depression. Sexual identity problems are related to either adolescent adjustment problems or homosexuality. Character disorders such as sociopathy, where problems with authority figures exist, result from unresolved parental conflict. ANALYSIS (PSYCHOSOCIAL, MENTAL HEALTH, PSYCHIATRIC PROBLEMS/ELATED-DEPRESSIVE BEHAVIOR)

83. **#2.** A regular schedule provides structure and removes the burden of making decisions from the depressed client. Giving him only 1 activity a day will reinforce his feelings of inadequacy and withdrawal. A depressed client's thinking processes are too slowed to allow him to choose activities or take the initiative in participating. He is in the hospital for the structure he could not provide for himself. IMPLEMENTATION (PSYCHOSOCIAL, MENTAL HEALTH, PSYCHIATRIC PROBLEMS/ELATED-DEPRESSIVE BEHAVIOR)

84. **#1.** Nonverbal ommunication may be necessary with a severely depressed client. The presence of the nurse indicates to him that he is regarded as a worthwhile person. Option #2 assumes that he is self-destructive. At this point, Mr. Chung lacks the energy to hurt himself. #3 is a judgmental response. The nurse needs to accept his discomfort and not place demands on Mr. Chung when he does not feel comfortable around others. IMPLEMENTATION (PSYCHOSOCIAL, MENTAL HEALTH, PSYCHIATRIC PROBLEMS/ELATED-DEPRESSIVE BEHAVIOR)

85. **#1.** A tricyclic is used first, because there are fewer side effects with this class of drugs. The dosage for imipramine is correct. Elavil has more sedative effects and the dose given is too high for starting dose. The MAO inhibitors, Marplan and Nardil, are generally contraindicated in the elderly and would be used only if the tricyclics do not work. IMPLEMENTATION (PSYCHOSOCIAL, MENTAL HEALTH, PSYCHIATRIC PROBLEMS/ELATED-DEPRESSIVE BEHAVIOR)

86. **#4.** When depression is severe, the client has insufficient energy to plan and execute a suicide attempt. When improvement begins, the risk of suicide is the greatest. If he is ready to go home, he is not suicidal. When his family goes on vacation, he might feel more depressed because he is being left behind, but would not necessarily become suicidal. ANALYSIS (PSYCHOSOCIAL, MENTAL HEALTH, PSYCHIATRIC PROBLEMS/ELATED-DEPRESSIVE BEHAVIOR)

87. **#2.** Keeping the suicidal client under constant close observation is mandatory protection from self-inflicted harm. Tranquilizers are contraindicated while taking antidepressants and will not eliminate the suicidal ideation. Suicidal feelings should be talked about and worked through until the internalized feelings of hostility are resolved. Other clients could be helpful in monitoring a suicidal client's behavior by lending support and increasing concern regarding the client's whereabouts. PLAN (PSYCHOSOCIAL, MENTAL HEALTH, PSYCHIATRIC PROBLEMS/ ELATED-DEPRESSIVE BEHAVIOR)

88. **#4.** The nurse is demonstrating a positive attitude and reassurance with the offer to accompany and remain with him. Mr. Chung did not say he changed his mind; he is indicating he has anxiety about the unknown and option #1 does not address the unknown aspects of the ECT procedure. It is true Mr. Chung does not have to go, but at his age of 60 years, ECT would be safer than MAO inhibitors in helping him overcome his depression. IMPLEMENTATION (PSYCHOSOCIAL, MENTAL HEALTH, PSYCHIATRIC PROBLEMS/ELATED-DEPRESSIVE BEHAVIOR)

89. **#3.** The most common post-ECT effects are confusion and memory loss for recent events. It is reassuring to the client to know this is a temporary condition. Headaches and dizziness are common side effects of MAO inhibitors. Nausea and vomiting are common side effects of many drugs. Diarrhea and urinary incontinence are common side effects of tricyclic antidepressants. ASSESSMENT (PSYCHOSOCIAL, MENTAL HEALTH, PSYCHIATRIC PROBLEMS/ELATED-DEPRESSIVE BEHAVIOR)

90. **#4.** All these drugs are used for the safest and most effective administration of ECT. ECT causes seizures so a muscle relaxant is given. An anesthetic is used to reduce sensations of the seizure. Atropine sulfate is used to decrease secretions and to relax smooth muscles. IMPLEMENTATION (PSYCHOSOCIAL, MENTAL HEALTH, PSYCHIATRIC PROBLEMS/ELATED-DEPRESSIVE BEHAVIOR)

91. **#4.** Group members provide feedback for each other through a variety of responses and reactions. This improves insight and self-knowledge. Group therapy's aim is not to increase socialization skills, because the focus is to work on one's own problems. Improved reality orientation is done through the use of calendars, clocks, and name tags. Universality or the feeling that other people have the same problem does provide comfort that one is not alone, but does not provide insight into the nature of depression. EVALUATION (PSYCHOSOCIAL, MENTAL HEALTH, PSYCHIATRIC PROBLEMS/ELATED-DEPRESSIVE BEHAVIOR)

92. **#2.** Currently, the most frequent use of electroconvulsive therapy (ECT) is to treat severe depression that has not responded to medication or psychotherapy. Following ECT, the client often becomes more accessible to psychotherapy. A shortened hospital stay is a benefit of ECT but not the chief benefit. After the client has had some psychotherapy, the length of hospitalization may be shortened, but follow-up care is usually required. ECT does not necessarily lessen the need for medication. PLAN (PSYCHOSOCIAL, MENTAL HEALTH, PSYCHIATRIC PROBLEMS/ELATED-DEPRESSIVE BEHAVIOR)

93. **#4.** Ordinarily, hospital policies and procedures require that the physician administer the shock to the client. Some of the nurse's responsibilities during ECT are cited in options #1 through #3. IMPLEMENTATION (PSYCHOSOCIAL, MENTAL HEALTH, PSYCHIATRIC PROBLEMS/ ELATED-DEPRESSIVE BEHAVIOR)

94. **#2.** Immediately following ECT, the client is given the same nursing care as that of any unconscious client. The client will experience drowsiness and confusion upon awakening. Orienting the client will decrease anxiety or fears. There is no reason for the client to remain in bed after vital signs have stabilized. Resumption of normal activity on the unit by the client soon after treatment places ECT in its proper perspective as one of a number of therapeutic modalities. IMPLEMENTATION (PSYCHOSOCIAL, MENTAL HEALTH, PSYCHIATRIC PROBLEMS/ ELATED-DEPRESSIVE BEHAVIOR)

95. **#3.** Mrs. Bell exhibits behaviors or symptoms that are considered at high risk for suicide: severe depression, history of suicidal ideation, hopelessness, anger at hospitalization, and a suicidal plan. Her age, sex, divorced and unemployed status also place her at high risk. ANALYSIS (PSYCHOSOCIAL, MENTAL HEALTH, PSYCHIATRIC PROBLEMS/ELATED-DEPRESSIVE BEHAVIOR)

96. **#4.** The elderly, adolescents, alcoholics, and drug abusers are statistically high-risk groups for suicidal behavior; people in their 30s are not. ASSESSMENT (PSYCHOSOCIAL, MENTAL HEALTH, PSYCHIATRIC PROBLEMS/ELATED-DEPRESSIVE BEHAVIOR)

97. **#4.** Suicidal clients often have problems talking about painful feelings; they need encouragement to express their feelings and concerns about suicide and hopelessness. Options #1, #2, and #3 are the responsibilities of a nurse when caring for a client with high risk of suicide. IMPLEMENTATION (PSYCHOSOCIAL, MENTAL HEALTH, PSYCHIATRIC PROBLEMS/ELATED-DEPRESSIVE BEHAVIOR)

98. **#2.** The *DSM-III* classifies depression as an affective disorder. Somatoform disorders are conditions characterized by complaints of physical distress. Mild depressions may take this form, but severe depressions do not. Anxiety disorders are conditions characterized by feelings of fear and symptoms such as palpitations, tachycardia, and tremors. Personality disorders are conditions characterized by long-standing problems with relationships and mood swings. ANAYLSIS (PSYCHOSOCIAL, MENTAL HEALTH, PSYCHIATRIC PROBLEMS/ELATED-DEPRESSIVE BEHAVIOR)

99. **#1.** A mild depression is primarily affective in nature (sadness, dejection, discouragement), while severe depression includes severe affective signs as well as a decrease in activity, thought patterns, communication, and socialization, and an increase in somatic symptoms and vegetative signs. Suicidal ideation can be associated with any level of depression. Duration of symptoms and age do not indicate severity, and mild depression can be lengthy. ASSESSMENT (PSYCHOSOCIAL, MENTAL HEALTH, PSYCHIATRIC PROBLEMS/ELATED-DEPRESSIVE BEHAVIOR)

100. **#3.** Napping in the daytime encourages increased withdrawal from social activity and also prevents the client from being tired enough to sleep through the night. Encouraging discussion of feelings and concerns will reduce anxiety associated with lack of sleep. Option #2 will engage client in participating in self-care. #4 provides structure and normalization of routine for client. PLAN (PSYCHOSOCIAL, MENTAL HEALTH, PSYCHIATRIC PROBLEMS/ELATED-DEPRESSIVE BEHAVIOR)

101. **#4.** Assisting the client to establish bedtime routines to promote rest and sleep will be a learning situation to practice in the hospital and to use at home; success builds hope and self-esteem. It would not be therapeutic to ignore sleep patterns and complaints because that discounts a client's concerns. Reassurance is rarely therapeutic. Option #3 would defeat the goal of normalization of sleep patterns. IMPLEMENTATION (PSYCHOSOCIAL, MENTAL HEALTH, PSYCHIATRIC PROBLEMS/ELATED-DEPRESSIVE BEHAVIOR)

102. **#1.** Tofranil is a tricyclic antidepressant. IMPLEMENTATION (PSYCHOSOCIAL, MENTAL HEALTH, PSYCHIATRIC PROBLEMS/ELATED-DEPRESSIVE BEHAVIOR)

103. **#1.** Tofranil causes urinary retention rather than urinary frequency. It may produce dry mouth, not increased salivation. Tofranil cannot be taken on an as-needed basis since it requires a blood concentration to be effective, which takes 2-4 weeks to establish itself. IMPLEMENTATION (PSYCHOSOCIAL, MENTAL HEALTH, PSYCHIATRIC PROBLEMS/ELATED-DEPRESSIVE BEHAVIOR)

104. **#4.** This option is a closed-ended, judgmental question and is not appropriate. The remaining options all assist the nurse to establish a useful data base. ASSESSMENT (PSYCHOSOCIAL, MENTAL HEALTH, PSYCHIATRIC PROBLEMS/ELATED-DEPRESSIVE BEHAVIOR)

105. **#4.** Denying feelings and complaints would not be helpful. Sharing painful feelings is vital in learning to cope with them. PLAN (PSYCHOSOCIAL, MENTAL HEALTH, PSYCHIATRIC PROBLEMS/ELATED-DEPRESSIVE BEHAVIOR)

106. **#1.** Focusing on the positive aspects of life has merit but is the least effective of the 4 actions given to meet the stated goal. Options #2 and #3 are basic to the nurse-client relationship no matter what the client problems may be. They are considered to be effective in assisting clients to cope. Option #4 is an effective method of providing alternatives, which assists in coping and decision-making. IMPLEMENTATION (PSYCHOSOCIAL, MENTAL HEALTH, PSYCHIATRIC PROBLEMS/ELATED-DEPRESSIVE BEHAVIOR)

107. **#1.** This action allows Mrs. Bell to maintain control and self-direction in her life and yet focus on concerns of discharge. Options #2 and #4 work against the nurse-client relationship and undermine client's control over her life. #3 fosters denial of the problem areas of her life and does not accomplish therapeutic goals. IMPLEMENTATION (PSYCHOSOCIAL, MENTAL HEALTH, PSYCHIATRIC PROBLEMS/ELATED-DEPRESSIVE BEHAVIOR)

108. **#2.** Rumination is psychotic behavior, and telling a client to stop does little good. Introducing communication that expands her narrow frame of reference will enhance interaction and redirect her thinking. Providing opportunities for activity and exercise will provide structure, redirection, and utilization of energy for clients who ruminate. Option #4 enhances self-awareness and self-esteem. IMPLEMENTATION (PSYCHOSOCIAL, MENTAL HEALTH, PSYCHIATRIC PROBLEMS/ELATED-DEPRESSIVE BEHAVIOR)

109. **#4.** Angry outbursts are a positive behavior for depressed clients and should never be ignored. Options #1, #2, and #3 are all appropriate communication techniques and strategies for working with all clients. IMPLEMENTATION (PSYCHOSOCIAL, MENTAL HEALTH, PSYCHIATRIC PROBLEMS/ELATED-DEPRESSIVE BEHAVIOR)

110. **#3.** Most individuals who are intent on suicide still wish very much to be rescued. The fact that Mrs. King tried to eliminate the possibility of rescue indicates the seriousness of the attempt and should alert the staff to the possibility of another attempt. A client may be unconscious as a result of a suicide gesture that was not intended to be serious. Many clients who are not serious use a potentially lethal method and kill themselves accidentally. Not leaving a suicide note may indicate nonintent; however, it may also indicate impulsive and serious intent. ASSESSMENT (PSYCHOSOCIAL, MENTAL HEALTH, PSYCHIATRIC PROBLEMS/ELATED-DEPRESSIVE BEHAVIOR)

111. **#2.** The client's response does not indicate remorsefulness about the suicide attempt, but disappointment at her ineffectiveness in carrying it out successfully. She is depressed and feeling hopeless, so the potential for another suicide attempt is great. As with most suicidal people, she is probably ambivalent about whether she wants to live or die. ANALYSIS (PSYCHOSOCIAL, MENTAL HEALTH, PSYCHIATRIC PROBLEMS/ ELATED-DEPRESSIVE BEHAVIOR)

112. **#1.** Although all the options are appropriate, the first priority is to protect the client from suicidal gestures. Options #2 and #3 are correct actions; however, they are not the highest priority when dealing with a high-potential suicide risk. #4 is of a higher priority and would be implemented as soon as the safety needs addressed in option #1 were accomplished. IMPLEMENTATION (PSYCHOSOCIAL, MENTAL HEALTH, PSYCHIATRIC PROBLEMS/ELATED-DEPRESSIVE BEHAVIOR)

113. **#3.** Any change in behavior may mean that the client has worked out a suicide plan. The apparent lifting of her depression may mean that Mrs. King now has the energy to carry out her plan. While any client's first weekend at home is stressful, for this client and her history, a weekend pass at this time is contraindicated, premature, and potentially dangerous. Depressed clients may have mood swings; however, the abruptness of this client's change and her request for a weekend pass must be explored and considered cautiously. ANALYSIS (PSYCHOSOCIAL, MENTAL HEALTH, PSYCHIATRIC PROBLEMS/ELATED-DEPRESSIVE BEHAVIOR)

114. **#1.** In treating low self-esteem, it is important to begin by giving clients minimal tasks that they can accomplish without failure. All the other suggestions contain the possibility of failure or are too stressful when the client is feeling helpless, or both. IMPLEMENTATION (PSYCHOSOCIAL, MENTAL HEALTH, PSYCHIATRIC PROBLEMS/ELATED-DEPRESSIVE BEHAVIOR)

115. **#3.** These clients need the security of being allowed to build a trusting relationship with a staff member. Dependence on the staff can more appropriately be dealt with by firm limit setting and encouragement to be more independent. Providing only the help needed and encouraging problem-solving would foster independence on the part of the client. Option #4 is an early attempt to reduce dependent behavior. IMPLEMENTATION (PSYCHOSOCIAL, MENTAL HEALTH, PSYCHIATRIC PROBLEMS/ELATED-DEPRESSIVE BEHAVIOR)

116. **#3.** Anxiousness, hopelessness, somatic complaints, depressions, suicidal behavior, and a sense of loss are symptoms of involutional states classified as psychotic depression. Middle age, a life centered on family and home, and children "leaving the nest" are other clues. Paranoid schizophrenia is characterized by a concrete and pervasive delusional system that is generally persecutory. No data is presented to suggest a history of mood swings, manic behavior, or substance abuse. ANALYSIS (PSYCHOSOCIAL, MENTAL HEALTH, PSYCHIATRIC PROBLEMS/ELATED-DEPRESSIVE BEHAVIOR)

117. **#2.** This client has already attempted suicide. Observation and protective measures should be instituted immediately. While food intake is a concern with clients expressing depression, it is not the most important nursing action listed. Data suggests that this client has already exhibited a high involvement with her family. The nursing intervention strategies would best be addressed to diversifying her interests at this time. Reassurance is rarely therapeutic. Based on the data presented, it would be presumptive to indicate that physical complaints are unwarranted. IMPLEMENTATION (PSYCHOSOCIAL, MENTAL HEALTH, PSYCHIATRIC PROBLEMS/ELATED-DEPRESSIVE BEHAVIOR)

118. **#3.** During times of deepest depression, the client lacks the energy to plan and carry out a suicide attempt. When depression lessens, the client has energy to act on self-destructive thoughts and impulses. ASSESSMENT (PSYCHOSOCIAL, MENTAL HEALTH, PSYCHIATRIC PROBLEMS/ELATED-DEPRESSIVE BEHAVIOR)

119. **#4.** Serious drug interactions occur when MAO inhibitors are given in combination with tricyclics, narcotics, alcohol, anticholinergics, antidiabetic agents, barbiturates, reserpine, sympathomimetics, and dibenzepin derivatives. Option #1 is incorrect since these drugs are slower to act than other antidepressants. While tachycardia may sometimes occur, the most common side effect of MAO inhibitors is hypertensive crisis. MAO inhibitors do not increase appetite; in fact, they may cause nausea and vomiting. Certain dietary restrictions are required when taking them. ASSESSMENT (PSYCHOSOCIAL, MENTAL HEALTH, PSYCHIATRIC PROBLEMS/ELATED-DEPRESSIVE BEHAVIOR)

120. **#3.** This comment by the nurse acknowledges the client's fear. Staying with the client also tends to allay anxiety. To tell the client who expresses fear to not be afraid discourages expression of the feelings. Options #2 and #4 are incorrect because they minimize the importance of these feelings. IMPLEMENTATION (PSYCHOSOCIAL, MENTAL HEALTH, PSYCHIATRIC PROBLEMS/ELATED-DEPRESSIVE BEHAVIOR)

121. **#4.** Their agitation causes these clients to be hyperactive, and they usually have difficulty getting sufficient sleep. Agitated depression is characterized by psychomotor restlessness, pacing, and handwringing. ASSESSMENT (PSYCHOSOCIAL, MENTAL HEALTH, PSYCHIATRIC PROBLEMS/ELATED-DEPRESSIVE BEHAVIOR)

122. **#1.** Elavil (amitriptyline HC1) is a tricyclic antidepressant. Although the monoamine oxidase inhibitors (MAOI) are also antidepressants, the MAOI mode of action is distinctly different from the tricyclics. Phenothiazines are antipsychotic medications. Antihistamines combat the side effects of the antipsychotic medications. ANALYSIS (PSYCHOSOCIAL, MENTAL HEALTH, PSYCHIATRIC PROBLEMS/ELATED-DEPRESSIVE BEHAVIOR)

123. **#3.** Dry mouth, constipation, and blurred vision are anticholinergic responses, indicative of side effects upon the autonomic nervous system. Cardiovascular and endocrine system side effects such as dysrhythmias and impotence can occur with Elavil but are not mentioned in this question. Respiratory system reactions are uncommon. ANALYSIS (PSYCHOSOCIAL, MENTAL HEALTH, PSYCHIATRIC PROBLEMS/ELATED-DEPRESSIVE BEHAVIOR)

124. **#3.** This is a major reason for noncompliance with tricyclic antidepressants. Symptomatic relief does not usually occur until after 2-4 weeks of therapy and clients often become noncompliant unless instructed about this time lag. Three days is an insufficient length of time to judge clinical effectiveness. Twenty-five milligrams TID is a therapeutic dose of Elavil. ANALYSIS (PSYCHOSOCIAL, MENTAL HEALTH, PSYCHIATRIC PROBLEMS/ELATED-DEPRESSIVE BEHAVIOR)

125. #2. The side effects of tricyclic antidepressant medications are most apparent during initiation of treatment and diminish as therapy progresses. Drug therapy requires regularity of administration for effectiveness. Although the client may discuss the side effects with her physician, it is appropriate for the nurse to discuss them also. It is nontherapeutic to threaten clients with electroconvulsive therapy. IMPLEMENTATION (PSYCHOSOCIAL, MENTAL HEALTH, PSYCHIATRIC PROBLEMS/ELATED-DEPRESSIVE BEHAVIOR)

126. #3. This indicates to the client that her distress was heard and permits exploration of feelings she is experiencing now. The second option asks for an explanation that the client is probably unable to give. The first option may make the client feel the nurse is minimizing or unaware of her feelings. The client with a major depression will not feel better about herself within a few days. IMPLEMENTATION (PSYCHOSOCIAL, MENTAL HEALTH, PSYCHIATRIC PROBLEMS/ELATED-DEPRESSIVE BEHAVIOR)

127. #2. One theory regarding the etiology of major depressive episodes is that symptoms reflect the individual's response to a severe threat to security (a loss). The loss may be real or imagined and is perceived by an individual, such as Mrs. Perkins, as a threat to her very being. A psychotic depression is not a normal response regardless of the severity of the precipitating stress. The incident described is a situational, not maturational, crisis. Major depressions may last for a long time and require hospitalization. ANALYSIS (PSYCHOSOCIAL, MENTAL HEALTH, PSYCHIATRIC PROBLEMS/ELATED-DEPRESSIVE BEHAVIOR)

128. #3. Focusing on making small decisions such as "Do you want to wear the blue blouse or red blouse?" is a first step in building self-esteem. The client may be unable to make decisions at this time and will need assistance. Explaining the importance of decision making is premature and likely to make her feel worse. Making all decisions for her will keep the client regressed and dependent. IMPLEMENTATION (PSYCHOSOCIAL, MENTAL HEALTH, PSYCHIATRIC PROBLEMS/ELATED-DEPRESSIVE BEHAVIOR)

129. #3. Short, frequent contacts, as tolerated, will assist in establishing the nurse-client relationship. Once this is accomplished, the client can be encouraged to participate in activities on the unit. Depressed clients need human contact. Aloneness will cause further alterations in the client's thought processes. However, she may be unable to attend activities yet. Explanations about the therapeutic value of activities is not a motivator for the depressed person. IMPLEMENTATION (PSYCHOSOCIAL, MENTAL HEALTH, PSYCHIATRIC PROBLEMS/ELATED-DEPRESSIVE BEHAVIOR)

130. #1. The preparation is basically the same as for any procedure where general anesthesia is used, since electroconvulsive therapy (ECT) produces a loss of consciousness. Include all measures (e.g., NPO, removal of dentures) necessary to preserve the safety of the client. There is continuing controversy about the use of ECT and many myths about it persist. Clients who have not responded to adequate trials of antidepressant medication may experience a reduction of symptoms following ECT. Short-term side effects of ECT are confusion, transient memory loss, and headache. ANALYSIS (PSYCHOSOCIAL, MENTAL HEALTH, PSYCHIATRIC PROBLEMS/ELATED-DEPRESSIVE BEHAVIOR)

131. #4. The human contact provided by remaining with her and conversing with her at her level of readiness will help to lighten the anxiety she is feeling. Valium and deep breathing lessen anxiety, but more important is the client's need to express her fears and to be given proper reassurance by the nurse. Mrs. Perkins must not eat or drink because an anesthetic will be administered. IMPLEMENTATION (PSYCHOSOCIAL, MENTAL HEALTH, PSYCHIATRIC PROBLEMS/ELATED-DEPRESSIVE BEHAVIOR)

132. #4. Prompt reorientation lessens the anxiety generated by the confusion. Some degree of confusion may persist during the day; however, observations by staff can take place in the dayroom. The client will remain in bed or on a stretcher until she is oriented, her vital signs stabilize, and she can safely join ward activities. There is no data to indicate the need for a physician. IMPLEMENTATION (PSYCHOSOCIAL, MENTAL HEALTH, PSYCHIATRIC PROBLEMS/ELATED-DEPRESSIVE BEHAVIOR)

133. **#2.** The working phase is characterized by the client's confronting problems and learning alternative methods of coping and problem solving. The initiating phase may also be called the orientating phase. In the terminating phase, the client and nurse summarize and evaluate the work of the relationship and express feelings and thoughts about termination. ANALYSIS (PSYCHOSOCIAL, MENTAL HEALTH, PSYCHIATRIC PROBLEMS/ELATED-DEPRESSIVE BEHAVIOR)

134. **#2.** The first priority with any depressed client is to ensure safety because of a high risk of suicide. Promoting self-esteem, reducing cognitive distortion, and presenting reality consistently to the client are very important, but safety is the highest priority. PLAN (PSYCHOSOCIAL, MENTAL HEALTH, PSYCHIATRIC PROBLEMS/ELATED-DEPRESSIVE BEHAVIOR)

135. **#2.** Encourage the client to express feelings in a realistic manner. Do not accept irrational statements. Do not argue with her, imply her beliefs are true, or dismiss her. The client will become more tenacious in holding on to this delusion if the nurse tries to argue her out of it. Option #3 implies that the client's delusion is true. #4 evades the issue and dismisses the client's concern. IMPLEMENTATION (PSYCHOSOCIAL, MENTAL HEALTH, PSYCHIATRIC PROBLEMS/ELATED-DEPRESSIVE BEHAVIOR)

136. **#4.** Prior to electroconvulsive therapy, give the client accurate information in a way that does not increase anxiety. Options #1, #2, and #3 are accurate but raise the client's anxiety by failing to provide any reassurance. IMPLEMENTATION (PSYCHOSOCIAL, MENTAL HEALTH, PSYCHIATRIC PROBLEMS/ELATED-DEPRESSIVE BEHAVIOR)

137. **#2.** It is normal for the client to fall asleep, and she does not need to be disturbed. There is no reason to wake the client, give a stimulant, or call the physician. IMPLEMENTATION (PSYCHOSOCIAL, MENTAL HEALTH, PSYCHIATRIC PROBLEMS/ELATED-DEPRESSIVE BEHAVIOR)

138. **#4.** Assist the client in doing activities of daily living until she is able to do them on her own. Depressed clients have psychomotor retardation and need help in mobilizing themselves. It may be beyond Mrs. Moskovitz's control to be punctual every day. ECT clients should be integrated into the unit routines and milieu as soon as possible to obtain maximum benefit. IMPLEMENTATION (PSYCHOSOCIAL, MENTAL HEALTH, PSYCHIATRIC PROBLEMS/ELATED-DEPRESSIVE BEHAVIOR)

139. **#1.** Acknowledge the client's feelings without implying that they are true or shared by the nurse. The depressed client cannot alter her way of thinking at this point in treatment. Mrs. Moskovitz may feel devalued and unimportant by options #3 and #4. IMPLEMENTATION (PSYCHOSOCIAL, MENTAL HEALTH, PSYCHIATRIC PROBLEMS/ELATED-DEPRESSIVE BEHAVIOR)

140. **#1.** When a client shows a change in behavior, the nurse should assess the behavior to understand the nature of the change and how to respond. Such a change might imply suicidal intent, but this cannot be determined without further questioning. There is insufficient data to warrant suicide precautions, increased participation in ward activities, or to suggest denial of her depression. IMPLEMENTATION (PSYCHOSOCIAL, MENTAL HEALTH, PSYCHIATRIC PROBLEMS/ELATED-DEPRESSIVE BEHAVIOR)

141. **#4.** Expressions of guilt often conceal unexpressed resentment and anger. The client needs to have the opportunity to identify and verbalize such feelings. Option #1 focuses on the children rather than the client. #2 and #3 make a universal conclusion about parenting and give false reassurance. IMPLEMENTATION (PSYCHOSOCIAL, MENTAL HEALTH, PSYCHIATRIC PROBLEMS/ELATED-DEPRESSIVE BEHAVIOR)

142. **#1.** Using reflection helps to identify feelings and gives the client the opportunity to express them directly. Options #2 and #4 may be perceived by Mrs. Moskovitz as punitive or as reprimands. The nurse should first help the client identify and deal with her feelings before focusing on dealing with separation and the transition. IMPLEMENTATION (PSYCHOSOCIAL, MENTAL HEALTH, PSYCHIATRIC PROBLEMS/ELATED-DEPRESSIVE BEHAVIOR)

143. **#4.** The first 3 options are all correct. A pure medical-biologic model does not address social and environmental conditions. However, some physicians may consider that these conditions have some influence on the illness. The medical-biologic model assumes mental illnesses are disease entities. A disease can be classified, diagnosed, and labeled, and is within the purview of the physician. ANALYSIS (PSYCHOSOCIAL, MENTAL HEALTH, PSYCHIATRIC PROBLEMS/ELATED-DEPRESSIVE BEHAVIOR)

144. #4. Manic behavior in manic-depressive illness (bipolar disorder) is the result of denial of underlying depression. The client copes with these feelings by demonstrating excessive activity. The other defense mechanisms listed, repression, suppression, and displacement, may also be utilized; but #4 is most characteristic of manic-depression. ANALYSIS (PSYCHOSOCIAL, MENTAL HEALTH, PSYCHIATRIC PROBLEMS/ ELATED-DEPRESSIVE BEHAVIOR)

145. #4. The presence of the nurse will promote client adjustment to new surroundings and personnel. A decrease in environmental stimulation is necessary for its calming effect. The overactivity of Mrs. Brooks should not be rewarded, because these clients are prone to self-injury and burnout. Involving the client in activities and introducing her to new people will increase her psychomotor activity. IMPLEMENTATION (PSYCHOSOCIAL, MENTAL HEALTH, PSYCHIATRIC PROBLEMS/ELATED-DEPRESSIVE BEHAVIOR)

146. #1. A short attention span is characteristic of manic behavior, and she would be unable to manage activities requiring extended concentration. Decreasing stimulation, channeling energy, and using distraction techniques are calming and therapeutic for manic clients. IMPLEMENTATION (PSYCHOSOCIAL, MENTAL HEALTH, PSYCHIATRIC PROBLEMS/ELATED-DEPRESSIVE BEHAVIOR)

147. #1. The therapeutic blood-level range of lithium is 0.5 to 1.5 mEq/liter. Lithium levels are not measured in mg/ml, but rather in mEq/liter. ASSESSMENT (PSYCHOSOCIAL, MENTAL HEALTH, PSYCHIATRIC PROBLEMS/ELATED-DEPRESSIVE BEHAVIOR)

148. #4. The therapeutic level and toxic level of lithium are so close, blood levels must be carefully monitored. The therapeutic level is 0.5 to 1.5 mEq/liter. Above 1.5 mEq/liter, significant side effects occur. The toxicity level is 2.0 to 3.0 mEq/liter. Options #1, #2, and #3 are not the reasons for determining lithium levels. ANALYSIS (PSYCHOSOCIAL, MENTAL HEALTH, PSYCHIATRIC PROBLEMS/ELATED-DEPRESSIVE BEHAVIOR)

149. #4. These are symptoms of mild lithium toxicity. Options #1, #2, and #3 are not characteristic of lithium toxicity. ASSESSMENT (PSYCHOSOCIAL, MENTAL HEALTH, PSYCHIATRIC PROBLEMS/ELATED-DEPRESSIVE BEHAVIOR)

150. #2. Once the therapeutic blood level is achieved, it should be monitored at least monthly for outpatients. The prognosis for manic-depressive episode is good, so Mrs. Brooks probably does not need anyone to stay with her. Genetic research studies suggest there is a dominant X-linked factor present for the transmission of manic-depressive illness. This factor is thought to occur in families in which 1 or more members have had manic as well as depressive episodes. However, the couple decides whether to have children. Tranquilizers are not indicated. IMPLEMENTATION (PSYCHOSOCIAL, MENTAL HEALTH, PSYCHIATRIC PROBLEMS/ELATED-DEPRESSIVE BEHAVIOR)

151. #1. Vomiting and diarrhea may be signs of lithium toxicity or may be due to other causes. Loss of fluid will increase the concentration of medicine in the blood and may produce toxicity. Dryness of the mouth, while a side effect of lithium, is not serious. Swollen lymph nodes and upper respiratory symptoms would be associated with a health problem (e.g., infection) rather than with lithium toxicity. EVALUATION (PSYCHOSOCIAL, MENTAL HEALTH, PSYCHIATRIC PROBLEMS/ELATED-DEPRESSIVE BEHAVIOR)

152. #4. There is thought to be a hereditary component to manic-depressive illness. Manic-depressive illness is a biochemical imbalance and is not related to childhood illnesses. There is no relationship to the abuse of alcohol during adolescence and the onset of manic-depressive illness in adulthood. Parents divorcing during childhood could contribute to an unresolved grief reaction and thus chronic depression, but this past history is usually not the cause of manic excitement. ASSESSMENT (PSYCHOSOCIAL, MENTAL HEALTH, PSYCHIATRIC PROBLEMS/ELATED-DEPRESSIVE BEHAVIOR)

153. #4. Clang associations occur in schizophrenia, not in manic-depressive disorders. Vegetative behavior is seen during the depressive phase of manic-depressive illness. Hypomanic behavior is seen during the acute manic phase of manic-depressive illness. A thought disorder is present during mania and depression and usually consists of morbid self-blame. ASSESSMENT (PSYCHOSOCIAL, MENTAL HEALTH, PSYCHIATRIC PROBLEMS/ELATED-DEPRESSIVE BEHAVIOR)

154. #4. The mania seen in such clients is thought to be an attempt to ward off an underlying depression. These clients characteristically sleep very little during a manic episode. The other options describe manifestations of hyperactivity, confused thinking, aggressiveness, and poor judgment that are characteristic of manic behavior. ASSESSMENT (PSYCHOSOCIAL, MENTAL HEALTH, PSYCHIATRIC PROBLEMS/ELATED-DEPRESSIVE BEHAVIOR)

155. #2. Providing empathy and indicating to the son that his actions will help his father are indicated. It would not be beneficial to the son to hear that his father is worse than anyone else the staff has dealt with or implying that he is not capable of caring for his father. Interpreting the father's behavior will not help at this point. Option #3 assumes that the son is embarrassed by his father's illness. IMPLEMENTATION (PSYCHOSOCIAL, MENTAL HEALTH, PSYCHIATRIC PROBLEMS/ELATED-DEPRESSIVE BEHAVIOR)

156. #3. Although Mr. Peters may be overly talkative, irritable, and have a short attention span, his remark specifically typifies the delusion of grandeur that is a disorder of thought. ANALYSIS (PSYCHOSOCIAL, MENTAL HEALTH, PSYCHIATRIC PROBLEMS/ELATED-DEPRESSIVE BEHAVIOR)

157. #3. Administer the upcoming dose, since the normal serum-level range is 0.6-1.5 mEq/liter. The nurse would ask for the test to be repeated or withhold the next dose if the client showed signs of toxicity. If pressured speech were still present, the nurse would record the observation and indicate to the physician that perhaps the client needed more lithium. IMPLEMENTATION (PSYCHOSOCIAL, MENTAL HEALTH, PSYCHIATRIC PROBLEMS/ELATED-DEPRESSIVE BEHAVIOR)

158. #3. With insufficient sodium, lithium is retained and the client becomes toxic. The body needs sodium in order to excrete lithium. Insufficient fat and carbohydrates will lead to weight reduction, and eventually the dosage may need to be readjusted; but these foods are not critical to the proper absorption and elimination of lithium. Potassium is necessary when taking diuretics and iron is important when anemia exists. Proteins are critical when damaged tissue is present. ANAYLSIS (PSYCHOSOCIAL, MENTAL HEALTH, PSYCHIATRIC PROBLEMS/ELATED-DEPRESSIVE BEHAVIOR)

159. #1. Kidney damage does occur in association with lithium treatment in some clients. If the client already has a problem of this type, it is more appropriate to try other medication prior to use of lithium. Lithium may be helpful in controlling suicidal urges when the client is coming out of the depression. Physically active clients should be advised to watch fluid and sodium intake. Lithium is known to decrease the amount of circulating thyroid hormones. ASSESSMENT (PSYCHOSOCIAL, MENTAL HEALTH, PSYCHIATRIC PROBLEMS/ELATED-DEPRESSIVE BEHAVIOR)

160. #2. Manic clients are very disruptive, usually hyperirritable, and often very hostile to other clients. Mr. Peters may or may not need restraints or seclusion on admission, but throughout his hospitalization, he needs an atmosphere of decreased stimuli, which is best achieved in a private room. In addition, client rights necessitate as unrestrictive an atmosphere as possible. Therefore, seclusion and restraints are not used unless absolutely necessary. IMPLEMENTATION (PSYCHOSOCIAL, MENTAL HEALTH, PSYCHIATRIC PROBLEMS/ELATED-DEPRESSIVE BEHAVIOR)

161. #3. By having the client speak more slowly, hopefully he will be able to focus and identify some of his difficulties. Having him verbalize his feelings will only increase his anger and his mania. Giving him insight into the nature of his illness will not be absorbed because he is not able to hear too many details at this point. Therefore, he needs to have support rather than insight. IMPLEMENTATION (PSYCHOSOCIAL, MENTAL HEALTH, PSYCHIATRIC PROBLEMS/ELATED-DEPRESSIVE BEHAVIOR)

162. #1. Competitive games are stimulating and escalate aggression; therefore, physical exercise of a noncompetitive nature is the more constructive way to aid the client to discharge aggressive and angry feelings. Reduction of stimuli and ventilation of feelings are also therapeutic interventions for the client during the manic phase. IMPLEMENTATION (PSYCHOSOCIAL, MENTAL HEALTH, PSYCHIATRIC PROBLEMS/ELATED-DEPRESSIVE BEHAVIOR)

163. **#1.** Recognizing signs and symptoms of escalating excited behavior will enable the client and his son to seek early treatment of a recurrent episode of mania. By making most major decisions, the son would increase his father's feelings of worthlessness. Option #2 has been the client's pattern anyway, especially during a hypomanic state; he needs to learn assertive behavior. Teaching the family about possible side effects of lithium is important; but if the client can recognize symptomatology of hypomanic behavior, he can inform the doctor that the medication can be increased. PLAN (PSYCHOSOCIAL, MENTAL HEALTH, PSYCHIATRIC PROBLEMS/ELATED-DEPRESSIVE BEHAVIOR)

164. **#3.** This kind of behavior is apt to be seen on admission, not discharge. In order for a client to be deemed ready for discharge, he must be able to perform activities of daily living. Options #2 and #3 indicate that he has changed his behavioral pattern of aggressiveness to one of assertiveness, and that the client believes in himself and feels worthy of asking for his needs directly. EVALUATION (PSYCHOSOCIAL, MENTAL HEALTH, PSYCHIATRIC PROBLEMS/ELATED-DEPRESSIVE BEHAVIOR)

165. **#3.** Although at some point options #1, #2, and #4 must be assessed, the most important initial determination is the degree of compliance with the medication regimen. ASSESSMENT (PSYCHOSOCIAL, MENTAL HEALTH, PSYCHIATRIC PROBLEMS/ELATED-DEPRESSIVE BEHAVIOR)

166. **#2.** Overactivity in motor behavior, speech, and thought patterns is characteristic of manic-depressive, manic-phase clients. Mr. White is not psychotic; therefore, he does not have withdrawal from reality, associative looseness, or inappropriate affect. ASSESSMENT (PSYCHOSOCIAL, MENTAL HEALTH, PSYCHIATRIC PROBLEMS/ELATED-DEPRESSIVE BEHAVIOR)

167. **#1.** Thought processes of the hypomanic client move rapidly. Focusing on inappropriate language only prolongs it. Mr. White is unable to grasp the meaning of his behavior at this time or to control it even when threatened or ordered to stop. Seclusion is a drastic measure for abusive language and not helpful in reducing its occurrence. IMPLEMENTATION (PSYCHOSOCIAL, MENTAL HEALTH, PSYCHIATRIC PROBLEMS/ELATED-DEPRESSIVE BEHAVIOR)

168. **#3.** Hyperactivity is a behavior seen in the manic client. Option #1 indicates a psychotic depression with guilty delusions. #2 would be typical behavior of a paranoid schizophrenic and #4 is a possibility but is unlikely. If he were not hyperactive, he would experience his hunger and request other food. ANALYSIS (PSYCHOSOCIAL, MENTAL HEALTH, PSYCHIATRIC PROBLEMS/ELATED-DEPRESSIVE BEHAVIOR)

169. **#4.** It is unrealistic to expect Mr. White to sit and eat large quantities of food. Providing nutritious snack foods will increase his overall intake. Keeping him company may only intensify his feelings of dependency, causing him to be angry and more hyperactive. IMPLEMENTATION (PSYCHOSOCIAL, MENTAL HEALTH, PSYCHIATRIC PROBLEMS/ELATED-DEPRESSIVE BEHAVIOR)

170. **#2.** High calorie finger foods and drinks can be consumed easily while standing or moving. He is not able to sit long enough to eat and will become irritated at your suggestion of putting off his work. Option #4 will put him on the defensive and not facilitate his eating. IMPLEMENTATION (PSYCHOSOCIAL, MENTAL HEALTH, PSYCHIATRIC PROBLEMS/ELATED-DEPRESSIVE BEHAVIOR)

171. **#3.** Large motor skills such as painting, drawing, and rug making on a loom provide for appropriate discharge of energy and tension. Occupational therapy is designed to teach people hobbies so they have other resources for relaxing; it is not the place to teach social skills, nor is it the appropriate environment for reality testing and confrontation. PLAN (PSYCHOSOCIAL, MENTAL HEALTH, PSYCHIATRIC PROBLEMS/ELATED-DEPRESSIVE BEHAVIOR)

172. **#3.** The most important determinant of abuse by parents is whether they were abused as children. Child abuse is a learned behavior. Education, age of menarche, and socioeconomic status are not of themselves indicators of potential or actual child abuse. ASSESSMENT (PSYCHOSOCIAL, MENTAL HEALTH, PSYCHIATRIC PROBLEMS/SOCIALLY MALADAPTIVE BEHAVIOR)

173. #2. The most important factor in the current situation is to determine if the abuse has already occurred. If this has happened, then more protective measures are necessary. This is the most important fact to determine when planning care. Being pregnant, not wanting her baby at the time of birth, and previous experience in caring for children do not indicate potential or actual child abuse. ASSESSMENT (PSYCHOSOCIAL, MENTAL HEALTH, PSYCHIATRIC PROBLEMS/ SOCIALLY MALADAPTIVE BEHAVIOR)

174. #1. Most teenage pregnancies result because the teenager thinks her unmet needs for love and affection can be provided by a baby. These expectations are unrealistic and lead to anger, frustration, and possible abuse, when the mother realizes the child cannot fulfill her needs. Teenagers often have a lack of knowledge about patterns of growth and development, child care, nutrition, and health needs of a baby. The pregnant teenager may not have an excellent role model for parenting from her own parents. PLAN (PSYCHOSOCIAL, MENTAL HEALTH, PSYCHIATRIC PROBLEMS/SOCIALLY MALADAPTIVE BEHAVIOR)

175. #3. The most helpful initial interventions are to support the mother in the process of learning about realistic growth and development of the child and to teach her appropriate child-care and parenting skills. The information given does not address whether contraception, nutritional counseling, first aid, or cardiopulmonary resuscitation are referral needs. IMPLEMENTATION (PSYCHOSOCIAL, MENTAL HEALTH, PSYCHIATRIC PROBLEMS/SOCIALLY MALADAPTIVE BEHAVIOR)

176. #3. The most appropriate response is to acknowledge Mrs. Lane's feelings and then explore the incident directly. By acknowledging the sadness, the nurse shows respect for her feelings and empathizes with Mrs. Lane's pain. By exploring the issue directly, the nurse conveys concern and caring and reduces Mrs. Lane's embarrassment and shame over the incident. It is important that the nurse indicate that it is acceptable to talk about this problem. Talking directly about the problem conveys confidence and a sense of control. Mrs. Lane has acknowledged, not denied, that she has a problem. Option #2 fails to address the client's feelings and will increase her shame and low self-esteem. Assessment about battering is an appropriate role and responsibility of nurses. A referral for psychotherapy can be made at a later point if the client wishes. IMPLEMENTATION (PSYCHOSOCIAL, MENTAL HEALTH, PSYCHIATRIC PROBLEMS/SOCIALLY MALADAPTIVE BEHAVIOR)

177. #2. The most common feelings experienced by the nurse are that of frustration and disappointment that the woman continues to remain in the destructive situation. These feelings influence the nurse's ability to remain nonjudgmental and objective. If the nurse is not aware of these feelings, it is easy to give up or avoid engaging the client in problem solving and exploration of alternate methods of dealing with the situation. It is unlikely that a nurse would experience apathy or ignore the behavior. Guilt, shame, denial, and repression are feelings that usually occur in battered women, rather than being a response of the nurse. ANALYSIS (PSYCHOSOCIAL, MENTAL HEALTH, PSYCHIATRIC PROBLEMS/ SOCIALLY MALADAPTIVE BEHAVIOR)

178. #4. Blaming the victim is a most common response to victims of battering. When this attitude is conveyed, the victim becomes reluctant to share the details of her experience or to discuss her feelings or engage in problem solving. This attitude often leaves the victim feeling helpless and powerless. Although indifference in the nurse is nontherapeutic, blaming the victim is a more powerful deterrent to self-disclosure by battered women. Some degree of concern over the detail of the situation may promote self-disclosure by the battered woman. Inquiring into the client's history should not affect self-disclosure. ANALYSIS (PSYCHOSOCIAL, MENTAL HEALTH, PSYCHIATRIC PROBLEMS/ SOCIALLY MALADAPTIVE BEHAVIOR)

179. **#1.** The most important information to provide is the numbers of the crisis center and the battered-women's shelter, so the victim has resources available to her if the incident occurs again or if the battered woman needs support to help her come to a decision regarding the situation. Assertiveness training classes and psychotherapy are usually beneficial; however, the most important and highest priority referrals are #1. It is neither professional nor ethical to withhold information needed by the client. Battering recurs and needs no witnesses for proof. IMPLEMENTATION (PSYCHOSOCIAL, MENTAL HEALTH, PSYCHIATRIC PROBLEMS/SOCIALLY MALADAPTIVE BEHAVIOR)

180. **#3.** Teasing is a way of testing the ability of staff to handle acting-out behavior. If staff are consistent and can control his behavior, the client will learn trust. He will need to know, also, that staff members understand his underlying fears. If these two components are present, the adolescent will be in a climate conducive to helping him learn new behavior patterns. The client's pattern of behavior is acting out and will continue until firm limits are set. None of the information indicates that he will want to be alone much of the time. Good interpersonal skills require more self-control than Thomas's behavior demonstrates. ASSESSMENT (PSYCHOSOCIAL, MENTAL HEALTH, PSYCHIATRIC PROBLEMS/SOCIALLY MALADAPTIVE BEHAVIOR)

181. **#1.** The acting-out behavior can provide a diversion from the overwhelming fears the adolescent experiences. It can also be a way of channeling feelings or a way of asking adults for help. Conduct disorders, however, are not a normal part of adolescence. The data does not indicate that the client perceives problems in social or intellectual functioning. ANALYSIS (PSYCHOSOCIAL, MENTAL HEALTH, PSYCHIATRIC PROBLEMS/SOCIALLY MALADAPTIVE BEHAVIOR)

182. **#3.** The adolescent will first need to decrease his acting-out behavior. He will then be ready to move on to other treatment goals. Acting out also pushes staff and peers away, so he will be unable to interact effectively with others until he can control his behavior. Acting-out behavior is an indication of anxiety. Initially, Tom would not be able to tolerate sitting and talking for 30 minutes daily. The client is very self-involved at this point and may not be able to empathize or be aware of his family's feelings. PLAN (PSYCHOSOCIAL, MENTAL HEALTH, PSYCHIATRIC PROBLEMS/SOCIALLY MALADAPTIVE BEHAVIOR)

183. **#3.** Limit setting is the method staff can use to provide the necessary control over acting-out behavior. Visits from friends could be disruptive. Such a visit could be used as a reward for showing self-control. The therapy should focus on the client at this time rather than his family because he may not understand nor want to know why his family is upset with him. Limit-setting should extend to control of abusive language. IMPLEMENTATION (PSYCHOSOCIAL, MENTAL HEALTH, PSYCHIATRIC PROBLEMS/SOCIALLY MALADAPTIVE BEHAVIOR)

184. **#3.** Delirium tremens is characteristic of the late stage of alcoholism. In the early stage, insomnia and tremors occur. In the middle stage, blackouts, amnesia, and physical changes such as chronic gastritis and fatty infiltration of the liver occur. A recovering alcoholic is not drinking and may be able to reduce some of the health problems that occurred as a consequence of alcohol ingestion. ANALYSIS (PSYCHOSOCIAL, MENTAL HEALTH, PSYCHIATRIC PROBLEMS/SOCIALLY MALADAPTIVE BEHAVIOR)

185. **#3.** Options #1, #2, and #4 are appropriate interventions. Identifying feelings, encouraging expression, and setting limits are therapeutic. Sitting close to the client would be avoided, since many potentially violent clients perceive closeness as an invasion of their territory and as a controlling maneuver on the part of staff. In response, the client is even more likely to assault the person who comes close. IMPLEMENTATION (PSYCHOSOCIAL, MENTAL HEALTH, PSYCHIATRIC PROBLEMS/SOCIALLY MALADAPTIVE BEHAVIOR)

186. **#1.** Unless options #2 through #4 are carried out, the staff or the client may be at greater risk of injury. Rarely would a physician refuse to write this order after the fact. Such an order can also be included as part of an institution's protocol for care of the potentially violent client. Tossing a sheet or blanket over a potentially violent client is another technique often included in standard protocols for control of potentially or actually violent behavior. IMPLEMENTATION (PSYCHOSOCIAL, MENTAL HEALTH, PSYCHIATRIC PROBLEMS/SOCIALLY MALADAPTIVE BEHAVIOR)

187. **#4.** Clients who have ingested barbiturates, opiates, or Valium would present with a general, depressant-withdrawal syndrome. PCP ingestion is associated with vivid hallucinations and persecutory delusions. ANALYSIS (PSYCHOSOCIAL, MENTAL HEALTH, PSYCHIATRIC PROBLEMS/SOCIALLY MALADAPTIVE BEHAVIOR)

188. **#4.** The behaviors listed in options #1 through #3 indicate that the client is regaining control. The behavior in #4 is more likely a way to manipulate staff. In short, the client is promising to behave in an unlikely way, considering her history of alcohol abuse. EVALUATION (PSYCHOSOCIAL, MENTAL HEALTH, PSYCHIATRIC PROBLEMS/SOCIALLY MALADAPTIVE BEHAVIOR)

189. **#2.** Determination of the victim's perception of the rape is of value initially. Marital status and identity of rapist may be contributory but not the most important information. To inquire about abortion is premature unless client indicates a wish to talk about this possibility. ASSESSMENT (PSYCHOSOCIAL, MENTAL HEALTH, PSYCHIATRIC PROBLEMS/SOCIALLY MALADAPTIVE BEHAVIOR)

190. **#1.** Rape is not considered a crime of passion, but rather one of violent aggression. Bestiality refers to sexual relations with an animal. Exposing one's sexual organs when socially inappropriate is called exhibitionism. Venting anger and hostility and exercising power and control are what motivate the rapist, rather than sexual passion. ANALYSIS (PSYCHOSOCIAL, MENTAL HEALTH, PSYCHIATRIC PROBLEMS/SOCIALLY MALADAPTIVE BEHAVIOR)

191. **#3.** It is very often a crisis for the significant other as well as for the victim. It is difficult for the significant other to perceive the victim as unchanged. Although option #4 is a possibility, #3 is more likely. ANALYSIS (PSYCHOSOCIAL, MENTAL HEALTH, PSYCHIATRIC PROBLEMS/SOCIALLY MALADAPTIVE BEHAVIOR)

192. **#4.** This will have the most significant effect in decreasing the trauma. Some victims develop post-traumatic stress disorder following a severe trauma like rape. Counseling and support from nursing colleagues and hospital administrators who are aware of Mrs. Smith's plight is also important. IMPLEMENTATION (PSYCHOSOCIAL, MENTAL HEALTH, PSYCHIATRIC PROBLEMS/SOCIALLY MALADAPTIVE BEHAVIOR)

193. **#4.** The client who has been raped is very anxious and fears being harmed. Being touched is very likely to be anxiety producing. First, establish rapport, then assess the level of anxiety. Attention to lacerations, wounds, and obtaining a semen specimen can be done later in the visit. The decision to notify a family member can be made later in conjunction with the client. IMPLEMENTATION (PSYCHOSOCIAL, MENTAL HEALTH, PSYCHIATRIC PROBLEMS/SOCIALLY MALADAPTIVE BEHAVIOR)

194. **#3.** Miss Long is in crisis and she is experiencing many changes. Nursing actions that focus on behavior deal with immediate needs. The symptoms will abate as her anxiety decreases. Her diagnosis and intellectual capacity have implications for care, but actions that address her presenting behaviors are most important initially. PLAN (PSYCHOSOCIAL, MENTAL HEALTH, PSYCHIATRIC PROBLEMS/SOCIALLY MALADAPTIVE BEHAVIOR)

195. **#2.** During the early stages of crisis intervention, the client will be unable to clearly understand the crisis situation; the understanding will come later. If frightening events are identified, Miss Long will be able to regain some feelings of control. Talking relieves anxiety for many people. A rape victim feels much shame and repulsion for what has happened to her body. Sometimes, the victim may feel the rape was her fault and suicidal thoughts may follow. Support systems and resource identification are necessary components of crisis intervention. IMPLEMENTATION (PSYCHOSOCIAL, MENTAL HEALTH, PSYCHIATRIC PROBLEMS/SOCIALLY MALADAPTIVE BEHAVIOR)

196. #4. Crisis theory is founded on the assumption that all plans will be developed in collaboration with the client. The underlying philosophy is that people have the resources to help themselves. The growth-and-development philosophy that is part of crisis theory is undermined when clients are not involved in their own decision making. The client's self-esteem will be lowered and she can feel devalued if decisions are made for her. Options #1, #2, and #3 describe important and necessary aspects of crisis intervention. IMPLEMENTATION (PSYCHOSOCIAL, MENTAL HEALTH, PSYCHIATRIC PROBLEMS/ SOCIALLY MALADAPTIVE BEHAVIOR)

197. #2. He has symptoms of a persecutory delusional system. The idea that his brother is attempting to steal his property is almost certainly a false belief, a misunderstanding of reality. An hallucination is an imagined sensory perception that occurs without an external stimulus. An illusion is a misinterpretation of a sensory stimulus of a real experience. A phobia is a persistent, irrational, obsessive, intense fear of a situation or an object that results in increased tension and anxiety. ANALYSIS (PSYCHOSOCIAL, MENTAL HEALTH, PSYCHIATRIC PROBLEMS/SUSPICIOUS BEHAVIOR)

198. #1. Denial and projection are most common in paranoia. In denial, a person treats obvious reality factors as though they do not exist because these factors are intolerable to the conscious mind. In projection, a person attributes his/her own unacceptable emotions and qualities to others. Repression is the involuntary, unconscious forgetting of unacceptable or painful impulses, thoughts, feelings, or acts. Displacement refers to the transferring of unacceptable feelings aroused by an object or situation to a more acceptable substitute. ANALYSIS (PSYCHOSOCIAL, MENTAL HEALTH, PSYCHIATRIC PROBLEMS/SUSPICIOUS BEHAVIOR)

199. #3. As the client becomes more socially adapted, delusions are utilized less. Structuring activities will assist in decreasing delusions. Ability for group participation comes slowly, if at all. Cheerful behavior on the part of others increases the suspiciousness of the paranoid client. These clients tend to misinterpret the touch, experiencing it as control, anger, or invasion of their territory or person. IMPLEMENTATION (PSYCHOSOCIAL, MENTAL HEALTH, PSYCHIATRIC PROBLEMS/SUSPICIOUS BEHAVIOR)

200. #2. Psychotropic drugs are used to lessen symptoms (e.g., paranoia, delusions, anxiety, psychomotor excitement) so that clients can benefit more from milieu therapy and psychotherapy. Initially, psychotropic drugs may sedate a client. However, sedation is not the intention. Psychotropic medications do not, of themselves, assist clients in gaining insights. They only contribute indirectly to improved self-esteem by enabling the client to benefit from therapy. ANALYSIS (PSYCHOSOCIAL, MENTAL HEALTH, PSYCHIATRIC PROBLEMS/SUSPICIOUS BEHAVIOR)

201. #1. Although the symptoms listed may all be side effects of chlorpromazine, protection from photosensitivity is most appropriate because the picnic is outdoors. Constipation, dry mouth, and stuffy nose occur because of the anticholinergic effect of Thorazine. Fatigue is usually transient and relieved as dosage is adjusted and individualized for each client. Cholestatic jaundice is a rare side effect that is usually benign, self-limiting, and reversible. Jaundice is not caused by exposure to light. IMPLEMENTATION (PSYCHOSOCIAL, MENTAL HEALTH, PSYCHIATRIC PROBLEMS/SUSPICIOUS BEHAVIOR)

202. #4. His statement demonstrates insight into past behavior. This response will help him to work on patterns of more acceptable behavior. The nurse's response also gives him the opportunity to tell her about the people and situations in which he thinks he was tolerant. Generally, it is better to avoid ''why'' questions since many clients feel put on the spot or do not know ''why.'' It is more therapeutic to focus on ways to change behavior rather than a particular person. The approach in option #3 is too broad and unfocused. Mr. Bonono needs help in learning ways to make his behavior more acceptable to others. IMPLEMENTATION (PSYCHOSOCIAL, MENTAL HEALTH, PSYCHIATRIC PROBLEMS/SUSPICIOUS BEHAVIOR)

203. #1. The first priority in working with a suspicious client is to establish a trusting relationship, so that other goals can be accomplished. The reality of the situation cannot be dealt with until a trusting relationship is established. Mr. Dooley's self-esteem should improve at a later point in his treatment. Mr. Dooley's social functioning should also improve as a result of improved self-esteem and as the client discontinues behaviors that disrupt his social relationships. PLAN (PSYCHOSOCIAL, MENTAL HEALTH, PSYCHIATRIC PROBLEMS/SUSPICIOUS BEHAVIOR)

204. **#4.** Ask questions that encourage the client to explore his situation and come to his own realization of his problems. Option #1 would be too confronting and threatening to the client. If his anxiety is kept within reasonable control, he will be better able to explore his difficulties. In #2, the nurse sides with the wife, which the client may experience as accusatory. Option #3 is likely to cause the client to hold more firmly to his delusions. IMPLEMENTATION (PSYCHOSOCIAL, MENTAL HEALTH, PSYCHIATRIC PROBLEMS/ SUSPICIOUS BEHAVIOR)

205. **#2.** An explanation for the lateness is most important. Establishing trust requires giving accurate information about what is happening in the client's environment. This avoids the problem of the client drawing conclusions that support a misinterpretation of events. If the nurse merely acknowledges lateness, the client's suspiciousness may lead him to conclude s/he does not want to see him. The nurse will not be viewed as a reliable person if s/he cancels the appointment after the delay. An apology rather than an explanation could be misinterpreted. IMPLEMENTATION (PSYCHOSOCIAL, MENTAL HEALTH, PSYCHIATRIC PROBLEMS/SUSPICIOUS BEHAVIOR)

206. **#1.** Communications with clients should always be honest. This is even more important with suspicious clients, so as not to contribute to the suspicious delusions. Options #2, #3, and #4 may raise the client's anxiety needlessly, reinforce his delusional system, and increase his suspicions of others. IMPLEMENTATION (PSYCHOSOCIAL, MENTAL HEALTH, PSYCHIATRIC PROBLEMS/SUSPICIOUS BEHAVIOR)

207. **#3.** When a suspicious client is willing to share feelings with a nurse, this is evidence that a trusting relationship is being formed. His delusions are an indication of anxiety and increase with greater anxiety. Trust with the nurse is not related to an explanation of the client's delusions by the nurse. Although desirable, the nurse's feeling at ease does not necessarily indicate that Mr. Dooley is developing a trusting relationship with the nurse. EVALUATION (PSYCHOSOCIAL, MENTAL HEALTH, PSYCHIATRIC PROBLEMS/SUSPICIOUS BEHAVIOR)

208. **#2.** The highest priority in assessment of a psychotic client is to evaluate physical well-being. Such a client may be suffering from an illness, fluid and/or electrolyte imbalances. She may also have physical injuries either self-inflicted or from an assault. Her perception of reality is also important to assess potential safety risks and reality testing, and to begin to set goals and plan the client's care. Observations at the bus station may or may not provide some useful information. Speech patterns may provide useful information, yet #2 has the highest priority. ASSESSMENT (PSYCHOSOCIAL, MENTAL HEALTH, PSYCHIATRIC PROBLEMS/WITHDRAWN BEHAVIOR)

209. **#3.** Establishing a therapeutic relationship with psychotic clients requires communicating, even when they seem out of touch with reality. Make directions and expectations as clear and unambiguous as possible. The client is regressed and baby talk or gibberish is part of her regression. It would not be therapeutic or effective to deal with her speech problem at this time. Therapeutic verbal and nonverbal communication by a professional person is a critical need of this client. Therapeutic communication and medication, not a speech therapist, will help the client. IMPLEMENTATION (PSYCHOSOCIAL, MENTAL HEALTH, PSYCHIATRIC PROBLEMS/ WITHDRAWN BEHAVIOR)

210. **#4.** The most common side effect of antipsychotic drugs is hypotension. Monitoring the blood pressure is necessary to ensure that appropriate measures can be taken if blood pressure falls below safe levels. Lying and standing blood pressures should be taken to test for orthostatic hypotension prior to each dose. A blood specimen and neurologic checks are not necessary prior to administering each dose of medication. Observation of parkinsonian side effects is important throughout hospitalization but is not necessary prior to each of these 3 doses. Fluids do not need to be offered. ASSESSMENT (PSYCHOSOCIAL, MENTAL HEALTH, PSYCHIATRIC PROBLEMS/WITHDRAWN BEHAVIOR)

211. #1. Control of psychotic symptoms may require as many as 10 doses of the medication within a matter of 5 to 6 hours. If the client is not experiencing any untoward side effects, further doses will probably be ordered by the physician. A nurse cannot administer any more haloperidol without a physician's order or a protocol. The nurse must always record the results of the medication. The point of this question is the nurse's next action. It is not necessary to observe the client for an hour but rather to assess intermittently and to ensure the client is safe. IMPLEMENTATION (PSYCHOSOCIAL, MENTAL HEALTH, PSYCHIATRIC PROBLEMS/WITHDRAWN BEHAVIOR)

212. #1. Mild hypotension may be present with haloperidol and may cause light-headedness when the client arises. This symptom usually disappears after 2 to 3 weeks. The drug controls psychotic symptoms. It is unlikely that the client will experience considerable drowsiness. Option #3 is inaccurate; the medication does have some major side effects, and the second part of the remark could be misunderstood by the client. The client will need medication for an extended period of time; the current psychotic episode was precipitated when she discontinued her medication. IMPLEMENTATION (PSYCHOSOCIAL, MENTAL HEALTH, PSYCHIATRIC PROBLEMS/WITHDRAWN BEHAVIOR)

213. #4. The nurse must make an assessment before assuming a client is hallucinating. A client should not be medicated prior to the nursing assessment and nursing diagnosis. The nurse must not jump to conclusions. It is not helpful to the client for the nurse to ignore the behavior; assessment is necessary. If hallucinating, clients may become worse if secluded, unless someone stays with them. IMPLEMENTATION (PSYCHOSOCIAL, MENTAL HEALTH, PSYCHIATRIC PROBLEMS/WITHDRAWN BEHAVIOR)

214. #4. Acknowledge that hallucinations are real to the client, but encourage her to communicate with staff present on the unit. Although option #1 does present reality, it is not therapeutic to the client at this time. #2 does not address a relevant issue and does not provide the client with the direction she needs, i.e., to talk with the nurse. In option #3, the nurse makes an assumption but has no data on which to base her conclusion. IMPLEMENTATION (PSYCHOSOCIAL, MENTAL HEALTH, PSYCHIATRIC PROBLEMS/WITHDRAWN BEHAVIOR)

215. #2. A psychotic client is unable to make choices and will not be able to engage in activities with other clients without support. Assigning a staff member gives the client an opportunity to build a relationship. The client may not be able to tell you what sports she enjoys, make choices, engage in activities with others, or develop an interest and initiate activity yet. IMPLEMENTATION (PSYCHOSOCIAL, MENTAL HEALTH, PSYCHIATRIC PROBLEMS/WITHDRAWN BEHAVIOR)

216. #3. Involving the aunt will enable the nurse to assess the aunt's ability to promote continued progress for the client. The nurse needs to assess the client's support system. The nurse needs to be more actively involved in the decision-making process because Miss Dumas may not be able to determine or make her needs known at this time. The nurse has not yet assessed the extent to which the aunt is helpful to Miss Dumas. There is no data on which to base the conclusion in option #4. PLAN (PSYCHOSOCIAL, MENTAL HEALTH, PSYCHIATRIC PROBLEMS/WITHDRAWN BEHAVIOR)

217. #2. Building a one-to-one relationship with the schizophrenic client is very important since this is a problem for her. A relationship with 1 staff member can lead to relationships with others if the client is able to increase trust. Usually it is not feasible for the client to work with 1 staff person for a 24-hour day, but the client should be assigned to as few staff members as possible. The new marriage and accompanying lifestyle changes may have precipitated this crisis and psychologic decompensation. An assessment of the relationship would be necessary before concentrating on helping her relate to her husband. Options #3 and #4 are important aspects of care but can only be successful after the client develops a trusting relationship with the nursing staff. PLAN (PSYCHOSOCIAL, MENTAL HEALTH, PSYCHIATRIC PROBLEMS/WITHDRAWN BEHAVIOR)

218. #4. Perseverance and patience are essential when working with a schizophrenic client. The nurse must continue to demonstrate interest and sincerity until the client feels able to trust the nurse in increasing ways. The other options demand more verbalization and changes in behavior that are not appropriate at this time. IMPLEMENTATION (PSYCHOSOCIAL, MENTAL HEALTH, PSYCHIATRIC PROBLEMS/WITHDRAWN BEHAVIOR)

219. **#3.** The schizophrenic client's mistrust and inability to interpret reality accurately inhibit the ability to make sense of what is happening. Here the nurse is orienting the client to the environment. Immediate involvement in unit activities may be too stimulating or demanding at this time and may cause the client's anxiety to escalate unnecessarily. IMPLEMENTATION (PSYCHOSOCIAL, MENTAL HEALTH, PSYCHIATRIC PROBLEMS/WITHDRAWN BEHAVIOR)

220. **#1.** The nurse should cast doubt on the client's perceptions, while at the same time not denying the validity of the perceptions to the client. Attempts to reason with the client or argue about, challenge, or reinforce the ideas only serve to entrench them more firmly. IMPLEMENTATION (PSYCHOSOCIAL, MENTAL HEALTH, PSYCHIATRIC PROBLEMS/WITHDRAWN BEHAVIOR)

221. **#3.** As above. Options #1, #2, and #4 could precipitate an increase in the client's level of anxiety. ANALYSIS (PSYCHOSOCIAL, MENTAL HEALTH, PSYCHIATRIC PROBLEMS/WITHDRAWN BEHAVIOR)

222. **#3.** Anxiety is one of the most crucial elements in the development of schizophrenia. As anxiety decreases, clients become more reality oriented and more approachable, and their behavior becomes more appropriate. Insight and receptivity to psychotherapy are usually not seen when there is an increase in anxiety. Option #4 may be true; however, she probably initially would exhibit an attention or memory deficit. ASSESSMENT (PSYCHOSOCIAL, MENTAL HEALTH, PSYCHIATRIC PROBLEMS/WITHDRAWN BEHAVIOR)

223. **#1.** Establishing a trusting relationship will decrease the client's anxiety and make it possible for the nurse to work toward other goals such as increasing communication and improving social skills. PLAN (PSYCHOSOCIAL, MENTAL HEALTH, PSYCHIATRIC PROBLEMS/WITHDRAWN BEHAVIOR)

224. **#1.** Sitting quietly will promote interpersonal contact without pressuring the client to communicate beyond his level of readiness. Options #2, #3, and #4 will probably result in further retreat from socialization because the client is frightened about the level of interaction the nurse is attempting. IMPLEMENTATION (PSYCHOSOCIAL, MENTAL HEALTH, PSYCHIATRIC PROBLEMS/WITHDRAWN BEHAVIOR)

225. **#3.** A picnic on the hospital grounds provides the opportunity for interaction with other clients and staff in a noncompetitive, nondemanding setting. Options #1, #2, and #4 are either physically demanding or require a high level of perceptual and cognitive awareness and may result in failure, further inhibiting socialization. IMPLEMENTATION (PSYCHOSOCIAL, MENTAL HEALTH, PSYCHIATRIC PROBLEMS/WITHDRAWN BEHAVIOR)

226. **#4.** Parkinsonian side effects are common with phenothiazine drugs. Unless severe, their presence is not an indication to stop the drug. Option #1 would be an excellent intervention if the client were experiencing orthostatic hypotension, another side effect of thorazine. #2 will not assist the client who is experiencing extrapyramidal effects of the antipsychotic agent. A neurologic consult would only be indicated if there were additional focal symptoms and if an antiparkinson agent did not alleviate the extrapyramidal symptoms. IMPLEMENTATION (PSYCHOSOCIAL, MENTAL HEALTH, PSYCHIATRIC PROBLEMS/WITHDRAWN BEHAVIOR)

227. **#3.** People tend to respond to current or anticipated losses as they have responded to losses in the past. Schizophrenic clients have difficulty dealing with closeness; however, a relationship has been established and there is an impending absence of the client's primary nurse, which the client internalizes as loss and abandonment. Schizophrenia does not have a pattern of cyclic exacerbation as in manic-depressive illness; this client is responding to a well-defined precipitating event. He apparently does feel he needs the relationship and is subsequently withdrawing from the nurse to get ready for the perceived loss of the relationship. ANALYSIS (PSYCHOSOCIAL, MENTAL HEALTH, PSYCHIATRIC PROBLEMS/WITHDRAWN BEHAVIOR)

228. #1. A diet with extra protein and C and B vitamins is indicated to compensate for the poor nutritional state present in many substance abusers. The addition of chlordiazepoxide will decrease anxiety and assist in detoxification. Cirrhosis of the liver, a common side effect of chronic alcoholism, necessitates a low-fat diet. Vitamin E, a fat soluble vitamin, is stored in the body and may not be depleted. Thorazine is contraindicated in withdrawal states from alcohol. While fluids are important to counteract dehydration, emphasis should be on high protein intake to build up depleted nutritional state. Demerol is an analgesic and is contraindicated with impaired hepatic function. While Dilantin is an important consideration to eliminate the possibility of seizures, as are fluids to counteract dehydration, Librium is the first drug of choice to reduce initial symptoms of anxiety in the acute phase. IMPLEMENTATION (PSYCHOSOCIAL, MENTAL HEALTH, PSYCHIATRIC PROBLEMS/SUBSTANCE USE DISORDERS)

229. #2. Poor dietary habits of many substance abusers cause marked deficiency in thiamine. This results in symptoms of Korsakoff's syndrome. Encephalamalacia, convulsions, and dystonia are consequences of impaired CNS functioning, not the causative factors of Korsakoff's. ANALYSIS (PSYCHOSOCIAL, MENTAL HEALTH, PSYCHIATRIC PROBLEMS/SUBSTANCE USE DISORDERS)

230. #3. These symptoms are accompanied by nausea and increased pulse rate and blood pressure. Alcohol withdrawal results in psychomotor agitation. The symptoms in option #1 are a result of autonomic nervous system depression. #2 lists manifestations of alcohol withdrawal but they are not the first symptoms observed. The symptoms in option #4 would not be a direct result of alcohol withdrawal but may occur as a secondary consequence (e.g., from seizures). ASSESSMENT (PSYCHOSOCIAL, MENTAL HEALTH, PSYCHIATRIC PROBLEMS/SUBSTANCE USE DISORDERS)

231. #1. Provide an environment with as few stimuli as possible. Remaining with the client provides reassurance. While bed rest and fluids, excluding caffeine products, are indicated, soft music is an environmental stimulation and would, therefore, be contraindicated. Caffeine, a stimulant found in tea, and high fat content, found in ice cream, are contraindicated in alcohol withdrawal. Restraints are only necessary if client is a safety threat to himself or others. Use of restraints should be avoided as they tend to agitate and confuse the client who is disoriented. Vital signs need to be monitored as necessary, but the nurse needs to minimize intrusions to maintain a quiet and calm environment. IMPLEMENTATION (PSYCHOSOCIAL, MENTAL HEALTH, PSYCHIATRIC PROBLEMS/ SUBSTANCE USE DISORDERS)

232. #1. The nurse gives information but leaves the opportunity for Mrs. Maling to ventilate her feelings and decide for herself. Option #2 implies that only the alcoholic is affected by the disease whereas it is insidious to the family system. Although many find Al-Anon helpful, participation is not mandatory and should be an individual consideration. IMPLEMENTATION (PSYCHOSOCIAL, MENTAL HEALTH, PSYCHIATRIC PROBLEMS/SUBSTANCE USE DISORDERS)

233. #2. The client must acknowledge the illness and be motivated to change his pattern of living. Atonement for past behavior is not nearly as important as motivation for change of future behavior. A strong support system is helpful in facilitating recovery; however, recovery is self-dependent. EVALUATION (PSYCHOSOCIAL, MENTAL HEALTH, PSYCHIATRIC PROBLEMS/SUBSTANCE USE DISORDERS)

234. #2. Most cough medicines contain varying amounts of alcohol and would cause him to become ill if he were to combine them with disulfiram. Aspirin, Tylenol, antacids, and laxatives are over-the-counter drugs that do not contain alcohol and, therefore, would not cause adverse effects. Heart and blood pressure medications, which are also prescribed by the physician, may be medically indicated. IMPLEMENTATION (PSYCHOSOCIAL, MENTAL HEALTH, PSYCHIATRIC PROBLEMS/SUBSTANCE USE DISORDERS)

235. #2. Alcoholics Anonymous is run entirely by alcoholics who have achieved sobriety. It is not group therapy nor is it led by professionals. It does not discourage relationships but instead recognizes the need for support. ANALYSIS (PSYCHOSOCIAL, MENTAL HEALTH, PSYCHIATRIC PROBLEMS/SUBSTANCE USE DISORDERS)

236. #3. A client who achieves sobriety after alcohol abuse is considered a recovering alcoholic. Alcoholism is not curable but can be controlled. Options #2 and #4 imply a resolved disease state whereas the potential for active alcoholism remains throughout the client's life. ANALYSIS (PSYCHOSOCIAL, MENTAL HEALTH, PSYCHIATRIC PROBLEMS/SUBSTANCE USE DISORDERS)

237. #3. Encourage the client to talk about feelings utilizing techniques such as reflection. Avoid judgmental responses such as #2 that close off communication. Neither option #1 or #4 allows for exploration of Mr. Trysdale's feelings on drinking. IMPLEMENTATION (PSYCHOSOCIAL, MENTAL HEALTH, PSYCHIATRIC PROBLEMS/SUBSTANCE USE DISORDERS)

238. #1. Clear explanations about treatment are appropriate. The nurse would then assess the client's status. Option #2 sounds judgmental. Sedation may not be indicated. While it is good to provide explanations to a client, #4 does not allow the nurse to explore the reason why Mr. Trysdale undid his traction. IMPLEMENTATION (PSYCHOSOCIAL, MENTAL HEALTH, PSYCHIATRIC PROBLEMS/SUBSTANCE USE DISORDERS)

239. #4. Reflection encourages the client to describe how he is feeling, so the nurse can assess, analyze, and plan care appropriately. Option #1 is a closed question and does not encourage exploration of client's feelings. #2 does not allow the nurse to explore with the client what he is experiencing and, therefore, does not provide the nurse with the necessary information to make a complete assessment. In option #3, the nurse is making an assumption that could make the client feel judged and prevent further exploration. IMPLEMENTATION (PSYCHOSOCIAL, MENTAL HEALTH, PSYCHIATRIC PROBLEMS/SUBSTANCE USE DISORDERS)

240. #1. Collaborate with the physician in order to plan appropriately. Adequate assessment has been obtained by the nurse over the course of a shift. Option #3 is not a nursing decision. The physician will make this decision based on the diagnosis. If the client's condition has changed, the sedative may be medically contraindicated. The physician should be alerted to any dramatic changes in client status. IMPLEMENTATION (PSYCHOSOCIAL, MENTAL HEALTH, PSYCHIATRIC PROBLEMS/SUBSTANCE USE DISORDERS)

241. #2. Point out reality to persons who are having hallucinations from substance withdrawal. Reassure and orient them frequently. Option #1 serves to reinforce his hallucinations. A physician's order is required to apply restraints and reassurance may be all that is needed as an initial nursing action. Nursing measures to calm and orient Mr. Trysdale should be done first. If the behavior continues, the administration of the prescribed tranquilizer may later be necessary. IMPLEMENTATION (PSYCHOSOCIAL, MENTAL HEALTH, PSYCHIATRIC PROBLEMS/SUBSTANCE USE DISORDERS)

242. #3. Persons in withdrawal need reassurance that they will be taken care of and will not be left alone. The client is unable to control himself at this time, and it is an inappropriate time to question him about his drinking habits. IMPLEMENTATION (PSYCHOSOCIAL, MENTAL HEALTH, PSYCHIATRIC PROBLEMS/SUBSTANCE USE DISORDERS)

243. #2. The highest priority is to prevent dehydration but caffeine drinks would increase agitation. This client has a physical problem that makes ambulation impossible. Keep the environment as quiet and distraction free as possible. IMPLEMENTATION (PSYCHOSOCIAL, MENTAL HEALTH, PSYCHIATRIC PROBLEMS/SUBSTANCE USE DISORDERS)

244. #4. The client has already admitted he has a problem. The most realistic and highest priority goal for him is to accept the help of others. Options #2 and #3 are long-term goals, not the first or immediate concern. PLAN (PSYCHOSOCIAL, MENTAL HEALTH, PSYCHIATRIC PROBLEMS/SUBSTANCE USE DISORDERS)

245. #1. Handle lapses nonjudgmentally and in a way that encourages the client to use the help of others to find new ways of coping. Option #2 is a judgment statement. The fact that Mr. Trysdale is drinking does not imply that he is unwilling to change. The client needs to be reassured that it is difficult, rather than to be chastised for his lapse. The focus should be on the client's needs and behaviors. He must assume responsibility and motivation for his recovery. IMPLEMENTATION (PSYCHOSOCIAL, MENTAL HEALTH, PSYCHIATRIC PROBLEMS/SUBSTANCE USE DISORDERS)

246. #1. Identify the difficulties associated with trying to stop alcohol intake, so that the client does not continue to fall back on superficiality and denial. Continue to encourage the client to seek help from others. #2 supports the client's denial of the difficulty involved with abstaining from alcohol. Value judgments and threats are contraindicated, and deny Mr. Trysdale the necessary support he needs at this time. IMPLEMENTATION (PSYCHOSOCIAL, MENTAL HEALTH, PSYCHIATRIC PROBLEMS/SUBSTANCE USE DISORDERS)

247. #3. Hallucinogenics cause an individual to lose contact with reality and hallucinate. Opiates are a class of drug that contain or are derived from opium. Barbiturates are a group of powerful sedative drugs that bring about relaxation and sleep. Stimulants are a class of drug whose major effect is to provide energy and alertness. ANALYSIS (PSYCHOSOCIAL, MENTAL HEALTH, PSYCHIATRIC PROBLEMS/SUBSTANCE USE DISORDERS)

248. #1. There is no evidence that LSD is physically addicting. Tolerance develops rapidly to hallucinogens with the client experiencing an overpowering desire to continue taking the drug. Heightened sensory perception can lead to an acute panic state. ANALYSIS (PSYCHOSOCIAL, MENTAL HEALTH, PSYCHIATRIC PROBLEMS/SUBSTANCE USE DISORDERS)

249. #4. No treatment modality has been very effective with drug abusers, and the relapse rate is about 90%. Treatment by former addicts has had the best results, because these persons, through their own experiences, are familiar with the behaviors of the drug abuser. The aim of psychoanalysis is to restructure the personality. Behavior modification uses learning principles to improve behavior and has not proven to be very effective in treating drug dependence. Family therapy does not focus on the drug abuser but instead treats family roles and attitudes. ANALYSIS (PSYCHOSOCIAL, MENTAL HEALTH, PSYCHIATRIC PROBLEMS/SUBSTANCE USE DISORDERS)

250. #2. One of the effects of LSD is heightened sensory perceptions, which can be very frightening to the client and cause an acute panic state in which the client can hurt himself and others. Seclusion will help to reduce environmental stimulation and protect both this client and others. Turning off the television and restraining the client are not sufficient. Client safety and dignity must be maintained. An order for sedation can be gotten later. IMPLEMENTATION (PSYCHOSOCIAL, MENTAL HEALTH, PSYCHIATRIC PROBLEMS/SUBSTANCE USE DISORDERS)

251. #4. Clients should be observed constantly when in seclusion, and seclusion should be used only when it is the most effective therapy for the client at that time. The client needs a quiet and calm environment to counteract heightened sensory perception. The use of seclusion to protect the client from harming self or others is legitimate, as safety is always an utmost concern. PLAN (PSYCHOSOCIAL, MENTAL HEALTH, PSYCHIATRIC PROBLEMS/SUBSTANCE USE DISORDERS)

252. #3. The nurse must help the client sort out what is real and what is not by giving reality-based feedback. Option #1 belittles the client's feelings and is condescending. #2 does not help the client determine what is real and what is hallucination. Discussing the hallucination, as suggested in option #4, will give it credence and increase the likelihood of recurrence. What the nurse discusses with a client reinforces it in the client's mind. IMPLEMENTATION (PSYCHOSOCIAL, MENTAL HEALTH, PSYCHIATRIC PROBLEMS/SUBSTANCE USE DISORDERS)

253. **#2.** Mr. Clements is having a delusion. Delusions are created in the mind to make up for or meet an underlying need. Option #2 responds to the possible need underlying this client's delusion. #1 and #3 foster his grandiose and aberrant thinking and do not orient him to reality. The presence of visual hallucinations does not necessitate the use of seclusion. IMPLEMENTATION (PSYCHOSOCIAL, MENTAL HEALTH, PSYCHIATRIC PROBLEMS/SUBSTANCE USE DISORDERS)

254. **#1.** Haloperidol is a major tranquilizer, the purpose of which is to treat psychosis or thought disorders. Lithium carbonate is the drug of choice for manic-depressive disorders. Diazepam is an antianxiety drug. Maprotiline is an antidepressant. ANALYSIS (PSYCHOSOCIAL, MENTAL HEALTH, PSYCHIATRIC PROBLEMS/SUBSTANCE USE DISORDERS)

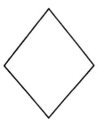

Reprints
Nursing Care of the Client with Psychosocial,
Psychiatric/Mental Health Problems

A M E R I C A N   J O U R N A L   O F   N U R S I N G

BORDERLINE PERSONALITY DISORDER

A THERAPEUTIC APPROACH

BY LOIS M. PLATT-KOCH

Reprinted from American Journal of Nursing, December, 1983

*Good/bad, love/hate, gratification/frustration—
the borderline patient's world is one of dichotomies.
The task: to 'heal the split' into a realistic whole.*

In my first therapy session with Susan, she could tell me nothing about herself or what she enjoyed in life. What she did say struck me as being what she thought I wanted to hear.

An attractive 18-year-old mother of two, Susan lived with her mother, grandmother, and siblings in a low-income urban neighborhood. She had completed the seventh grade and then, by chronically running away, had drifted out of school.

According to her mother, Susan was now periodically leaving home and her children to live with her boyfriend, who physically and sexually abused her. Her mother insisted that she seek treatment and threatened to give her children "to the state" if she did not.

When I asked her to tell me about her home life, she said it was fine, except for her boyfriend who occasionally "kidnapped" her, kept her prisoner in his home, and forced her to perform various sexual acts. She passively accepted his treatment of her and had little anxiety about it. It would soon become clear that Susan had borderline

Lois M. Platt-Koch, RN, MS, is a clinical specialist in adolescent psychiatry at Cook County Hospital, Chicago, Ill.

personality disorder, one of the most difficult personality problems to treat.

THE UNDERLYING ISSUES

The behavior of borderline patients stems from problems in two major areas: identity and intimacy. According to Erikson, individuals who successfully complete early adolescence have a sense of who they are, of what they like and do not like, what they value, and what is important to them(1).

Clients who have borderline personality disorder lack this personal identity. My first clue that Susan might have the disorder was her inability to tell me anything substantial about herself. Further evidence was my sense that she was telling me what she thought I wanted to hear. I could not get a feeling for who she really was. Often these patients are experienced by others as "chameleonlike." They seem to take on the values and characteristics of whomever they are with. They may even give the impression of being fairly well adjusted, but because their behavior is based on imitation, it does not appear genuine. Helene Deutsch called this the "as if" personality(2). It is "as if" they were like other people.

As treatment with Susan progressed,

it became increasingly clear that she had no sense of personal identity. She had no idea of what she wanted to do with her life, and whatever happened to her happened because someone else acted. She was in treatment, for example, because her mother had insisted upon it. Susan told me that she wanted to finish school, but she had not registered in over two years.

In the area of intimacy, clients who have borderline personality disorder have an approach-avoidance conflict. They long for intimacy, but are afraid of being engulfed and destroyed by the other person. They also fear that they themselves will engulf and destroy anyone with whom they are intimate. Because they both long for and fear intimacy, feeling close to another person causes them to do something to drive that person away. When that succeeds, the resulting feeling of alienation causes the person with borderline personality disorder to panic and to then try to draw the other person back. Obviously, such behavior creates stormy interpersonal relationships.

When I began to express concern about Susan's self-destructive lifestyle, my warmth and caring stimulated longing, fear, and rage in her. To put dis-

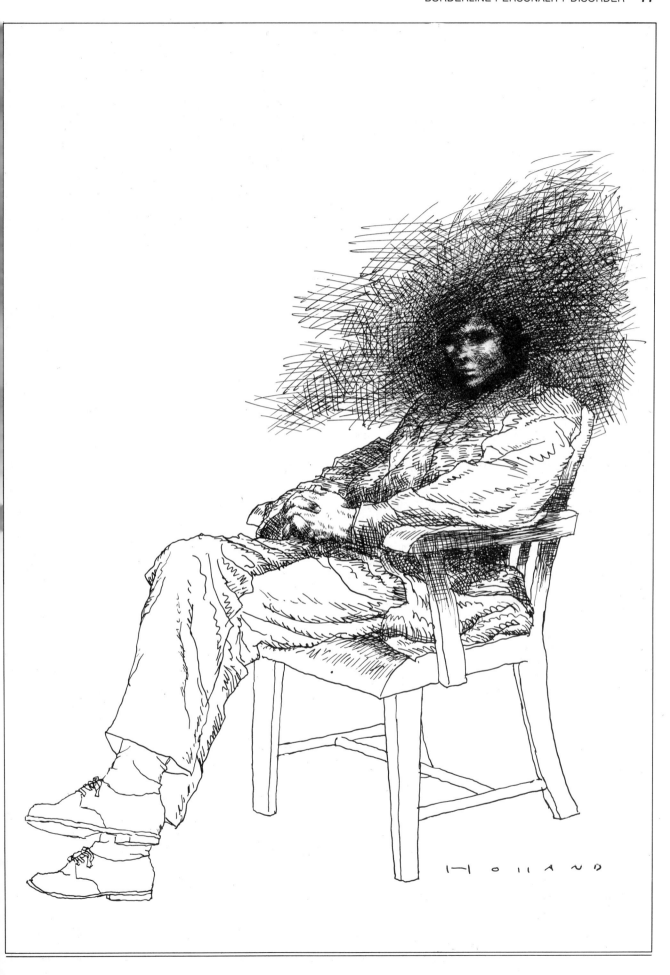

tance between us and thereby protect us both from the feared engulfment and annihilation, she began devaluing me. It started subtly: She would yawn and repeatedly look at the clock. With time, she became openly hostile and sarcastic, saying such things as, "I can't stand you" and "You need your butt kicked."

Such behavior can confuse and exhaust the therapist. Just when you think you are making progress, the patient does something to hurt you, leaving you discouraged and usually angry. And of course that is exactly what happens in all the patient's close relationships. The only intimacy Susan could tolerate was contaminated by violence, as demonstrated by her relationship with her boyfriend.

A useful technique for dealing with hostility is to ask patients who had treated them with hostility in the past. This causes patients to reflect on their feelings and behavior and to see that there is an historical reason for the rage. Understanding that their intense anger is not caused by the current treatment relationship, but rather by what has happened in the past helps patients take responsibility for their behavior. It also changes the therapist from passive victim of a raging onslaught to an active, helping person.

Throughout treatment, the therapist must modulate the amount of warmth shown to the patient. Too much warmth and closeness frighten the patient and stimulate rage and destructive feelings. But gradually, patients learn that they can care about others without destroying them or being destroyed.

Because people with borderline personality disorder desperately need relationships, they may at first be charming, which will attract others, but then they become manipulative and demanding. Although they often succeed in manipulating others, frequently through suicidal gestures and threats, it is usually at the expense of making the others furious and resentful.

EGO DEFENSES

One of the most common ego defenses employed by these patients is primitive dissociation—or splitting(3,4). In their view, people are either all bad or all good. It is believed the patient has "split" his world into these two extremes for fear that, if combined, the bad could overwhelm and destroy the good. These patients work hard at keeping good and bad separate,

but their estimation of the goodness or badness of anyone can change from week to week, even minute to minute.

In practice, you will notice that the patient alternates between idealization and devaluation of you and others. For example, the patient may tell you that you are the most wonderful person in the world, or, conversely, that you are absolutely the worst. Depending on which of these views the patient is projecting, the inexperienced therapist may feel either gifted or incompetent. Probably neither view is correct.

Patients with borderline personality disorder cannot integrate the negative and positive characteristics of people they care about. They lack "object constancy"—they do not have a consistent, well-rounded concept of another's personality. Therefore, when you gratify them, you are wonderful, and when you frustrate them, you are an abomination. The danger is that the inexperienced therapist will try only to gratify, never to frustrate.

In order to get better, patients who have borderline personality disorder need to experience both love and hate for the therapist. Thus, the work of therapy involves helping patients learn that the same person can nurture and gratify as well as frustrate and anger them. The technique used to unite the patient's fragmented and conflicting views of others into a realistic whole is called "healing the split."

Suppose Mr. James says, "I can never talk to any of the other nurses the way I can talk to you. You always make me feel better. No one else cares like you do." A helpful response from you would be, "I'm glad our sessions make you feel better, but I know that Mr. Allen sat with you for over an hour last night when you were upset and that he helped you quite a bit. It would be good for you to talk with him and some of the other staff members about your feelings." This answer challenges the patient's idealization of you.

Now suppose that later in the day Mr. James says to you, "I can't believe this place actually pays you to work here. Where did you get your license, in a Cracker Jack box? I always feel worse after you come to see me."

You might respond appropriately with: "You are angry with me now, and it's okay to feel that way. But remember this morning when you told me that I made you feel very good? I'm still the same person now as I was then." By

reminding him of what happened earlier, you challenge his devaluation. Having discrepancies in their behavior pointed out literally thousands of times helps patients begin to understand that other people have both positive and negative qualities, and that these qualities can coexist in the same person.

Projective identification is another ego defense frequently used by patients with borderline personality disorder. Because of their insatiable longing for love, these patients begin to hate any person who elicits such longings. But because it is unbearable to both hate and love the same person, the patients project their hatred onto the other person, especially the therapist. They then see the therapist as hateful and malicious and therefore worthy of abuse. The patient has projected his negative feelings, identified with the hatred he sees in the therapist, and feels justified in protecting himself from an imagined attack by abusing the therapist.

Susan, for example, accused me of hating her and wanting to hurt her. She could then feel justified in "hating me back" and wanting to hurt me. When you notice patients projecting their feelings onto you, tell them that you do not feel the way they imagine you to feel (if that is truly the case).

It may be, however, that the therapist does begin to hate the patient, because going hand in hand with projective identification is provocation. Patients will try to provoke your anger and will search for evidence that you do indeed hate them. Immediately confront such tactics. While communicating that you believe the patient can learn more satisfying ways of relating to others, say what has made you angry and draw a parallel between how you respond to the patient and how other people are likely to respond.

For example, I said to Susan, "When you sneer at me and refuse to talk, you make me very angry. If you do that to your boyfriend, I can see how it could provoke him into beating you. I am not saying that he is right in beating you, but your behavior is extremely provoking. I know you can learn to behave differently and to be happier in your life, and my job is to help you do that by talking to you about your behavior."

Certainly, it takes experience to immediately analyze the dynamics of an interaction and to express them to the patient in a helpful way. For that reason, a patient with borderline personality disorder needs a therapist who has access to good supervision.

ACTING OUT

Depression alternates with rage in borderline clients. The quality of the depression is not guilty and self-deprecatory, but empty and lonely. These patients feel, and are, left out of genuine reciprocal human interactions(5). The emptiness stems from the patients' lack of identity, which leaves a frightening inner void that they try to fill with impulsive, self-destructive act-

DIAGNOSTIC CRITERIA

The term borderline came into being because a group of patients seemed to fall on the border between neurosis and psychosis. Superficially, these patients appeared neurotic, but close inspection showed impaired thought, emotions, and behavior; and they did sometimes decompensate into psychosis. They did not have classic symptoms of schizophrenia, but there was similarity enough to warrant the label of pseudoneurotic schizophrenia(1).

In 1980 the American Psychiatric Association, in its effort to clarify and standardize psychiatric diagnostic labels, officially classified the borderline patient as having a personality disorder. Hence, in DSM III, borderline personality disorder is listed among 11 other personality disorders(2).

To be diagnosed as having a personality disorder, the patient must have a core of stable, maladaptive personality traits that consistently cause serious problems in relating to other people. Personality traits are fairly stable patterns of perceiving, thinking about, and interacting with the world. Traits can become rigid under stress, but are usually not maladaptive and usually do not cause problems in relating.

For example, a person with compulsive personality traits might be well organized and successful. Patients with compulsive personality disorder have rigid, maladaptive traits that cause them many problems. For instance they may be preoccupied with trivia, rules, and order; perfectionistic to the point of inability to make decisions for fear of making a mistake; or so insistent that things be done their way that others refuse to work or live with them.

The criteria for making the diagnosis of borderline personality disorder are listed below as they appear in DSM III(2).

Diagnostic criteria for borderline personality disorder. The following are characteristic of the individual's current and long-term functioning, are not limited to episodes of illness, and cause either significant impairment in social or occupational functioning or subjective distress.

A. At least five of the following are required:

1. impulsivity or unpredictability in at least two areas that are potentially self-damaging; e.g., spending, sex, gambling, substance use, shoplifting, overeating, physically self-damaging acts;

2. a pattern of unstable and intense interpersonal relationships; e.g., marked shifts of attitude, idealization, devaluation, manipulation (consistently using others for one's own ends);

3. inappropriate, intense anger or lack of control of anger; e.g., frequent displays of temper, constant anger;

4. identity disturbance manifested by uncertainty about several issues relating to identity, such as self-image, gender identity, long-term goals or career choice, friendship patterns, values, and loyalties; e.g., "Who am I?", "I feel like I am my sister when I am good";

5. affective instability: marked shifts from normal mood to depression, irritability, or anxiety, usually lasting a few hours and only rarely more than a few days, with a return to normal mood;

6. intolerance of being alone; e.g., frantic efforts to avoid being alone, depressed when alone;

7. physically self-damaging acts; e.g., suicidal gestures, self-mutilation, recurrent accidents or physical fights;

8. chronic feelings of emptiness or boredom.

B. If under 18, does not meet the criteria for Identity Disorder.

REFERENCES

1. Hoch, P. H., and others. The course and outcome of pseudoneurotic schizophrenia. *Am.J.Psychiatry* 119:106–115, Aug. 1962.
2. American Psychiatric Association. *Diagnostic and Statistical Manual of Mental Disorders*, 3rd ed. Washington, D.C., the Association, 1980, pp. 321-323.

ing out—sex, gambling, substance use, suicidal gestures.

Susan defended herself against emptiness by her involvement with an exciting, violent man who "kidnapped" her and "forced" her to perform aberrant sexual acts. Her sexual behavior was colored by sadism, aggression, and loss of control to a violent man, suggesting fixation at a pregenital level of sexuality. In other words, she was unable to enjoy affectionate, mutually satisfying, genital sex with an adult. The term polymorphous perverse sexuality is often used to describe the sexual behavior of borderline patients. It refers to sexual behavior that is not *primarily* directed toward genital intercourse, but rather includes behavior that would be considered sexually immature or perverse. The behavior interferes with the patient's ability to have reciprocal, affectionate sexual relationships.

Anhedonia is also characteristic of these patients. They cannot enjoy life. In spite of their intense quest for gratification, as in sexual acting out and substance abuse, they experience little, if any, pleasure(5). They also lack the capacity for self-soothing, that is, the ability to calm themselves down(6). People with healthier personalities can tell themselves to take it easy, that everything will be all right. In contrast, when patients with borderline personality disorder are under stress, they cannot maintain emotional equilibrium and therefore act out impulsively.

Because of their impulsiveness, unpredictability, and acting out, these patients usually lead chaotic lives. The therapist must guard against being seduced by the excitement of the chaos and allowing the patient's predicaments to become the focus of the therapy session. Otherwise, the patient and therapist may unconsciously collude to avoid dealing with the real issue—the patient's emptiness and depression.

In treatment, patients need to be confronted with the ways in which they deny themselves pleasure, and to be continually educated about how the "average person" lives. All the while, the therapist empathizes with the patient's depression and emptiness and continues to stress that the patient can change. In effect, through therapy, the patient learns "how to be."

DISTORTIONS OF REALITY

Patients with borderline personality disorder cannot tolerate being alone. Because they lack personal identity, they need other people to make them feel complete. They often describe feelings of depersonalization (feeling unreal or strange) and derealization (the sense that the environment is unreal and strange). Much delicate wrist-cutting—multiple superficial incisions—is done to counteract these feelings. Because these patients often do not initially feel pain when they cut themselves, they continue to cut until they finally do feel pain(7,8). Going to such extremes to feel "something" demonstrates the panic patients feel when in a depersonalized state. Seeing blood and feeling pain reassures them that they really do exist.

Because of their lack of object constancy, patients may believe the therapist ceases to exist when no longer physically present. I give patients a transitional object—an appointment card or a postcard when I'm on vacation—to help them remember me. One patient told me she was comforted by seeing my name written in a book I lent her. Many of the "pesky" phone calls therapists receive from their borderline clients serve to reassure the patient that the therapist still exists.

Although splitting, depersonalization, and derealization all represent serious distortions of reality, actual psychosis is the exception rather than the rule for borderline clients(5). When these patients do decompensate into psychosis, however, the psychotic episode has several distinctive features: It is stress-induced, brief, reversible, and ego-alien (i.e., the individual finds it an uncomfortable state).

NEGATIVE COUNTERTRANSFERENCE

One of the most difficult aspects of treating borderline clients is handling negative countertransference—a negative emotional reaction of the therapist to the patient. These patients can be hateful, stirring up many unpleasant feelings in the therapist, who must identify and accept the feelings and then use them in therapy.

In their excellent article on the subject, Maltsberger and Buie identify two feelings that the therapist will inevitably have when working with a "hateful" patient: malice and aversion(9). Feelings of malice translate into a desire to make the patient suffer. The therapist might wish to administer a sound thrashing to show who's boss. When the therapist feels aversion, the general de-

A COMMENT ON HOSPITALIZATION

BY LINDA L. LACY / WESLEY M. PITTS, JR.

The patient with borderline personality disorder is truly an enigma: First, engaging, socially skilled, and projecting a strong sense of inner strength; then suddenly immature, whiny, angry, negative, and possibly violent and self-destructive.

An increasing number of borderline clients have been admitted to psychiatric inpatient settings. Reasons for hospitalization include control of impulsivity and acting out, evaluation and control of suicidal or homicidal thoughts and activity, treatment and evaluation of a psychotic episode, drug or alcohol detoxification, and diagnostic evaluation. Often, admission is precipitated by conflict in an important relationship.

These patients also may be admitted to medical or surgical services because of overdoses, wrist slashing, and unexplained automobile accidents. In such situations, patients usually have not been diagnosed as borderline, but the nursing staff will identify them as difficult and demanding.

Linda L. Lacy, RN, MS, MEd, is head nurse of a psychiatric ward at the Houston Veteran's Administration Medical Center, Tex., where Wesley M. Pitts, Jr., MD, is director of the Clinical Psychiatric Research Unit.

The authors thank Margaret Dodson for her help in preparing this article.

When patients are admitted to our facility, our first concern is whether or not they have self-destructive, suicidal, or homicidal tendencies. We consider the patients' history of such behavior and their current feelings, keeping in mind that they often use flippancy and a light affect to minimize or discount their pain and desperation. If the patient has a well-thought-out plan on when, where, and how self-destructive or other destructive acts would occur, a protective environment is indicated. The more considered the plan, the more lethal the individual.

Clients who are assessed as self-destructive or homicidal are placed on closed psychiatric wards. Those who describe feelings of aloneness, isolation, or alienation need an open ward that permits them to express their feelings, but at the same time offers security. It is not uncommon for a borderline client to be moved back and forth between open and closed wards during hospitalization.

We find that our borderline clients are likely to have unrealistic expectations of therapy and hospitalization. For example, they may believe that medication or unlimited time with a skilled therapist will rapidly and forever solve their problems, or that they will leave the hospital cured. When patients express such beliefs, we stress that hos-

pitalization will be for a limited time and that psychotherapy will need to be continued long after discharge.

Once the person with borderline personality disorder enters the hospital, regression should be expected, if it has not already occurred. Hospitalization fosters regression because it promises quick, intense relationships with nurturing people. Regression usually takes the form of clinging and demanding behavior, multiple somatic complaints, suicide threats, and/or self-destructive acts.

To contain and prevent regression, we set limits. From the day of admission the patient is told what is and is not acceptable and what is expected. For example, we stress that the client is not psychotic or organically impaired, and thus will be held accountable for all behavior, that suicidal activity or psychosis will result in transfer to a closed ward, that assaulting other patients or staff will result in discharge, and that substance abuse will result in disciplinary action.

In addition to fostering regression, the hospital environment is an ideal breeding ground for the clients' use of projective identification and splitting (they tend to see members of the staff as all good or all bad). These patients are expert at dividing the staff through labeling and manipulation. For exam-

sire is to get away from the patient.

As unpleasant as it is to feel malice toward a patient, the patient is safer when the therapist's feelings of malice are stronger than feelings of aversion. When the therapist feels malice, the patient receives the unconscious message that the therapist wants to torture him. This implies a continuation of the relationship and therefore continued existence of both people. When the therapist feels aversion, the unconscious message is that the therapist wants the patient to go away. The danger is that the patient may act out the therapist's wish by attempting suicide. Thus, when aversion begins to predominate, the therapist has the very difficult task of striving to stay in touch with feelings of malice so that the patient remains in therapy.

It is essential that those who choose to work with borderline clients understand themselves, have a good deal of patience, and be able to tolerate the uncomfortable countertransference feelings that are an inevitable part of therapy. They must be able to receive satisfaction from tiny bits of progress and remain as therapist for a difficult patient for a long period of time—a ten-year treatment goal is not unrealistic.

Working with borderline clients can be compared to working in physical rehabilitation. The work is frustrating and the road is long, but the potential for personal and professional growth is enormous.

REFERENCES

1. Erikson, E. H. *Childhood and Society*. 2nd ed. New York, W.W. Norton & Co. 1964, pp. 261–263.
2. Deutsch, Helene. Some forms of emotional disturbance and their relationship to schizophrenia. *Psychoanal.Q.* 11:301–321, 1942.
3. Kernberg, O. F. A psychoanalytic classification of character pathology. *J.Am.Psychoanal.Assoc.* 18:800–822, Oct. 1970.
4. _____ . The treatment of patients with borderline personality organization. *Int.J.Psychoanal.* 49:600–619, Oct. 1968.
5. Gunderson, J. G., and Singer, M. T. Defining borderline patients: an overview. *Am.J.Psychiatry* 132:1–10, Jan. 1975.
6. Blanck, Gertrude, and Blanck, Rubin. *Ego Psychology II; Psychoanalytic Developmental Psychology*. New York, Columbia University Press, 1979.
7. Kafka, J. S. The body as a transitional object: a psychoanalytic study of a self-mutilating patient. *Br.J.Med.Psychol.* 42(3):207–212, 1969.
8. Pao, P.N. The syndrome of delicate self-cutting. *Br.J.Med.Psychol.* 42:195–206, Aug. 1969.
9. Maltsberger, J. T., and Buie, D. H. Countertransference hate in the treatment of suicidal patients. *Arch.Gen.Psychiatry* 30:625–633, May 1974.

---

ple, a borderline patient might say, "You're no nurse; if you were a decent nurse like Ms. Repitti you would get me some stronger medication." Or, "Ms. Sloan is all right; she let me go out after the doors were locked last night."

To work successfully with this group of patients, staff must know each other well, set limits, and enforce them consistently. Frequent staff meetings are essential to counteract the patient's divisive attempts.

Our approach is empathic and supportive, but firm and direct. Nevertheless, enforcement of limits will frustrate the borderline client, who will react with verbal or, if permitted, physical aggression. Helping the patient to handle anger therefore becomes an important staff function. Throughout hospitalization, ways of tolerating delay and frustration are explored with the client; the goal being to help the person learn to put anger into words rather than action (acting out or regressing). We encourage verbal expression of anger, and positively reinforce it.

At some point, most staff members will respond negatively to these patients. When that happens, the feelings need to be acknowledged and the patient should be confronted with what he has done and how it has made the staff member feel. Care should be taken, however, not to express "countertransference hate," which would result in the staff member trying to avoid the patient, or setting punitive, repressive limits. Limit setting is therapeutic when done to help clients learn that there are consequences for their actions, not when it is simply punishment for making a staff member angry.

Learning to act within limits helps the borderline client in two ways: It prevents the vicious circle of frustration-acting out-anxiety-frustration. And learning to handle frustration strengthens the client's ego, paving the way for the emotional discomfort of psychotherapy and/or somatic therapies.

CASE EXAMPLE

Mike, after a stay on the alcohol detoxification unit, was transferred to our open general psychiatric unit. Although vague about specific changes he wished to make, his goals were to "get my life straightened out" and to "get my head together."

While on the detoxification unit, he had been angry and irritable, had demanded more frequent and heavier medication than was prescribed, and had had difficulties with other patients and staff. The first three days on our unit he seemed the model patient. But then he became critical and hostile, complained of boredom and that no one was helping him, and verbal y abused staff and patients. He also resisted participating in ward activities, including various therapies, and he expressed numerous somatic complaints.

On a one-to-one basis, staff members assessed his symptoms and offered support and understanding, but at the same time informed him of what was expected while he was a patient on the unit. His response was to become more angry and critical and to stomp away from the staff member.

After about two weeks of his demanding and regressive behavior, we decided to set his discharge date, and to move it up one day for each day that he refused to participate in group and other therapies. Suddenly, his behavior changed. He did remain somewhat hostile and sarcastic, but he was where he was supposed to be, and on time.

As his discharge date approached, he became more receptive to therapy and he began to look for a job. When his prospects for finding and holding a job began to look favorable, he was able to state and focus on his goals. He wanted, for instance, to rent an apartment instead of living with his mother.

He requested an extension of his discharge date, which was granted, and in the final weeks of hospitalization he worked toward his objective of independent living. He also accepted the need for ongoing therapy as an outpatient.□

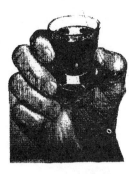

Hospital Dialogues

Reprinted from American Journal of Nursing, December 1982

By Jean Krajicek Weist
 Marlene G. Lindeman
 Marian Newton

As many as 64 percent of hospital admissions have been reported to be alcohol-related(1). Although nurses—and medical-surgical nurses in particular— are in an ideal position to assist the alcoholic patient, they are usually hesitant to intervene because they simply don't know what to say.

Here are some guidelines, illustrated by four clinical situations. In each case, the nurse timed the verbal intervention so that the patient was neither too physically ill to respond nor so well that he could ignore evidence of the effects of alcohol. In each situation, the nurse had established a relationship with the patient.

Connecting Alcohol To the Problems

John, a 25-year-old man with a college degree in a health profession, was hospitalized for treatment of fractures of the orbit of the eye, the humerus, and the femur. The injuries were the result of a motorcycle accident.

What Was Said	Why It Was Said
Nurse: "When I read the admission note, John, I noticed that your friend said that you two were drinking very heavily on the night of the accident. He also said you were 'serious' drinking buddies." John: "I do a fair amount of drinking, but only on weekends, and never during the day. I'm single again and taking courses. Weekends are my only time to get wild. I haven't had any problems because of drinking."	• Because alcoholics often deny that they have problems with alcohol, the nurse should present the facts early. Since the patient may not remember events leading to his admission, the nurse can begin by talking with him about his drinking in general(2). In dealing directly with the drinking problem, the nurse shows that she is not afraid of what the patient has to say(3). • In early interactions, the nurse should avoid using the word *alcoholism* or labeling the patient *alcoholic*. Such terms can increase the patient's denial and evoke a defensive response. "Drinking patterns" or "problems with drinking" are less threatening(2).
Nurse: "It interests me that you say that, John, because I see a possible relationship between the drinking and your accident. Also, heavy weekend drinking can be a sign of a serious problem. You aren't safe from problems because drinking is confined to weekends." John was silent for a long period of time before he responded: "I have never made any connection between the accident and the drinking. The highway was rough where I wrecked. I felt I lost control because of the sudden change in condition of the surface."	• Identifying a learning need—in this case, the patient's apparent lack of awareness of the nature and implications of alcoholism—provides the nurse with a concrete way to begin to talk and give information about alcohol and alcoholism(4). • Many patients, especially those with early-stage alcoholism, do not associate certain incidents (e.g., accidents, injury) with their abuse of alcohol until the relationship is made clear to them(5).
Nurse: "Maybe the alcohol made you more apt to lose control when the surface roughened. It's a possibility." John: "I don't think so, but I get your message." Nurse: "It's something to consider, John. There is plenty of help available if you ever decide that drinking is a problem for you."	• The alcoholic must admit that there may be a connection between alcohol intake and problems in living before he will accept assistance in recovery. • The alcoholic patient responds to cues in voice and manner that reveal feelings and attitudes of the caregiver. The nurse needs to make sure he or she is not taking a judgmental or hostile tone; it is important to show genuine caring, concern, and interest(6).

Moving Beyond Denial and Defensiveness

Mr. Anton, 52 years old, was admitted because of a fractured humerus incurred when he fell over some furniture in his home. He had had previous hospital admissions related to alcohol abuse. Intoxicated at the time of admission, he developed signs of alcohol withdrawal and needed to be detoxified. The following interchange with the nurse took place when he improved physically and was moving about in his room.

What Was Said	Why It Was Said
Nurse: "You look much better. You had some difficult days last week." Mr. Anton became guarded: "What do you mean?" Nurse: "You required a lot of care." Mr. Anton: "It's rough when you break your arm." Nurse: "We cared for your arm, but you needed care in other ways, too. You became ill because being hospitalized suddenly stopped your intake of alcohol. Do you remember that just this morning your physician told you that he's concerned about your drinking?" Mr. Anton responded abruptly: "I don't drink."	• The essential elements in a relationship with an alcoholic patient are knowledge about the disease, a nonjudgmental attitude, and the ability to confront an individual with alcoholism with the same professional acceptance that one would adopt toward a patient with any other disease(7).
The nurse allowed a long period of silence. Mr. Anton: "What did the nurses have to do?"	• If the nurse anticipates defensiveness, knowing that it is part of the symptomatology of alcoholism, he or she can monitor the patient's responses, taking care not to become involved in reciprocal defensiveness(5).
Nurse: "We had to bathe you, turn you frequently and give you IVs. We had to bathe you often because you lost control of your bowels." (Nurse continued with descriptions of care.)	• The alcoholic patient often perceives the nurse as the least threatening of all the health team members and typically relates well to the nurse who has cared for him. This contact unquestionably enhances the nurse's potential, if he or she is willing to tap it, for influencing the alcoholic's life(8). A caring and honest directness is the approach that seems to have the best chance of reaching the alcoholic and keeping him engaged(9). • The alcoholic patient must be treated with respect and consideration. To establish trust and confidence, the nurse must answer the patient's questions about his health and his care frankly and completely(10).
Nurse: "Nurses really care about your health, Mr. Anton. There are ways to help you prevent illness and injury like this in the future. I can spend some time with you now or talk more about this later if you wish." Mr. Anton motioned for the nurse to leave.	• By addressing patients by name, making eye contact, and encouraging patient decision-making, the nurse demonstrates sincere interest in promoting the patient's self-esteem and sense of well-being(11). • An essential tool in successful treatment is respect for the patient as a unique person who can be helped, but who must be allowed the dignity of choice(12).

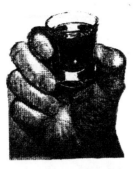

Developing A Specific Plan

Mary, a 28-year-old obese client with a young daughter, was in skeletal traction for treatment of a self-inflicted gunshot wound to the leg. She had been hospitalized for weeks. Her friends visited frequently and there always seemed to be a party in Mary's room. The staff's discussions with Mary never went beyond the healing of the wound or the decorations that hung on the traction.

What Was Said	Why It Was Said
Nurse: "Mary, I've noticed that almost everybody who comes into your room focuses on your leg or on activities to keep you happy. No one is looking at the problem that started it all—the drinking."	• The initial confrontation is rarely pleasant but it's worth investing the effort because it is often the turning point(10).
Nurse: "You were drinking when you shot yourself. That's really serious, and I'm worried that you might do it again when you leave the hospital. I'm also concerned that drinking might interfere with your ability to care for your little girl." To the nurse's astonishment, Mary admitted that she had attended an outpatient treatment center. She saw an alcoholism counselor regularly for about six months and then stopped.	• The nurse may find that focusing on the problems in everyday living caused by alcohol is more helpful than concentrating solely on the drinking behaviors(3).
Nurse: "There must have been a reason that you stopped going. What would you think if I called your counselor and asked her to come and see you? I would like to meet her, too." Mary: "That's okay." Nurse: "I get the idea that you had some of the same concerns I had. Am I correct in saying that?" Mary: "Yes." Nurse: "Since there's no phone here, I'll call your counselor and come back to tell you what she says."	• A broad, open-ended clarifying statement may elicit the patient's willingness to look at the problem. Asking a "why" question often blocks communication. • The plans for alcoholism treatment or referrals should be personal, supportive, specific, and action-oriented. Speaking in generalities hinders the development of a working plan. A plan that will foster change needs to be mutually developed and agreed upon by both nurse and patient(10).

The authors are all at the University of Nebraska College of Nursing in Omaha and are members of the Alcoholism Nursing Research Team there.

JEAN KRAJICEK WEIST, RN, MSN, is assistant professor and project director of the research team.

MARLENE G. LINDEMAN, RN, MSN, is an instructor.

MARIAN NEWTON, RN, MN, is an assistant professor.

References

1. Stark, M. J., and Nichols, H. G. Alcohol-related admissions to a general hospital. *Alc.Health Res. World* 1:11-14, Summer 1977.
2. Bluhm, Judy. When you face the alcoholic patient. *Nursing '81* 11:70-73, Feb. 1981.
3. Burgess, A. W., and Lazure, Aaron. *Psychiatry in the Hospital and the Community.* 2nd ed. Englewood Cliffs, N. J., Prentice-Hall, 1976, pp. 463-464. (3rd ed., 1981).

Confronting the Relapsed Patient

Jake, age 50, was hospitalized for therapy for muscle weakness related to a previous traumatic injury that occurred during a drinking episode. His medical record stated that he was a recovering alcoholic.

What Was Said	**Why It Was Said**
Nurse: "Jake, the nursing student caring for you told me that the thermos in your room has liquor in it. This concerns me very much because the admission information on your chart states that you are a recovering alcoholic. We really do care about your sobriety." Jake looked startled, but not angry: "A lot of things have happened at home lately that made me feel sort of down. My wife is ill; my daughter got pregnant. All the noise and problems of teenagers got to me. I'm worried myself that I've been sneaking drinks. Would you believe that just this morning I was sitting here thinking that I've got to quit this foolishness and get back into AA?"	• When the nurse keeps in mind that alcoholism is a chronic disease often associated with relapses, she can approach the alcoholic patient with an attitude of professional acceptance and caring. Confrontation can be an effective technique, but only if the patient does not sense feelings of hostility, condescension, or disgust(13).
Nurse: "I'm glad I didn't hesitate to talk to you like this and that you were able to share those concerns about your drinking with me. You know I can ask AA to send a hospital visitor." Jake: "All I want right now is to get some alcoholism materials to read. Don't send anyone to see me. And will you get some Al-Anon information for my wife? She can't go, but she will read it."	• During the crisis of hospitalization and illness, the patient is more ready than at any other time to reflect upon his use of alcohol and is more open to considering alternatives to drinking(4). • Depression is a common feature of alcoholism. The nurse listens to the patient's expressions of depression, but also helps him to focus on treatment rather than on his feelings of low self-esteem and guilt.
Nurse: "I'll get the leaflets right away. Obviously, you are aware of the problem. Now you need to decide what you are going to do about it."	• The nurse should avoid making an issue over or standing in judgment of the method of recovery selected by the alcoholic. In fact, the nurse should give immediate encouragement to any realistic goal the patient sets for himself.

The skillful use of words in promoting recovery from alcoholism is indeed a profound nursing intervention. The nurse conveys an important message—that she knows the serious problems related to alcoholism and cares enough to tell the patient when she detects a relationship between the patient's drinking and his health. A nurse may never know the long-range success of the words she chooses to use when the patient's problem is alcoholism. However, as Reed writes, "she will till the soil, readying the patient's mind and spirit for personal growth and restoration of health"(4). There are always benefits, even when there is no storybook ending.

4. Reed, S. W. Symposium on alcoholism and drug addiction. Assessing the patient with an alcohol problem. *Nurs.Clin.North Am.* 11:483-492, Sept. 1976.
5. Estes, N. J., and others. *Nursing Diagnosis of the Alcoholic Person.* St. Louis, the C. V. Mosby Co., 1980, pp. 125-136.
6. Chafetz, M. E. Alcohol and alcoholism. *Am.Sci.* 67:293-299, May-June 1979.
7. Parks, Gladys. Alcoholism primer for nurses. *Penn.Nurse* 34:7-11, Feb. 1979.
8. Schwerdtfeger, T. H. Developing a nursing staff in an alcoholism treatment center. *Superv.Nurse* 11:43-45, Feb. 1980.
9. Mitchell, C. E., Assessment of alcohol abuse. *Nurs.Outlook* 24:511-515, Aug. 1976.
10. Green, D. E. Alcoholism and the nurse. *N.Z.Med.J.* 87:287-288, Apr. 26, 1978.
11. Chavigny, Katherine. Self-esteem for the alcoholic: an epidemiologic approach. *Nurs.Outlook* 24:636-639, Oct. 1976.
12. Gilmour, Vera. How do nurses feel about alcoholism? *N.Z.Nurs.J.* 66:31-32, Sept. 1973.
13. Burkhalter, P. K. *Nursing Care of the Alcoholic and Drug Abuser.* New York, McGraw-Hill Book Co., 1975, pp. 14-15.

A M E R I C A N   J O U R N A L   O F   N U R S I N G

THE AGITATED AGGRESSIVE PATIENT

BY CYNTHIA BRIGMAN/CAROL DICKEY/LOUISE JIMM ZEGEER

Reprinted from American Journal of Nursing, October 1983

One of the most vexing problems that can develop during recovery from a head injury is agitated-aggressive behavior. Not only does such behavior pose difficulties for nursing care, it can, if it persists, impair rehabilitation efforts and the patient's subsequent ability to live independently.

Agitated-aggressive patients may be uncooperative, incoherent, abusive, and/or irritable. They lack self-control, and short-term recall, and are often unable to discriminate between people and objects.

These patients need assistance with activities of daily living because their short attention spans make it difficult for them to complete tasks. Furthermore, they are likely to injure themselves or others; sometimes deliberately, but usually because they cannot control their behavior. They fall out of bed, wander away from the unit, and injure their arms and legs by bumping against walls, wheelchairs, bedrails, and, some-

Cynthia Brigman, RN, BSN, is brain injury unit coordinator at Cardinal Hill Rehabilitation Hospital. Carol A. Dickey, RN, MSN, is director of nursing at Cardinal Hill Rehabilitation Hospital, Lexington, KY. Louise Jimm Zegeer, RN, MSN, is professor of clinical nursing at the University of Kentucky College of Nursing.

> ## Recovery from head injury may involve a period of disorientation and violent behavior.

times, other people.

Although all this can frustrate even the experienced nurse, there is a positive way of looking at agitated behavior—that is, as a stage in the process of recovering from head injury. While not all patients go through an agitated stage and not all patients progress beyond it, the usual sequence of recovery from severe head injury is as follows: First there is coma, then a period of hypokinesia (lethargy, stupor, or passivity), then a period of hyperactivity (agitation). As recovery progresses, an almost lucid phase with automatism may occur—the patient automatically and unconsciously performs previously learned movements that are inappro-

priate to the situation. Examples are picking at bedclothes, or buttoning and unbuttoning shirts. Finally, if full recovery occurs, the patient returns to the preinjured state.

How long it takes for patients in coma to reach the agitated state and how long they remain in it varies with the individual, the depth and duration of coma, and the person's age. Agitated behavior may appear in the acute care setting or not until the patient is transferred to a rehab setting. It may last a few hours or persist indefinitely because of permanent cortical damage. Children usually recover from head injury faster than adults because of the plasticity of the immature nervous system.

HOW TO PROMOTE PATIENT SAFETY

Although it is tempting—as well as common practice—to use physical or chemical restraints to control agitated-aggressive behavior, we do not advise it. Body jackets, wrist and leg restraints tend to potentiate agitation, and patients can injure themselves while fighting restraints. Sedation inhibits the patient's ability to learn, interrupts the recovery process, and may lengthen the period of agitation.

To protect restless patients and still allow them to move freely, we use floor

PETER FIORE

A M E R I C A N   J O U R N A L   O F   N U R S I N G

> *Sedation is a last resort because it inhibits the patient's ability to learn, interrupts recovery, and may lengthen the period of agitation.*

beds. (See photo, next page.) Families and visitors are carefully prepared about the purpose of floor beds so that they understand the benefits.

Patients with tracheostomies and feeding tubes can be managed on the floor beds, but indwelling catheters are removed because the drainage bag cannot be placed below the level of the bladder. Urinary incontinence is managed with external catheters, incontinence briefs, and toileting regimens.

Although it is awkward to care for patients while kneeling on mattresses, the benefits of patient safety far outweigh that disadvantage, and on any given day we usually do not have more than two patients using floor beds.

For patients who attempt to remove trach or feeding tubes, mitts are as effective as wrist restraints. Even though patients could pull out feeding tubes by grasping the tube with both mitted hands, most are not mentally alert enough to do it. The only disadvantage of mitts is reduced range of motion of the fingers; to overcome this we remove the mitts and exercise the patients' fingers at least every eight hours.

To ensure that ambulatory patients or those who are independent in wheelchairs do not wander into unsupervised areas, we keep the unit locked. Although the unit can be entered without a key, a key is required to get out. Staff carry keys to provide visitors and approved patients easy egress and to open fire doors during fire drills or alarms. Close supervision is still required because a patient could wander out when someone else enters.

In fact, frequent observation, necessitating adequate staffing, is essential in preventing accidents.

HOW TO PROTECT YOURSELF

To manage the assaultive patient, the staff needs to be taught appropriate techniques. Some of our nursing staff have attended workshops on the management of aggressive patients, and we also have a videotape ("Prevention and Management of Disturbed Behavior," available from the Ministry of Health, Ontario, Canada) that we use to orient new staff and to re-educate existing staff.

A calm, quiet, confident, but firm attitude will minimize most assaultive episodes. But for those situations in which the patient does become physically abusive, enough staff members—usually two or three—must respond promptly, effectively, and in the least stimulating manner. Without avoiding the patient, they need to protect themselves from being kicked, hit, or bitten.

One of our extremely aggressive patients was Allen, 37 years old, who had sustained a closed head injury in an automobile accident. When Allen was admitted to our unit three weeks postinjury, he was confused and agitated. A violent kicker and hitter, he was also frequently incontinent of urine. Because Allen was strong, it took three of us to change his clothes. Two staff members held his hands while staying clear of his legs. The third staff member, who approached from the side and worked quickly, explained the procedure to him while changing his clothes. Allen was like many of our patients in that if more than one staff member talked to him during the procedure his agitation would increase.

In order to work effectively with a potentially assaultive patient, you need to convey an attitude of being in control of the situation. If a patient grabs your arm, remove the patient's hand, make eye contact, and say, "I am not going to allow you to hurt me." Then direct the patient's attention to another activity. During episodes of severe agitation, the most effective staff member should be assigned to work with the patient on a one-to-one basis.

In some instances, chemical restraints are necessary, but only as a last resort. Most sedatives are ordered PRN and the nurses decide when they are truly needed.

Agitation can be heightened by an overload of stimuli. Too much stimulation can also precipitate agitation, as demonstrated by Joyce, a 28-year-old who had sustained a closed head injury that rendered her immediately unconscious. By the time she was admitted to our unit, although confused and disoriented she was docile, cooperative, and able to move about without assistance.

The day after her admission, we had a fire drill. As soon as the alarm sounded, she screamed, "You are all witches and are going to let me burn!" Then she began to hit and scratch anyone near her. Though fire alarms can and do stimulate aggressive behavior, patients are more commonly overstimulated by too many visitors, excessive television, loud noises, numerous demands, or even the frequent touch involved in nursing care.

HOW TO REDUCE STIMULATION

To control stimulation, our unit has been located out of the main traffic flow of visitors and staff. Closed double doors deter casual entry into the unit and help reduce noise. After our experience with Joyce, we turned down the fire alarm speaker.

Unit nurses are particularly sensitive to patients' signals of overstimulation—increased talkativeness, pacing, rapid eye movements, abusive behavior, and irritability. When a patient's agitation begins to increase, there are several techniques to be tried. Not every patient responds to the same approach. Some need to be transferred to a private room so they are not overstimulated by roommates. Others need to have their visitors restricted for a period of time. Still others respond well to a "time-out" room; a room specifically set aside to allow patients a little time away from the stimulating activities of the unit.

One patient who responded well to the "time-out" room was Richard, a 15-year-old who, six months before admission to our unit, suffered a head injury after being struck by an automobile. On admission, Richard was wheelchair-bound and alert, but oriented only to person. During his stay with us he would occasionally become combative and verbally abusive. When such be-

A M E R I C A N   J O U R N A L   O F   N U R S I N G

havior occurred, the staff member working with him would take him to the "time out" room, where he usually remained for about five minutes under staff observation; afterward, he was able to resume his previous activity.

To control agitation, whatever technique works most effectively for the individual must be used consistently by all staff and family. Thus, we always explain the approach to family members, since without their cooperation, our efforts to calm the patient cannot be successful.

HOW TO MINIMIZE CONFUSION

Because agitated patients can also be confused and disoriented, we provide continuous reality orientation. Located on the main corridor is the " real-ity-orientation board," on which we post the date, the next meal, the day of the week, and the weather. Staff continually reinforce this information throughout the day. Recent photographs and names of staff are also posted so patients and family members can learn to associate names and faces.

Confused patients are particularly disturbed by a constantly changing staff. Thus we try to arrange the schedule so that patients have contact with as few staff members as possible. Float personnel are not usually assigned to the unit. Some nurses clearly have a talent for relating to confused patients; whenever possible, these nurses are assigned accordingly.

Consistent scheduling of patient activities also minimizes confusion, allow-ing the patients to anticipate coming events. Thus, we never vary our daily schedule for mealtimes, therapies, rest periods, recreational activities, visiting hours, baths, and bedtime. Our patients carry their daily schedule with them in what we call a memory book. We also have a large master schedule board posted where patients can easily see it. Confusion is further minimized by reducing the number of locations for patient activities. All therapies, meals, and recreational activities take place in one large room within the unit.

Certain communication techniques also reduce confusion. We use, and teach the family to use, short sentences and simple words. We present the patient with one thought or command at a time. If the patient does not respond

A staff member demonstrates the use of the floor bed and mitts. These alternatives to restraints offer protection while still allowing the restless patient freedom to move about the bed.

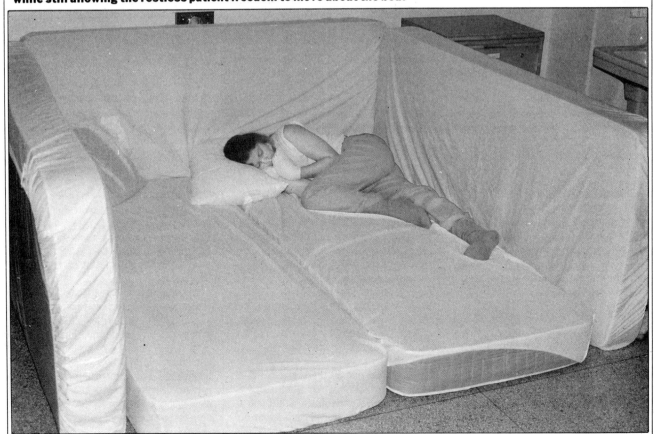

Patients often are aware of their behavior: Once they move beyond the period of agitation, they are embarrassed about things they have done.

or seem to understand, we restate the idea, using exactly the same words, to help the patient reprocess the thought. Whenever the patients express confused thoughts or ideas, we correct them rather than letting them go by without comment. For example, if the patient seems to think the nurse is his wife, she tells him her name and that she is a nurse.

HOW TO DEAL WITH INAPPROPRIATE BEHAVIOR

The techniques for reducing agitation and confusion usually are effective for socially inappropriate behavior as well. But inappropriate behavior may be persistent, especially in patients with irreversible brain damage. Inappropriate behavior can take the form of asking to use the toilet every five minutes, constant rapid eating, sexual preoccupation, temper tantrums, spitting and crying, or aggressive-assaultive behavior.

Behavior modification techniques can be of help in many instances. Our approach is to be kind and gentle, while firmly conveying that we expect the patient to behave appropriately. Twenty-two-year-old David, for example, was admitted to the unit two and one-half weeks after receiving a gunshot wound to his left frontal lobe. He was oriented to time, inconsistently oriented to person and place, and had severe short- and long-term memory loss. Although he was ambulatory, he would lie in bed with his curtain pulled and the television on, missing therapies and meals. To change his behavior, we did not give him the option of going to meals or therapies. Instead, we directed him to the correct location and praised him when he voluntarily attended scheduled activities. We have found that lectures, reprimands, and punishment do not improve inappropriate behavior, and may, in fact, make it worse.

Setting limits is another effective way to change certain kinds of inappropriate behavior. Because consistency is essential to its success, we use nursing care conferences and case conferences to plan the exact approach. Doris was a patient who constantly asked to be taken to the bathroom to urinate. Once we had established that there was no physiologic basis for her requests, we, together with Doris, planned a voiding schedule which was posted where she and the staff could see it. Whenever she asked to urinate, she was told to check the schedule to see if it was time. The approach reduced her preoccupation with voiding and resulted in longer intervals between requests.

When patients act inappropriately as a way of seeking attention, it is best to just ignore the behavior, unless it is destructive. Chuck, a 26-year-old, was admitted six weeks after sustaining a closed head injury. He was hemiplegic, moderately agitated, and he perseverated on sexual topics. He usually sat in the hall making lewd comments to all who walked past. At first, we scolded him, but that approach just increased the inappropriate behavior. Instead, we decided to ignore the sexual comments, but to spend extra time with him when he was behaving appropriately. We also used diversion with Chuck. Sometimes he would inappropriately put his hand on a female staff member. If he did, the nurse would matter-of-factly remove his hand and redirect his attention to something else. Gradually his inappropriate sexual behavior diminished.

Diversion can also be effective in preventing or stopping destructive behavior. On the day of admission, Stan, a young teenager who had suffered a closed head injury nine days earlier, paced the halls and threw his basketball violently against the unit doors. One of the nurses discovered that Stan was fascinated by Rubik's cube. Playing with the cube diverted his attention from the basketball and calmed him. We stopped another patient from pacing and yelling by playing cards with her. Remember that because the head-injured patient's attention span is frequently short, you'll need a variety of activities on hand.

A final piece of advice: It may seem an obvious point, but it is important for staff to resist the temptation to laugh at or joke about odd behavior in front of the patient. Aside from the fact that laughing at a patient is thoughtless, we find that the patients often are aware of their behavior so that once they move beyond the period of agitation and confusion they are embarrassed about things they have said and done. It is not uncommon for them to apologize to the nurses, and we have noticed that they often feel empathy for other patients who are still agitated.

HOW TO REDUCE THE FAMILY'S ANXIETY

Immediately following the head injury and once the patient's survival is assured, families expect that their loved one will return to his usual level of function, and that normal personality will be restored. They therefore need to be prepared for the possibility of agitated-aggressive behavior. Families who are unprepared suffer unnecessary embarrassment at the language and behavior of the patient. Typical comments are: "I don't believe she is saying that!" or "He was not brought up to act like that." Families not only need to understand that the patient is not in control of the behavior, they also need support from the staff in order to manage unaccustomed problems.

Each primary nurse assesses the family's as well as the patient's needs, encourages family members to call if they have any questions, and makes an appointment for a family conference. All management strategies—limit setting or use of the floor bed, for example—are discussed with the family prior to use. The family conference, scheduled about two weeks after admission, is set aside specifically for the family to learn about the patient's care. Families spend one day going with the patient through all his daily activities.

We have found that some families can serve as support for other families. Therefore, families who choose to do so meet weekly as a group to learn about brain injury sequelae and to express their feelings. Attendance at these meetings is excellent, and many families develop friendships that continue long after discharge. □

Nursing Care of the Adult

Coordinator

Paulette D. Rollant, MSN, RN, CCRN

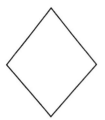

Questions

A nurse comes upon an auto accident and discovers a young man lying beside the road. He has a carotid pulse but does not seem to be breathing.

1. Which action would be *incorrect*?
   - ○ 1. Clear the mouth.
   - ○ 2. Hyperextend the neck.
   - ○ 3. Pull the mandible forward by resting the fingertips near the thyroid cartilage.
   - ○ 4. Inhale deeply and deliver several rapid breaths smoothly.

2. If the victim had oral injuries, the nurse would deliver mouth-to-nose resuscitation. Which of the following would be correct for mouth-to-nose resuscitation but *not* correct for mouth-to-mouth?
   - ○ 1. More force is required.
   - ○ 2. The victim's mouth is closed during inspiration.
   - ○ 3. The victim's mouth is open during expiration.
   - ○ 4. The victim's neck is extended.

3. An Ambu bag is available. If used with one hand, how many milliliters of air can be delivered?
   - ○ 1. 1,000
   - ○ 2. 800
   - ○ 3. 600
   - ○ 4. 400

4. The victim has a blood pressure of 60/0 mm Hg, and a pulse of 140. Following adequate ventilation, the first treatment priority is
   - ○ 1. sodium bicarbonate.
   - ○ 2. range of motion.
   - ○ 3. turn, cough, deep breathe.
   - ○ 4. fluid infusion.

5. The victim is admitted to the emergency room with chest injuries. Which piece of information will be the most helpful to the physician in assessing blood loss and deciding what action to take?
   - ○ 1. What was the cause of the injury
   - ○ 2. History of mentation since the accident
   - ○ 3. Time of injury
   - ○ 4. Sex of the victim

6. A thoracentesis is performed, but no fluid or air is found. Blood is administered IV, but his vital signs do not improve. A central venous pressure line is inserted and the initial reading is 20 cm. The nurse notes distension of the jugular vein. The most likely cause of these findings is
   - ○ 1. spontaneous pneumothorax.   *pericardial tamponade compression of the heart*
   - ○ 2. ruptured diaphragm.
   - ○ 3. hemothorax.   *D₂ collection of fluid or blood in the pericardium*
   - ○ 4. pericardial tamponade.

Carl Bates, a 75-year-old man, underwent abdominal surgery for a bowel obstruction. In the immediate post-op period, he developed signs and symptoms of hypovolemic shock.

7. Below what systolic blood pressure level is perfusion to the vital organs markedly compromised in a usually normotensive client?
   - ○ 1. 100 mm Hg
   - ○ 2. 90 mm Hg
   - ○ 3. 80 mm Hg
   - ○ 4. 70 mm Hg

8. Blood levels of angiotensin and renin are increased during shock. What triggers this response?
   - ○ 1. Adrenal response to antidiuretic hormone (ADH)
   - ○ 2. Renal response to ischemia   *(response ↓ flo vol ischemia → A + R)*
   - ○ 3. Cardiac response to catacholamines
   - ○ 4. Central nervous system response to diminished blood pressure

9. Why is dopamine frequently used to treat shock?   *Vaso supressor.*
   - ○ 1. It is a powerful vasodilator.
   - ○ 2. It has no untoward side effects.
   - ○ 3. Cardiac function is not affected.
   - ○ 4. Kidney perfusion is maintained.

10. What is the best parameter for adequate fluid replacement in a client who is in shock?
    - ○ 1. Systolic blood pressure above 100 mm Hg
    - ○ 2. Systolic blood pressure above 90 mm Hg
    - ○ 3. Urine output of 30 ml/hour
    - ○ 4. Urine output of 20 ml/hour

11. A fluid challenge is begun on Mr. Bates. Which assessment will give the best indication of client response to this treatment?
   ○ 1. Swan-Ganz readings, hourly urine outputs
   ○ 2. Blood pressure, apical rate checks
   ○ 3. Lung sounds, arterial blood gases
   ○ 4. Electrolytes, BUN, creatinine result

12. Why are adrenergic agents particularly useful in treating hypotension and controlling superficial bleeding?
   ○ 1. They cause dilatation of peripheral vessels.
   ○ 2. They cause constriction of peripheral vessels.
   ○ 3. They decrease the cardiac output.
   ○ 4. They block the effects of acetylcholine.

13. Adrenergic drugs, such as epinephrine (Adrenalin), are given in emergency situations for what primary reason?
   ○ 1. To increase cardiac output by increasing the rate and strength of myocardial contraction
   ○ 2. To increase tone and motility of the gastrointestinal tract
   ○ 3. To prevent spasm and constriction of peripheral vessels
   ○ 4. To prevent cardiac dysrhythmias

14. The most serious side effect of the adrenergic drugs is
   ○ 1. dilated pupils.
   ○ 2. headache.
   ○ 3. cardiac dysrhythmias.
   ○ 4. nervousness.

15. Mr. Bates's arterial blood gas results are: pH 7.30, pO$_2$ 58, pCO$_2$ 34, HCO$_3$. What acid-base imbalance would these results most likely indicate?
   ○ 1. Metabolic acidosis   ↓ pH ↓ HCO$_3$
   ○ 2. Metabolic alkalosis
   ○ 3. Respiratory acidosis
   ○ 4. Respiratory alkalosis

16. Why are acid-base imbalances life threatening?
   ○ 1. Enzyme activity is inhibited. Δ pH ≥ ΔEnzy N≥
   ○ 2. Increased catecholamines cause cardiac ↓ Body fx stimulation.
   ○ 3. Increased metabolites depress nerve activity.
   ○ 4. Increased enzyme activity causes a hypermetabolic state.

17. Mr. Bates's first line of defense when his body is attempting to compensate for his acid-base problem would be which of the following?
   ○ 1. Hormonal activity
   ○ 2. Increased alveolar CO$_2$
   ○ 3. Retention of bicarbonate by the kidneys 2 take 24°
   ○ 4. Blood-buffering systems   1°

Ted Fontaine has done well in surgery and returns to the unit, postcholecystectomy. During the night, the nurse discovers his incisional area has become hard and elevated, his blood pressure is 80/60, and his pulse is 124. Blood studies show his hematocrit and hemoglobin are both low, his platelet count is 100,000/mm^3, and his prothrombin time is prolonged. Whole blood is administered, but Mr. Fontaine does not improve. The nursing history reveals Mr. Fontaine took prednisone for a year prior to admission.

18. Information is obtained from clients regarding previous use of corticosteroids to help identify
   ○ 1. related adrenocortical insufficiency.
   ○ 2. Addison's disease.
   ○ 3. severe adrenocortical insufficiency.
   ○ 4. azotemia.

19. Mr. Fontaine is most likely exhibiting signs of
   ○ 1. acute tubular necrosis.
   ○ 2. azotemia.
   ○ 3. disseminated intravascular coagulation (DIC). c̄ microcoagulation
   ○ 4. Waterhouse-Friderichsen syndrome.

20. Drug therapy for Mr. Fontaine will probably include
   ○ 1. tranquilizers.
   ○ 2. vitamins.
   ○ 3. adrenocorticosteroids.
   ○ 4. adrenocorticosteroids and pressor agents.

21. Additionally, Mr. Fontaine will most likely need which of the following treatments?
   ○ 1. Heparin and whole blood
   ○ 2. Whole blood
   ○ 3. Peritoneal dialysis
   ○ 4. Antibiotics

22. If not successfully treated, Mr. Fontaine's condition could result in
   ○ 1. addisonian crisis.
   ○ 2. renal failure.
   ○ 3. hemophilia.
   ○ 4. neutropenia.

23. Mr. Fontaine's fever climbs to 104.6°F (40.3°C). His physician orders hypothermia equipment and asks the nurse to maintain his body temperature at 99.6°F (37.5°C). At what body temperature would the nurse discontinue the hypothermia treatment?
   ○ 1. 97.6°F (36.4°C)
   ○ 2. 98.6°F (37°C)
   ○ 3. 99.6°F (37.5°C)
   ○ 4. 100.6°F (38.1°C) recommend 1°↑

Sinja Mung, a 55-year-old Korean, is employed as a cook in a local restaurant. He is awakened one night with crushing substernal chest pain, diaphoresis, and nausea. His wife calls the paramedics, and Mr. Mung is taken to the closest emergency room. He has the classic signs of myocardial infarction.

24. Mr. Mung arrives in the emergency room, still in pain; he is quickly assessed by the nurse and the physician. The best initial nursing action is to
   ○ **1.** start an IV.
   ○ **2.** give the pain medication as ordered by the physician.
   ○ **3.** prepare him for immediate transfer to the coronary care unit.
   ○ **4.** get a complete history from his wife.

25. The pain experienced by Mr. Mung is probably due to
   ○ **1.** vasoconstriction because of arterial spasms.
   ○ **2.** myocardial ischemia.
   ○ **3.** fear of death.
   ○ **4.** irritation of nerve endings in the cardiac plexus.

26. Which area of the heart most frequently suffers the most damage in a myocardial infarction?
   ○ **1.** Conduction system
   ○ **2.** Heart valves
   ○ **3.** Left ventricle
   ○ **4.** Right ventricle

27. Which of the following should also be included in the admission process?
   ○ **1.** Contact client's place of employment.
   ○ **2.** Ensure someone stays with significant others.
   ○ **3.** Keep family and significant others informed of progress and status.
   ○ **4.** Secure information about client's medical insurance status.

28. When the nurse talks to Mr. Mung's wife, she reports that he had experienced some angina for months prior to admission but had not sought medical attention. What is the probable reason for his neglect?
   ○ **1.** He has a high threshold for pain.
   ○ **2.** He lacks knowledge about health maintenance.
   ○ **3.** He denied the significance of the pain.
   ○ **4.** He was afraid it would be interpreted as psychosomatic.

29. Mr. Mung experiences a cardiac arrest. What should be the first nursing action in this situation?
   ○ **1.** Call the physician on duty.
   ○ **2.** Establish an airway.
   ○ **3.** Start closed-chest massage.
   ○ **4.** Give a bolus of sodium bicarbonate.

30. What initial nursing assessment would best indicate that Mr. Mung had been resuscitated?
   ○ **1.** Skin warm and dry
   ○ **2.** Pupils equal and react to light
   ○ **3.** Palpable carotid pulse
   ○ **4.** Positive Babinski reflex

31. Mr. Mung was transferred to the coronary care unit after an ECG indicated a posterior-wall infarction. Upon arriving at the unit, he complained of chest pain. In assessing the pain, which of the following is *not* characteristic of the pain of an acute myocardial infarction.
   ○ **1.** Intense, crushing
   ○ **2.** Relieved by nitroglycerin *(Angina)*
   ○ **3.** May radiate to one or both arms, neck, or jaw
   ○ **4.** Is of long duration, not relieved by rest

32. What is the narcotic of choice in this situation?
   ○ **1.** Morphine sulfate
   ○ **2.** Meperidine (Demerol)
   ○ **3.** Codeine sulfate
   ○ **4.** Hydromorphone chloride (Dilaudid)

33. Upon his admission to the coronary care unit, oxygen was ordered. The primary purpose of oxygen administration in this situation is to
   ○ **1.** relieve dyspnea.
   ○ **2.** relieve cyanosis.
   ○ **3.** increase oxygen concentration in the myocardium.
   ○ **4.** supersaturate the red blood cells.

34. The most dangerous period for a client following a myocardial infarction is
   ○ **1.** the first 24 to 48 hours
   ○ **2.** the first 72 to 96 hours
   ○ **3.** 4 to 10 days post-myocardial infarction.
   ○ **4.** from time of symptom onset until treatment is begun.

35. What is the most lethal complication in the post-MI period?
   ○ **1.** Cardiogenic shock
   ○ **2.** Ventricular dysrhythmias
   ○ **3.** Pulmonary embolus
   ○ **4.** Cardiac tamponade

36. Which fact is accurate about cardiogenic shock?
    - ○ 1. It is easily treated with drugs.
    - ○ 2. It can be prevented with close monitoring.
    - ○ 3. The mortality rate is very high. *80%*
    - ○ 4. it is difficult to identify high-risk clients.

37. Cardiac-enzyme studies are helpful in diagnosing a myocardial infarction. These studies are most indicative of *∴ tissue death*
    - ○ 1. cardiac ischemia.
    - ○ 2. location of the myocardial infarction.
    - ○ 3. cardiac necrosis.
    - ○ 4. size of the infarct.

38. Which drug is a first choice to reduce premature ventricular contractions? *(PVC)*
    - ○ 1. Procainamide (Pronestyl) *2°*
    - ○ 2. Phenytoin (Dilantin)
    - ○ 3. Xylocaine (Lidocaine) *1° ↓ vent cond ∴ ↓ pvc*
    - ○ 4. Digoxin (Lanoxin)

39. Which of the following is a common side effect of this drug?
    - ○ 1. Tachycardia
    - ○ 2. Decreased respirations
    - ○ 3. Seizures
    - ○ 4. Sedation *→ ↓ CNS*

40. Valsalva's maneuver can result in bradycardia, which can be very dangerous for the myocardial infarction client. Which nursing action will prevent Valsalva's maneuver?
    - ○ 1. Administer oral laxatives prn.
    - ○ 2. Teach the client to hold his breath when changing position.
    - ○ 3. Service liquids at room temperature.
    - ○ 4. Encourage the client to cough and deep breathe frequently.

41. Mrs. Mung tells the nurse she is afraid her husband is going to die. Anticipatory grieving is important for her to experience at this time. Which of the following nursing actions would probably *hinder* her experiencing anticipatory grieving?
    - ○ 1. Have her participate in her husband's care when possible.
    - ○ 2. Let her express her fears about the possibility of his dying.
    - ○ 3. Give her frequent reports about her husband's condition.
    - ○ 4. Tell her that the nurses are very competent.

42. Mr. Mung, now considerably improved, wants to talk about his sexual activity after he has been discharged from the hospital. What should be the nurse's initial approach?
    - ○ 1. Give him some written materials and then answer questions.
    - ○ 2. Plan a teaching session with Mr. Mung and his wife.
    - ○ 3. Answer his questions accurately and directly.
    - ○ 4. Provide enough time and privacy so that he can express his concerns fully.

43. Mr. Mung is to be discharged on a low cholesterol diet. Which of the following foods is lowest in cholesterol?
    - ○ 1. Liver
    - ○ 2. Tuna fish
    - ○ 3. Shellfish
    - ○ 4. Rice

44. Which of the following would *not* contribute to Mr. Mung's risk of another myocardial infarction?
    - ○ 1. His brother had a myocardial infarction 2 years ago.
    - ○ 2. He had diabetes.
    - ○ 3. He smokes a pack of cigarettes daily.
    - ○ 4. He takes 4 aspirins daily.

45. Mr. Mung lives in a 2-story house but has bathrooms upstairs and down. Which of the following is the most correct teaching for him with regard to activity after discharge?
    - ○ 1. "Do what you feel like."
    - ○ 2. "Do not do any walking except to the bathroom from bed. Take your meals in the bedroom."
    - ○ 3. "Walk around in the house; do not walk up or down steps until you have seen the doctor."
    - ○ 4. "Do all the walking you wish inside and outside. You can climb stairs inside the house."

Michelle Allen, aged 32, is admitted to the critical care unit in atrial fibrillation; she has not been taking any drugs.

46. Which of the following treatments is most appropriate?
    - ○ 1. Cardiac pacing
    - ○ 2. Cardioversion *or Countershock*
    - ○ 3. Mitral commissurotomy
    - ○ 4. Coronary artery bypass

47. If the primary treatment fails, which drug would be best to use?
- ○ **1.** Isoproterenol (Isuprel)
- ○ **2.** Epinephrine (Adrenalin)
- ○ **3.** Propranolol (Inderal)
- ○ **4.** Xylocaine (Lidocaine)

48. Which of the following drugs would be used to treat heart block when the blood pressure is also low?
- ○ **1.** Propranolol (Inderal)
- ○ **2.** Epinephrine
- ○ **3.** Atropine *safest Rx for heart block ass 2nd/3R*
- ○ **4.** Procainamide (Pronestyl)

49. Which drug is *not* used for a hypotensive client?
- ○ **1.** Norepinephrine (Levophed)
- ○ **2.** Procainamide (Pronestyl) *∋↓ C.O. ?*
- ○ **3.** Dopamine (Intropin)
- ○ **4.** Metaraminol (Aramine)

50. When Miss Allen is transferred to an observational unit, the nurse notes the following normal cardiac rhythm during a routine check: each P wave is followed by a QRS complex; each QRS complex is followed by a
- ○ **1.** U wave.
- ○ **2.** R wave.
- ○ **3.** Q wave.
- ○ **4.** T wave.

Mai Ling Chang, aged 25, was taken to the emergency room by her mother. Miss Chang, a nursing student, was studying for a final examination when she started complaining of a "pounding heart," syncope, diaphoresis, and diarrhea. An electrocardiogram indicated she had atrial tachycardia.

51. What is the most common cause of this condition?
- ○ **1.** Depression
- ○ **2.** Stress
- ○ **3.** Hypothyroidism
- ○ **4.** Anemia

52. What would be the most appropriate medical treatment in this situation?
- ○ **1.** Antidysrhythmic drug
- ○ **2.** Hospital admission for further observation
- ○ **3.** Mild sedative and discharge
- ○ **4.** Beta-adrenergic blocking agent

53. What would be the most appropriate nursing action?
- ○ **1.** Advise Miss Chang to take the examination at a later date.
- ○ **2.** Help her seek psychologic counseling.
- ○ **3.** Refer her to a stress-management counselor.
- ○ **4.** Teach her stress-management skills.

Henry Duboff, a 50-year-old white man, awakes in the middle of the night with severe dyspnea, bilateral basilar rales, and expectoration of frothy, blood-tinged sputum. He is brought to the hospital in congestive heart failure complicated by pulmonary edema.

54. Dyspnea is a characteristic sign of congestive heart failure. This is due primarily to
- ○ **1.** accumulation of serous fluid in alveolar spaces. *circ. conj. ; rale*
- ○ **2.** obstruction of bronchi by mucoid secretions.
- ○ **3.** compression of lung tissue by a dilated heart.
- ○ **4.** restriction of respiratory movement by ascites.

55. In congestive heart failure, edema develops primarily because
- ○ **1.** diffusion is inhibited.
- ○ **2.** the capillary bed dilates.
- ○ **3.** venous pressure increases. *→ stasis*
- ○ **4.** ostomic pressure increases.

56. Edema caused by cardiac failure tends to be
- ○ **1.** painful.
- ○ **2.** dependent.
- ○ **3.** periorbital.
- ○ **4.** nonpitting.

57. Left-sided congestive heart failure is most often associated with which sign or symptom? *L side → pulmo prob.*
- ○ **1.** Dyspnea *LS*
- ○ **2.** Distended neck veins *RS*
- ○ **3.** Hepatomegaly *RS*
- ○ **4.** Pedal edema *RS*

58. Force of cardiac contraction (systole) is *decreased* by which of the following?
- ○ **1.** Calcium ions
- ○ **2.** Chloride ions
- ○ **3.** Potassium ions *K effect neuro musc. activity K>5.5 > V fib.*
- ○ **4.** Sodium ions

59. Respirations of the client with congestive heart failure are usually
- ○ **1.** rapid and shallow.
- ○ **2.** deep and stertorous.
- ○ **3.** rapid and wheezing. *↓ wheez*
- ○ **4.** Cheyne-Stokes.

60. What is the optimal bed position for the client with congestive heart failure?
- ○ **1.** Position of comfort, to relax the client
- ○ **2.** Semirecumbent, to ease dyspnea and metabolic demands on the heart *= Fowlers / Semi Fowlers*
- ○ **3.** Upright, to decrease danger of pulmonary edema
- ○ **4.** Flat, to decrease edema formation in the extremities

61. Why are IV drugs more effective in a client with congestive heart failure than IM or oral administration?
    ○ 1. Altered circulation slows the action of IM and ingested drugs.
    ○ 2. Altered circulation speeds the action of IM and ingested drugs.
    ○ 3. An enlarged heart needs a stronger dose.
    ○ 4. There is no difference between IV, IM, and PO drug absorption in clients with congestive heart failure.

62. The nurse's main concern when caring for the digitalized client receiving furosemide (Lasix) is to ↓K →↑ dig effect ↓↑ dig tox.
    ○ 1. take central venous pressure readings.
    ○ 2. observe for decreased edema.
    ○ 3. observe for dysrhythmias caused by hypokalemia.
    ○ 4. force fluids.

63. How do rotating tourniquets relieve the symptoms of acute pulmonary edema?
    ○ 1. Cause vasoconstriction
    ○ 2. Cause vasodilation
    ○ 3. Decrease the amount of circulating blood ↓Ven Return
    ○ 4. Increase the amount of circulating blood

64. When tourniquets are applied to extremities to relieve the symptoms of pulmonary edema, one tourniquet is rotated, in order, every
    ○ 1. 5 minutes. (for elderly)
    ○ 2. 15 minutes.
    ○ 3. 30 minutes.
    ○ 4. 60 minutes.

65. Mr. Duboff is restricted to a 2,000 mg sodium diet. He is instructed to not salt his food and to avoid
    ○ 1. whole milk.
    ○ 2. canned tuna.
    ○ 3. plain nuts.
    ○ 4. eggs.

66. Mr. Duboff is counseled regarding his potassium intake while he is receiving diuretics. Which of the following foods have very low levels of potassium?
    ○ 1. Meats and milk
    ○ 2. Citrus fruits
    ○ 3. Potatoes
    ○ 4. Cereals and breads

Rosalind Avery is being admitted with a diagnosis of thrombophlebitis.

67. Which of the following signs and symptoms would the nurse most expect to find when assessing Mrs. Avery?
    ○ 1. A negative Homans' sign
    ○ 2. Pallor of the legs
    ○ 3. Shiny, atrophic skin on the legs
    ○ 4. Unilateral leg swelling

68. Which of the following actions is most appropriate for Mrs. Avery?
    ○ 1. Apply warm, dry packs to the involved site. moist
    ○ 2. Elevate her legs 45°.
    ○ 3. Maintain her on bed rest for 10 to 14 days. 5-10
    ○ 4. Provide range-of-motion to both legs at least twice every shift. (unaffected leg)

69. Mrs. Avery starts receiving heparin sodium. Which of the following rationales for heparin therapy is most correct?
    ○ 1. It dissolves existing thrombi.
    ○ 2. It inactivates thrombin that forms.
    ○ 3. It inactivates thrombin that forms and dissolves existing thrombi.
    ○ 4. It interferes with vitamin K absorption.

70. Which of the following lab tests needs to be monitored while Mrs. Avery is being given heparin?
    ○ 1. Bleeding time
    ○ 2. Partial thromboplastin time (PTT)
    ○ 3. Prothrombin consumption test (PCT)
    ○ 4. Prothrombin time (PT) (for Coumadin)

71. Which of the following would *not* be a sign or symptom of overdosage of heparin?
    ○ 1. Rectal bleeding
    ○ 2. Positive Homans' sign (= phlebitis)
    ○ 3. Smokey, dark urine
    ○ 4. Epistaxis

72. Which of the following drugs blocks the action of heparin?
    ○ 1. AquaMEPHYTON
    ○ 2. Atropine sulfate
    ○ 3. Protamine sulfate
    ○ 4. Vitamin K

73. Mrs. Avery is to take warfarin sodium (Coumadin) at home. Which of the following should be included in her discharge instruction?
    ○ 1. "Keep a vial of vitamin A available at all times."
    ○ 2. "Report any blood in your stools or urine to your doctor."
    ○ 3. "Take aspirin for headaches."
    ○ 4. "Use a firm toothbrush."

Shara Ahmed was admitted to the hospital with chest pain and shortness of breath. She stated that she was treated for thrombophlebitis of the left thigh 3 months ago and is not taking any medicines for it. Her admitting diagnosis possible pulmonary embolism. Her arterial blood gases on admission were: pH 7.52, pCO$_2$ 27, HCO$_3$ 22, base excess 0, pO$_2$ 53, O$_2$ saturation 91%.

74. The above values suggest that on admission Mrs. Ahmed was exhibiting
    - ○ 1. respiratory alkalosis.
    - ○ 2. respiratory acidosis.
    - ○ 3. metabolic alkalosis.
    - ○ 4. metabolic acidosis.

75. By examining her arterial blood gas (ABGs), the nurse knows that Mrs. Ahmed is most probably
    - ○ 1. breathing slowly and shallowly.
    - ○ 2. breathing rapidly and deeply.
    - ○ 3. restless and in obvious oxygen hunger.
    - ○ 4. comatose.

76. Which of the following would be the most serious symptom for Mrs. Ahmed?
    - ○ 1. Resonance over the chest on percussion
    - ○ 2. Expirations 1½ times longer than inspirations
    - ○ 3. Central cyanosis
    - ○ 4. Peripheral cyanosis

77. What is the normal ratio of pCO$_2$ to HCO$_3$?
    - ○ 1. 1:10
    - ○ 2. 1:20
    - ○ 3. 10:1
    - ○ 4. 20:1

Gordon McLaughlin has a history of chronic obstructive pulmonary disease, but presents with edema of the legs and feet, distended neck veins, and a large, palpable liver.

78. What is Mr. McLaughlin most likely suffering from?
    - ○ 1. Atelectasis
    - ○ 2. Pulmonary embolus
    - ○ 3. Cor pulmonale
    - ○ 4. Pleurisy

79. As the nurse enters Mr. McLaughlin's room, his oxygen is running at 6 liters/minute, his color is pink, and his respirations are 9/minute. What is the best initial action?
    - ○ 1. Take his vital signs.
    - ○ 2. Call the physician.
    - ○ 3. Lower the oxygen rate.
    - ○ 4. Put the client in Fowler's position.

80. What is the primary purpose of instructing Mr. McLaughlin to use pursed-lip breathing?
    - ○ 1. Prolonged exhalation helps prevent air trapping.
    - ○ 2. This trains the diaphragm to aid inspiration.
    - ○ 3. It improves the delivery of oral and nasal inhaler medications.
    - ○ 4. It facilitates the movement of thick mucus.

81. Percussion is ordered for Mr. McLaughlin to facilitate the movement of thick mucus out of the lungs. In which of the following situations would percussion be *contraindicated*?
    - ○ 1. Hemoptysis
    - ○ 2. Pneumonia
    - ○ 3. Cystic fibrosis
    - ○ 4. Atelectasis

82. What should the nurse expect Mr. McLaughlin's potassium level to be?
    - ○ 1. Normal
    - ○ 2. Elevated
    - ○ 3. Low
    - ○ 4. Unrelated to the pH

Mike Pierce, a 45-year-old steel-mill worker, is admitted through the emergency room with complaints of stabbing chest pain that becomes worse with coughing, chills, diaphoresis, and rust-colored sputum. He states "It came on suddenly."

83. What is the most probable diagnosis associated with these symptoms?
    - ○ 1. Angina
    - ○ 2. Congestive heart failure
    - ○ 3. Pneumonia
    - ○ 4. Pulmonary edema

84. What is very likely the causative factor of this diagnosis?
    - ○ 1. Chemical irritant
    - ○ 2. Coronary artery disease
    - ○ 3. Fluid overload
    - ○ 4. Pneumococci

85. Mr. Pierce's diagnosis is pneumonia of the right lower lobe. What should the nurse expect to find on physical assessment?
    - ○ 1. Bradycardia
    - ○ 2. Shallow respirations
    - ○ 3. Diminished breath sounds on the left
    - ○ 4. Pericardial rub

86. A chest x-ray confirms consolidation in right lower lobe. When percussing this area, what sound should the nurse most expect to hear?
    - ○ 1. Tympany
    - ○ 2. Resonance
    - ○ 3. Dullness
    - ○ 4. Hyperresonance

87. While inspecting Mr. Pierce's thorax, the nurse observes that the client is splinting. What is this?
    ○ 1. Client exhales with pursed lips.
    ○ 2. Client holds his chest rigid.
    ○ 3. Client uses neck and shoulder muscles to exhale.
    ○ 4. Client flares the nares on inspiration.

88. Which of the following should be included in a nursing plan for Mr. Pierce?
    ○ 1. Cough and deep breathe TID to minimize chest discomfort. 9 2°-4°
    ○ 2. Give intermittent positive pressure breathing treatments without percussion to minimize chest discomfort.
    ○ 3. Give 3 to 4 liters of fluid/day.
    ○ 4. Avoid analgesics so as not to suppress respirations.

89. What is the major advantage of the Venturi mask ordered for Mr. Pierce?
    ○ 1. It can be used while the client eats.
    ○ 2. Precise, high or low flow rates of oxygen can be delivered.
    ○ 3. Humidification of oxygen is unnecessary.
    ○ 4. It administers oxygen in concentrations of 95% to 100%.

90. Gentamicin (Garamycin) 60 mg PO q8h is ordered for Mr. Pierce. Which of the following should the nurse monitor most closely when this drug is given. aminoglycoside are nephrotoxic
    ○ 1. BUN and serum creatinine
    ○ 2. Hemoglobin and hematocrit
    ○ 3. SGOT and SGPT
    ○ 4. PT and PTT

91. Atelectasis develops in Mr. Pierce's right lower lobe. What is this?
    ○ 1. Edematous fluid in the alveoli
    ○ 2. Residual consolidation
    ○ 3. Purulent exudate in the pleura
    ○ 4. Collapsed, airless alveoli

92. When suctioning Mr. Pierce, which of the following nursing actions would *not* be appropriate?
    ○ 1. Lubricate the catheter tip.
    ○ 2. Use sterile technique.
    ○ 3. Suction 40 to 60 seconds at one time.
    ○ 4. Hyperoxygenate the client.

Horace Brown is skin tested for tuberculosis using PPD.

93. Which of the following types of organisms cause tuberculosis?
    ○ 1. Bacteria
    ○ 2. Fungus
    ○ 3. Virus
    ○ 4. Spore

94. When the visiting nurse reads Mr. Brown's skin test, it is positive. Which of the following indicates a positive tuberculin test?
    ○ 1. Induration is 15 mm or larger.
    ○ 2. Induration is 5 to 9 mm.
    ○ 3. Induration is 0 to 4 mm.
    ○ 4. Induration is 10 mm or larger.

95. A positive reaction to PPD indicates that
    ○ 1. the client has active tuberculosis.
    ○ 2. the client has been exposed to *Mycobacterium tuberculosis*.
    ○ 3. the client will never have tuberculosis.
    ○ 4. the client has never been infected with *Mycobacterium tuberculosis*.

96. The health team meets and reviews Mr. Brown's history. Because of the positive skin test and a history of pulmonary disease, the physician prescribes oral rifampin (Rimactane) and isoniazid (INH) for at least 9 months. When informing Mr. Brown of this decision, the nurse knows that the purpose of this choice of treatment is to
    ○ 1. cause less irritation to the gastrointestinal tract.
    ○ 2. destroy resistant organisms and promote proper blood levels of the drugs.
    ○ 3. gain a more rapid systemic effect.
    ○ 4. delay resistance and increase the tuberculostatic effect.

97. Which of these occurrences in Mr. Brown would probably be indicative of an untoward effect of isoniazid (INH)?
    ○ 1. Purpura
    ○ 2. Peripheral neuritis most common D. V_B6 d
    ○ 3. Hyperuricemia
    ○ 4. Optic neuritis

98. To prevent the untoward effect of isoniazid (INH), another drug is added to Mr. Brown's chemotherapy. Which drug is this likely to be?
    ○ 1. Vitamin B_{12}
    ○ 2. Vitamin B_1 (thiamine)
    ○ 3. Vitamin C (ascorbic acid)
    ○ 4. Vitamin B_6 (pyridoxine)

99. Mr. Brown is taught that a fairly common side effect of the drug rifampin (Rimactane) is
    - ○ 1. reddish orange color of urine, sputum, and saliva.
    - ○ 2. ectopic dermatitis.
    - ○ 3. eighth cranial nerve damage.
    - ○ 4. vestibular dysfunction.

100. Mrs. Brown is skin tested for tuberculosis and has a negative result. However, because of her husband's newly diagnosed tuberculosis, the physician recommends chemotherapy for her. What is the drug of choice for preventive therapy of tuberculosis?
    - ○ 1. Streptomycin
    - ○ 2. Para-aminosalicylic acid (PAS)
    - ○ 3. Isoniazid (INH) *preventive therapy*
    - ○ 4. Ethambutol (Myambutol)

101. Before starting on preventive drug therapy for tuberculosis, Mrs. Brown will probably receive
    - ○ 1. serum creatinine and BUN.
    - ○ 2. SGOT and SGPT. *(INH can cause hepatitis)*
    - ○ 3. dexamethasone suppression test.
    - ○ 4. serum cortisol level.

102. Mr. Brown also received a skin test for histoplasmosis. Histoplasmosis is often mistaken for
    - ○ 1. lung cancer. *a fungus*
    - ○ 2. pneumonia.
    - ○ 3. tuberculosis.
    - ○ 4. bronchitis.

103. The drug of choice in the treatment of histoplasmosis is
    - ○ 1. isoniazid (INH).
    - ○ 2. amphotericin B.
    - ○ 3. para-aminosalicylic acid (PAS).
    - ○ 4. streptomycin.

Steven Nelson undergoes a left thoracotomy and a partial pneumonectomy. Chest tubes are inserted and 1-bottle, water-seal drainage is instituted in the operating room.

104. Postoperatively, Mr. Nelson is positioned in Fowler's position on either his right side or back in order to achieve
    - ○ 1. reduction of incisional pain.
    - ○ 2. facilitation of ventilation of the left lung.
    - ○ 3. equalization of pressure in the pleural space.
    - ○ 4. promotion of drainage by gravity.

105. Which of the following would be considered most normal within the first 24 hours postoperatively with 1-bottle, water-deal drainage?
    - ○ 1. No fluctuation in the water-seal tube
    - ○ 2. Intermittent slight bubbling from the water-seal tube
    - ○ 3. Bright red bloody drainage
    - ○ 4. Orders to maintain suction at 30 cm H$_2$O

106. Water-seal chest drainage involves attaching the chest tube to a
    - ○ 1. bottle at a level above the bed.
    - ○ 2. tube that is submerged under water.
    - ○ 3. tube that is open to the air.
    - ○ 4. drainage bottle.

107. Fluid oscillating in the tubing in the water-seal bottle indicates
    - ○ 1. the equipment is working well.
    - ○ 2. the chest tube is clogged.
    - ○ 3. the end of the tube is not under water.
    - ○ 4. air has leaked into the chest cavity.

Miguel Orlando, a 50-year-old construction worker, is admitted to the unit with a tentative diagnosis of cancer of the lung.

108. Which of the following symptoms is a common, presenting symptom of bronchogenic carcinoma?
    - ○ 1. Dyspnea on exertion
    - ○ 2. Foamy, blood-tinged sputum
    - ○ 3. Wheezing sound on inspiration
    - ○ 4. Cough or change in a chronic cough

109. Several diagnostic tests have been ordered. Bronchoscopy and bronchial washings have been scheduled. When teaching Mr. Orlando what to expect postoperatively, what would be the nurse's highest priority?
    - ○ 1. Food and fluids will be withheld for at least 2 hours. *NPO until gag reflex pres*
    - ○ 2. Warm saline gargles will be done q2h.
    - ○ 3. Coughing and deep breathing exercises will be done q2h.
    - ○ 4. Only ice chips and cold liquids will be allowed for 2 hours.

110. Mr. Orlando has a left upper lobectomy. Which action by the nurse would best facilitate effective coughing and deep breathing postoperatively?
    ○ 1. Encourage him to take a day at a time and do his best to cough and deep breathe.
    ○ 2. Give him a back rub in order to relax him prior to coughing and deep breathing.
    ○ 3. Administer pain medication 20 minutes prior to coughing and deep breathing.
    ○ 4. Position him for postural drainage with cupping and vibration 10 minutes prior to coughing and deep breathing.

111. What is the purpose of the long glass tube that is immersed 3 cm below the water level in Mr. Orlando's water-seal bottle?
    ○ 1. To humidify the air leaving the pleural space
    ○ 2. To allow the drainage to mix with sterile water
    ○ 3. To monitor the respirations by visualizing the fluctuations
    ○ 4. To prevent atmospheric air from entering the chest tube

112. Continuous bubbling in the water-seal bottle is observed during morning rounds. Which of the following factors best accounts for this phenomenon?
    ○ 1. The system is functioning adequately.
    ○ 2. There is an air leak in the system.
    ○ 3. The lung has reexpanded.
    ○ 4. The suction pressure is low.

113. Mr. Orlando's vital signs have been stable, and he has been alert and oriented. Today, however, he has had several periods of confusion. His physician orders arterial blood gases. The respiratory therapist draws the blood but asks the nurse to apply pressure to the area, so that she can leave and take the specimen to the lab. How long does the nurse apply pressure to the area?
    ○ 1. 2 minutes
    ○ 2. 5 minutes
    ○ 3. 8 minutes
    ○ 4. 10 minutes

114. The arterial blood gas values are pH 7.5, pCO_2 33.5, pO_2 45.7, oxygen saturation 86.7%. Which value is within normal limits?
    ○ 1. Oxygen saturation
    ○ 2. pO_2
    ○ 3. pCO_2
    ○ 4. None of these values are normal.

115. At the end of the hour, Mr. Orlando's arterial blood gases are pH 7.45, pCO_2 34.7, pO_2 71.8, oxygen saturation 95.6%. The nurse will most likely expect Mr. Orlando to be
    ○ 1. combative.
    ○ 2. less confused.
    ○ 3. more confused.
    ○ 4. about the same.

John Baker, aged 50, has experienced bouts of retrosternal burning and pain for 6 months. His condition has recently been diagnosed as esophagitis related to reflux of gastric contents into the esophagus with resultant mucosal injury.

116. When documenting Mr. Baker's health history, the nurse would most likely expect him to report that his symptoms are worse
    ○ 1. when he is active and busy.
    ○ 2. while lying down.
    ○ 3. while sitting.
    ○ 4. when he is upset and under stress.

117. In assessing the client's dietary habits, the nurse finds that he has increased symptoms with foods that are associated with lowered esophageal-sphincter pressure. What are those foods?
    ○ 1. Poultry, yogurt
    ○ 2. Fruits, vegetables
    ○ 3. Fatty foods, chocolate
    ○ 4. High-fiber foods, vanilla

118. Esophageal problems associated with reflux may necessitate a change in life-style such as which of the following?
    ○ 1. Increase the amount of exercise
    ○ 2. Discontinue smoking and alcohol
    ○ 3. Increase body weight
    ○ 4. Raise the foot of bed to sleep

119. Cancer of the esophagus occurs more commonly in men over age 50 and is associated with esophageal obstructions. Why does it have a poor prognosis?
    ○ 1. Histologically, the cells are very malignant.
    ○ 2. Symptoms develop late, and lymphatic spread occurs early.
    ○ 3. Ulceration and hemorrhage occur.
    ○ 4. Malnutrition and aspiration are present.

120. How can gastric regurgitation best be reduced?
    ○ 1. Eat small, frequent meals; avoid overeating.
    ○ 2. Have a small evening meal, followed by a bedtime snack.
    ○ 3. Belch frequently.
    ○ 4. Swallow air.

Vernon Crabtree, 47 years old, is admitted with a diagnosis of possible gastric ulcer.

121. Mr. Crabtree undergoes an endoscopy. When may food and fluids be given following this examination?
○ 1. Upon the client's request
○ 2. When the gag reflex returns
○ 3. Within 30 minutes after the test
○ 4. As soon as the client returns to the ward

122. The physician's orders instruct guaiac tests of all stools to determine the presence of
○ 1. hydrochloric acid.
○ 2. undigested food.
○ 3. occult blood.
○ 4. inflammatory cells.

123. Unlike Mr. Crabtree, the client with a duodenal ulcer is most likely to complain of pain
○ 1. during a meal.
○ 2. 15 minutes after eating.
○ 3. 1 to 4 hours after meals.
○ 4. about 30 minutes after eating.

124. When Mr. Crabtree requests a cigarette, the best response of the nurse would be which of the following?
○ 1. "One cigarette a day is all that is permitted."
○ 2. "Nicotine increases gastric acid and stomach activity."
○ 3. "Nicotine decreases gastric acid and lessens stomach activity."
○ 4. "Cigars are less harmful than cigarettes."

125. Mr. Crabtree is advised by his physician not to drink coffee. The nurse explains that coffee
○ 1. increases mental stress.
○ 2. stimulates gastric secretions.
○ 3. increases smooth muscle tone.
○ 4. elevates systolic blood pressure.

126. Mr. Crabtree does not respond to medical treatment for his peptic ulcer. He is advised to have a subtotal gastrectomy. In preparing for patient teaching the nurse knows this procedure involves removal of what?
○ 1. Cardiac sphincter and upper half of the stomach
○ 2. Pyloric region of the stomach and duodenum
○ 3. Entire stomach and associated lymph nodes
○ 4. Lower one half to two thirds of the stomach

127. A vagotomy is done as part of the surgical treatment for peptic ulcers in order to
○ 1. decrease secretion of hydrochloric acid.
○ 2. improve the tone of the gastrointestinal muscles.
○ 3. increase blood supply to the jejunum.
○ 4. prevent the transmission of pain impulses.

128. Which of the following facts best explains why the duodenum is not removed during a subtotal gastrectomy?
○ 1. The head of the pancreas is adherent to the duodenal wall.
○ 2. The common bile duct empties into the duodenal lumen.
○ 3. The wall of the jejunum contains no intestinal villi.
○ 4. The jejunum receives its blood supply through the duodenum.

129. During Mr. Crabtree's immediate post-op care, why must the nurse be particularly conscientious to encourage him to cough and deep breathe at regular intervals?
○ 1. Marked changes in intrathoracic pressure will stimulate gastric drainage.
○ 2. The high abdominal incision will lead to shallow breathing to avoid pain.
○ 3. The phrenic nerve will have been permanently damaged during the surgical procedure.
○ 4. Deep breathing will prevent post-op vomiting and intestinal distension.

130. Mr. Crabtree has an nasogastric tube. It will be removed when there is
○ 1. inflammation of the pharyngeal mucosa.
○ 2. absence of bile in gastric drainage.
○ 3. return of bowel sounds to normal.
○ 4. passage of numerous liquid stools.

131. Mr. Crabtree is told about the dumping syndrome. It is the result of
○ 1. the body's absorption of toxins produced by liquefaction of dead tissue.
○ 2. formation of an ulcer at the margin of the gastrojejunal anastomosis.
○ 3. obstruction of venous flow from the stomach into the portal system.
○ 4. rapid emptying of food and fluid from the stomach into the jejunum.

132. Aluminum hydroxide gel (Amphogel) is preferred to sodium bicarbonate in treating hyperacidity, because unlike sodium bicarbonate, aluminum hydroxide gel
    ○ 1. is not absorbed from the bowel.
    ○ 2. does not predispose to constipation.
    ○ 3. dissolves rapidly in all body fluids.
    ○ 4. has no effect on phosphorus excretion.

133. In which of the following drug classifications does propantheline bromide (Pro-Banthine) fall?
    ○ 1. Sedative
    ○ 2. Antacid
    ○ 3. Astringent
    ○ 4. Anticholinergic

134. The pharmacologic effect of propantheline bromide (Pro-Banthine) is to
    ○ 1. neutralize hydrochloric acid.
    ○ 2. inhibit gastrointestinal motility and gastric secretions.
    ○ 3. depress the cerebral cortex.
    ○ 4. coat and soothe mucous membranes.

135. Which of the following side effects of propantheline bromide (Pro-Banthine) is most dose limiting?
    ○ 1. Dry mouth
    ○ 2. Hiccoughs
    ○ 3. Visual blurring
    ○ 4. Urinary retention

Aretha Gamble, a 65-year-old retired teacher, is admitted for tests. Her major complaints include crampy, lower abdominal pain and frequent, bloody stools with mucus.

136. Which of the following diagnoses is likely to manifest the above signs and symptoms?
    ○ 1. Appendicitis
    ○ 2. Cholecystitis
    ○ 3. Diverticulitis
    ○ 4. Pancreatitis

137. When assessing Mrs. Gamble, the nurse should observe for
    ○ 1. jaundice, clay-colored stools.
    ○ 2. rigid, tender abdomen; absence of bowel sounds.
    ○ 3. nausea, vomiting, pruritus.
    ○ 4. dyspnea, chest pain.

138. Which of the following diagnostic examinations is most likely to be ordered for Mrs. Gamble?
    ○ 1. Lower gastrointestinal series, barium enema, colonoscopy
    ○ 2. Upper gastrointestinal series, gastric analysis
    ○ 3. Cholecystogram, abdominal CT scan
    ○ 4. Schilling test, sigmoidoscopy

139. Mrs. Gamble receives a diagnosis of diverticulitis. Prior to her discharge, which of the following would be *inappropriate* to include in a teaching session?
    ○ 1. Practice stress-management techniques.
    ○ 2. Eat a high-residue diet.
    ○ 3. Take psyllium hydrophilic mucilloid (Metamucil).
    ○ 4. Eat foods that are highly refined.

Don Sharp, a 17-year-old college student, was stricken with periumbilical pain while playing baseball. Because the pain increased rapidly in intensity during the next few hours, his fraternity brothers took him to the dispensary. The nurse put Don to bed and called the physician. The physician made a diagnosis of acute appendicitis and ordered that Don be admitted to the university hospital immediately for an emergency appendectomy.

140. Which of the following is the most common precipitating cause of acute appendicitis?
    ○ 1. Chemical irritation by digestive juices
    ○ 2. Mechanical obstruction of the lumen of the appendix
    ○ 3. Mechanical irritation of overlying pelvic viscera
    ○ 4. Ischemic damage from mesenteric thrombosis

141. Peritonitis resulting from rupture of an inflamed appendix is primarily the result of
    ○ 1. chemical irritation by digestive juices.
    ○ 2. bacterial contamination by intestinal organisms.
    ○ 3. mechanical pressure exerted by the distended bowel.
    ○ 4. ischemic damage from mesenteric thrombosis.

142. In order to promote capillary proliferation and formation of scar tissue, Don may be given a supplementary dose of which vitamin?
    ○ 1. A
    ○ 2. B_1
    ○ 3. C
    ○ 4. D

Tina Cortez was admitted to the hospital because of nausea and abdominal pain after having eaten a fatty meal. Her condition was diagnosed as cholelithiasis (gallstones). A cholecystectomy with common bile duct exploration was performed.

143. Mrs. Cortez has arrived in the postanesthesia room. She is semiconscious. Her vital signs are within normal limits. Which of the following nursing actions would be *inappropriate*?
    ○ 1. Apply a warm blanket to her body.
    ○ 2. Place her in semi-Fowler's position.
    ○ 3. Attach her T tube to gravity drainage.
    ○ 4. Set up low, intermittent suction for her nasogastric tube.

144. Mrs. Cortez had an uneventful stay in the postanesthesia room and has returned to her room. She complains of abdominal pain. Her physician has ordered meperidine (Demerol) 50 to 100 mg, q3h, prn for pain. Which of the following is an *inappropriate* criterion when deciding how much to administer?
    ○ 1. Mrs. Cortez's vital signs
    ○ 2. Anesthetics and drugs used during surgery
    ○ 3. The amount of discomfort Mrs. Cortez is exhibiting
    ○ 4. The time and amount of any previous doses of Demerol

145. When planning Mrs. Cortez's care for the next 24 hours, the nurse should select which of the following as the primary goal?
    ○ 1. To prevent respiratory complications
    ○ 2. To assess level of consciousness
    ○ 3. To maintain range of joint motion
    ○ 4. To promote normal bowel function

146. Which of the following would be most indicative of complications during the first 24 hours postoperatively?
    ○ 1. Serous drainage on the surgical dressing
    ○ 2. Golden-colored fluid draining from the T tube
    ○ 3. Urinary output of 20 ml/hour
    ○ 4. Body temperature of 99.8°F (37.6°C)

147. Mrs. Cortez, like many people who require a cholecystectomy, is obese. Because of her obesity, she would be most closely observed for which of the following complications?
    ○ 1. Clay-colored, fatty stools
    ○ 2. Inadequate blood clotting
    ○ 3. Cardiac irregularities
    ○ 4. Delayed wound healing

148. The nurse knows that Mrs. Cortez needs further discharge teaching if she states which of the following?
    ○ 1. "I will not climb stairs for a month."
    ○ 2. "I will make a follow-up appointment with my surgeon."
    ○ 3. "Eating fatty foods may cause me some discomfort for awhile."
    ○ 4. "Redness or swelling in the incision must be reported to my surgeon immediately."

Joan Belzer, a 45-year-old obese stockbroker and mother of 3, is admitted with a diagnosis of possible cholecystitis.

149. Which of the following signs and symptoms are most likely to be included in the initial assessment of Mrs. Belzer?
    ○ 1. Abdominal pain, usually in the left upper quadrant
    ○ 2. Dyspepsia following carbohydrate ingestion
    ○ 3. Fullness and eructation following protein ingestion
    ○ 4. Nausea and vomiting

150. Mrs. Belzer is having severe pain. Morphine sulfate 10 mg IM every 3 to 4 hours prn for severe pain, or morphine sulfate 6 mg IM every 3 to 4 hours prn for moderate pain has been ordered. What should the nurse do?
    ○ 1. Ask her if she is allergic to morphine.
    ○ 2. Give 6 mg of morphine sulfate IM.
    ○ 3. Give 10 mg of morphine sulfate IM.
    ○ 4. Verify the order with the physician who wrote it.

151. Since Mrs. Belzer is scheduled for a cholecystogram, which of the following questions is best to ask her?
    ○ 1. "Are you on a low-sodium diet?"
    ○ 2. "Have you ever had a barium study?"
    ○ 3. "Have you ever had a nasogastric tube inserted?"
    ○ 4. "Are you allergic to any drugs?"

152. Two days later Mrs. Belzer has a cholecystectomy and is now ready to return to her room from the recovery room. Mrs. Belzer has an IV of 5% dextrose in 0.45% normal saline infusing at 100 ml/hour, a T tube connected to gravity drainage, and a nasogastric tube connected to low intermittent suction. What does the T tube indicate?
    ○ 1. Stones were removed from the cystic bile duct.
    ○ 2. Stones were removed from the gallbladder.
    ○ 3. The common bile duct was explored.
    ○ 4. The cystic duct was removed.

153. During the first 2 hours postoperatively, Mrs. Belzer's nasogastric tube drains greenish liquid; then the drainage suddenly stops. What is the first action to take?
    ○ **1.** Irrigate it as ordered with distilled water.
    ○ **2.** Irrigate it as ordered with normal saline.
    ○ **3.** Notify her physician.
    ○ **4.** Reposition it.

154. Mrs. Belzer asks you how long it will be before she can have something to eat. The nurse replies
    ○ **1.** "Are you hungry already?"
    ○ **2.** "Since you are slightly overweight, now would be a good time for you to begin reducing."
    ○ **3.** "The doctor makes that decision."
    ○ **4.** "Usually patients start clear liquids 72 hours after this kind of surgery."

155. On Mrs. Belzer's second post-op day, the T tube drains 30 ml during the morning shift the nurse is working. What is the best action?
    ○ **1.** Irrigate the T tube with 50 ml normal saline.
    ○ **2.** Irrigate the T tube with 50 ml distilled water.
    ○ **3.** Nothing, this is normal.
    ○ **4.** Notify the physician.

156. Mrs. Belzer asks when the T tube will be removed? What would be best to tell her?
    ○ **1.** usually 3 to 4 days after surgery
    ○ **2.** usually 6 to 8 days after surgery, and following an x-ray of the cystic duct
    ○ **3.** usually 10 to 12 days after surgery, and following a T-tube cholangiogram
    ○ **4.** When the drainage exceeds 500 ml/day

Joseph Morris, a 40-year-old man, is admitted to the hospital with severe, left, midepigastric pain, and nausea and vomiting. This is his second admission for acute pancreatitis.

157. In assessing Mr. Morris, the nurse knows that common causes of pancreatitis are
    ○ **1.** alcohol abuse and congestive heart failure.
    ○ **2.** alcohol abuse and gallbladder disease.
    ○ **3.** epileptic seizures and pancreatic fibrosis.
    ○ **4.** pancreatic fibrosis and chronic obstructive pulmonary disease.

158. Which of the following is an exocrine function of the pancreas?
    ○ **1.** Secrete insulin and glucagon
    ○ **2.** Secrete digestive enzymes
    ○ **3.** Promote glucose uptake by the liver
    ○ **4.** Facilitate glucose transport into the cells

159. What is the initial treatment plan for acute pancreatitis?
    ○ **1.** Keep the gastrointestinal tract at rest to prevent pancreatic stimulation.
    ○ **2.** Provide adequate nutrition to enhance healing.
    ○ **3.** Prevent secondary complications such as peritonitis.
    ○ **4.** Maintain adequate fluid and electrolyte balance.

160. Which of the following drugs may best be used in conjunction with analgesics to decrease the pain of pancreatitis?
    ○ **1.** Magnesium hydroxide (Maalox)
    ○ **2.** Prochlorperazine (Compazine)
    ○ **3.** Propantheline bromide (Pro-Banthine)
    ○ **4.** Pancreatin (Viokase)

161. Which diagnostic test best measures the response to treatment in the client with pancreatitis?
    ○ **1.** Serum amylase
    ○ **2.** Abdominal CAT scan
    ○ **3.** Serum glutamic-oxaloacetic transaminase (SGOT)
    ○ **4.** Erythrocyte sedimentation rate (ESR)

Carol Hansen, aged 19, is admitted to the hospital with a diagnosis of infectious hepatitis.

162. Initially, what laboratory test shows elevated values in viral hepatitis?
    ○ **1.** Serum ammonia
    ○ **2.** Serum bilirubin
    ○ **3.** Prothrombin time
    ○ **4.** Serum transaminase

163. Which of the following goals would be given highest priority?
    ○ **1.** Prevent decubitus ulcers.
    ○ **2.** Limit physical activity.
    ○ **3.** Eliminate emotional stress.
    ○ **4.** Promote activity and diversion.

164. Which of the following diets will most probably be prescribed for Miss Hansen?
    ○ **1.** High fat
    ○ **2.** Low sodium
    ○ **3.** High calorie
    ○ **4.** Low carbohydrate

Albert Gates is a 48-year-old transient, unskilled laborer, who has a 33-year-old history of alcohol abuse and a 12-year history of cirrhosis. He was admitted with the complaint of hematemesis and rectal bleeding. While in the emergency room, he had a bright red emesis of approximately 400 ml, which was positive for blood. His admission diagnosis is bleeding esophageal varices with ascites. His blood pressure is 100/50 mm Hg, pulse 112, respirations 24, temperature 99°F (37.2°C) rectally. His breath smells of alcohol and he reports having drunk whiskey within the past 3 hours. He has an IV of 5% dextrose and water running at 125 ml/hour.

165. Which of the following is an *incorrect* statement about cirrhosis?
    ○ 1. It is a chronic disease resulting in inflammation, degeneration, and necrosis of the liver.
    ○ 2. It causes obstruction of the venous and sinusoidal channels of the liver.
    ○ 3. It is frequently caused by alcohol abuse.
    ○ 4. It causes decreased resistance to blood flow through the liver.

166. Mr. Gates's initial care plan should include which of the following?
    ○ 1. Elicit an alcohol consumption history.
    ○ 2. Obtain a social service referral.
    ○ 3. Secure a visit from an Alcoholics Anonymous representative.
    ○ 4. Plan for a psychiatric evaluation.

167. Which of these actions should the nurse be prepared to institute for the client who is experiencing delirium tremens?
    ○ 1. Provide a dark, quiet room, restraints, and side rails.
    ○ 2. Arrange a room away from the nurse's station and keep the TV on continuously.
    ○ 3. Keep the client's room door closed and a bright light on in the room.
    ○ 4. Provide a room with lighting that decreases shadows and have someone in constant attendance.

168. Which of the following would most likely be observed during an assessment of Mr. Gates?
    ○ 1. Spider angiomas, palmar erythema, headache, lower abdominal pain
    ○ 2. Peripheral edema, right upper quadrant pain, hemorrhoids, decreased urine output
    ○ 3. Hepatomegaly, decreased peripheral pulses, cool extremities, intermittent claudication
    ○ 4. Dyspnea, pruritus, inspiratory stridor, intermittent jaundice

169. Which of the following laboratory results would *not* be expected with the diagnosis of cirrhosis?
    ○ 1. Decreased serum folic acid and albumin
    ○ 2. Decreased platelets and increased bilirubin
    ○ 3. Decreased prothrombin time and leukocytes
    ○ 4. Elevated SGPT, SGOT, and LDH

170. The most important pathologic factor contributing to the formation of esophageal varices that the nurse needs to consider when planning care for Mr. Gates is
    ○ 1. increased platelet count.
    ○ 2. portal hypertension.
    ○ 3. increased pulmonary artery pressure.
    ○ 4. renal failure.

171. In assessing Mr. Gates, the nurse knows that portal hypertension usually does *not* cause
    ○ 1. esophageal varices.
    ○ 2. pulmonary edema.
    ○ 3. ascites.
    ○ 4. hemorrhoids.

172. Mr. Gates continues to bleed from the esophageal varices. Prior to the insertion of a Sengstaken Blakemore tube, what will the nurse need to do?
    ○ 1. Check each balloon for leaks and label all tube ports.
    ○ 2. Clamp the lumen of the nasogastric tube.
    ○ 3. Insert ice water into the gastric balloon.
    ○ 4. Insert mercury into the esophageal balloon.

173. The nurse needs to do additional preparation prior to the insertion of the Sengstaken-Blakemore tube. Which of the following would be *inappropriate* prior to insertion?
    ○ 1. Place the client in a high-Fowler's position.
    ○ 2. Administer a neomycin enema.
    ○ 3. Instruct the client about the procedure.
    ○ 4. Lubricate the tube with water-soluble lubricant.

174. The tube has been inserted and the balloons have been inflated. An *incorrect* action would be which of the following?
    ○ 1. Insert a nasogastric tube above the esophageal balloon and connect it to intermittent suction.
    ○ 2. Tape the tube to provide some traction and decrease movement.
    ○ 3. Place the client in a supine position.
    ○ 4. Tape a scissors to the bedside to be used to cut the tube in the event of severe respiratory distress.

175. Complications resulting from the Sengstaken-Blakemore tube can occur. As the nurse caring for Mr. Gates, the priority complication to monitor for would be
    ○ 1. ulceration of the esophagus and gastric mucosa.
    ○ 2. esophageal perforation.
    ○ 3. upward dislodgment of the gastric balloon.
    ○ 4. downward dislodgment of the esophageal balloon.

176. If Mr. Gates's bleeding is not controlled by the Sengstaken-Blakemore tube, the nurse should be prepared to administer which of the following?
    ○ 1. Hydralazine (Apresoline)
    ○ 2. Vasopressin (Pitressin)
    ○ 3. Meprobamate (Miltown)
    ○ 4. Diazepam (Valium)

177. In caring for Mr. Gates with the Sengstaken-Blakemore tube in place, which of the following actions is *inappropriate*?
    ○ 1. Monitor intake and output carefully.
    ○ 2. Give frequent oral hygiene.
    ○ 3. Maintain bed rest.
    ○ 4. Sedate client.

178. Several days later, the Sengstaken-Blakemore tube is gradually deflated and removed, because Mr. Gates's bleeding has subsided. When teaching Mr. Gates about prevention of esophageal bleeding, what should he be instructed to do?
    ○ 1. Eat a well-balanced, highly nutritious, bland, low-sodium diet.
    ○ 2. Eat a low-protein, high-carbohydrate diet.
    ○ 3. It is OK to maintain alcohol intake if diet is balanced.
    ○ 4. Eat a general diet with no restrictions.

Mr. Gates was discharged. Four months later he is readmitted in a comatose state.

179. Knowing Mr. Gates's past history, what condition would the nurse most likely suspect?
    ○ 1. Brain tumor
    ○ 2. Hepatic encephalopathy
    ○ 3. Respiratory failure
    ○ 4. Parkinson's disease

180. While caring for Mr. Gates, the nurse must consider that the most important pathophysiologic factor contributing to his current state is which of the following?
    ○ 1. Increased prothrombin time
    ○ 2. Portal hypertension
    ○ 3. Increased serum ammonia levels
    ○ 4. Increased serum bilirubin

181. Mr. Gates's urine output falls below 20 ml/hour and a central venous pressure (CVP) line is placed in his subclavian vein. What should be done after the insertion, calibration, and zeroing of the line?
    ○ 1. Check vital signs.
    ○ 2. Check CVP reading.
    ○ 3. Check his intake for the last 12 hours.
    ○ 4. Measure output for 1 more hour.

182. Which of the following is an unlikely assessment for clients with a diagnosis of hepatic encephalopathy?
    ○ 1. Asterixis
    ○ 2. Decreased level of consciousness
    ○ 3. Muscle twitching
    ○ 4. Exophthalmos

183. Which of the following should the nurse be prepared to administer to Mr. Gates?
    ○ 1. Neomycin and lactulose (Cephulac) enema
    ○ 2. Protein tube feeding
    ○ 3. Phenobarbital (Luminal)
    ○ 4. Phenytoin sodium (Dilantin)

184. What is the therapeutic effect of this treatment?
    ○ 1. To decrease muscular twitching
    ○ 2. To induce sedation
    ○ 3. To provide nutrition that promotes healing
    ○ 4. To prevent formation of ammonia

185. In planning care for Mr. Gates, which of the following statements best describes the necessary dietary alterations?
    ○ 1. High carbohydrate, protein, fat
    ○ 2. Low protein
    ○ 3. Low carbohydrate, fat
    ○ 4. High fiber

186. Mr. Gates's condition improves. In planning discharge health teaching, which of the following is *inappropriate* for the nurse to include?
    ○ 1. The need for a balance between activity and rest
    ○ 2. How to avoid constipation
    ○ 3. What kinds of foods to avoid
    ○ 4. The need to drink 3 to 4 liters of water each day

James Yamamoto, aged 45, is an unemployed carpenter who drinks heavily. He has been hospitalized on 4 occasions for acute alcoholism. He was admitted to the hospital after having vomited a large quantity of bright red blood and smaller quantities of coffee-ground emesis.

187. On admission, which one of the following clinical manifestations of a liver pathologic condition *cannot* be observed by the nurse?
    ○ **1.** Ascites
    ○ **2.** Mild jaundice
    ○ **3.** Purpuric spots on his arms and legs
    ○ **4.** Esophageal varices

188. Following are the most probable causes of Mr. Yamamoto's cirrhosis. Which has the most important implications for long-term nursing care plans?
    ○ **1.** Obstruction of major bile ducts
    ○ **2.** Chronic ingestion of alcoholic beverages
    ○ **3.** Long-term nutritional inadequacy
    ○ **4.** Viral inflammation of liver cells

189. Immediately following Mr. Yamamoto's admission to the hospital, which of the following should be provided in order to make him more comfortable?
    ○ **1.** Vigorous backrub
    ○ **2.** Scrupulous mouth care
    ○ **3.** Complete tub bath
    ○ **4.** Shave and haircut

190. With esophageal varices, the priority assessment focus would be
    ○ **1.** portal hypertension.
    ○ **2.** hemorrhage.
    ○ **3.** jaundice.
    ○ **4.** ascites.

191. Accurate observation of Mr. Yamamoto's jaundice would be recorded, as which of the following might likely be expected to develop?
    ○ **1.** Hiccoughs
    ○ **2.** Pruritus
    ○ **3.** Anuria
    ○ **4.** Diarrhea

192. Why would Mr. Yamamoto be weighed daily?
    ○ **1.** To allow correction of a nutritional deficiency
    ○ **2.** To monitor accumulation of edema and ascites
    ○ **3.** To assess breakdown of tissue protein
    ○ **4.** To monitor enlargement of the liver and spleen

193. Because of his chronically poor physiologic state, assessments and nursing actions would *not* be directed toward prevention of which of the following?
    ○ **1.** Pneumonia
    ○ **2.** Decubitus ulcers
    ○ **3.** Cystitis
    ○ **4.** Gynecomastia

Larry Pearson, 38 years old, is admitted with complaints of headache and lethargy. After extensive diagnostic tests, acromegaly is diagnosed.

194. Which of the following statements about acromegaly is most accurate regarding Mr. Pearson?
    ○ **1.** It is caused by an excess of secretions from the neurohypophysis.
    ○ **2.** It is characterized by an increase in height.
    ○ **3.** It often causes visual deterioration to the point of blindness.
    ○ **4.** It can be treated with complete reversal of symptoms.

Maria Garcia, a 19-year-old woman, is admitted to the hospital with a diagnosis of possible pituitary tumor. She has been having headaches and galactorrhea.

195. Overproduction of which of the following pituitary hormones can cause galactorrhea?
    ○ **1.** Follicle-stimulating hormone (FSH)
    ○ **2.** Estrogen
    ○ **3.** Progesterone
    ○ **4.** Prolactin

196. Which of the following diagnostic tests would provide the *least* helpful information in diagnosing a pituitary tumor?
    ○ **1.** Hormonal assays
    ○ **2.** CT scan
    ○ **3.** Visual fields
    ○ **4.** Serum calcium

197. A hypophysectomy is planned for Miss Garcia. What would be the most important nursing action in the immediate post-op period?
    ○ **1.** Instruct her to cough and deep breathe.
    ○ **2.** Assess urinary output hourly.
    ○ **3.** Keep her in a semi-Fowler's position.
    ○ **4.** Perform nasotracheal suctioning frequently.

198. What long-term problem may result from having had a hypophysectomy?
    ○ **1.** Hypopituitarism
    ○ **2.** Acromegaly
    ○ **3.** Cushing's disease
    ○ **4.** Diabetes mellitus

199. Before Miss Garcia leaves the hospital, she confides to you that she is worried that, ''I'll never be able to have babies.'' What information relative to her case is most correct?
- ○ **1.** The surgery has had no effect on her reproductive hormones.
- ○ **2.** Her sexual libido may be decreased but not her ability to conceive.
- ○ **3.** A decrease in gonadal hormones is common, but replacements can be given.
- ○ **4.** The ovaries can function independently without the pituitary hormones.

Rose Schiller had a subtotal thyroidectomy today for removal of a nodule and is to return from the recovery room soon.

200. Which of the following questions is most important to ask Mrs. Schiller postoperatively?
- ○ **1.** ''Do you feel uncomfortable?''
- ○ **2.** ''Do you have any tingling of your toes, fingers, or around your mouth?''
- ○ **3.** ''Do your arms or legs seem heavier than usual?''
- ○ **4.** ''Please tell me your name and where you are?''

201. Which of the following positions would Mrs. Schiller be placed in when she returns from the recovery room?
- ○ **1.** High-Fowler's with the neck supported
- ○ **2.** Left lateral recumbent with the upper part of the back supported
- ○ **3.** Semi-Fowler's with the neck supported
- ○ **4.** Supine with sandbags at the head

202. Postoperatively, the nurse continues to assess for signs and symptoms of hypoparathyroidism; which of the following signs and symptoms are *not* indicative of hypoparathyroidism?
- ○ **1.** Abdominal cramping and convulsions
- ○ **2.** Dyspnea and cyanosis
- ○ **3.** Positive Chvostek's and Trousseau's signs
- ○ **4.** Muscular flaccidity and hypotension

203. Which of the following pieces of equipment should be kept on hand for Mrs. Schiller?
- ○ **1.** An arterial line
- ○ **2.** A nerve stimulator
- ○ **3.** A tracheostomy set
- ○ **4.** Rotating tourniquets

204. Which of the following drugs should be readily available for Mrs. Schiller?
- ○ **1.** Calcitonin
- ○ **2.** Calcium gluconate
- ○ **3.** Calcium chloride
- ○ **4.** Saturated solution of potassium iodine

205. Which of the following nursing actions is *inappropriate* for the post-op thyroidectomy client?
- ○ **1.** Encourage slight vocalization after surgery.
- ○ **2.** Support the head with at least 2 to 3 pillows.
- ○ **3.** Check the back of the neck for drainage.
- ○ **4.** Provide oral fluids as tolerated.

The nurse is preparing a care plan for Julia Canon, a 28-year-old, newly diagnosed diabetic.

206. What nursing action is vital to the implementation of this care plan for Miss Canon?
- ○ **1.** Determine if she is a ketosis-prone or a ketosis-resistant diabetic.
- ○ **2.** Assess her knowledge of the disease process.
- ○ **3.** Ask if her family has a history of diabetes.
- ○ **4.** Instruct Miss Canon that her life-style will never be the same.

207. Which of the following is true regarding diabetes?
- ○ **1.** Diabetes is an acute disorder that responds only to insulin treatment.
- ○ **2.** Diabetes is a curable illness.
- ○ **3.** Diabetes is characterized by an abnormality of carbohydrate metabolism.
- ○ **4.** Diabetes is not a significant cause of death in the United States.

208. From your understanding of diabetes, you know that Miss Canon's symptom of polyuria is most likely caused by what physiologic change?
- ○ **1.** Glucose, acting as a hypertonic agent, draws water from the extracellular fluid into the renal tubules.
- ○ **2.** Increased insulin levels promote a diuretic effect.
- ○ **3.** Electrolyte changes lead to the retention of sodium and potassium.
- ○ **4.** Microvascular changes alter the effectiveness of the kidneys.

209. The nursing care plan includes teaching Miss Canon how to prepare and give herself insulin injections. What is the most important reason for instructing her to rotate injection sites?
- ○ **1.** Lipodystrophy can result and is extremely painful and unsightly.
- ○ **2.** Poor rotation technique can cause superficial hemorrhaging.
- ○ **3.** Lipodystrophic areas can result, causing erratic insulin absorption rates.
- ○ **4.** Injection sites can never be reused.

210. Regular insulin is ordered for Miss Canon. The first dose is administered at 7:30 A.M. If a hypoglycemic reaction occurs, it would most likely occur at what time?
- ○ **1.** After breakfast
- ○ **2.** After lunch
- ○ **3.** After dinner
- ○ **4.** After bedtime

211. Which of the following are symptoms of hypoglycemia?
- ○ **1.** Polydipsia, polyuria
- ○ **2.** Elevated urine glucose
- ○ **3.** Rapid, deep respirations
- ○ **4.** Rapid, shallow respirations

212. Miss Canon is now prepared for discharge. She is concerned about continuing her aerobics program. What should the nurse suggest to her?
- ○ **1.** Aerobic exercise is too strenuous for diabetics.
- ○ **2.** An exercise program is an important part of diabetic management, when balanced with insulin and diet.
- ○ **3.** She should limit her activities to brisk walking.
- ○ **4.** Exercise increases the risk of diabetic complications (e.g., peripheral neuropathy).

Olga Schumacher, a 65-year-old woman, is admitted with the diagnosis of hyperglycemic, hyperosmolar, nonketotic coma. Her blood glucose level is 1,000 mg/100 ml.

213. Characteristic findings of diabetes do *not* include
- ○ **1.** polyuria caused by the excessive amounts of glucose in the urine.
- ○ **2.** polyphagia caused by starvation at the cellular level.
- ○ **3.** polydypsia caused by polyuria.
- ○ **4.** weight gain caused by excessive appetite.

214. Which terms would best describe the most likely condition of Mrs. Schumacher's skin on admission?
- ○ **1.** Warm, flushed, dry
- ○ **2.** Cool, clammy
- ○ **3.** Cool, dry
- ○ **4.** Warm, pale, clammy

215. The highest priority of care when Mrs. Schumacher is admitted is to
- ○ **1.** force fluids orally to 4 liters or more per 24 hours.
- ○ **2.** administer large doses of regular insulin as ordered.
- ○ **3.** administer 2 to 3 liters IV fluids in first 1 to 2 hours.
- ○ **4.** administer large doses of NPH or Lente insulin.

216. When Mrs. Schumacher regains consciousness, she is told she has diabetes. She replies, "I might as well be dead. I'll never be able to lead a normal life again." The best response to this is
- ○ **1.** "After I teach you everything you need to know, you'll find out you're wrong."
- ○ **2.** "Don't worry. Everything will be fine."
- ○ **3.** "The doctor gave you some medicine that will take care of everything."
- ○ **4.** "You will have to do some things differently to control this disease, but you can still lead a normal life."

Martha Carter, 65 years old, has had diabetes for 10 years. The diabetes has been controlled by diet and tolbutamide (Orinase). Recently, she has complained of discomfort in her left leg.

217. The classic sign/symptom of arterial insufficiency of the lower extremities is which of the following?
- ○ **1.** Intermittent claudication
- ○ **2.** Peripheral parasthesias
- ○ **3.** Shiny, atrophic skin over the tibia
- ○ **4.** Pain on dorsiflexion of the foot

218. Promoting arterial blood flow to Mrs. Carter's feet is a nursing goal. Which nursing action would best achieve this?
- ○ **1.** Encourage her to dorsiflex her toes frequently.
- ○ **2.** Keep her feet covered with socks at all times.
- ○ **3.** Apply external heat to the feet.
- ○ **4.** Massage the feet briskly TID.

219. Mrs. Carter is scheduled for a left femoral-popliteal bypass graft. The day before surgery, she says to you, ''I know this is only the beginning; soon they'll take my leg.'' Which response is most appropriate now?

○ **1.** ''Many persons who have had this surgery have not needed an amputation.''

○ **2.** ''That may be a possibility some day, but don't worry about it now.''

○ **3.** ''I see this is worrying you. What would losing your leg mean to you?''

○ **4.** ''There have been vast improvements in vascular surgery.''

220. During Mrs. Carter's first few post-op days, her diabetes can be best controlled by

○ **1.** restarting her oral agent as soon as possible.

○ **2.** administering an intermediate insulin daily.

○ **3.** ensuring she eats all the food on her trays.

○ **4.** administering short-acting insulin based on q4h blood sugars.

221. When the nurse goes into Mrs. Carter's room to give her morning care, she is very irritable and tells the nurse to get out of her room. What is the best initial action?

○ **1.** Assess her for other signs of hypoglycemia.

○ **2.** Ask her if she would like you to come back later.

○ **3.** Allow her to express her anger and stay with her.

○ **4.** Recognize she may be confused and orient her to her surroundings.

222. While Mrs. Carter is in the hospital, the nurse reviews a diabetic diet with her. Which fact is most accurate?

○ **1.** Recent research indicates fats should be eliminated.

○ **2.** Dietetic fruits may be eaten as free foods.

○ **3.** A regular meal pattern need not be followed since she is not taking insulin.

○ **4.** Complex carbohydrates such as breads and cereals should be included in her diet.

223. Mrs. Carter is to be discharged soon. Which of the following would be *inappropriate* to include in her teaching plan?

○ **1.** Change position hourly to increase circulation.

○ **2.** Inspect feet and legs daily for any changes.

○ **3.** Keep legs elevated on 2 pillows while sleeping.

○ **4.** Keep the incision clean dry.

Linda Adams, aged 70, has been diagnosed with Addison's disease.

224. As the completes the nursing history, Mrs. Adams would most likely complain of

○ **1.** weakness, decreased skin pigmentation, weight gain.

○ **2.** weakness, increased skin pigmentation, weight loss.

○ **3.** weakness, pallor, weight loss.

○ **4.** insomnia, weight loss, nervousness.

225. Which action would be most appropriate when administering care to Mrs. Adams?

○ **1.** Encourage exercise.

○ **2.** Protect from exertion.

○ **3.** Provide a variety of diversional activities.

○ **4.** Permit as much activity as she desires.

226. Which of the following nursing actions for the client with Addison's disease would be *inappropriate*?

○ **1.** Observe for fluid and electrolyte imbalances.

○ **2.** Administer varying amounts of cortisol as ordered.

○ **3.** Administer aldosterone as ordered.

○ **4.** Watch for symptoms of hypertension and tachycardia.

227. Which symptoms would alert the nurse to a deterioration in Mrs. Adams's condition (i.e., addisonian crisis)?

○ **1.** Increased blood pressure, polyuria, pulmonary edema

○ **2.** Increased blood pressure, oliguria

○ **3.** Decreased blood pressure, urine output of 35 ml/hour

○ **4.** Decreased blood pressure, oliguria

228. Mrs. Adams will be treated with replacement glucocorticoid, cortisone, and fludrocortisone acetate (Florinef). In developing the teaching plan, the nurse identifies which of the following as *inappropriate* to include?

○ **1.** The different types and actions of medications

○ **2.** The need to wear or carry medical alert identification of condition and medications

○ **3.** The use of hydrocortisone IM in an emergency

○ **4.** The need for a life-style change, even with the use of replacement medications

Jack Thomas, a 56-year-old personnel director, is admitted for a cystoscopy. While admitting him, you learn that he has a urinary tract infection, smokes half a pack of cigarettes a day, and had a hernia repaired 20 years ago. He takes chlorothiazide (Diuril) for high blood pressure and follows a mild sodium-restricted diet.

229. Which of the following factors most increases the risk of Mr. Thomas's developing septic shock postoperatively?
- ○ **1.** Cystoscopy in the presence of a urinary tract infection
- ○ **2.** High blood pressure
- ○ **3.** Sodium-restricted diet
- ○ **4.** Smoking

230. While the nurse is preparing Mr. Thomas for the procedure, he says, "I think I'm going to die." What is an appropriate nursing response?
- ○ **1.** "Don't worry, your doctor is one of the best."
- ○ **2.** "This procedure has a very low mortality rate."
- ○ **3.** "What ever gave you that idea?"
- ○ **4.** "You think you're going to die?"

231. Mr. Thomas returns from the recovery room at 9:00 A.M. alert and oriented, with an IV infusing. His pulse is 80, blood pressure is 120/80, respirations are 20, and all are within normal range. At 10:00 A.M. and at 11:00 A.M., his vital signs are stable. At noon, however, his pulse rate is 84, blood pressure is 110/74, and respirations are 24. What nursing action is most appropriate?
- ○ **1.** Increase the IV rate.
- ○ **2.** Notify his physician.
- ○ **3.** Take his vital signs again in 15 minutes.
- ○ **4.** Take his vital signs again in an hour.

232. Which of the following is an *early* sign of septic shock?
- ○ **1.** Cool, clammy skin
- ○ **2.** Hypotension
- ○ **3.** Increased urinary output
- ○ **4.** Restlessness

233. The nurse shows Mr. Thomas a list of foods and asks him to select any items included in his diet. His selection of which item probably indicates that he understand his dietary restrictions?
- ○ **1.** Beef broth
- ○ **2.** Cheese
- ○ **3.** Dried apricots
- ○ **4.** Peanut butter

234. Before Mr. Thomas is discharged, the nurse evaluates the effects of teaching. Which of the following statements best indicates that Mr. Thomas understands hypertension and his treatment?
- ○ **1.** "I only add a little salt while preparing my food, and salt my food lightly at the table."
- ○ **2.** "I have blurred vision once in a while, but high blood pressure doesn't cause that."
- ○ **3.** "I know smoking increases my blood pressure and that I should stop, but it's very hard to do."
- ○ **4.** "I take my blood pressure pill whenever I get a severe headache."

During her hospitalization for a cataract extraction, Martha Cook acquires a urinary tract infection.

235. Besides instructing Mrs. Cook on how, when, and why she should take her antibiotics, the nurse knows that the most important thing Mrs. Cook needs to learn to clear the infection is which of the following?
- ○ **1.** To drink up to 3 liters of fluid each day
- ○ **2.** How to cleanse her perineum after voiding
- ○ **3.** To limit fluids to increase the bacteriostatic activity of the urine
- ○ **4.** To acidify the urine by drinking cranberry juice

236. Because her urinary tract infection is still present several weeks after hospital discharge and following several courses of antibiotic therapy, she is scheduled for an intravenous pyelogram (IVP). If Mrs. Cook experiences any of the following reactions after injection of the contrast material for IVP, which one would have to be reported immediately?
- ○ **1.** Feeling of warmth
- ○ **2.** Flushing of the face
- ○ **3.** Salty taste in the mouth
- ○ **4.** Urticaria

237. The IVP reveals that Mrs. Cook has a renal calculus. She is believed to have a small stone that will pass spontaneously. To increase the chance of her passing the stone, the nurse should force fluids and do which of the following?
- ○ **1.** Teach her to strain all urine.
- ○ **2.** Have her ambulate.
- ○ **3.** Keep her on bed rest.
- ○ **4.** Give medications to relax her.

238. Which factor predisposes the development of renal calculi?
○ **1.** Bed rest for a client with multiple myeloma
○ **2.** Use of a tilt table for a client who has a spinal cord injury
○ **3.** Forcing fluids in a client on bed rest
○ **4.** Decreasing calcium in the diet of a client with Paget's disease

Randolph Parker, a 64-year-old carpenter, has a diagnosis of bladder cancer.

239. A risk factor of bladder carcinoma is
○ **1.** cigarette smoking.
○ **2.** family history.
○ **3.** low-bulk diet.
○ **4.** stress.

240. What is the most common clinical finding in carcinoma of the bladder?
○ **1.** Abdominal pain
○ **2.** Gross, painless hematuria
○ **3.** Palpable tumor
○ **4.** Melena

241. Mr. Parker is scheduled for a cystectomy with the creation of an ileal conduit in the morning. He is wringing his hand and pacing the floor when the nurse enters his room. What is the best approach?
○ **1.** "Good evening, Mr. Parker. Wasn't it a pleasant day, today?"
○ **2.** "Mr. Parker, you must be so worried, I'll leave you alone with your thoughts."
○ **3.** "Mr. Parker, you'll wear out the hospital floors and yourself at this rate."
○ **4.** "Mr. Parker, you appear anxious to me. How are you feeling about tomorrow's surgery?"

242. In addition to emotional support, range-of-motion (ROM) exercise is another nursing action that would be included in the nursing care plan for Mr. Parker. Why?
○ **1.** Ambulation will be restricted for 1 week postoperatively.
○ **2.** There is an increased risk of thrombophlebitis following pelvic surgery.
○ **3.** Cystectomies are extremely painful and limit the client's ability to move.
○ **4.** ROM helps to make the client feel he is involved in his care.

243. After surgery, Mr. Parker has a nasogastric tube in place but continues to complain of nausea. Which action should the nurse take?
○ **1.** Call the physician immediately.
○ **2.** Administer the prescribed antiemetic.
○ **3.** Irrigate the tube to check for patency.
○ **4.** Reposition the client.

244. Why is a nasogastric tube inserted postoperatively for Mr. Parker?
○ **1.** To administer tube feedings
○ **2.** To test gastric secretions for bacteria
○ **3.** To reduce the risk of paralytic ileus
○ **4.** To increase the abdominal girth

245. What color should Mr. Parker's urinary stoma be?
○ **1.** Brown
○ **2.** Dark red
○ **3.** Light brown
○ **4.** Pink to red

246. Mr. Parker's post-op vital signs are a blood pressure of 80/40 mm Hg, a pulse of 140, and respirations of 32. Suspecting shock, which of the following orders should the nurse question?
○ **1.** Put the client in modified Trendelenburg's position.
○ **2.** Administer oxygen at 100%.
○ **3.** Monitor urine output qh.
○ **4.** Administer morphine 10 mg IM q3–4h.

Gwen Harris is admitted to the unit with a diagnosis of acute renal failure. This is her first hospitalization for this disease. She is awake, alert, oriented, and complaining of severe back pain and abdominal cramps. Her vital signs are blood pressure 170/100 mm Hg, pulse 110, respirations 30, oral temperature 100.4°F (38°C). Her electrolytes are sodium 120 mEq/liter, potassium 7mEq/liter; her urinary output for the first 8 hours is 50 ml.

247. Mrs. Harris is displaying signs of which electrolyte imbalance?
○ **1.** Hyponatremia
○ **2.** Hyperkalemia
○ **3.** Hyperphosphatemia
○ **4.** Hypercalcemia

248. The normal medical management of Mrs. Harris's sodium imbalance is most likely to be
○ **1.** fluid restriction.
○ **2.** fluid replacement.
○ **3.** whole blood replacement.
○ **4.** sodium replacement.

249. When taking Mrs. Harris's blood pressure, you observe the presence of Trousseau's sign. This is an indication of
   ○ 1. hyponatremia.
   ○ 2. hyperkalemia.
   ○ 3. hypocalcemia.
   ○ 4. anemia.

250. Which of the following are the most appropriate nursing actions for Mrs. Harris?
   ○ 1. Intake and output, daily weight, routine cardiopulmonary assessment
   ○ 2. Intake and output, up ad lib, restrict fluids
   ○ 3. Daily weight, force fluids, daily measurement of dependent edema
   ○ 4. Daily weight, up ad lib, restrict fluids

251. Mrs. Harris's urinary output suddenly increases to 150 ml/hour. The nurse assesses that she has entered the second phase of acute renal failure. Nursing actions throughout this phase include observation for signs and symptoms of
   ○ 1. hypervolemia, hypokalemia, hypernatremia.
   ○ 2. hypervolemia, hyperkalemia, hypernatremia.
   ○ 3. hypovolemia, hypokalemia, hyponatremia.
   ○ 4. hypovolemia, hypokalemia, hypernatremia.

Stanley Kleszewski is admitted to the hospital in acute renal failure. His symptoms include oliguria, lethargy, and elevated blood urea nitrogen (BUN).

252. Which statement best explains the elevation in his BUN?
   ○ 1. Increased protein metabolism
   ○ 2. Hemolysis of red blood cells
   ○ 3. Damage to the kidney cells
   ○ 4. Decreased protein metabolism

253. A low-protein diet is ordered for Mr. Kleszewski. What is the rationale the nurse would give the client for this type of diet?
   ○ 1. Minimize protein breakdown
   ○ 2. Reduce the metabolic rate
   ○ 3. Decrease sodium intoxication
   ○ 4. Minimize the development of edema

254. The nurse's aide assists with Mr. Kleszewski's care. Which assignment to the aide would be the nurse's priority to check?
   ○ 1. Obtaining his vital signs
   ○ 2. Recording his intake and output
   ○ 3. Monitoring the amount of food he consumes
   ○ 4. Checking his bowel movements

Wilmont Brown is admitted to the unit with the diagnosis of chronic renal failure.

255. Assessing the laboratory findings, which of the following results would you most likely expect to find on Mr. Brown?
   ○ 1. BUN 10 to 30 mg/dl, potassium 4.0 mEq/liter, creatinine 0.5 to 1.5 mg/dl
   ○ 2. Decreased serum calcium, blood pH 7.2, potassium 6.5 mEq/liter
   ○ 3. BUN 15 mg/dl, increased serum calcium, creatinine 1.0 mg/dl
   ○ 4. BUN 35 to 40 mg/dl, potassium 3.5 mEq/liter, pH 7.35, decreased serum calcium

256. The most likely cause of the peaked T waves that appear on Mr. Brown's electrocardiogram is
   ○ 1. hypernatremia.
   ○ 2. hypervolemia.
   ○ 3. hypokalemia.
   ○ 4. hyperkalemia.

257. Mr. Brown starts having Kussmaul's respirations. Which of the following statements best describes the rationale for this occurrence?
   ○ 1. The kidneys cannot excrete the hydrogen ion or reabsorb bicarbonate.
   ○ 2. The kidneys cannot excrete the bicarbonate ion or reabsorb the hydrogen ion.
   ○ 3. The kidneys are unable to excrete the potassium ion, resulting in acidosis.
   ○ 4. The kidneys are unable to excrete sodium and phosphorus, resulting in alkalosis.

258. Laboratory studies on Mr. Brown reveal hyperkalemia, the most serious electrolyte problem associated with renal failure. Hyperkalemia occurs for all but one of the following reasons. Which explanation is *not* accurate?
   ○ 1. Hyperkalemia results from failure of the excretory ability of the kidneys.
   ○ 2. Hyperkalemia results from the breakdown of the cellular protein that releases potassium.
   ○ 3. Hyperkalemia results from acidosis, which causes the shift of potassium from the intracellular to the extracellular space.
   ○ 4. Hyperkalemia results from decreased serum calcium, because these electrolytes are inversely related.

259. Which of the following drugs would be *ineffective* in lowering Mr. Brown's serum potassium level?
   ○ 1. Glucose and insulin
   ○ 2. Polystyrene sulfonate (Kayexalate)
   ○ 3. Calcium gluconate
   ○ 4. Aluminum hydroxide

260. Peritoneal dialysis is considered as a possible means of treatment for Mr. Brown. Which of the following is the main *disadvantage* of peritoneal dialysis?
    ○ 1. Vascular access is required.
    ○ 2. The possibility of contracting hepatitis is great.
    ○ 3. It is a slow method of treatment.
    ○ 4. Fluid and electrolyte exchange is gradual.

261. The most common and severe complication that requires assessment during peritoneal dialysis is
    ○ 1. respiratory distress.
    ○ 2. peritonitis.
    ○ 3. hemorrhage.
    ○ 4. abdominal pain.

262. The physicians decide against peritoneal dialysis for Mr. Brown. Treatment with hemodialysis is ordered and an external shunt is created. Which of the following nursing actions would be of highest priority with regard to the external shunt?
    ○ 1. Heparinize it daily.
    ○ 2. Avoid taking blood pressure measurements or blood samples from the affected arm.
    ○ 3. Change the Silastic tube daily.
    ○ 4. Instruct the client not to use the affected arm.

263. During the hemodialysis procedure, Mr. Brown complains of nausea, vomits, and is disoriented. Which of the following should be the first nursing action?
    ○ 1. Slow the rate of dialysis.
    ○ 2. Administer protamine zinc.
    ○ 3. Reassure the client; anxiety frequently accompanies the procedure.
    ○ 4. Place the client in Trendelenburg's position.

Fredrick Rasmussen is a 69-year-old retired salesman. He is admitted with a diagnosis of urinary retention. His physician immediately inserts a Foley catheter. While being admitted Mr. Rasmussen tells the nurse that he is going to have his prostate "shaved," because it is enlarged.

264. Which of the following parameters should be monitored throughout Mr. Rasmussen's pre-op period?
    ○ 1. Fluid intake
    ○ 2. Intake and output
    ○ 3. Urinary output
    ○ 4. Urinary pH

265. Mr. Rasmussen is scheduled for a transurethral resection of the prostate (TURP) tomorrow. During pre-op teaching, he asks where his incision will be. What is the most appropriate response?
    ○ 1. "The incision is made in the abdomen."
    ○ 2. "The incision is made in the lower abdomen."
    ○ 3. "The incision is made in the perineum between the scrotum and the rectum."
    ○ 4. "There is no incision. The doctor inserts an instrument through the urethra, the opening in the penis."

266. When Mr. Rasmussen returns from the recovery room, he has an IV infusing at 100 ml/hour, a 3-way Foley catheter in place, and constant bladder irrigation. What should the nurse do first when increased blood in the urine is detected?
    ○ 1. Increase the speed of the irrigation.
    ○ 2. Release the traction on the Foley.
    ○ 3. Irrigate the catheter manually.
    ○ 4. Notify the physician.

267. Mr. Rasmussen complains of pain and bladder spasms. Which of the following nursing actions is most appropriate after determining that the drainage system is patent?
    ○ 1. Administer narcotics plus anticholinergic drugs, as ordered.
    ○ 2. Assist him to a sitz bath.
    ○ 3. Decrease the speed of the irrigation.
    ○ 4. Decrease the traction on the Foley.

268. Nursing strategies can help prevent which of the following complications associated with a transurethral resection of the prostate (TURP)?
    ○ 1. Epididymitis
    ○ 2. Incontinence
    ○ 3. Osteitis pubis
    ○ 4. Thrombophlebitis

269. Which of the following should be included in the discharge teaching for Mr. Rasmussen?
    ○ 1. "Avoid straining at stool."
    ○ 2. "Avoid heavy lifting for approximately 2 weeks after surgery."
    ○ 3. "Drive your car whenever you are ready to do so."
    ○ 4. "Refrain from sexual intercourse for 12 weeks."

270. Which of the following statements indicates that Mr. Rasmussen understands his discharge instruction?
- ○ **1.** "I know my urine may be slightly pink tinged."
- ○ **2.** "I know my urine should be clear all the time."
- ○ **3.** "I know my urine should be clear most of the time."
- ○ **4.** "I'll let my doctor know if I have any urinary dribbling."

John Halston, a retired bank manager, is admitted for evaluation of an enlarged prostate.

271. Which of the following is a common early symptom of prostate hypertrophy?
- ○ **1.** Difficulty urinating
- ○ **2.** Impotence
- ○ **3.** Urinary infection
- ○ **4.** Hematuria

272. The physician wants to examine Mr. Halston's prostate gland. What equipment will be necessary for the exam?
- ○ **1.** A Foley catheter
- ○ **2.** Lubricant and gloves
- ○ **3.** Urethral dilators
- ○ **4.** A rectal tube

273. Mr. Halston is scheduled to have an IV pyelogram (IVP) and cystoscopy. What nursing measure is essential to prepare him for the IVP?
- ○ **1.** Force fluids prior to the exam.
- ○ **2.** Insert a Foley catheter.
- ○ **3.** Administer cleansing enemas.
- ○ **4.** Administer iopanoic acid (Telepaque) tablets the evening before.

274. Mr. Halston undergoes a transurethral resection of the prostate (TURP) under spinal anesthesia. He returns to his room with continuous bladder irrigation (CBI). Which of these statements best explains the reason for the CBI?
- ○ **1.** To decrease bladder atony
- ○ **2.** To remove blood clots from the bladder
- ○ **3.** To maintain patency of the urethral catheter
- ○ **4.** To dilute the concentrated urine

275. The nursing assistant reports to the nurse that Mr. Halston is confused. "He keeps saying he has to urinate, but he has a catheter in place." Which of the following responses would be most appropriate for the nurse to make?
- ○ **1.** "His catheter is probably plugged. I'll irrigate is shortly."
- ○ **2.** "He may be confused. What else did he say or do?"
- ○ **3.** "That may be a sign of internal bleeding."
- ○ **4.** "The urge to urinate is usually caused by the catheter. He may also have bladder spasms."

276. Which of the following symptoms can be expected temporarily when Mr. Halston's Foley catheter is removed?
- ○ **1.** Urgency
- ○ **2.** Dribbling
- ○ **3.** Urinary retention
- ○ **4.** Decreased urinary output

Rennie Lacona, aged 78, is admitted to the hospital with the diagnosis of benign prostatic hypertrophy (BPH). He is scheduled for a transurethral resection of the prostate (TURP).

277. When planning for Mr. Lacona's care which of the following is *not* important to consider when evaluating his ability to withstand surgery?
- ○ **1.** Age
- ○ **2.** Nutritional status
- ○ **3.** Race
- ○ **4.** Function of the involved area

278. It would be *inappropriate* to include which of the following points in pre-op teaching?
- ○ **1.** TURP is the most common operation for BPH.
- ○ **2.** An explanation of the purpose and function of a 2-way irrigation system.
- ○ **3.** Expectation of bloody urine, which will clear as healing takes place.
- ○ **4.** He will be pain free.

279. If a client has had a perineal prostatectomy, which of the following is the most appropriate during the post-op period?
- ○ **1.** Take rectal temperatures, not only to determine body temperature but also to note the adequacy of perineal circulation.
- ○ **2.** A Foley catheter with a 30 ml inflation bag is is used to promote hemostasis.
- ○ **3.** For comfort, have the client sit on a semi-inflated air ring.
- ○ **4.** Have the client sit on a hard surface to support the perineal incision.

280. Which of the following is *inappropriate* to include in the nursing plan in the immediate post-op period?
    ○ 1. Monitor for signs and symptoms of shock (e.g., vital signs, level of consciousness).
    ○ 2. Monitor for hemorrhage.
    ○ 3. Observe patency of the catheter, color of the drainage.
    ○ 4. Assess sexual potency.

281. Which of the following daily nursing actions would it be *inappropriate* to include?
    ○ 1. Position the catheter to drain freely.
    ○ 2. Encourage adequate amount of fluids unless contraindicated by preexisting problems.
    ○ 3. Ambulate the client.
    ○ 4. Measure I&O.

282. Which one of the following is the most common complication following a prostatectomy that is pertinent to nursing assessment and action?
    ○ 1. Urinary tract infection
    ○ 2. Cardiac arrest
    ○ 3. Pneumonia
    ○ 4. Thrombophlebitis

283. When doing discharge planning for Mr. Lacona, what would be the high priority?
    ○ 1. Diet
    ○ 2. Fluid restriction
    ○ 3. Bladder training
    ○ 4. Resumption of sexual relations

Heidi Papps is a 25-year-old woman who has been experiencing intermittent bouts of diarrhea for the past 2 years. This condition has been becoming increasingly worse for the past 2 months. She is seeking medical attention, because her self-medication program is no longer working. Miss Papps is admitted to the hospital for diagnostic testing.

284. Which of the following is the most appropriate when preparing a client for a proctosigmoidoscopy?
    ○ 1. On the morning of the examination administer enemas until the returns are clear.
    ○ 2. Maintain the client NPO for 24 hours preceding the examination.
    ○ 3. Give a strong cathartic on both the evening before and the morning of the examination.
    ○ 4. Give sitz baths 3 times daily for 3 days preceding the examination.

285. What position is best for a client during a proctoscopic examination?
    ○ 1. Prone
    ○ 2. Right Sims'
    ○ 3. Lithotomy
    ○ 4. Knee-chest

286. Which nursing response is the most appropriate when preparing a client for a proctosigmoidoscopy?
    ○ 1. "You need have no anxiety concerning this procedure. You will experience no pain or discomfort."
    ○ 2. "You will experience a feeling of pressure and the desire to move your bowels during the brief time that the scope is in place."
    ○ 3. "You can reduce your discomfort during the procedure to a minimum by bearing down as the proctoscope is introduced."
    ○ 4. "You will experience no discomfort during the procedure, because a topical anesthetic will applies to the anus."

287. The physician wants a stool sample to check for amoebae. What is the correct procedure for obtaining a stool specimen for examination for amoebae?
    ○ 1. Deliver the specimen immediately to the laboratory while still warm and fresh.
    ○ 2. Mix the specimen with chlorinated lime solution before taking it to the laboratory.
    ○ 3. Refrigerate the specimen until it is picked up by a laboratory technician.
    ○ 4. Store the specimen in a warm water bath until time for delivery to the laboratory.

288. The tests confirm Miss Papps has ulcerative colitis. Which of the following is most characteristic of the stools in ulcerative colitis?
    ○ 1. Diarrhea with blood and mucus
    ○ 2. Clay-colored with blood and mucus
    ○ 3. Gray and foamy
    ○ 4. Semisolid, green with blood and mucus

289. Miss Papp's prothrombin time is considerably lowered. This most likely indicates
    ○ 1. decreased absorption of vitamin K.
    ○ 2. decreased absorption of vitamin C.
    ○ 3. decreased absorption of protein and potassium.
    ○ 4. decreased absorption of sodium, potassium, chloride, and fats.

290. Opiates and anticholinergic drugs are ordered for Miss Papps during her initial hospitalization, primarily to decrease
    ○ **1.** acute intestinal hypermotility and spasms.
    ○ **2.** gastric secretions.
    ○ **3.** irritability and nervousness.
    ○ **4.** pain.

291. Miss Papps does not respond to therapy. A colectomy and ileostomy are proposed. This surgery involves which of the following?
    ○ **1.** Removal of the rectum with a portion of the colon brought through the abdominal wall
    ○ **2.** Removal of the colon with a portion of the ileum brought through the abdominal wall
    ○ **3.** Removal of the ileum with a portion of the colon brought through the abdominal wall
    ○ **4.** A "pull through" procedure

292. Which of the following is *not* anticipated after this type of surgery?
    ○ **1.** Weight gain
    ○ **2.** Liquid stool
    ○ **3.** Reestablishment of a regular bowel pattern
    ○ **4.** Irritation of the skin around the stoma

Abel Hawkins, a 47-year-old computer programmer, is admitted with a suspected small-bowel obstruction. He is 5 ft 7 in tall and weighs 210 lb. An IV of 5% dextrose in 0.45% saline with 20 mEq KCl is to infuse at 150 ml/hour. A nasogastric tube is inserted and connected to continuous, medium suction; it immediately begins to drain large amounts of gastric drainage.

293. While taking a nursing history from Mr. Hawkins, the nurse should particularly monitor for an indication of a predisposition to bowel malignancy. Which disease of the bowel does *not* indicate such a predisposition?
    ○ **1.** Hemorrhoids
    ○ **2.** Colitis
    ○ **3.** Amebiasis
    ○ **4.** Polyps

294. When examining Mr. Hawkins's abdomen, which technique is performed last?
    ○ **1.** Auscultation
    ○ **2.** Inspection
    ○ **3.** Palpation
    ○ **4.** Percussion

295. Which of the following factors is most consistent with a small-bowel obstruction?
    ○ **1.** Diarrhea with blood and mucus
    ○ **2.** Increased flatus
    ○ **3.** Malnutrition
    ○ **4.** Projectile vomiting

296. What is the major problem for Mr. Hawkins if the intestinal blood supply is *not* compromised?
    ○ **1.** Alteration in body image
    ○ **2.** Decreased tissue perfusion
    ○ **3.** Fluid and electrolyte deficiency
    ○ **4.** Pain

297. Mr. Hawkins has a Miller-Abbott tube inserted in an effort to relieve the bowel obstruction. Which of the following is contraindicated?
    ○ **1.** Position the client on his right side until the tube passes the pyloric sphincter.
    ○ **2.** Tape the client's tube securely to the nose.
    ○ **3.** Connect the tube to suction.
    ○ **4.** Give mouth and nose care after any manipulation.

298. If Mr. Hawkins needed emergency surgery, precluding thorough pre-op teaching, which of the following would be the most important for the nurse to review with Mr. Hawkins?
    ○ **1.** Deep breathing exercises
    ○ **2.** Painless movement from side to side
    ○ **3.** Relaxation techniques
    ○ **4.** Use of an IPPB machine

Orville Kaufman, a 54-year-old business executive, was admitted for severe abdominal pain, nausea, and vomiting. His abdomen was rigid and tender to the touch; there were no bowel sounds, and his temperature was 101°F (38.3°C) rectally. Mr. Kaufman has a 4-year history of diverticulitis for which he has been treated medically. On admission, he needed emergency surgery for a ruptured diverticulum. He is now 3 days post-op and has a transverse colostomy.

299. Based upon the location of the colostomy, the nurse would most likely expect that Mr. Kaufman's normal stool consistency would be
    ○ **1.** liquid.
    ○ **2.** semiformed.
    ○ **3.** well formed.
    ○ **4.** hard and solid.

300. When teaching Mr. Kaufman how to irrigate his colostomy, which of the following points is *incorrect* to include?
    ○ **1.** Use a catheter with a shield or cone.
    ○ **2.** Hang the irrigation reservoir about 18 to 24 inches above the stoma.
    ○ **3.** Irrigate twice a day until regulated, then decrease to once a day.
    ○ **4.** Clear all air from the tubing prior to irrigation.

301. Skin care around the stoma is critical. In performing Mr. Kaufman's skin care, which of the following is *contraindicated*?
    ○ **1.** Observe for any excoriated areas.
    ○ **2.** Use karaya paste and rings around the stoma.
    ○ **3.** Apply mineral oil to the area for moisture.
    ○ **4.** Clean the area daily with soap and water before applying the bag.

302. Regulation of Mr. Kaufman's colostomy will be most enhanced if he
    ○ **1.** eats balanced meals at regular intervals.
    ○ **2.** irrigates after lunch each day.
    ○ **3.** restricts exercise to walking only.
    ○ **4.** eats fruit at all 3 meals.

303. When helping Mr. Kaufman to accept his colostomy, which of the following actions is *inappropriate*?
    ○ **1.** Encourage him to look at the stoma.
    ○ **2.** Emphasize his positive attributes.
    ○ **3.** Involve the family in his care.
    ○ **4.** Have him do his own irrigations right from the start.

The surgeon informed Jeff Oakes that he has cancer of the rectum and advised that he undergo surgery for the removal of the rectum and formation of a permanent colostomy.

304. A gastric suction tube was inserted before Mr. Oakes was sent to surgery, in order to
    ○ **1.** facilitate administration of high caloric, nutritious liquids immediately after completion of the procedure.
    ○ **2.** prevent accumulation of gas and fluid in the stomach both during and following surgical action.
    ○ **3.** provide a reliable means of detecting gastrointestinal hemorrhage during the operative procedure.
    ○ **4.** serve as a stimulus to restore normal peristaltic movement following recovery from anesthesia.

305. What is the primary purpose of inserting an indwelling Foley catheter before taking Mr. Oakes to the operating room?
    ○ **1.** To facilitate distension of the bladder with saline during surgery
    ○ **2.** To provide a ready check for renal function throughout surgery
    ○ **3.** To reduce the possibility of bladder injury during the procedure
    ○ **4.** To prevent contamination of the operative field resulting form incontinence

306. Sections of colon both above and below the site of tumor were removed in order to prevent
    ○ **1.** direct extension and metastatic spread of the tumor.
    ○ **2.** post-op paralysis and distension of the bowel.
    ○ **3.** accidental loosening of bowel sutures post-operatively.
    ○ **4.** pressure injury to the perineal suture line.

307. When considering whether Mr. Oakes will receive tube feedings postoperatively, the nurse remembers tube feedings are designed to provide adequate nutrition for all of the following clients *except*
    ○ **1.** those who have difficulty in swallowing.
    ○ **2.** those who are comatose.
    ○ **3.** those who do not have a functioning gastrointestinal tract.
    ○ **4.** those who are anorexic.

308. How should the nurse prepare Mr. Oakes for the first irrigation of his colostomy?
    ○ **1.** Explain that the procedure will be short and painless.
    ○ **2.** Give him a pamphlet to read that outlines the procedure.
    ○ **3.** Talk with his spouse.
    ○ **4.** Show him pictures, and have him talk briefly with a person who has a well-regulated colostomy.

309. Which of the following would be best suited for irrigation of Mr. Oakes's colostomy?
    ○ **1.** 10% saline solution
    ○ **2.** Mild soap solution
    ○ **3.** Warm tap water
    ○ **4.** Dilute hydrogen peroxide

310. Which of the following is the most likely to promote success when Mr. Oakes is irrigating his colostomy?
    ○ **1.** Size of the stoma
    ○ **2.** Excitement
    ○ **3.** Hunger
    ○ **4.** Relaxation

Alan Simms, a 56-year-old man, is admitted to the hospital with a tentative diagnosis of cancer of the colon.

311. The symptoms of colon cancer vary depending on where in the colon the lesion is located. Which would *not* be a classic symptom of colon cancer?
    ○ **1.** Change in bowel habits
    ○ **2.** Excessive flatus
    ○ **3.** Pain on the right side
    ○ **4.** Anorexia and nausea

312. Which of the following diagnostic tests will confirm the diagnosis of colon cancer most conclusively?
- ○ **1.** Carcinoembryonic antigen (CEA)
- ○ **2.** Barium enema
- ○ **3.** Biopsy of the lesion
- ○ **4.** Stool examination

313. Mr. Simms is found to have a lesion of the distal sigmoid colon and rectum. An abdominoperineal resection is planned. A bowel preparation is begun. After Mr. Simms has received 3 doses of neomycin, he complains of frequent stools. What should the nursing action be?
- ○ **1.** See if there is an order for antidiarrheal medication.
- ○ **2.** Explain to Mr. Simms that this is the desired result.
- ○ **3.** Ask Mr. Simms to record his stools.
- ○ **4.** Withhold the laxative that was ordered as part of the prep.

314. Mr. Simms and his wife have been taught about the nature of the surgery. The nurse asks Mr. Simms to repeat what he has learned. Which of the statements most indicates the need for follow-up by the nurse?
- ○ **1.** "Maybe my colostomy won't have to be permanent."
- ○ **2.** "My perineal wound may not be healed when I go home."
- ○ **3.** "I will be able to have normal bowel movements from my colostomy."
- ○ **4.** "I will have 3 incisions."

315. Mr. Simms recovers from surgery. He is scheduled to return to the hospital in a month for a course of chemotherapy. Before leaving, he says to you, "I'm not sure I want to come back. Maybe I'll just take my chances." What would be the best response be?
- ○ **1.** "It is your decision, and you should do what you feel is right."
- ○ **2.** "What concerns you the most about coming back?"
- ○ **3.** "Have you discussed this with your wife and doctor?"
- ○ **4.** "The survival rate with adjuvant chemotherapy is quite high."

316. Mr. Simms is to be started on a regimen of 5-fluorouracil (5-FU). During the time that he is receiving this drug, it is most important to
- ○ **1.** force fluids to maintain a good output.
- ○ **2.** practice good asepsis to prevent him from getting an infection.
- ○ **3.** give frequent mouth care with lemon swabs.
- ○ **4.** monitor his blood pressure during drug administration.

Peggy Swan, a 52-year-old woman, is admitted to the emergency room in an unconscious state. She is accompanied by a friend. Mrs. Swan passed out while shopping. The nurse notes that she is exhibiting Biot's respirations, her color is fair, blood pressure is 120/80, temperature is 99.6°F (37.5°C) rectally, and there are no cuts or bruises. Her pupils react sluggishly to light and are unequal. The friend informs the nurse that Mrs. Swan has a history of hypertension and complained of a headache while they were shopping.

317. What action should the nurse do first?
- ○ **1.** Prepare a lumbar puncture setup.
- ○ **2.** Insert a Levin tube.
- ○ **3.** Start an IV after taking a blood sample to check her glucose level.
- ○ **4.** Send her to x-ray for a chest film.

318. Routine procedure for an unconscious client who has just been admitted should include
- ○ **1.** vital signs q15min till stable.
- ○ **2.** lumbar puncture.
- ○ **3.** emergency tracheostomy.
- ○ **4.** nasogastric tube insertion, flexing client's neck to close the epiglottis.

319. Unequal pupillary light reflexes in the unconscious client is *not* likely to be a symptom of
- ○ **1.** ketoacidosis.
- ○ **2.** brain contusion.
- ○ **3.** epidural hematoma.
- ○ **4.** brain tumor.

320. Biot's respirations can be best described as
- ○ **1.** shallow, then increasingly deep, in a pattern.
- ○ **2.** extremely slow and fairly regular.
- ○ **3.** totally irregular in rate and depth.
- ○ **4.** rapid and deep.

321. Mrs. Swan now is displaying decerebrate posturing in response to pressure on the trapezius muscle. Decerebrate posturing is exhibited by which of the following?
- ○ **1.** Extension of lower and upper extremities
- ○ **2.** Extension of lower and flexion of upper extremities
- ○ **3.** Flexion of lower and upper extremities
- ○ **4.** Flexion of lower and extension of upper extremities

322. The most likely cause of Mrs. Swan's condition is
- ○ **1.** meningitis.
- ○ **2.** intracranial hematoma.
- ○ **3.** diabetic ketoacidosis.
- ○ **4.** cerebral concussion.

323. Mrs. Swan is scheduled for a craniotomy. What is the most important aspect of her pre-op care?
- ○ **1.** Notify her relatives.
- ○ **2.** Assess and establish a neurologic baseline.
- ○ **3.** Obtain a complete history and physical.
- ○ **4.** Find out where the lesion is located.

324. What will be most important to include in Mrs. Swan's post-op nursing?
- ○ **1.** Maintenance of adequate respiratory function
- ○ **2.** Frequent pupil and neurologic checks
- ○ **3.** Dressing checks q8h
- ○ **4.** Vital signs q4h

325. Mrs. Swan's breathing is assisted by a respirator and she requires suctioning. She has been lying on her right side for 2 hours. The nurse should follow which of he following procedures?
- ○ **1.** Turn her to her other side, then suction her.
- ○ **2.** Suction her; then turn her.
- ○ **3.** Turn her to her back; then suction her.
- ○ **4.** Just suction her; position does not affect the procedure.

326. Which of the following is the most correct statement?
- ○ **1.** If an endotracheal tube is to be left in for an extended time, a tracheostomy is usually performed.
- ○ **2.** An IPPB machine may be used for ventilation in cardiopulmonary resuscitation.
- ○ **3.** Stroking the trachea helps inhibiting coughing.
- ○ **4.** Postural drainage should be performed immediately following meals.

327. Which of the following steps would be *inappropriate* when suctioning a client?
- ○ **1.** Use a sterile catheter.
- ○ **2.** Instruct the client to cough before you insert the catheter into the trachea.
- ○ **3.** Instill 5 to 10 ml of sterile normal saline into the trachea, if secretions are thick.
- ○ **4.** Suction the trachea after suctioning the mouth.

328. Which of the following is most correct about cuffed tracheostomy tubes?
- ○ **1.** Deflate the cuff before suctioning.
- ○ **2.** Suction the pharynx before the cuff is deflated.
- ○ **3.** A hissing sound is desirable.
- ○ **4.** Sterile normal saline is used to inflate the cuff.

329. Respirators are *not* routinely used for
- ○ **1.** respiratory failure.
- ○ **2.** correction of acidosis.
- ○ **3.** improvement of tidal volume.
- ○ **4.** treatment of spinal shock.

330. If the client "fights" the respirator, which of the following actions would *not* be appropriate?
- ○ **1.** Remove the respirator, ventilate with an Ambu bag, and then reinstate the respirator.
- ○ **2.** Check the respiratory rate and air flow.
- ○ **3.** Give morphine sulfate or muscle relaxants as ordered.
- ○ **4.** Restrain the client.

331. Which group of drugs does *not* cause respiratory depression?
- ○ **1.** Sedatives
- ○ **2.** Tranquilizers
- ○ **3.** Anti-inflammatories
- ○ **4.** Narcotics

During the first 8 hours following a head injury, Jack Water, aged 25, excretes 3,000 ml of urine; his fluid intake has been 800 ml, and no diuretics have been given.

332. The above clinical signs are probably indicative of
- ○ **1.** cerebral edema.
- ○ **2.** diabetes insipidus.
- ○ **3.** cerebral contusion.
- ○ **4.** cerebral concussion.

333. The affected area of Mr. Water's brain is probably the
- ○ **1.** anterior pituitary lobe.
- ○ **2.** cerebral cortex.
- ○ **3.** posterior pituitary lobe.
- ○ **4.** thalamus.

334. Although not immediately life threatening, the condition from which Mr. Water is suffering, if not treated, will lead to
- ○ **1.** increased intracranial pressure.
- ○ **2.** hypovolemia and electrolyte imbalance.
- ○ **3.** cerebral infection.
- ○ **4.** retrograde amnesia.

335. What would you expect the specific gravity of Mr. Water's urine to be?
- ◯ **1.** Low
- ◯ **2.** High
- ◯ **3.** Normal
- ◯ **4.** Variable

Elizabeth Allen, 88 years old, was admitted to the hospital with the diagnosis of a head injury. She had fallen and hit her head after suffering a transient ischemic attack (TIA).

336. The admitting nurse, after completing her assessment, notes all the following in the nurses' notes. Which one is *not* commonly found in clients who have suffered a TIA?
- ◯ **1.** Paresthesias
- ◯ **2.** Vertigo
- ◯ **3.** Tachycardia
- ◯ **4.** Disorientation

337. In planning care, the nurse knows that noninvasive diagnostic tests may be ordered to evaluate the TIAs. Which one of the following is considered an invasive test?
- ◯ **1.** Electroencephalogram
- ◯ **2.** CT scan
- ◯ **3.** Echoencephalogram
- ◯ **4.** Arteriogram

338. Four days after Mrs. Allen's admission, the nurse assesses a change in her behavior. She has become combative, abusive, and generally more maladaptive. This behavior most likely suggests injury to which lobe of the brain?
- ◯ **1.** Temporal
- ◯ **2.** Frontal
- ◯ **3.** Occipital
- ◯ **4.** Parietal

339. What would be the best nursing approach for Mrs. Allen at this time?
- ◯ **1.** Devise a reorientation program.
- ◯ **2.** Request a psychiatric consultation.
- ◯ **3.** Decrease the environmental stimuli.
- ◯ **4.** Assign someone to stay with her to prevent any physical injury.

Emma Brandt, 59 years old, was eating dinner when she suddenly was unable to lift her fork or speak clearly. Her husband rushed her to the hospital, where the examining physician found her to be unconscious and diagnosed her condition as a cerebrovascular accident (CVA).

340. While caring for Mrs. Brandt during her unconscious, acute stage, the nurse routinely assesses her status. Which is the most important assessment the nurse should make?
- ◯ **1.** Patency of airway and adequacy of respirations
- ◯ **2.** Pupillary reflexes
- ◯ **3.** Level of awareness
- ◯ **4.** Response to sensory stimulation, such as a pinprick on a lower extremity

341. On admission, Mrs. Brandt's vital signs were temperature 99.4°F (37.4°C), pulse 97, respirations 27, blood pressure 260/140 mm Hg. Based on these assessments, what is the most probable cause of the CVA?
- ◯ **1.** Obesity
- ◯ **2.** Kidney disease
- ◯ **3.** Hypertension
- ◯ **4.** Hypercholesterolemia

342. Which of the following best represent assessment priorities during Mrs. Brandt's admission process?
- ◯ **1.** Religion, marital status, insurance
- ◯ **2.** Level of consciousness, vital signs, motor function
- ◯ **3.** Medical and social history
- ◯ **4.** Vital capacity of the lungs

343. When preparing a bed and equipment for Mrs. Brandt's use, which one of the following is most important to include?
- ◯ **1.** Footboard
- ◯ **2.** Suction machine
- ◯ **3.** Bed-linen cradle
- ◯ **4.** Sandbags and trochanter rolls

344. Why should Mrs. Brandt receive frequent mouth care?
- ◯ **1.** She will experience severe thirst during the time that she is unable to take liquids orally.
- ◯ **2.** Her oral mucosa will become dried and cracked because of mouth breathing during coma.
- ◯ **3.** Her mouth may contain dried blood from having bitten her tongue or lips during a seizure.
- ◯ **4.** Tactile stimulation of the tongue and buccal mucosa will facilitate the return of consciousness.

345. While Mrs. Brandt is hospitalized, the nurse is concerned with preventing the complications of prolonged bed rest. Mrs. Brandt already has a reddened area over the sacrum and coccyx. The nurse knows that the most important action to prevent a decubitus ulcer is to
   ○ 1. keep the skin area clean, dry, and free from urine, feces, and perspiration.
   ○ 2. place an alternating-air-pressure or water mattress on the bed.
   ○ 3. massage the reddened area with lotion or oil to stimulate circulation.
   ○ 4. turn and reposition the client at least q2h; avoid positioning her on the affected side if possible.

346. Which of the following is the most correct statement about positioning the stroke client?
   ○ 1. Flexor muscles are generally stronger than extensors.
   ○ 2. Extensor muscles are generally stronger than flexors.
   ○ 3. The fingers should be flexed tightly.
   ○ 4. The footboard should be flush with the mattress.

Two days after Mrs. Brandt's admission, she has a steady rise in her temperature accompanied by a slow pulse and labile respirations.

347. What do these symptoms most likely suggest?
   ○ 1. Absorption of the clot in the damaged area of the brain
   ○ 2. Injury to the vital centers in the brain stem
   ○ 3. Development of hypostatic pneumonia
   ○ 4. Bacterial infection of the central nervous system

348. A lumbar puncture is ordered for Mrs. Brandt. During the procedure, in order to maintain the client in the proper position, the nurse should
   ○ 1. discourage distracting conversation among personnel.
   ○ 2. restrain the client's arms in a folded position over her chest.
   ○ 3. prevent plantar flexion of both the feet and toes.
   ○ 4. hold the client on her side and keep the uppermost shoulder from falling forward.

349. After reviewing the lab results of the spinal fluid, the nurse notes the following. Which result is *abnormal*?
   ○ 1. Specific gravity 1.007
   ○ 2. Glucose 60 mg
   ○ 3. Red blood cell count 20 to 50
   ○ 4. White blood cell count 2 to 5

350. As Mrs. Brandt's condition improves and she regains consciousness, her behavior becomes erratic. She frequently swears at the nurse who provides her daily care and cries without apparent cause. Mr. Brandt is very upset about his wife's unpredictable and often unpleasant behavior. What should the nurse explain to Mr. Brandt?
   ○ 1. She is probably suffering from emotional lability characteristic of clients with CVA.
   ○ 2. She is reacting to medications such as hydrochlorothiazide, which frequently cause behavior changes.
   ○ 3. She seems to be hostile and angry because of her illness; to avoid upsetting her, it is wisest for the family not to visit so frequently.
   ○ 4. She is in need of long-term psychiatric therapy.

A 35-year-old man is admitted to the emergency room following an auto accident with a possible spinal injury. The client, Joseph Reed, is conscious. He is unable to move his legs or his arms on command.

351. When transferring a client with a possible spinal cord injury, what is the most important consideration for the nurse to remember?
   ○ 1. Support the lower extremities, since they are likely to be weak or paralyzed.
   ○ 2. Explain what you are about to do, so the client can assist you.
   ○ 3. Support the back with additional pillows to prevent further spinal trauma.
   ○ 4. Immobilize the head and neck to prevent further spinal trauma.

352. Which of the following would be *absent* if Mr. Reed has spinal shock?
   ○ 1. Hypotension
   ○ 2. Hypertension
   ○ 3. Hyperthermia
   ○ 4. Dry skin

353. Mr. Reed has complete destruction of the spinal cord at C3-4. Select the most important action for a nurse caring for this kind of client in the acute stage following injury.
   ○ 1. Turn and position at least q2h.
   ○ 2. Immobilize the head and neck.
   ○ 3. Maintain a patent airway and adequate ventilation.
   ○ 4. Monitor renal output.

354. Immediately after his injury, Mr. Reed's bladder will
○ **1.** be spastic.
○ **2.** be atonic.
○ **3.** empty with slightest stimulus.
○ **4.** be normal.

355. Which one of the following statements is correct concerning the relationship between the branches of the autonomic nervous system?
○ **1.** The parasympathetic branch excites all systems, and the sympathetic inhibits all systems.
○ **2.** The parasympathetic branch excites most systems except the gastrointestinal tract and urinary bladder, and the sympathetic has the opposite effect.
○ **3.** The sympathetic branch stimulates most systems but inhibits the gastrointestinal tract and urinary bladder; the parasympathetic branch inhibits most systems but stimulates the gastrointestinal tract and urinary bladder.
○ **4.** There is no relationship between the two branches.

356. What is characteristic of a reflex arc?
○ **1.** Always includes a sensory and motor neuron
○ **2.** Always terminates in a muscle or gland
○ **3.** Always has its center in the brain or spinal cord
○ **4.** All the above are characteristic of a reflex arc.

357. When should the nurse expect Mr. Reed to exhibit mass reflex activity?
○ **1.** Immediately
○ **2.** In a few days
○ **3.** In a few months
○ **4.** Never

358. A bowel and bladder routine is to be established for Mr. Reed. He has had a Foley catheter and it is being clamped for intervals to increase bladder capacity. The plan is to use an external catheter and to teach him to stimulate voiding by stimulating his thigh. After the catheter has been clamped for 1 hour, Mr. Reed complains of a headache, is sweating, and has an elevated blood pressure. The most probable cause of these signs and symptoms is
○ **1.** hyperreflexia of parasympathetic system.
○ **2.** hyperreflexia of sympathetic system.
○ **3.** hyperreflexia of sensory system.
○ **4.** septicemia resulting from lack of flushing of bacteria from the bladder.

359. The most probable stimulus for this episode is
○ **1.** bowel distension.
○ **2.** stimulation of urinary sphincter by Foley catheter.
○ **3.** bladder distension.
○ **4.** fear.

360. Mr. Reed is progressing well with rehabilitation. He tells you that the dietitian has cautioned him about the amount of milk he drinks and told him that this could contribute to his problems with kidney stones. He says he is drinking no more than he did before the accident and wonders why it would be a problem now. The nurse's response should include which of the following facts?
○ **1.** He probably is drinking more milk than before and just does not realize it.
○ **2.** He has better absorption of calcium now than before the accident.
○ **3.** His kidneys are not clearing calcium as well as before surgery.
○ **4.** The lack of stress on the long bones causes demineralization and increases the amount of calcium to be cleared by the kidneys.

361. Mr. Reed asks how the injury is going to affect his sexual function. The nurse's response should include which of the following?
○ **1.** Normal sexual function is not possible.
○ **2.** His sexual functioning should not be impaired at all.
○ **3.** He will probably be able to have erections.
○ **4.** Ejaculation will be normal.

Eunice Raye, a 30-year-old homemaker, fell asleep while smoking a cigarette. She sustained severe burns of the face, neck, anterior chest, and both arms and hands.

362. Using the "rule of nines," which of the following is the best estimate of total body-surface area burned?
○ **1.** 18%
○ **2.** 22%
○ **3.** 31%
○ **4.** 40%

363. The nurse determines that Mrs. Raye has second- and third-degree burns. Which of the following would be characteristic of a fresh, second-degree burn?
○ **1.** Absence of pain and pressure sense
○ **2.** White or dark, dry, leathery appearance
○ **3.** Large thick blisters
○ **4.** Visible, thrombosed small vessels

364. Because of the location of Mrs. Raye's burns, what is the nurse's primary concern?
    ○ 1. Debride and dress the wounds.
    ○ 2. Initiate and administer antibiotics.
    ○ 3. Frequently observe for hoarseness, stridor, and dyspnea.
    ○ 4. Obtain a thorough history of events leading to the accident.

365. A narcotic IV was ordered to control Mrs. Raye's pain. Why was the IV route selected?
    ○ 1. Burns cause excruciating pain, requiring immediate relief.
    ○ 2. Circulatory blood volume is reduce, delaying absorption from subcutaneous and muscle tissue.
    ○ 3. Cardiac function is enhanced by immediate action of the drug.
    ○ 4. Metabolism of the drug would be delayed because of decreased insulin production.

366. A major goal during the first 48 hours is to prevent hypovolemic shock. Which of the following would *not* be a useful guide to fluid restitution during this period?
    ○ 1. Elevated hematocrit
    ○ 2. Urine output of 30 ml/hour
    ○ 3. Change in sensorium
    ○ 4. Estimate of fluid loss through the burn eschar

367. Mafenide acetate (Sulfamylon) is applied to Mrs. Raye's wounds every 12 hours. The nurse's assessment would include observation for which of the following side effects of this drug?
    ○ 1. Metabolic acidosis
    ○ 2. Discoloration of the skin
    ○ 3. Maceration of the skin
    ○ 4. Dehydration and electrolyte loss

368. Eventually, autografts are done. Care of the donor site would *not* include
    ○ 1. changing the dressing every shift.
    ○ 2. reporting any odor to the physician.
    ○ 3. using a heat lamp to dry the wound.
    ○ 4. exposing the mesh-covered wound to the air.

369. Contractures are among the most serious of the long-term complications of a burn. Because of the location of these burns, which of the following nursing measures would most likely cause Mrs. Raye to have contractures
    ○ 1. Change the location of the bed or the TV set or both daily.
    ○ 2. Encourage her to chew gum and blow up balloons.
    ○ 3. Avoid using a pillow or place the head in a position of hyperextension.
    ○ 4. Assist her to assume a position of comfort.

370. What is the primary aim of all burn-wound care?
    ○ 1. To debride the wound of dead tissue and eschar
    ○ 2. To limit fluid loss through the skin
    ○ 3. To prevent growth of microorganisms
    ○ 4. To decrease formation of disfiguring scars

Arnold Hamilton, aged 63, has recently received a diagnosis of Parkinson's syndrome.

371. The pathophysiology in parkinsonism is commonly believed found in which part of the brain?
    ○ 1. Medulla oblongata
    ○ 2. Thalamus
    ○ 3. Basal ganglia
    ○ 4. Brain stem

372. Parkinsonism is best characterized by
    ○ 1. progressive weakness and atrophy of muscles.
    ○ 2. weakness, visual impairment, and slurred speech.
    ○ 3. involuntary, tremulous motion.
    ○ 4. masklike, dry face.

373. A client's motor function can be best assessed in which of the following ways?
    ○ 1. Check the Babinski's reflex.
    ○ 2. Have the client count backwards from 100 by sevens.
    ○ 3. Have the client walk the length of the room.
    ○ 4. Test the knee jerk.

374. There are several forms of parkinsonism. The most common etiologic classification is
    ○ 1. idiopathic.
    ○ 2. postencephalitic.
    ○ 3. atherosclerotic.
    ○ 4. drug induced.

375. The last symptom to improve when levodopa is administered to a client with Parkinson's syndrome is which of the following?
- ○ **1.** Festinating gait
- ○ **2.** Seborrhea
- ○ **3.** Sialorrhea
- ○ **4.** Tremor

Leonard Vernon is a 30-year-old, admitted with a diagnosis of multiple sclerosis and worsening of symptoms.

376. In taking a history, which of the following complaints would the nurse consider most *atypical*?
- ○ **1.** Tremors
- ○ **2.** Pain
- ○ **3.** Incontinence
- ○ **4.** Numbness of hands

377. Mr. Vernon is started on a prednisone regimen. He states he has never been treated with this drug before and asks for general information. Which of the following pieces of information would *not* be correct to give?
- ○ **1.** The drug should make him feel better.
- ○ **2.** He will be taking it the rest of his life.
- ○ **3.** It might be working by decreasing edema around involved areas of the nervous systems.
- ○ **4.** The way in which it improves symptoms in multiple sclerosis is unknown.

A nurse in a department store notices a group of people gathered around a person lying on the floor having a seizure.

378. The best immediate response would be to
- ○ **1.** cradle the person's head in your lap.
- ○ **2.** place something in the person's mouth.
- ○ **3.** hold the person's arms down.
- ○ **4.** move the person to a place of safety.

379. Which type of seizure is frequently preceded by an aura?
- ○ **1.** Jacksonian
- ○ **2.** Petit mal
- ○ **3.** Major
- ○ **4.** Focal

380. All but one of the following statements concerning epilepsy (recurrent seizures) are true. Identify the *false* statement.
- ○ **1.** Epilepsy is a disease that afflicts about 1 in every 200 Americans.
- ○ **2.** Epilepsy can be controlled by medications in all cases.
- ○ **3.** There is still a stigma connected with the term epilepsy.
- ○ **4.** The causes of most cases of epilepsy remain unknown.

381. Which of the following tests furnishes the best diagnostic information about seizures?
- ○ **1.** Pneumonencephalogram
- ○ **2.** Electroencephalogram
- ○ **3.** Cerebral angiogram
- ○ **4.** Cerebral tomography

382. What is the most common reason why clients suffer from sudden seizure recurrence?
- ○ **1.** Extreme physical or emotional stress
- ○ **2.** Alcoholic beverages in excess
- ○ **3.** Premenstrual fluid retention
- ○ **4.** Noncompliance with medication schedules

383. When one seizure after another occurs without the client's regaining consciousness between seizures, it is called
- ○ **1.** frequent seizures.
- ○ **2.** febrile seizures.
- ○ **3.** status epilepticus.
- ○ **4.** petit mal seizures.

Foster Williams, a 55-year-old black man, was admitted to the hospital in acute respiratory distress. His condition had previously been diagnosed as myasthenia gravis.

384. The emergency room treatment of a client with severe weakness related to myasthenia gravis should focus on
- ○ **1.** renal failure.
- ○ **2.** reversing coma.
- ○ **3.** restoring blood volume.
- ○ **4.** ventilation.

385. Which of the following is *not* a reliable assessment parameter for cyanosis in dark-skinned persons?
- ○ **1.** Conjunctiva and oral mucosa
- ○ **2.** Nail beds
- ○ **3.** Hard palate
- ○ **4.** Behavioral responses to hypoxia

386. What is the primary nursing approach in the care of Mr. Williams?
    ○ 1. Prevent contractures and atrophy of muscles.
    ○ 2. Decrease environmental stimuli.
    ○ 3. Maintain open and optimal respirations.
    ○ 4. Foster communication with significant others.

387. An IV was started on Mr. Williams in the emergency room, but he started to complain of pain at the site upon admission to the unit. Which of the following is not likely to be an indication of an infiltrated IV in this client?
    ○ 1. Pain on touch
    ○ 2. Redness at the IV site
    ○ 3. Edema at the site
    ○ 4. No blood return when lowering the IV bottle

388. The following day the physician orders hydrocortisone sodium succinate (Solu-Cortef). What is the purpose of this medication in this situation?
    ○ 1. Decrease hypercapnia
    ○ 2. Relax smooth muscle and produce diuresis
    ○ 3. Support the body through crisis by reducing the inflammatory response
    ○ 4. Decrease client anxiety

389. Cholinergic drugs act directly and indirectly to produce the same type of effects as which neurohormone?
    ○ 1. Norepinephrine
    ○ 2. Acetylcholine
    ○ 3. Epinephrine
    ○ 4. Acetylcholinesterase

390. Cholinergic agents act on effector organs to produce three of the following reactions. Which one is *not* an outcome of cholinergic drug administration?
    ○ 1. Increased motility and tone of smooth muscles in the gastrointestinal tract
    ○ 2. Increased mucus secretion, sweating, and salivation
    ○ 3. Increased heart rate and constriction of blood vessels
    ○ 4. Miosis and a reduction in intraocular pressure

The head nurse of an eye and ear clinic is orienting nursing students.

391. Normal visual acuity as measured with a Snellen eye chart is 20/20. What does a visual acuity of 20/30 indicate?
    ○ 1. At 20 feet, an individual can only read letters large enough to be read at 30 feet
    ○ 2. At 30 feet, an individual can read letters small enough to be read at 20 feet
    ○ 3. An individual can read 20 out of 30 total letters on the chart
    ○ 4. An individual can read 30 out of 50 total letters on the chart at 20 feet.

392. Damage to the visual area of the occipital lobe of the cerebrum, on the *left* side, would produce what type of visual loss?
    ○ 1. Left eye only
    ○ 2. Right eye only
    ○ 3. Medial half of the right eye and lateral half of the left eye
    ○ 4. Medial half of the left eye and lateral half of the right eye

393. The anterior chamber of the eye refers to all the space in what area?
    ○ 1. Anterior to the retina
    ○ 2. Between the iris and the cornea
    ○ 3. Between the lens and the cornea
    ○ 4. Between the lens and the iris

394. What condition results when rays of light are focused in front of the retina?
    ○ 1. Myopia
    ○ 2. Hyperopia
    ○ 3. Presbyopia
    ○ 4. Emmetropia

395. As the person grows older, the lens loses its elasticity, causing which kind of farsightedness?
    ○ 1. Emmetropia
    ○ 2. Presbyopia
    ○ 3. Diplopia
    ○ 4. Myopia

396. If a person has a foreign object of unknown material that is not readily seen in one eye, what should the first action be?
    ○ 1. Irrigate the eye with a boric acid solution.
    ○ 2. Examine the lower eyelid and then the upper eyelid.
    ○ 3. Irrigate the eye with copious amounts of water.
    ○ 4. Cover the eye with a tight eye patch and seek medical help.

397. A sudden loss of an area of vision, as if a curtain were being drawn, is a principal symptom of
○ **1.** retinal detachment.
○ **2.** glaucoma.
○ **3.** cataract.
○ **4.** keratitis.

398. Post-op care for a client following a stapedectomy would *not* include which of the following?
○ **1.** Out of bed as desired
○ **2.** No moisture in the affected ear
○ **3.** Avoid sneezing
○ **4.** No bending over or lifting of heavy objects

399. Dimenhydrinate (Dramamine) is given after a stapedectomy
○ **1.** to accelerate the auditory process.
○ **2.** to dull the pain experienced when the semicircular canal is disturbed.
○ **3.** to minimize the sensations of equilibrium disturbances and imbalance.
○ **4.** to prevent an increased tendency toward nausea.

400. Why is there no hearing loss after a myringotomy?
○ **1.** The procedure involves just washing out the ear.
○ **2.** The procedure involves removing fluid from the outer ear.
○ **3.** The procedure involves cutting the tympanic membrane, but it heals very quickly.
○ **4.** The procedure requires removing the tympanic membrane and putting a new membrane in.

401. A client with Ménière's syndrome is extremely uncomfortable because of which of
○ **1.** severe earache.
○ **2.** many perceptual difficulties.
○ **3.** vertigo and resultant nausea.
○ **4.** facial paralysis.

Ona Clark is admitted for cataract extraction.

402. What is a cataract of the eye?
○ **1.** Opacity of the cornea
○ **2.** Clouding of the aqueous humor
○ **3.** Opacity of the lens
○ **4.** Papilledema

403. Treatment of a cataract is primarily concerned with which of the following?
○ **1.** Instillation of miotics
○ **2.** Instillation of mydriatics
○ **3.** Removal of the lens
○ **4.** Enucleation

404. Pre-op instruction will *not* need to include
○ **1.** type of surgery.
○ **2.** how to use the call bell.
○ **3.** how to prevent paralytic ileus.
○ **4.** how to prevent respiratory infections.

405. In preparing to teach Mrs. Cook about adjustment to cataract lenses, the nurse needs to know that the lenses will
○ **1.** magnify objects one third with central vision.
○ **2.** magnify objects one third with peripheral vision.
○ **3.** reduce objects one third with central vision.
○ **4.** reduce objects one third with peripheral vision.

406. In the immediate post-op period, the one action that is contraindicated for Mrs. Clark compared with clients after most other operations is which of the following?
○ **1.** Coughing
○ **2.** Turning on the unoperative side
○ **3.** Measures to control nausea and vomiting
○ **4.** Eating after nausea passes

407. Immediate nursing care following cataract extraction is directed primarily toward preventing
○ **1.** atelectasis.
○ **2.** infection of the cornea.
○ **3.** hemorrhage.
○ **4.** prolapse of the iris.

408. Mrs. Clark is confused her first night after eye surgery. What should the nurse do?
○ **1.** Tell her to stay in bed.
○ **2.** Apply restraints to keep her in bed.
○ **3.** Explain why she can not get out of bed, keep side rails up, and check her frequently.
○ **4.** Give her the sedation.

409. Discharge teaching for Mrs. Clark would probably *not* need to include
○ **1.** staying in a darkened room as much as possible.
○ **2.** avoiding alcoholic drinks; limiting the use of tea and coffee.
○ **3.** using no eye washes or drops unless they were prescribed by the physician.
○ **4.** avoiding being excessively sedentary.

410. Mrs. Clark also needs to be instructed to limit
○ **1.** sewing.
○ **2.** watching TV.
○ **3.** walking.
○ **4.** weeding her garden.

Helen Kowalski visits her ophthalmologist and receives a mydriatric in order to facilitate the examination. After returning home, she experiences severe eye pain, nausea and vomiting, and blurred vision. During a visit to the emergency room, a diagnosis of acute glaucoma is made.

411. Mrs. Kowalski's glaucoma has been caused by
- ○ **1.** blockage of the outflow of aqueous humor by the dilation of the pupil.
- ○ **2.** blockage of the outflow of aqueous humor by the constriction of the pupil.
- ○ **3.** increased intraocular pressure resulting from the increased production of aqueous humor.
- ○ **4.** decreased intraocular pressure resulting from decreased production of aqueous humor.

412. Intraocular pressure is measured clinically by a tonometer. What tonometer reading would be indicative of glaucoma?
- ○ **1.** Pressure of 10 mm Hg
- ○ **2.** Pressure of 15 mm Hg
- ○ **3.** Pressure of 20 mm Hg
- ○ **4.** Pressure of 25 mm Hg

413. Which cranial nerve transmits visual impulses?
- ○ **1.** I
- ○ **2.** II
- ○ **3.** III
- ○ **4.** IV

414. Untreated or uncontrolled glaucoma damages the optic nerve. Three of the following signs and symptoms result from optic nerve atrophy; which one does *not*?
- ○ **1.** Colored halos around lights
- ○ **2.** Severe pain in the eye
- ○ **3.** Dilated and fixed pupils
- ○ **4.** Opacity of the lens

415. Glaucoma is conservatively managed with miotic eye drops. Mydriatic eye drops are contraindicated for glaucoma. Which of the following drugs is a mydriatic?
- ○ **1.** Neostigmine
- ○ **2.** Pilocarpine
- ○ **3.** Physostigmine
- ○ **4.** Atropine

416. Glaucoma may require surgical treatment. Preoperatively, the client should be taught to expect which of the following postoperatively?
- ○ **1.** Cough and deep breathe qh
- ○ **2.** Turn only to the unaffected side
- ○ **3.** Medication for severe eye pain
- ○ **4.** Restriction of fluids for the first 24 hours

Allen James, a 55-year-old man, is admitted to the hospital with wide-angle glaucoma.

417. What was the symptom that probably brought Mr. James to the ophthalmologist initially?
- ○ **1.** Decreasing vision
- ○ **2.** Extreme pain in the eye
- ○ **3.** Redness and tearing of the eye
- ○ **4.** Seeing colored flashes of light

418. The teaching plan for Mr. James should include which of the following?
- ○ **1.** Reduce fluid intake.
- ○ **2.** Add extra lighting in the home.
- ○ **3.** Wear dark glasses during the day.
- ○ **4.** Avoid exercise.

419. Miotics are used in the treatment of glaucoma. What is an example of a commonly used miotic?
- ○ **1.** Atropine
- ○ **2.** Pilocarpine
- ○ **3.** Acetazolamide (Diamox)
- ○ **4.** Scopolamine

420. What is the rationale for using miotics in the treatment of glaucoma?
- ○ **1.** They decrease the rate of aqueous humor production.
- ○ **2.** Pupil constriction increases outflow of aqueous humor.
- ○ **3.** Increased pupil size relaxes the ciliary muscles.
- ○ **4.** The blood flow to the conjunctiva is increased.

421. When instilling eye drops for a client with glaucoma, what procedure should the nurse follow?
- ○ **1.** Place the medication in the middle of the lower lid and put pressure on the lacrimal duct after instillation.
- ○ **2.** Instill the drug at the outer angle of the eye; have client tilt head back.
- ○ **3.** Instill the drug at the most inner angle; wipe with cotton away from inner aspect.
- ○ **4.** Instill medication in middle of eye; have client blink for better absorption.

422. Carbonic anhydrase inhibitors are sometimes used in the treatment of glaucoma because they
- ○ **1.** depress secretion of aqueous humor.
- ○ **2.** dilate the pupil.
- ○ **3.** paralyze power of accommodation.
- ○ **4.** increase the power of accommodation.

423. Teaching a client with glaucoma will *not* include which of the following?
- ○ **1.** Vision can be restored only if the client remains under a physician's care.
- ○ **2.** Avoid stimulants, e.g., caffeine.
- ○ **3.** Take all medications conscientiously.
- ○ **4.** Prevent constipation, and avoid heavy lifting and emotional excitement.

424. Glaucoma is a progressive disease that can lead to blindness. It can be managed if diagnosed early. Preventive health teaching would best include which of the following points?
- ○ **1.** Early surgical action may be necessary.
- ○ **2.** All clients over 40 years of age should have an annual tonometry exam.
- ○ **3.** The use of contact lens in older clients is not advisable.
- ○ **4.** Clients should seek early treatment for eye infections.

425. A client with progressive glaucoma may be experiencing sensory deprivation. Which of the following actions would best minimize this problem?
- ○ **1.** Speak in a louder voice.
- ○ **2.** Ensure that a sedative is ordered.
- ○ **3.** Orient the client to time, place, person.
- ○ **4.** Use touch frequently when providing care.

Brenda Bates is a 20-year-old college student, who is self-conscious about the appearance of her nose. She is admitted to the hospital for an elective rhinoplasty.

426. Nursing management following rhinoplasty will *not* include which of the following?
- ○ **1.** Elevate the head of the bed.
- ○ **2.** Check the gag reflex.
- ○ **3.** Observe for frequent swallowing.
- ○ **4.** Monitor the HemoVac suction.

427. While caring for Mrs. Bates, the nurse observes one small, tarry stool. What is the most appropriate nursing action?
- ○ **1.** Call the physician immediately.
- ○ **2.** Administer analgesics.
- ○ **3.** Observe for signs of fresh bleeding.
- ○ **4.** Check her gag reflex.

428. Prior to her discharge, the nurse should instruct Mrs. Bates to
- ○ **1.** "Avoid blowing your nose for 3 to 4 days."
- ○ **2.** "Resume your prior activities immediately."
- ○ **3.** "Limit your fluid intake for 1 week."
- ○ **4.** "Take aspirin if you observe increased pain and swelling."

Claude Rollins is seen in the emergency room with the diagnosis of epistaxis.

429. It is unlikely that Mr. Rollins's history will include
- ○ **1.** minor trauma to the nose.
- ○ **2.** a deviated septum.
- ○ **3.** acute sinusitis.
- ○ **4.** hypotension.

430. Which of the following medications would be used with Mr. Rollins in order to promote vasoconstriction and control bleeding?
- ○ **1.** Epinephrine
- ○ **2.** Lidocaine (Xylocaine)
- ○ **3.** Pilocarpine
- ○ **4.** Cyclopentolate HCl (Cyclogyl)

431. Which of the following positions would be most desirable for Mr. Rollins?
- ○ **1.** Trendelenburg's, to control shock
- ○ **2.** A sitting position, unless he is hypotensive
- ○ **3.** Side-lying, to prevent aspiration
- ○ **4.** Prone, to prevent aspiration

432. The physician decides to insert nasal packing. Of the following nursing actions, which would have the highest priority?
- ○ **1.** Encourage Mr. Rollins to breathe through his mouth, as he may feel panicky after the insertion.
- ○ **2.** Advise Mr. Rollins to expectorate the blood in the nasopharynx gently and not to swallow it.
- ○ **3.** Periodically check the position of the nasal packing, as airway obstruction can occur if the packing accidentally slips out of place.
- ○ **4.** Take rectal temperatures, as he must rely on mouth breathing and would be unable to keep his mouth closed on the thermometer.

433. After bleeding has been controlled, Mr. Rollins is taken to surgery to correct a deviated nasal septum. Which of the following is a likely complication of this surgery?
- ○ **1.** Loss of the ability to smell
- ○ **2.** Inability to breathe through the nose
- ○ **3.** Infection
- ○ **4.** Hemorrhage

434. Upon his discharge, the nurse instructs Mr. Rollins on the use of vasoconstrictive nose drops and cautions him to avoid too frequent and excessive use of these drugs. Which of the following provides the best rationale for this caution?
- ○ **1.** A rebound effect occurs in which stuffiness worsens after each successive dose.
- ○ **2.** Cocaine, a frequent ingredient in nose drops, may lead to psychologic addiction.
- ○ **3.** These medications may be absorbed systemically, causing severe hypotension.
- ○ **4.** Persistent vasoconstriction of the nasal mucosa can lead to alterations in the olfactory nerve.

Mary Hayes has had radical head and neck surgery for cancer of the larynx.

435. Mrs. Hayes has a tracheostomy. When suctioning the tracheostomy, which of the following is *not* correct?
- ○ **1.** Use sterile technique.
- ○ **2.** Turn head to right to suction left bronchus.
- ○ **3.** Suction for 10 to 15 seconds.
- ○ **4.** Observe for tachycardia.

436. Mrs. Hayes requires both nasopharyngeal suctioning and suctioning through the laryngectomy tube. When doing these two procedures at the same time, the nurse should *not* do which of the following?
- ○ **1.** Use a sterile suction setup.
- ○ **2.** Suction the nose first, then the laryngectomy tube.
- ○ **3.** Suction the laryngectomy tube first, then the nose.
- ○ **4.** Lubricate the catheter with saline.

437. A nasogastric tube is used to provide Mrs. Hayes with fluids and nutrients for approximately 10 days, for which of the following reasons?
- ○ **1.** To prevent pain while swallowing
- ○ **2.** To prevent contamination of the suture line
- ○ **3.** To decrease need for swallowing
- ○ **4.** To prevent need for holding head up to eat

438. Acidosis would most likely follow which condition?
- ○ **1.** Excessive loss of sodium and potassium ions in diarrhea
- ○ **2.** Loss of hydrogen and chloride ions in vomiting
- ○ **3.** Excessive conservation of bicarbonate in urine
- ○ **4.** Increased loss of carbon dioxide with hyperventilation

439. Mrs. Hayes's children are concerned about their own risk of developing cancer. All but one of the following are facts that describe malignant neoplasia and must be considered by the nurse in her responses. Which one is *incorrect*?
- ○ **1.** Familial factors may influence an individual's susceptibility to neoplasia.
- ○ **2.** Long-term use of corticosteriods enhances the body's defense against the development of cancer.
- ○ **3.** Sexual differences influence an individual's susceptibility to specific neoplasms.
- ○ **4.** Living in industrialized areas increases an individual's susceptibility to a malignant neoplasm.

440. When would Mrs. Hayes best begin speech rehabilitation?
- ○ **1.** When she leaves the hospital
- ○ **2.** When the esophageal suture line is healed
- ○ **3.** Three months after surgery
- ○ **4.** When she regains all her strength

David Wilson, a 24-year-old client, sustained a compound fracture of the shaft of the right femur in a motorcycle accident. Paramedics reach the scene and administer emergency treatment, which includes the application of a splint.

441. How should the splint be applied?
- ○ **1.** Apply it while the limb is in good alignment
- ○ **2.** Apply it to the limb in the position in which it is found
- ○ **3.** Extending from the fracture site downward
- ○ **4.** Extending from the fracture site upward

442. Mr. Wilson is brought to the emergency room. What is the first thing the emergency room nurse should do?
- ○ **1.** Cover the open wounds.
- ○ **2.** Take his blood pressure.
- ○ **3.** Clean the fracture site.
- ○ **4.** Assess his respiratory status.

443. After an open reduction of his fracture, Mr. Wilson displayed the following symptoms postoperatively: an increase in blood pressure, signs of confusion, and increased restlessness. Which one of the following would the nurse most likely suspect?
- ○ **1.** Concussion
- ○ **2.** Impending shock
- ○ **3.** Fat emboli
- ○ **4.** Anxiety

Henry Kahn, aged 45, was in an auto accident and suffered a fracture of the tibia and fibula. He was taken to surgery for an open reduction with internal fixation. He arrived in the orthopedic unit with a cast extending from above the knee to below the ankle.

444. Mr. Kahn is cautioned to be careful of the cast until it is dry. A dry cast has which of the following characteristics?
- ○ **1.** Gray, dull, a musty odor
- ○ **2.** Gray, shiny, a musty odor
- ○ **3.** White, shiny, odorless
- ○ **4.** White, dull, tends to flake off when scratched

445. Which of the following is the recommended method of drying Mr. Kahn's cast?
- ○ **1.** Place a radiation heat lamp about 1 foot from the cast.
- ○ **2.** Cover the extremity with an electric heat cradle.
- ○ **3.** Place an electric fan at the food of the bed.
- ○ **4.** Leave the cast uncovered in a well-ventilated room.

446. Which of the following is an *inappropriate* nursing action during the first 24 to 48 hours?
- ○ **1.** Handle the cast with the palms of the hand.
- ○ **2.** Place the casted extremity in normal alignment.
- ○ **3.** Place rubber-covered pillows under the cast.
- ○ **4.** Elevate the entire extremity.

447. When Mr. Kahn returned from surgery, there were 2 small blood stains on the cast. Four hours later the stains double in size. What should the nurse do?
- ○ **1.** Call the physician.
- ○ **2.** Outline the spots with a pencil; note the time and date on the cast.
- ○ **3.** Cut a window in the cast to observe the site.
- ○ **4.** Record the amount of bleeding in the nurses' notes only.

448. On the first post-op day, Mr. Kahn complains of a burning pain in one spot under the cast. The nurse should suspect which of the following as the source of the discomfort?
- ○ **1.** Skin irritation from a pressure spot
- ○ **2.** A burn from the cast
- ○ **3.** An infection in the operative site
- ○ **4.** Hemorrhage from the incision

449. The first indication of an infection in Mr. Kahn's leg would most likely be
- ○ **1.** an elevated temperature.
- ○ **2.** an unpleasant odor.
- ○ **3.** redness and heat above and below the cast.
- ○ **4.** purulent drainage on the cast.

450. Mr. Kahn is at risk for peroneal nerve palsy. Which of the following is *not* characteristic of this complication?
- ○ **1.** Inability to dorsiflex the foot and extend the toes
- ○ **2.** Numbness in the webbed space between the first and second toe
- ○ **3.** Inability to touch the heel to the floor when standing
- ○ **4.** Cyanotic toes

451. Before discharge, Mr. Kahn asks how to clean his cast. How should the nurse reply?
- ○ **1.** ''Cover the soiled area with shoe polish.''
- ○ **2.** ''Spray the cast with shellac.''
- ○ **3.** ''Wipe the soiled area with a cloth moistened with alcohol.''
- ○ **4.** ''Clean soiled areas with a small amount of Bon Ami and a damp cloth.''

Megan Carey slipped on some grease on her kitchen floor and fractured the proximal end of the ulna. There was extensive soft tissue damage in the fracture area. A cast was applied in the emergency department.

452. Because of the location and type of fracture, Mrs. Carey is most at risk for the complication of compartment syndrome. Which of the following would be the earliest indication of this phenomenon?
- ○ **1.** Absence of the pulse distal to the fracture
- ○ **2.** Pallor of the extremity
- ○ **3.** Paralysis of the hand
- ○ **4.** Progressive pain unrelieved by analgesics

453. If Mrs. Carey experiences the symptoms of compartment syndrome, which of the following is the recommended course of action?
- ○ **1.** Bivalve the cast and wrap it loosely with an elastic bandage.
- ○ **2.** Apply hot packs to improve venous circulation.
- ○ **3.** Administer diuretics to reduce edema.
- ○ **4.** Encourage flexion and extension of the fingers on the affected arm.

454. If compartment syndrome is not recognized and treated early, what is the probable outcome?
- ○ **1.** Gangrene will develop.
- ○ **2.** A paralyzed and deformed arm with a claw-like hand results.
- ○ **3.** Healing of the fracture is delayed.
- ○ **4.** Cast syndrome will result.

Elaina Balinski is a 78-year-old woman who was admitted because of dehydration. In the hospital, she was reaching for a glass of water when she fell out of bed and fractured the neck of the femur.

455. Mrs. Balinski is at risk of suffering serious complications. What assessments are characteristic of a fat embolus after a fracture?
- ○ **1.** Severe, stabbing chest pain 10 days post-fracture
- ○ **2.** Frothy sputum
- ○ **3.** Petechiae across the chest and shoulders 24 hours postfracture
- ○ **4.** Hypertension and coma

456. What is the most common reason why elderly women sustain hip fractures?
- ○ **1.** Decreased intake of calcium
- ○ **2.** Lack of muscles
- ○ **3.** Decreased production of bone marrow
- ○ **4.** Osteoporosis

457. Buck's extension was applied to Mrs. Balinski's fractured leg. Which of the following is an *inappropriate* reason for using Buck's traction?
- ○ **1.** Reduces muscle spasms and pain
- ○ **2.** Prevents further soft-tissue damage
- ○ **3.** Reduces the fracture
- ○ **4.** Immobilizes the leg while the dehydration is being treated

458. Buck's traction would be contraindicated if Mrs. Balinski experienced which of the following?
- ○ **1.** Arthritis
- ○ **2.** Bilateral lower leg ulcers
- ○ **3.** Pelvic pain
- ○ **4.** Deformity of the affected leg

459. A plan of care for Mrs. Balinski would include which of the following?
- ○ **1.** Remove the traction every shift to observe for pressure areas and provide skin care.
- ○ **2.** Turn her to the unaffected side for back care.
- ○ **3.** Elevate the head of the bed to apply countertraction.
- ○ **4.** Raise the knee gatch to prevent her sliding down in bed.

460. When a client is immobilized, what is the most appropriate plan to prevent constipation?
- ○ **1.** Encourage daily laxative use.
- ○ **2.** Limit fluid intake.
- ○ **3.** Encourage frequent periods of sitting on the bedpan.
- ○ **4.** Increase the fiber in the client's diet.

461. Which of the following is an *inappropriate* statement concerning avascular necrosis of the femoral head?
- ○ **1.** It is often a complication of total hip replacement.
- ○ **2.** It results from impaired circulation.
- ○ **3.** Pain in the groin may be the first symptom in adults.
- ○ **4.** Restriction of abduction and internal rotation can occur.

Arnold Jessup had a standard above-the-knee amputation (AKA) with an immediate prosthesis fitting.

462. The surgeon's final decision on the level of Mr. Jessup's amputation is based on
- ○ **1.** saving all possible length and tissue of the extremity.
- ○ **2.** results of diagnostic tests such as an arteriography.
- ○ **3.** observation of vascularity of tissue on the operating table.
- ○ **4.** the best level to facilitate fitting with a prosthesis.

463. During Mr. Jessup's fifth post-op day, his rigid dressing falls off. What is the nurse's first course of action?
- ○ **1.** Call the physician.
- ○ **2.** Apply an elastic bandage firmly.
- ○ **3.** Apply a saline dressing.
- ○ **4.** Elevate the limb on a pillow.

464. The nurse includes the important measures for stump care in the teaching plan for Mr. Jessup. Which measures would be *inappropriate* for the teaching plan?
- ○ **1.** Wash, dry, and inspect the stump daily.
- ○ **2.** Treat superficial abrasions and blisters promptly.
- ○ **3.** Apply a "shrinker" bandage with tighter turns around the proximal end of the affected limb.
- ○ **4.** Toughen the stump by pushing it against a progressively harder substance (e.g., pillow on a footstool).

Ron Gillman's left arm was badly mutilated in a boating accident and has been amputated just below the shoulder.

465. While the nurse is checking Mr. Gillman's dressing, he says he is anxious and asks to have both his hands held. Which of the following is the nurse's best response?
- ○ **1.** "Mr. Gillman, I'm holding your hand."
- ○ **2.** "Your left hand and arm were amputated the day of the boating accident."
- ○ **3.** "Your dressing is dry and clean where the doctors removed your arm."
- ○ **4.** "Many persons think their missing extremity is still present immediately after surgery."

466. How can the nurse best help Mr. Gillman adapt to his new body image?
- ○ **1.** Have him think of how he would like to look.
- ○ **2.** Talk to his wife about his change in body image.
- ○ **3.** Have him write about his feelings.
- ○ **4.** Have him touch and reorient himself to his body.

Alice Balio, 65 years old, came to the clinic for a routine checkup. She is 5 ft 4 in tall and weighs 180 lb. Her major complaint is pain in her joints. She is retired and has had to give up her volunteer work because of her discomfort. She was told her diagnosis was osteoarthritis about 5 years ago.

467. Which of the following is *least* characteristic of osteoarthritis?
- ○ **1.** It most commonly affects the weight-bearing joints.
- ○ **2.** Stiffness lasts about 15 minutes after a period of inactivity.
- ○ **3.** Joint effusion and crepitus are often present.
- ○ **4.** Inflammation and systemic symptoms are apparent.

468. Which of the following would be *inappropriate* to include on the care plan for Mrs. Balio?
- ○ **1.** Decrease the calorie count of her daily diet.
- ○ **2.** Take warm baths when arising.
- ○ **3.** Slide items across the floor rather than lift them.
- ○ **4.** Place items so that it is necessary to bend or stretch to reach them.

469. The drug of choice for the treatment of arthritis is aspirin. Mrs. Balio's knowledge concerning aspirin is correct if she repeats which of the following?
- ○ **1.** Avoid enteric-coated aspirin if gastrointestinal discomfort occurs.
- ○ **2.** Take as many as 12 to 16 tablets every day on a regularly scheduled basis.
- ○ **3.** Increase the amount taken if there is ringing in the ears.
- ○ **4.** Absence of sensitivity to aspirin over time ensures continued safety.

Matt Flore is a young adult admitted from the emergency department with severe pain and edema in the right foot. His diagnosis is gouty arthritis.

470. Which of the following is most characteristic of gout?
- ○ **1.** It is a familial metabolic disorder of purine metabolism.
- ○ **2.** Ninety-five percent of the clients with gout are men between 18 and 30.
- ○ **3.** Urate crystal deposits cause a foreign body reaction in the plasma.
- ○ **4.** It usually occurs in previously traumatized joints.

471. When developing a plan of care, which of the following would have the highest priority?
- ○ **1.** Apply hot compresses to the affected joints.
- ○ **2.** Stress the importance of maintaining good posture to prevent deformities.
- ○ **3.** Administer salicylates to minimize the inflammatory reaction.
- ○ **4.** Ensure an intake of at least 3,000 ml fluid/day.

472. Which of the following dietary practices would be most appropriate for Mr. Flore?
- ○ **1.** Permanently restrict foods high in purine.
- ○ **2.** Restrict foods high in purine only during the acute phase.
- ○ **3.** Permanently restrict ingestion of alcohol and all rich foods.
- ○ **4.** Ingest foods that will keep the urine acidic.

The nurse in a cancer-prevention and screening clinic is responsible for health education.

473. Which of the following is *not* one of the 7 warning signs of cancer cited by the American Cancer Society?
- ○ **1.** Indigestion or difficulty swallowing
- ○ **2.** Unusually slow healing sore
- ○ **3.** Unusual bleeding or discharge
- ○ **4.** Unusual tenderness in breast tissue

474. In the education class, the 7 safeguards against cancer are discussed. Which response from a group member best indicates correct understanding of the guidelines from the American Cancer Society?
    ○ 1. "Both men and women should check their breasts for thickening or lumps at least every 3 months."
    ○ 2. "Lots of sunshine is healthy for me, as long as I wear a sunscreening tanning lotion."
    ○ 3. "I should have my mouth and teeth examined once a year."
    ○ 4. "Adults should have an annual physical examination and chest x-ray."

475. A 40-year-old woman in the class asks what part of her body the cell sample is taken from for her yearly Pap smear. The nurse replies that the cells are scraped from the
    ○ 1. cervix.
    ○ 2. uterus.
    ○ 3. vagina.
    ○ 4. fallopian tubes.

476. If a client receives a Pap smear report that is Class I, what should the nurse advise?
    ○ 1. Call the physician for more specific results.
    ○ 2. Prepare to go to the hospital for surgery.
    ○ 3. Refrain from sexual activity.
    ○ 4. Return for another Pap smear in 1 year.

477. One of the best screening procedures for colorectal cancer is a
    ○ 1. barium enema for change in bowel pattern.
    ○ 2. home Hemoccult test.
    ○ 3. yearly proctosigmoidoscopy.
    ○ 4. digital rectal self-examination.

478. The most useful screening method for bronchogenic carcinoma is which of the following?
    ○ 1. Chest x-ray
    ○ 2. Sputum examination for cytology
    ○ 3. Bronchoscopy
    ○ 4. Scalene-node biopsy

479. Three of the following statements are true about bronchogenic carcinoma. Which one is *incorrect*?
    ○ 1. Diagnosis is difficult to make, because symptoms are often exactly like those of benign respiratory disease.
    ○ 2. Diagnosis is difficult, because the earliest signs are bizarre and unrelated to respiratory insufficiency.
    ○ 3. Of those treated surgically, 40% reach 5-year survival.
    ○ 4. Treatment is nearly exclusively palliative.

Robert Varella is 54 years old and is admitted to the hospital for suspected colon cancer.

480. During the pre-op period, what is the most important aspect of Mr. Varella's nursing care?
    ○ 1. Assure Mr. Varella that he will be cured of cancer.
    ○ 2. Assess understanding of the procedure and expectation of bodily appearance after surgery.
    ○ 3. Maintain a cheerful and optimistic environment.
    ○ 4. Keep visitors to a minimum, so that he can have time to think things through.

481. Mr. Varella is found to have adenocarcinoma of the rectum. An abdominoperineal resection with a colostomy will be done. What surgical principle is applied when surgery is performed to cure or control cancer?
    ○ 1. A margin of normal, healthy tissue must surround the tumor at the time of resection.
    ○ 2. More tissue than necessary is removed to ensure that the cancer does not spread.
    ○ 3. Surgery is usually done only as a last resort, after failure of radiation and chemotherapy.
    ○ 4. The more radical the surgery, the better the prognosis.

482. During surgery, it was found that Mr. Varella had positive peritoneal lymph nodes. The next most likely site of metastasis would be the
    ○ 1. brain.
    ○ 2. bone.
    ○ 3. liver.
    ○ 4. mediastinum.

483. A chemotherapeutic agent, 5-fluorouracil (5-FU) is ordered for Mr. Varella as an adjunct measure to surgery. Which of the following statements about chemotherapy is true?
    ○ 1. It is a local treatment affecting only tumor cells.
    ○ 2. It is a systemic treatment affecting both tumor and normal cells.
    ○ 3. It has not yet been proven an effective treatment for cancer.
    ○ 4. It causes few if any side effects.

484. Mr. Varella develops stomatitis during his course of 5-FU. Nursing care for this problem should include
    ○ 1. a soft, bland diet.
    ○ 2. restricting fluids to decrease salivation.
    ○ 3. avoiding topical anesthetics, because they alter taste sensations.
    ○ 4. encouraging the client to drink hot liquids.

485. Mr. Varella asks the nurse why these sores developed in his mouth. What is the most appropriate response?
- ○ **1.** "Don't worry; it always happens with chemotherapy."
- ○ **2.** "Your oral hygiene needs improvement."
- ○ **3.** "It is a sign that the medication is working effectively."
- ○ **4.** "The sores result because the cells in the mouth are sensitive to the chemotherapy."

Susan Allen is a 24-year-old woman who has a diagnosis of acute granulocytic leukemia. She presented with an acute upper respiratory infection and bleeding gums.

486. When Mrs. Allen's husband is told that she has leukemia, he insists that she not be told her diagnosis. Which approach is best?
- ○ **1.** Tell her husband that it is her right to be told.
- ○ **2.** Suggest that he talk with the hospital chaplain.
- ○ **3.** Allow him to express his feelings and explain how his wife can benefit from being told.
- ○ **4.** Be patient with him, hoping he will feel differently when his anger subsides.

487. Mrs. Allen is started in a regimen of chemotherapy. Her platelet count begins to fall to critical levels. Which action is *not* necessary at this time?
- ○ **1.** Frequent turning to prevent skin breakdown
- ○ **2.** Assessing her level of consciousness
- ○ **3.** Giving oral hygiene with a soft toothbrush
- ○ **4.** Providing her with soft, bland foods

488. High uric acid levels may develop in clients who are receiving chemotherapy. This is caused by
- ○ **1.** the inability of the kidneys to excrete the drug metabolites.
- ○ **2.** rapid cell catabolism.
- ○ **3.** toxic effects of the prophylactic antibiotics that are given concurrently.
- ○ **4.** the altered blood pH from the acid medium of the drugs.

489. The drug of choice to decrease uric acid levels is
- ○ **1.** prednisone.
- ○ **2.** allopurinol (Zyloprim).
- ○ **3.** indomethacin (Indocin).
- ○ **4.** hydrochlorothiazide (HydroDIURIL).

490. Nursing care for the client undergoing chemotherapy includes assessment for signs of bone-marrow depression. Which of the following accounts for some of the symptoms related to bone-marrow depression?
- ○ **1.** Erythrocytosis
- ○ **2.** Leukocytosis
- ○ **3.** Polycythemia
- ○ **4.** Thrombocytopenia

Upon admission to the hospital, Joanne Day describes symptoms of intermenstrual bleeding and a foul-smelling vaginal discharge. An outpatient punch biopsy confirms cervical cancer.

491. Which of the following is *not* a predisposing factor for cervical cancer?
- ○ **1.** Early sexual experience with multiple partners
- ○ **2.** History of herpes genitalis, chronic cervicitis, or venereal disease
- ○ **3.** Family history of cervical cancer
- ○ **4.** Multiple pregnancies at an early age

492. Medical treatment for Mrs. Day will include a hysterectomy followed by internal radiation. Although she is 32 years old and has 3 children, Mrs. Day tells the nurse that she is anxious regarding the impending treatment and loss of her femininity. Which of the following interactions is most appropriate?
- ○ **1.** Tell Mrs. Day that now she does not have to worry about pregnancy.
- ○ **2.** Provide Mrs. Day with adequate information about the effects of treatment on sexual functioning.
- ○ **3.** Refer her to the physician.
- ○ **4.** Avoid the question. Nurses are not specialists in providing sexual counseling.

493. Mrs. Day receives a radium implant. She would be closely observed for any untoward side effects. What are they?
- ○ **1.** Nausea, vomiting, diarrhea, and malaise
- ○ **2.** Disorientation related to isolation
- ○ **3.** Severe pain and discomfort
- ○ **4.** Difficulty in urinating and cystitis

Phyllis Newsberg, a 34-year-old client, has recently had a mastectomy.

494. Prior to discharge from the hospital, the nurse encourages Mrs. Newsberg to look at the incision. She turns her head and cries, "It is horrible." How should the nurse respond?
- ○ **1.** "I know, I'd feel the same way too."
- ○ **2.** "It's OK, you can look at it anytime."
- ○ **3.** "Your feelings are normal; it's all right to cry."
- ○ **4.** "I know this is depressing, but it's not that terrible."

495. An important part of Mrs. Newsberg's long-term rehabilitation is teaching her the techniques of breast self-examination (BSE). Why is this important?
- ○ **1.** Breast cancer can be bilateral.
- ○ **2.** It will help the client confront the deformity.
- ○ **3.** It helps the client to focus on the possibility of future metastasis.
- ○ **4.** Teaching BSE really is not important as long as the client visits her physician regularly.

Two days before 65-year-old Delores Wu and her husband were to leave on a trip to Florida, she found a lump in her breast. She is admitted for a biopsy of the right breast with possible mastectomy and node dissection. While the nurse is doing pre-op teaching, Mrs. Wu says, "I'm sure this surgery will make me look like half a woman."

496. What is the most appropriate nursing response?
- ○ **1.** "I'm sure no one will know you've had a mastectomy."
- ○ **2.** "Today's prosthetic devices are very realistic."
- ○ **3.** "You're concerned about how you'll look after surgery?"
- ○ **4.** "You're going to be the same person after surgery that you are now."

497. What does the nurse do after having premedicated Mrs. Wu for surgery?
- ○ **1.** Check her vital signs and document them on the chart.
- ○ **2.** Have Mrs. Wu sign the operative permit.
- ○ **3.** Have Mrs. Wu void.
- ○ **4.** Put the side rails up.

498. Mrs. Wu's post-op diagnosis is breast cancer, treated with a right, modified mastectomy. She returns from the recovery room in supine position, with an IV infusing, an elastic bandage wrapped around her chest, and a HemoVac in place. The nurse monitors Mrs. Wu's vital signs and her dressing. Which part of the dressing does the nurse particularly observe for drainage?
- ○ **1.** Back
- ○ **2.** Front
- ○ **3.** Left side
- ○ **4.** Right side

499. Which of the following discharge instructions is essential for the nurse to give Mrs. Wu?
- ○ **1.** "Don't shave your right axilla."
- ○ **2.** "Don't wear your bra until after the first visit to your doctor's office."
- ○ **3.** "Increase your sodium and fluid intake."
- ○ **4.** "Wash the incision every day with a soft cloth and an antiseptic solution."

Forty-year-old Rita Goldfarb recently visited her gynecologist for her annual examination. During the visit, the nurse practitioner palpated a lump in Mrs. Goldfarb's right breast. She has now been admitted to the hospital for a breast biopsy.

500. Which of the following is *not* necessary to include in the admission assessment data?
- ○ **1.** Prior sexual relationships
- ○ **2.** Quality of present sexual relationship
- ○ **3.** Body image
- ○ **4.** Occupational role

501. During her admission interview, Mrs. Goldfarb states, "This is really nothing to worry about. After all, I had a normal checkup last year. I expect to be back home tomorrow night." Mrs. Goldfarb is most likely experiencing which of the following?
- ○ **1.** Anger
- ○ **2.** Denial
- ○ **3.** Depression
- ○ **4.** Loss

502. After the biopsy, it is clear that Mrs. Goldfarb has breast cancer. Her physician discusses her case with the hospital tumor board and reports the tumor to be stage IV with the following classification: $T_2N_3M_1$. What does this mean?
○ **1.** The tumor is large, but does not involve the axillary or other nodes.
○ **2.** The tumor is small with extensive axillary involvement and no distant metastasis.
○ **3.** The tumor is fixed to the chest wall with supraclavicular nodal involvement and distant metastasis.
○ **4.** The tumor is small, but involves 3 nodes.

503. Depression may follow the mastectomy. Which of the following observations would most alert the nurse to depression in this client?
○ **1.** Disorientation during afternoon hours
○ **2.** Increased agitation or restlessness
○ **3.** Verbalization of hopelessness or helplessness
○ **4.** Increased desire to sleep

504. Which of the following nursing diagnoses is this client most likely to have following her mastectomy?
○ **1.** Disturbance in self-concept
○ **2.** Self-care deficit
○ **3.** Impaired verbal communication
○ **4.** Alteration in cardiac output

505. Lymphedema is the most common post-op complication following axillary lymph node dissection. Which of the following actions would minimize this problem?
○ **1.** Avoid injections in and blood pressure measurements and constrictive clothing on the affected arm.
○ **2.** Place the affected arm in a sling.
○ **3.** Discourage feeding, washing, or hair combing with the affected arm.
○ **4.** Place the affected arm in a dependent position, below the level of the heart.

506. It has been decided that Mrs. Goldfarb will have antineoplastic chemotherapy after surgery. Which of the following purposes of this chemotherapy will also help best explain to the client the possible side effects of the therapy?
○ **1.** It offers the only hope of cure.
○ **2.** It attacks the fastest growing cells of the body.
○ **3.** It is always indicated postmastectomy.
○ **4.** It is a new treatment with few side effects.

507. Since Mrs. Goldfarb's left breast is free of tumor, the nurse reviews the technique of self-breast examination with her before discharge. When would be the most appropriate time for this client to perform this examination?
○ **1.** Just prior to the time of menstruation
○ **2.** The day menstruation begins
○ **3.** One week after the start of each menstrual period
○ **4.** Varying times throughout the month

Jean Chambers has had a mammogram and biopsy for bleeding from the nipple of her left breast. The physician diagnosed intraductal breast cancer and explained a modified mastectomy is necessary. Miss Chambers has agreed to the surgery, which is scheduled for the following morning.

508. What would be the most important aspect of the nurse's pre-op teaching?
○ **1.** Discuss with the client how her sexual relations will be altered.
○ **2.** Discuss the skin graft that will be necessary.
○ **3.** Explore the client's feelings and expectations about the surgery and correct any misconceptions.
○ **4.** Explain that most breast masses are benign, and hers will most likely be nonmalignant.

509. A HemoVac suction apparatus is in place at the surgical site postoperatively. Which of the following nursing actions would be *incorrect* when caring for the HemoVac?
○ **1.** Report bright red bloody drainage to the physician immediately.
○ **2.** Maintain aseptic technique.
○ **3.** Curl the tubing and tape firmly against the skin.
○ **4.** Check the HemoVac drum frequently and empty it when half full.

510. In the early post-op period, the surgeon has encouraged Mrs. Chambers to begin using her left arm. She tells the nurse it hurts too much to move. What would be the best nursing action to reinforce the physician's instructions?
○ **1.** Put the left arm in a sling to provide support.
○ **2.** Initiate slow, passive, range-of-motion exercises.
○ **3.** Teach the client full active range of motion.
○ **4.** Have the client do stretching exercises.

511. Which of the following nursing actions is *least* appropriate in planning for Mrs. Chamber's discharge from the hospital?
○ **1.** Provide information on a local "Reach-to-Recovery" group.
○ **2.** Discuss plans for obtaining a permanent prosthesis.
○ **3.** Discuss the possibility of a breast reconstruction in the future.
○ **4.** Discuss activities the client will need to discontinue.

References

Brunner, N. (1983). *Orthopedic nursing—A programmed approach.* St. Louis: Mosby.

Carini, G., & Birmingham, J. (1980). *Traction made manageable.* New York: McGraw-Hill.

Farrell, J. (1982). *Illustrated guide to orthopedic nursing.* Philadelphia: Lippincott.

Gordon, M. (1982). *Manual of nursing diagnosis.* New York: McGraw-Hill.

Govoni, L., & Hayes, J. (1985). *Drugs and nursing implications* (5th ed.). Norwalk, CT: Appleton-Century-Crofts.

Green, M., & Harry, J. (1981). *Nutrition in contemporary nursing practice.* New York: Wiley.

Haber, J., Leach, A., Schudy, S., & Sideleau, B. (1982). *Comprehensive psychiatric nursing* (2nd ed.). New York: McGraw-Hill.

Lewis, S., & Collier, I. (1983). *Medical-surgical nursing: Assessment and management of clinical problems.* New York: McGraw-Hill.

Luckmann, J., & Sorensen, K. (Eds.). (1986). *Medical-surgical nursing: A psychophysiologic approach* (3rd ed.). Philadelphia: Saunders.

Marino, L. (1981). *Cancer nursing.* St. Louis: Mosby.

Mims, F., & Simenson, M. (1980). *Sexuality: A nursing perspective.* New York: McGraw-Hill.

Nurse's Reference Library. (1982). *Diagnostics.* Springhouse, PA: Intermed.

Phipps, W., Long, B., & Woods, N. (1983). *Medical-surgical nursing: Concepts and clinical practice* (2nd ed.). St. Louis: Mosby.

Price, S., & Wilson, L. (1982). *Pathophysiology: Clinical concepts of disease processes.* New York: McGraw-Hill.

Reckling, J. (1982). Safeguarding the renal transplant patient. *Nursing82, 12*(12), 46–55.

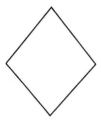

Section 3
Correct Answers

1. #2.	47. #3.	93. #1.	139. #4.
2. #2.	48. #3.	94. #4.	140. #2.
3. #4.	49. #2.	95. #2.	141. #2.
4. #4.	50. #4.	96. #4.	142. #3.
5. #1.	51. #2.	97. #2.	143. #2.
6. #4.	52. #3.	98. #4.	144. #3.
7. #3.	53. #3.	99. #1.	145. #1.
8. #2.	54. #1.	100. #3.	146. #3.
9. #4.	55. #3.	101. #2.	147. #4.
10. #3.	56. #2.	102. #3.	148. #1.
11. #1.	57. #1.	103. #2.	149. #4.
12. #2.	58. #3.	104. #2.	150. #4.
13. #1.	59. #1.	105. #2.	151. #4.
14. #3.	60. #2.	106. #2.	152. #3.
15. #1.	61. #1.	107. #1.	153. #2.
16. #1.	62. #3.	108. #4.	154. #4.
17. #4.	63. #3.	109. #1.	155. #4.
18. #1.	64. #2.	110. #3.	156. #3.
19. #3.	65. #2.	111. #4.	157. #2.
20. #4.	66. #4.	112. #2.	158. #2.
21. #1.	67. #4.	113. #2.	159. #1.
22. #2.	68. #2.	114. #4.	160. #3.
23. #4.	69. #2.	115. #2.	161. #1.
24. #2.	70. #2.	116. #2.	162. #4.
25. #2.	71. #2.	117. #3.	163. #2.
26. #3.	72. #3.	118. #2.	164. #3.
27. #3.	73. #2.	119. #2.	165. #4.
28. #3.	74. #1.	120. #1.	166. #1.
29. #2.	75. #2.	121. #2.	167. #4.
30. #3.	76. #3.	122. #3.	168. #2.
31. #2.	77. #2.	123. #3.	169. #3.
32. #1.	78. #3.	124. #2.	170. #2.
33. #3.	79. #3.	125. #2.	171. #2.
34. #1.	80. #1.	126. #4.	172. #1.
35. #2.	81. #1.	127. #1.	173. #2.
36. #3.	82. #2.	128. #2.	174. #3.
37. #3.	83. #3.	129. #2.	175. #3.
38. #3.	84. #4.	130. #3.	176. #2.
39. #4.	85. #2.	131. #4.	177. #4.
40. #1.	86. #3.	132. #1.	178. #1.
41. #4.	87. #2.	133. #4.	179. #2.
42. #4.	88. #3.	134. #2.	180. #3.
43. #4.	89. #2.	135. #4.	181. #2.
44. #4.	90. #1.	136. #3.	182. #4.
45. #3.	91. #4.	137. #2.	183. #1.
46. #2.	92. #3.	138. #1.	184. #4.

185. #2.	**240.** #2.	**295.** #4.	**350.** #1.
186. #4.	**241.** #4.	**296.** #3.	**351.** #4.
187. #4.	**242.** #2.	**297.** #2.	**352.** #2.
188. #2.	**243.** #3.	**298.** #1.	**353.** #3.
189. #2.	**244.** #3.	**299.** #2.	**354.** #2.
190. #2.	**245.** #4.	**300.** #3.	**355.** #3.
191. #2.	**246.** #4.	**301.** #3.	**356.** #4.
192. #2.	**247.** #2.	**302.** #1.	**357.** #3.
193. #4.	**248.** #1.	**303.** #4.	**358.** #2.
194. #3.	**249.** #3.	**304.** #2.	**359.** #3.
195. #4.	**250.** #1.	**305.** #3.	**360.** #4.
196. #4.	**251.** #3.	**306.** #1.	**361.** #3.
197. #2.	**252.** #3.	**307.** #3.	**362.** #3.
198. #1.	**253.** #1.	**308.** #4.	**363.** #3.
199. #3.	**254.** #2.	**309.** #3.	**364.** #3.
200. #2.	**255.** #2.	**310.** #4.	**365.** #2.
201. #3.	**256.** #4.	**311.** #2.	**366.** #4.
202. #4.	**257.** #1.	**312.** #3.	**367.** #1.
203. #3.	**258.** #4.	**313.** #2.	**368.** #1.
204. #2.	**259.** #4.	**314.** #1.	**369.** #4.
205. #2.	**260.** #3.	**315.** #2.	**370.** #3.
206. #2.	**261.** #1.	**316.** #2.	**371.** #3.
207. #3.	**262.** #2.	**317.** #3.	**372.** #3.
208. #1.	**263.** #1.	**318.** #1.	**373.** #3.
209. #3.	**264.** #2.	**319.** #1.	**374.** #1.
210. #1.	**265.** #4.	**320.** #3.	**375.** #4.
211. #4.	**266.** #1.	**321.** #1.	**376.** #2.
212. #2.	**267.** #1.	**322.** #2.	**377.** #2.
213. #4.	**268.** #4.	**323.** #2.	**378.** #1.
214. #1.	**269.** #1.	**324.** #1.	**379.** #3.
215. #3.	**270.** #2.	**325.** #2.	**380.** #2.
216. #4.	**271.** #1.	**326.** #1.	**381.** #2.
217. #1.	**272.** #2.	**327.** #4.	**382.** #4.
218. #2.	**273.** #3.	**328.** #2.	**383.** #3.
219. #3.	**274.** #2.	**329.** #2.	**384.** #4.
220. #4.	**275.** #4.	**330.** #4.	**385.** #3.
221. #1.	**276.** #2.	**331.** #3.	**386.** #3.
222. #4.	**277.** #4.	**332.** #2.	**387.** #2.
223. #3.	**278.** #4.	**333.** #3.	**388.** #3.
224. #2.	**279.** #2.	**334.** #2.	**389.** #2.
225. #2.	**280.** #4.	**335.** #1.	**390.** #3.
226. #4.	**281.** #3.	**336.** #3.	**391.** #1.
227. #4.	**282.** #1.	**337.** #4.	**392.** #3.
228. #4.	**283.** #3.	**338.** #2.	**393.** #3.
229. #1.	**284.** #1.	**339.** #4.	**394.** #1.
230. #4.	**285.** #4.	**340.** #1.	**395.** #2.
231. #3.	**286.** #2.	**341.** #3.	**396.** #4.
232. #4.	**287.** #1.	**342.** #2.	**397.** #1.
233. #3.	**288.** #1.	**343.** #2.	**398.** #1.
234. #3.	**289.** #1.	**344.** #2.	**399.** #3.
235. #1.	**290.** #1.	**345.** #4.	**400.** #3.
236. #4.	**291.** #2.	**346.** #1.	**401.** #3.
237. #2.	**292.** #3.	**347.** #2.	**402.** #3.
238. #1.	**293.** #1.	**348.** #4.	**403.** #3.
239. #1.	**294.** #3.	**349.** #3.	**404.** #3.

405. #1.	**432.** #3.	**459.** #1.	**486.** #3.
406. #1.	**433.** #4.	**460.** #4.	**487.** #4.
407. #4.	**434.** #1.	**461.** #1.	**488.** #2.
408. #3.	**435.** #4.	**462.** #3.	**489.** #2.
409. #1.	**436.** #2.	**463.** #2.	**490.** #4.
410. #4.	**437.** #2.	**464.** #3.	**491.** #3.
411. #1.	**438.** #1.	**465.** #2.	**492.** #2.
412. #4.	**439.** #2.	**466.** #4.	**493.** #1.
413. #2.	**440.** #2.	**467.** #4.	**494.** #3.
414. #4.	**441.** #2.	**468.** #4.	**495.** #1.
415. #4.	**442.** #4.	**469.** #2.	**496.** #3.
416. #2.	**443.** #3.	**470.** #1.	**497.** #4.
417. #1.	**444.** #3.	**471.** #4.	**498.** #1.
418. #2.	**445.** #4.	**472.** #2.	**499.** #1.
419. #2.	**446.** #3.	**473.** #4.	**500.** #1.
420. #2.	**447.** #2.	**474.** #3.	**501.** #2.
421. #1.	**448.** #1.	**475.** #1.	**502.** #2.
422. #1.	**449.** #2.	**476.** #4.	**503.** #3.
423. #1.	**450.** #4.	**477.** #2.	**504.** #1.
424. #2.	**451.** #4.	**478.** #1.	**505.** #1.
425. #4.	**452.** #4.	**479.** #3.	**506.** #2.
426. #4.	**453.** #1.	**480.** #2.	**507.** #3.
427. #3.	**454.** #2.	**481.** #1.	**508.** #3.
428. #1.	**455.** #3.	**482.** #3.	**509.** #3.
429. #4.	**456.** #4.	**483.** #2.	**510.** #2.
430. #1.	**457.** #3.	**484.** #1.	**511.** #4.
431. #2.	**458.** #2.	**485.** #4.	

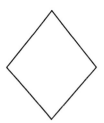

Correct Answers with Rationales

Editors note:

Two pieces of information are supplied at the end of each rationale. First we tell you what part of the nursing process the question addresses. Second, in parentheses, you will find a reference to a section in the *AJN Nursing Boards Review* where a more complete discussion of the topic may be found should you desire more information.

1. **#2.** Hyperextending the neck can cause a spinal injury, if the vertebrae have been fractured. IMPLEMENTATION (ADULT/OXYGENATION)

2. **#2.** The mouth is kept closed during inspiration. No more force than normal is required. IMPLEMENTATION (ADULT/OXYGENATION)

3. **#4.** Using one hand, only approximately 400 ml of air can be delivered. Almost 1,000 ml can be delivered if both hands are used. ANALYSIS (ADULT/OXYGENATION)

4. **#4.** Fluid volume is the first priority after adequate ventilation. The blood pressure and pulse indicate the client is in a volume-depleted state. PLAN (ADULT/OXYGENATION)

5. **#1.** The type of instrument involved (blunt versus sharp) and where it hit is information of the most value, since it will help define the type of injury. ASSESSMENT (ADULT/OXYGENATION)

6. **#4.** With a negative thoracentesis and a rising central venous pressure, the only reasonable conclusion is that cardiac tamponade is the cause. Bleeding into the pericardial sac causes both decreased blood pressure and increased central venous pressure. ANALYSIS (ADULT/OXYGENATION)

7. **#3.** When the systolic blood pressure falls below 80 mm Hg, circulation to the vital organs is markedly compromised. ASSESSMENT (ADULT/OXYGENATION)

8. **#2.** The renal response to decreased fluid volume in the kidneys (resulting in ischemia) initiates this response. ANALYSIS (ADULT/OXYGENATION)

9. **#4.** Although dopamine is a potent vasopressor, kidney perfusion can be maintained in the mild to moderate dosage range. ANALYSIS (ADULT/OXYGENATION)

10. **#3.** A urine output of 30 ml/hour indicates there is adequate kidney perfusion. In selected cases systolic pressure of 90 or 100 mm Hg would not ensure adequate renal perfusion. 30 ml/hour is the minimum for adequate urine output. ASSESSMENT (ADULT/OXYGENATION)

11. **#1.** The most precise measurement of hemodynamic status would be used, particularly in an older client. A Swan-Ganz catheter would best reflect response to treatment as well as hourly urine output. EVALUATION (ADULT/OXYGENATION)

12. **#2.** As sympathomimetics, adrenergic agents cause vasoconstriction. Options #1 and #3 are incorrect and not desirable in the client in shock. ANALYSIS (ADULT/OXYGENATION)

13. **#1.** Adrenalin is a potent cardiac stimulant. It does not cause the effects listed in the other options. ANALYSIS (ADULT/OXYGENATION)

14. **#3.** As sympathomimetics, adrenergics can cause overstimulation of the heart and dysrhythmias. The other side effects listed are not considered serious. ASSESSMENT (ADULT/OXYGENATION)

15. **#1.** These values indicate metabolic acidosis, as evidenced by low pH, normal pCO_2, low bicarbonate level. pO_2 has no bearing on determining type of acidosis or alkalosis. ANALYSIS (ADULT/OXYGENATION)

16. **#1.** Any extreme in pH will inhibit enzyme activity with resulting loss of total body functioning. ANALYSIS (ADULT/OXYGENATION)

17. **#4.** The blood buffers (oxyhemoglobin, phosphates, carbonates) are the first line of defense. Retention of bicarbonate by the kidneys is a slow process; this usually takes at least 24 hours to be effective. ANALYSIS (ADULT/OXYGENATION)

18. **#1.** A client on chronic steroid therapy is very prone to a relative insufficiency when stressed, since the adrenals cannot produce extra amounts of cortisol as required. ANALYSIS (ADULT/NUTRITION AND METABOLISM)

19. **#3.** These symptoms are typical of disseminated intravascular coagulation. ANALYSIS (ADULT/OXYGENATION)

20. **#4.** This client will have a relative deficiency of glucocorticoids and mineralocorticoids when under stress, requiring replacement drugs. ANALYSIS (ADULT/NUTRITION AND METABOLISM)

21. **#1.** Although hemorrhage is a symptom seen in disseminated intravascular coagulation, the problem is really one of microcoagulation. Heparin would be cautiously used. ANALYSIS (ADULT/OXYGENATION)

22. **#2.** The first phase of disseminated intravascular coagulation, hypercoagulation, results in the formation of microthrombi. Renal failure can result from thrombosis of the microcirculation of the kidneys. ANALYSIS (ADULT/OXYGENATION)

23. **#4.** Remove hypothermia equipment when the client is one degree above the recommended temperature, because an additional temperature drop may occur after discontinuance. IMPLEMENTATION (ADULT/OXYGENATION)

24. **#2.** Decreasing his pain is the most important priority at this time. As long as the pain is present, there is the danger of extension of the infarcted area. Starting an IV is a second action, especially if the medication is ordered IV. IMPLEMENTATION (ADULT/OXYGENATION)

25. **#2.** An infarction results in anoxia of the involved tissue, which irritates the nerve endings in the infarcted area resulting in pain. ANALYSIS (ADULT/OXYGENATION)

26. **#3.** The left ventricle of the heart, which contributes most to contraction, is most frequently the site of the myocardial infarction. ANALYSIS (ADULT/OXYGENATION)

27. **#3.** Keeping family and significant others informed of client progress is of paramount importance and therapeutic for the client. IMPLEMENTATION (ADULT/OXYGENATION)

28. **#3.** Denial is the most common reason for not seeking medical attention. The client may fear the consequences, and thus uses denial as a defense mechanism. ANALYSIS (ADULT/OXYGENATION)

29. **#2.** Establishment of an airway is the primary objective and action in any emergency, especially in a cardiopulmonary arrest. Initiating cardiac massage and calling a physician follow quickly. IMPLEMENTATION (ADULT/OXYGENATION)

30. **#3.** Presence of a cartoid pulse represents adequate vascular perfusion and oxygenation. EVALUATION (ADULT/OXYGENATION)

31. **#2.** Chest pain in an acute myocardial infarction is intense and severe and is not relieved by nitroglycerin. Nitroglycerin is the drug of choice for angina pectoris. ASSESSMENT (ADULT/OXYGENATION)

32. **#1.** Morphine sulfate is the drug of choice in this situation, because it has a rapid action, is potent, has a diuretic effect, results in slight coronary vasodilation, and is helpful in relieving anxiety. These are all particularly beneficial outcomes for the myocardial infarction client. ANALYSIS (ADULT/OXYGENATION)

33. **#3.** With an infarction, anoxia of the myocardium occurs. Administration of oxygen will help relieve dyspnea and cyanosis associated with the pain, but the primary purpose is to increase oxygen concentration in the damaged tissue of the myocardium. ANALYSIS (ADULT/OXYGENATION)

34. **#1.** The first 24 to 48 hours is a very dangerous period, because of the extreme irritability of the heart. The irritability comes from the ischemic area surrounding the infarcted area, or from dead cells. ANALYSIS (ADULT/OXYGENATION)

35. **#2.** The heart is very irritable at this time, and ventricular dysrhythmias are quite common and very serious. The other options listed are serious but not as commonly associated with myocardial infarction as dysrhythmias. ANALYSIS (ADULT/OXYGENATION)

36. **#3.** The mortality rate is 80% for all clients who go into cardiogenic shock. Even sophisticated drugs and intra-aortic-balloon pumping cannot help the client who has lost the pumping action of the heart. ANALYSIS (ADULT/OXYGENATION)

37. **#3.** Whenever there is tissue death, certain enzymes are released. Creatine phosphokinase (CPK) and lactate dehydrogenase (LDH) isoenzymes are specific for cardiac muscle. ANALYSIS (ADULT/OXYGENATION)

38. **#3.** Xylocaine decreases ventricular irritability and thereby reduces premature ventricular contractions. Procainamide and phenytoin are second-choice drugs if lidocaine is ineffective. ANALYSIS (ADULT/OXYGENATION)

39. **#4.** Sedation is a frequent side effect of lidocaine. It actually may be a positive action, since it helps the client to relax; however, it must be assessed so that central nervous system depression does not progress. ASSESSMENT (ADULT/OXYGENATION)

40. **#1.** Administration of laxatives can prevent straining on defection. Straining results in Valsalva's maneuver. IMPLEMENTATION (ADULT/OXYGENATION)

41. **#4.** There is a high probability that her husband may die, and she needs to prepare for that. Letting her know the nurses are competent may reassure her but will not help with anticipatory grieving. IMPLEMENTATION (ADULT/OXYGENATION)

42. **#4.** Allowing Mr. Mung to express his concerns is the initial priority. When he feels comfortable, a teaching session with his wife may be planned. PLAN (ADULT/OXYGENATION)

43. **#4.** Liver is an organ meat high in cholesterol; tuna and shellfish have minimal cholesterol. Rice has the lowest amount. ANALYSIS (ADULT/OXYGENATION)

44. **#4.** Taking aspirin daily prevents platelet aggregation and may decrease the risk of myocardial infarction. Family history of cardiovascular disease, diabetes, and smoking increases the risk. ASSESSMENT (ADULT/OXYGENATION)

45. **#3.** This represents the most reasonable amount of activity. Walking up stairs significantly increases the workload of the heart. The physician will determine how and when the client can undertake this activity. IMPLEMENTATION (ADULT/OXYGENATION)

46. **#2.** Cardioversion or countershock can readily convert atrial fibrillation in a client with no other cardiac problems. ANALYSIS (ADULT/OXYGENATION)

47. **#3.** Propranolol (Inderal) is often given alone or with digoxin to slow the atrial rate while increasing the strength of contractions. Isoproterenol and epinephrine increase the atrial and ventricular irritability. Xylocaine has a direct effect only on irritable ventricles. ANALYSIS (ADULT/OXYGENATION)

48. **#3.** Atropine is the safest drug to use for heart block associated with hypotension. ANALYSIS (ADULT/OXYGENATION)

49. **#2.** Procainamide (Pronestyl) may decrease cardiac output, especially when given IV. All the other drugs are vasopressors. ANALYSIS (ADULT/OXYGENATION)

50. **#4.** A normal cardiac cycle contains P, QRS, and T waves, respectively. ASSESSMENT (ADULT/OXYGENATION)

51. **#2.** In the young adult years, stress can result in atrial tachycardia and subsequent signs and symptoms. ASSESSMENT (ADULT/OXYGENATION)

52. **#3.** The diagnosis is not serious enough to warrant options #1, #2, or #4. ANALYSIS (ADULT/OXYGENATION)

53. **#3.** Realistically, teaching stress-management skills is not appropriate for the limited emergency room visit; in addition, Miss Chang is likely to be anxious and, thus, less receptive to teaching. Referral is most appropriate. IMPLEMENTATION (ADULT/OXYGENATION)

54. **#1.** Congestive heart failure results from circulatory congestion and the characteristic symptom is dyspnea. ANALYSIS (ADULT/OXYGENATION)

55. **#3.** Venous pressure increases and stasis occurs, promoting the extravasation of fluid from the vascular space into the tissue. ANALYSIS (ADULT/OXYGENATION)

56. **#2.** Because of gravity, dependent edema, especially in the feet, occurs in cardiac failure. The edema is pitting and nonpainful in nature. Periorbital edema usually occurs as a result of head trauma or renal failure. ASSESSMENT (ADULT/OXYGENATION)

57. **#1.** *Left-sided* congestive heart failure produces pulmonary symptoms because the blood is in the pulmonary system before entering the left heart chambers. The other symptoms listed are systemic ones associated with *right-sided* congestive heart failure. ASSESSMENT (ADULT/OXYGENATION)

58. **#3.** Potassium affects neuromuscular activity. Hyperkalemia (serum potassium greater than 5.5 mEq) often results in ventricular fibrillation, leading to death. ANALYSIS (ADULT/OXYGENATION)

59. #1. Respirations in congestive heart failure are rapid and shallow because a shift of fluid from extravascular to the vascular space results in increased venous return and greater work load on the heart and lungs. Wheezing does not occur from heart failure alone; however, if a client also has chronic obstructive pulmonary disease, then wheezing might be heard. ASSESSMENT (ADULT/OXYGENATION)

60. #2. The client with congestive heart failure can breathe with more ease in a Fowler's or semi-Fowler's position as gravity promotes drainage of secretions from the pulmonary bed and pooling of blood in the extremities. Also maximal lung expansion is permitted, because there is less pressure from the abdominal organs. IMPLEMENTATION (ADULT/OXYGENATION)

61. #1. Circulation is decreased in congestive heart failure; thus drug absorption and distribution are slowed. ANALYSIS (ADULT/OXYGENATION)

62. #3. Furosemide (Lasix) causes loss of potassium. Hypokalemia increases the effect of digoxin and increases the risk of digitalis toxicity. PLAN (ADULT/OXYGENATION)

63. #3. Rotating tourniquets are used to decrease venous return to the right side of the heart, thus relieving some of the congestion in the heart and lungs. ANALYSIS (ADULT/OXYGENATION)

64. #2. This ensures that no single extremity is compressed for more than 45 minutes. In the elderly client, this procedure may be modified by rotating tourniquets at 5-minute intervals rather than 15-minute intervals. IMPLEMENTATION (ADULT/OXYGENATION)

65. #2. Canned tuna is highly salted (628 mg sodium/3¼ oz). Unsalted nuts are not contraindicated on a sodium-restricted diet. Whole milk and eggs are not allowed on a low-cholesterol, low-polysaturated-fat diet, but they are allowed on a 2,000-mg sodium diet. Low-sodium milk is used only on a *severely* sodium-restricted diet (200 to 500 mg sodium). IMPLEMENTATION (ADULT/OXYGENATION)

66. #4. Breads and cereals contain almost no potassium. IMPLEMENTATION (ADULT/OXYGENATION)

67. #4. Thrombophlebitis is the occlusion of a vessel with inflammation and thrombus formation. It results in such signs and symptoms as a positive Homans' sign, history of leg pain, redness, and unilateral swelling. ASSESSMENT (ADULT/OXYGENATION)

68. #2. In order to prevent dislodgment of a thrombus, maintain bed rest for 5 to 10 days, elevate the legs, apply warm, moist packs to the involved site, and provide range-of-motion exercises to the *unaffected* extremity at least 2 times per shift. PLAN (ADULT/OXYGENATION)

69. #2. Heparin inactivates thromboplastin and thrombin that forms. Neither parenteral nor oral anticoagulants affect existing thrombi. ANALYSIS (ADULT/OXYGENATION)

70. #2. Monitor the partial thromboplastin time (PTT) when clients are receiving parenteral anticoagulants. Prothrombin times are monitored when a client is on warfarin (Coumadin) or dicumerol. IMPLEMENTATION (ADULT/OXYGENATION)

71. #2. A positive Homans' sign is pain in the calf when the foot is dorsiflexed. It is a sign of phlebitis. ASSESSMENT (ADULT/OXYGENATION)

72. #3. Protamine sulfate is the antidote for heparin sodium; vitamin K is the antidote for warfarin (Coumadin). ANALYSIS (ADULT/OXYGENATION)

73. #2. Mrs. Avery should avoid using any product that increases anticoagulation (e.g., aspirin) or causes bleeding (e.g., a hard toothbrush). She should notify her physician at once of any signs and symptoms of bleeding such as hematuria or melena. IMPLEMENTATION (ADULT/OXYGENATION)

74. #1. A pulmonary embolus causes hyperventilation. This lowers the pCO_2 and produces respiratory alkalosis. ANALYSIS (ADULT/OXYGENATION)

75. #2. Hyperventilation and lowered pCO_2 are common after a pulmonary embolus. ASSESSMENT (ADULT/OXYGENATION)

76. #3. Central cyanosis would indicate a serious drop in the pO_2. It is the most significant sign of hypoxia. ASSESSMENT (ADULT/OXYGENATION)

77. #2. The ratio is 1 part of carbonic acid (pCO_2) to 20 parts of base bicarbonate (HCO_3). ANALYSIS (ADULT/OXYGENATION)

78. #3. Cor pulmonale is a complication of obstructive pulmonary disease. It is hypertrophy of the right side of the heart because of pulmonary hypertension. Resulting are the signs and symptoms of right-sided heart failure. ANALYSIS (ADULT/OXYGENATION)

79. #3. For clients with a long-standing history of chronic obstructive pulmonary disease, hypoxemia is the major stimulus to respiration. If oxygen is administered in high concentrations, it will eliminate this hypoxic drive, and the rate and depth of respirations will decrease. IMPLEMENTATION (ADULT/OXYGENATION)

80. #1. Pursed-lip breathing prevents bronchiolar collapse, resulting in air trapping. ANALYSIS (ADULT/OXYGENATION)

81. #1. Hemoptysis indicates bleeding, and percussion could exacerbate this condition. ANALYSIS (ADULT/OXYGENATION)

82. #2. Hyperkalemia always occurs with acidemia. ASSESSMENT (ADULT/OXYGENATION)

83. #3. Pneumonia is characterized by these symptoms. Anginal pain is not usually influenced by coughing nor associated with a productive cough. Pulmonary edema is associated with frothy pink, blood-tinged sputum. ANALYSIS (ADULT/OXYGENATION)

84. #4. The pneumococcal bacteria account for the majority of pneumonia cases, and the resulting infection is characterized by rust-colored sputum. Sputum color varies with different types of organisms. ASSESSMENT (ADULT/OXYGENATION)

85. #2. Respirations are usually rapid and shallow in pneumonia, because of pain on deep inspiration. Tachycardia often occurs with the fever; breath sounds would be diminished on the right side; and a pleural friction rub would be auscultated. ASSESSMENT (ADULT/OXYGENATION)

86. #3. Dullness is of medium-intensity pitch and is elicited over areas of mixed solid and lung tissues, as with the consolidated lung tissue in pneumonia. ASSESSMENT (ADULT/OXYGENATION)

87. #2. Splinting occurs when the chest is held rigid to prevent pain on respiratory movement. ASSESSMENT (ADULT/OXYGENATION)

88. #3. Increased fluids are needed to help liquefy secretions; no history of cardiac problems has been given which would contraindicate this action. Analgesics (though not necessarily narcotics) are given so the discomfort associated with coughing, deep breathing, percussion, and postural drainage every 2 to 4 hours can be tolerated. PLAN (ADULT/OXYGENATION)

89. #2. Venturi masks can control oxygen delivery at 24%, 28%, 31%, 35%, and 40% with a great deal of accuracy. ANALYSIS (ADULT/OXYGENATION)

90. #1. Gentamicin is an aminoglycoside. This group of antibiotics is nephrotoxic, and BUN and creatinine must be monitored to assess for any decrease in renal function as shown by an increase in BUN and creatinine. ASSESSMENT (ADULT/OXYGENATION)

91. #4. Atelectasis is a complication of pneumonia; it is treated with tracheal suctioning, effective coughing, and deep breathing. ANALYSIS (ADULT/OXYGENATION)

92. #3. Measures to prevent hypoxemia during suctioning include preoxygenation and limiting each suctioning to 10 to 15 seconds. IMPLEMENTATION (ADULT/OXYGENATION)

93. #1. Tuberculosis is an infectious disease caused by the bacteria *Mycobacterium tuberculosis*. ANALYSIS (ADULT/OXYGENATION)

94. #4. The PPD skin test is specific for tuberculosis and is considered positive when there is induration of 10 mm or larger. ASSESSMENT (ADULT/OXYGENATION)

95. #2. The PPD skin test is used to determine presence of tuberculous antibodies; it indicates, when positive, that a person has been exposed to *Mycobacterium tuberculosis*. Further studies are needed to determine the presence of an active infection. ANALYSIS (ADULT/OXYGENATION)

96. #4. In the treatment of tuberculosis, drugs are often given in combination with other drugs to delay development of resistance and to increase tuberculostatic effects. ANALYSIS (ADULT/OXYGENATION)

97. #2. The most common and important untoward effect of isoniazid (INH) is peripheral neuritis. ASSESSMENT (ADULT/OXYGENATION)

98. #4. The peripheral neuritis that occurs with isoniazid therapy can be controlled with the administration of vitamin B_6 (pyridoxine), because the neuritis is a result of pyridoxine deficiency. ANALYSIS (ADULT/OXYGENATION)

99. #1. A fairly common side effect of rifampin (Rimactane) therapy is reddish-orange urine, saliva, and sputum. IMPLEMENTATION (ADULT/OXYGENATION)

100. #3. Isoniazid (INH) is used as preventive therapy in household members of newly diagnosed clients. It is effective and inexpensive and is given orally. ANALYSIS (ADULT/OXYGENATION)

101. #2. Because isoniazid (INH) is known to cause hepatitis in some persons, liver function tests may be done before the client starts taking the drug. ASSESSMENT (ADULT/OXYGENATION)

102. #3. Histoplasmosis has many of the same symptoms as tuberculosis, but is caused by a fungus. ANALYSIS (ADULT/OXYGENATION)

103. #2. The fungus is responsive to amphotericin B, not to the other drugs listed. ANALYSIS (ADULT/OXYGENATION)

104. #2. This position promotes maximal ventilation of the affected lung. Positioning on the operative side would inhibit thoracic excursion and, therefore, ventilation. Fowler's position increases the intrathoracic space, which allows maximal ventilation. PLAN (ADULT/OXYGENATION)

105. #2. Continuous bubbling could indicate an air leak in the system. Bubbling should be intermittent, and it indicates the expulsion of air from the pleural space. There should be fluctuation in the water-seal tube with respiration. Suction is not used in a one-bottle setup. ASSESSMENT (ADULT/OXYGENATION)

106. #2. Water-seal drainage means that the chest tube is under a water seal to prevent air from entering the chest cavity. ANALYSIS (ADULT/OXYGENATION)

107. #1. The fluid in the tube oscillates with inspiration and expiration when the water-seal apparatus is functioning properly. On inspiration the fluid will rise; on expiration the fluid will fall. ANALYSIS (ADULT/OXYGENATION)

108. #4. The most common symptom of bronchogenic carcinoma is the development of a cough or change in the severity of a chronic cough. There are no early signs of lung cancer. ASSESSMENT (ADULT/OXYGENATION)

109. #1. The client will be kept NPO until the gag reflex returns in 2 to 4 hours. PLAN (ADULT/OXYGENATION)

110. #3. The less pain the client experiences, the more effectively he can cough and deep breathe. IMPLEMENTATION (ADULT/OXYGENATION)

111. #4. The long tube submerged 3 to 5 cm below the fluid level acts as a one-way valve, permitting air and fluid to drain out of the pleural space while preventing influx of air. ANALYSIS (ADULT/OXYGENATION)

112. #2. Continuous bubbling in the water-seal bottle during inspiration and expiration may indicate an air leak. Bubbling should be intermittent. ANALYSIS (ADULT/OXYGENATION)

113. #2. After the specimen is obtained, apply pressure to the area for 5 minutes to prevent bleeding and hematoma formation. IMPLEMENTATION (ADULT/OXYGENATION)

114. #4. Normal values are as follows: pH 7.35 to 7.45, pO_2 80 to 100 mm Hg, pCO_2 35 to 45 mm Hg, oxygen saturation 95% to 98%. ASSESSMENT (ADULT/OXYGENATION)

115. #2. The client should be less confused because all the blood gas values have improved. Confusion usually results when the pO_2 falls below 50. EVALUATION (ADULT/OXYGENATION)

116. #2. Effects of gravity are lost when lying or bending, and gastric reflux occurs more easily. ASSESSMENT (ADULT/NUTRITION AND METABOLISM)

117. #3. Esophagus-sphincter pressure is increased by gastrin in the stomach and decreased by fatty foods, secretin, and cholecystokinin from the small intestine. ASSESSMENT (ADULT/NUTRITION AND METABOLISM)

118. #2. Smoking and alcohol aggravate and contribute to the condition. The head of the bed should be raised. PLAN (ADULT/NUTRITION AND METABOLISM)

119. #2. The late development of symptoms, coupled with early lymphatic spread, means that metastasis has probably occurred by the time the disease is diagnosed. ANALYSIS (ADULT/NUTRITION AND METABOLISM)

120. #1. Clients are advised to eat small meals to prevent excessive gastric distension, and to avoid eating prior to going to bed or lying down. IMPLEMENTATION (ADULT/NUTRITION AND METABOLISM)

121. **#2.** A local anesthetic is given to deaden the gag reflex. Do not give oral fluids until this reflex returns. Without a gag reflex, risk of aspiration is high. IMPLEMENTATION (ADULT/NUTRITION AND METABOLISM)

122. **#3.** Guaiac testing is done to detect presence of occult (not visible) blood. ANALYSIS (ADULT/NUTRITION AND METABOLISM)

123. **#3.** Duodenal ulcer pain occurs when excess hydrochloric acid irritates an empty stomach. ASSESSMENT (ADULT/NUTRITION AND METABOLISM)

124. **#2.** Nicotine stimulates the secretory cells and increases gastric acidity thus enhancing symptoms. IMPLEMENTATION (ADULT/NUTRITION AND METABOLISM)

125. **#2.** Caffeine also stimulates gastric acidity. IMPLEMENTATION (ADULT/NUTRITION AND METABOLISM)

126. **#4.** A subtotal gastrectomy (Bilroth I or II) involves removal of ½ to ⅔ of the lower stomach. ANALYSIS (ADULT/NUTRITION AND METABOLISM)

127. **#1.** The vagus nerve stimulates secretion of hydrochloric acid. The other options do not describe functions of the vagus nerve. ANALYSIS (ADULT/NUTRITION AND METABOLISM)

128. **#2.** The secretion of bile is blocked if the duodenum is removed. ANALYSIS (ADULT/NUTRITION AND METABOLISM)

129. **#2.** The high incision causes pain that, in turn, limits chest expansion. ANALYSIS (ADULT/NUTRITION AND METABOLISM)

130. **#3.** When bowel sounds return to normal, peristalsis has returned and the nasogastric tube can be removed. ANALYSIS (ADULT/NUTRITION AND METABOLISM)

131. **#4.** Post-subtotal gastrectomy, food can move quickly into the jejunum in a highly concentrated form, causing what is known as the dumping syndrome. ANALYSIS (ADULT/NUTRITION AND METABOLISM)

132. **#1.** Amphogel coats the gastrointestinal mucosa, but is not absorbed systemically. Constipation may result from the aluminum. Phosphorus excretion is enhanced; it binds the phosphorus from the serum and is lost in the stool. Both constipation and phosphorus excretion may be dose related. ANALYSIS (ADULT/NUTRITION AND METABOLISM)

133. **#4.** Propantheline bromide (Pro-Banthine) is an anticholinergic drug. ANALYSIS (ADULT/NUTRITION AND METABOLISM)

134. **#2.** The primary function of propantheline is to decrease acid secretion; decreasing motility results in slowed emptying. ANALYSIS (ADULT/NUTRITION AND METABOLISM)

135. **#4.** Urinary retention can be a serious side effect of propantheline bromide. ANALYSIS (ADULT/NUTRITION AND METABOLISM)

136. **#3.** Diverticulitis is an inflammatory condition manifested by crampy lower quadrant pain, diarrhea with blood and mucus, weakness, and anemia. ANALYSIS (ADULT/NUTRITION AND METABOLISM)

137. **#2.** Diverticula often perforate. These are signs and symptoms of perforation and peritonitis. ASSESSMENT (ADULT/NUTRITION AND METABOLISM)

138. **#1.** Diverticula are usually located in the sigmoid colon. Because a diagnosis of diverticulitis has not been previously established, the entire lower gastrointestinal tract will be x-rayed and the entire colon examined to rule out other abnormalities. ANALYSIS (ADULT/NUTRITION AND METABOLISM)

139. **#4.** Clients with diverticulitis should have a high-residue diet and avoid foods that are highly refined and processed, as they predispose the clients to this condition. IMPLEMENTATION (ADULT/NUTRITION AND METABOLISM)

140. **#2.** A fecalith obstructs the lumen of the appendix leading to inflammation. ANALYSIS (ADULT/NUTRITION AND METABOLISM)

141. **#2.** The colon is filled with bacteria that invade the peritoneal cavity after the appendix ruptures. ANALYSIS (ADULT/NUTRITION AND METABOLISM)

142. **#3.** Vitamin C is important in the formation of granulation and collagen tissue. ANALYSIS (ADULT/NUTRITION AND METABOLISM)

143. **#2.** Until the client is responsive, she should be maintained in a side-lying position to prevent aspiration of secretions or vomitus. IMPLEMENTATION (ADULT/NUTRITION AND METABOLISM)

144. #3. Pain is a subjective experience. Clients' reactions to pain vary widely, depending upon such factors as training, culture, and previous experiences. How a client exhibits pain is not always a reliable indicator of how much pain s/he is experiencing. ASSESSMENT (ADULT/NUTRITION AND METABOLISM)

145. #1. Cholecystectomy clients have an increased susceptibility to respiratory complications. Because of the subcostal incision and the discomfort associated with the incision site, they tend to breathe shallowly. PLAN (ADULT/NUTRITION AND METABOLISM)

146. #3. An output of 30 ml or less per hour is indicative of inadequate fluid-volume replacement after surgery. Options #1, #2, and #4 are expected outcomes after this surgery. ASSESSMENT (ADULT/NUTRITION AND METABOLISM)

147. #4. Factors that contribute to delayed wound healing in obese clients are limited vascularity of adipose tissue, dead spaces in adipose tissue left during suturing, and increased tension on sutures. ASSESSMENT (ADULT/NUTRITION AND METABOLISM)

148. #1. Following discharge, the client who has had abdominal surgery is usually permitted activity as tolerated. The only restriction is to avoid heavy lifting, pushing, and pulling. EVALUATION (ADULT/NUTRITION AND METABOLISM)

149. #4. Signs and symptoms consistent with a diagnosis of cholecystitis include fullness, eructation, and dyspepsia following fat ingestion; abdominal pain, usually in the right upper quadrant; and nausea and vomiting. ASSESSMENT (ADULT/NUTRITION AND METABOLISM)

150. #4. You would verify the order with the physician who wrote it. Meperidine (Demerol) is usually ordered, because morphine causes spasms of the bile ducts, which may result in increased pain. IMPLEMENTATION (ADULT/NUTRITION AND METABOLISM)

151. #4. A cholecystogram is an x-ray visualization of the gallbladder and biliary tract following oral ingestion of iodine dye. An allergy history is important. If she is allergic to any shellfish, she may be allergic to iodine. ASSESSMENT (ADULT/NUTRITION AND METABOLISM)

152. #3. A T tube is inserted whenever the common bile duct is explored. The other options describe a standard cholecystectomy, which does not require placement of a T tube. ANALYSIS (ADULT/NUTRITION AND METABOLISM)

153. #2. You would irrigate a nasogastric tube only with normal saline and as ordered to keep it patent. Using distilled water can cause electrolyte depletion. IMPLEMENTATION (ADULT/NUTRITION AND METABOLISM)

154. #4. This answer provides Mrs. Belzer with specific information. IMPLEMENTATION (ADULT/NUTRITION AND METABOLISM)

155. #4. You would notify her physician, because drainage should be 200 to 500 ml per day for the first several days. IMPLEMENTATION (ADULT/NUTRITION AND METABOLISM)

156. #3. A T tube is usually removed 10 to 12 days after surgery, following a T-tube cholangiogram, to determine the status of the common bile duct, which should be patent. ANALYSIS (ADULT/NUTRITION AND METABOLISM)

157. #2. Common causes of pancreatitis are trauma, infection, alcohol abuse, and gallbladder disease. These disorders can cause fibrosis of the pancreas, which results in inadequate digestion of fats and proteins. ASSESSMENT (ADULT/NUTRITION AND METABOLISM)

158. #2. The exocrine function of the pancreas is to secrete amylase, lipase, and trypsin. Secretion of insulin is an endocrine function. ANALYSIS (ADULT/NUTRITION AND METABOLISM)

159. #1. By keeping the client NPO, digestive activity is decreased, and there is less pancreatic stimulation. The other options are appropriate secondary goals. PLAN (ADULT/NUTRITION AND METABOLISM)

160. #3. Propantheline bromide (Pro-Banthine) is an anticholinergic drug useful as an antispasmodic to relieve pancreatic pain. ANALYSIS (ADULT/NUTRITION AND METABOLISM)

161. #1. The serum amylase is the first of the pancreatic enzymes to rise in pancreatitis, and the level is used most frequently to diagnose and to evaluate response to treatment. EVALUATION (ADULT/NUTRITION AND METABOLISM)

162. #4. The serum transaminases are the first to show an elevation. Abnormal serum ammonia or bilirubin or prothrombin time are all indicative of more advanced, more serious disease. ASSESSMENT (ADULT/NUTRITION AND METABOLISM)

163. **#2.** Bed rest with bathroom privileges is recommended to promote liver regeneration. PLAN (ADULT/NUTRITION AND METABOLISM)

164. **#3.** Adequate calories either in the diet or through intravenous therapy are necessary for the liver to regenerate. PLAN (ADULT/NUTRITION AND METABOLISM)

165. **#4.** In cirrhosis, the liver cells develop fatty infiltrates and degenerate by an inflammatory process. Therefore, there are fewer liver cells available to accommodate the volume of blood. The inflammatory process also increases the congestion in the liver, which inhibits blood flow. This results in venous back-up causing dilation of the esophageal vessels. ANALYSIS (ADULT/NUTRITION AND METABOLISM)

166. **#1.** It is important for the nurse to elicit an alcohol-consumption history from the client in order to accurately observe withdrawal. PLAN (ADULT/NUTRITION AND METABOLISM)

167. **#4.** A quiet, calm environment with even lighting minimizes the chance of creating shadows and reactions such as alcoholic hallucinations. Unusual noise or lighting may increase or stimulate agitation. IMPLEMENTATION (ADULT/NUTRITION AND METABOLISM)

168. **#2.** Portal hypertension is common in cirrhosis and causes these problems. ASSESSMENT (ADULT/NUTRITION AND METABOLISM)

169. **#3.** Prothrombin time increases in clients with cirrhosis; it takes blood longer to clot when there is liver failure. ASSESSMENT (ADULT/NUTRITION AND METABOLISM)

170. **#2.** Portal hypertension causes blood to accumulate in the weaker vessels of the esophagus, causing them to become distended. These vessels can rupture, if the distension becomes too great. ANALYSIS (ADULT/NUTRITION AND METABOLISM)

171. **#2.** Portal hypertension will not cause pulmonary edema. Pulmonary edema is usually due to left-sided heart failure. ANALYSIS (ADULT/NUTRITION AND METABOLISM)

172. **#1.** Insertion of any tube through the esophagus traumatizes the distended vessels making reinsertion for a faulty tube undesirable. Therefore, checking the balloons for leaks prior to insertion is a priority. Labeling the lumens of the tube prevents confusion after the tube has been inserted. Both balloons are always inflated with air, never fluid, and are inflated after placement. IMPLEMENTATION (ADULT/NUTRITION AND METABOLISM)

173. **#2.** The administration of a neomycin enema may be done at a later time to decrease ammonia production in the bowel and to prevent hepatic coma. IMPLEMENTATION (ADULT/NUTRITION AND METABOLISM)

174. **#3.** The client should be placed in a semi-Fowler's position (not supine) to promote ventilation and prevent gastric reflux and aspiration. Side lying with the head up is also acceptable. IMPLEMENTATION (ADULT/NUTRITION AND METABOLISM)

175. **#3.** Upward dislodgment of the gastric balloon may result in respiration obstruction. ANALYSIS (ADULT/NUTRITION AND METABOLISM)

176. **#2.** Vasopressin is a potent vasopressor; optimally, it results in constriction of the esophageal veins. It can be given IV or via a nasogastric tube. IMPLEMENTATION (ADULT/NUTRITION AND METABOLISM)

177. **#4.** Clients with Sengstaken-Blakemore tubes should be sedated cautiously because of the risk of aspiration and respiratory insufficiency. PLAN (ADULT/NUTRITION AND METABOLISM)

178. **#1.** This client needs a bland diet to reduce the amount of hydrochloric acid in the stomach; he needs a low-sodium diet to decrease his ascites. IMPLEMENTATION (ADULT/NUTRITION AND METABOLISM)

179. **#2.** Hepatic encephalopathy occurs frequently in clients with severe liver disease. ANALYSIS (ADULT/NUTRITION AND METABOLISM)

180. **#3.** In hepatic encephalopathy, the liver is unable to detoxify ammonia and convert it to urea. The ammonia levels build and ammonia crosses the blood-brain barrier, causing decreased mentation. ANALYSIS (ADULT/NUTRITION AND METABOLISM)

181. **#2.** The central venous pressure will give the best and quickest indication of circulating volume. A baseline reading immediately after insertion of the line is a priority. This information is an indirect assessment of adequacy of renal perfusion. IMPLEMENTATION (ADULT/NUTRITION AND METABOLISM)

182. **#4.** Exophthalmos occurs primarily with hyperthyroidism; it is not a sign or symptom of hepatic encephalopathy. ASSESSMENT (ADULT/NUTRITION AND METABOLISM)

183. #1. Neomycin decreases the ammonia-forming bacteria in the intestinal tract, thus decreasing the serum ammonia level. Lactulose decreases the pH of the colon, which allows ammonias to diffuse into the colon from the blood to form nonabsorbable ammonium ions. These are then eliminated in the stool. ANALYSIS (ADULT/NUTRITION AND METABOLISM)

184. #4. Normal bacteria found in the gastrointestinal tract cause ammonia to form. The antibacterial effect of neomycin reduces the intestinal flora. The client's level of consciousness will improve when serum ammonia levels are reduced. PLAN (ADULT/NUTRITION AND METABOLISM)

185. #2. Proteins (amino acids) break down in the body to form ammonia; therefore, a low-protein diet will help prevent the build up of ammonia. PLAN (ADULT/NUTRITION AND METABOLISM)

186. #4. Water intake is restricted to control ascites. IMPLEMENTATION (ADULT/NUTRITION AND METABOLISM)

187. #4. Esophageal varices are observed only with an x-ray or by direct visualization through an endoscope. ASSESSMENT (ADULT/NUTRITION AND METABOLISM)

188. #2. The nutritional inadequacies are easier to correct by teaching about nutrition and diet. Long-term substance-abuse problems are difficult to control. ANALYSIS (ADULT/NUTRITION AND METABOLISM)

189. #2. He was admitted after having vomited large quantities of blood. Oral hygiene is most likely to make him comfortable. IMPLEMENTATION (ADULT/NUTRITION AND METABOLISM)

190. #2. Rupture of varices causes hemorrhage that can be life threatening. ASSESSMENT (ADULT/NUTRITION AND METABOLISM)

191. #2. Pruritus is a result of bile salt excretion through the skin. It has major implications for nursing care. ASSESSMENT (ADULT/NUTRITION AND METABOLISM)

192. #2. Weight loss or gain directly reflects water loss or gain. ASSESSMENT (ADULT/NUTRITION AND METABOLISM)

193. #4. Gynecomastia is an endocrine problem commonly seen in cirrhosis of the liver, but it is not preventable with nursing actions. ANALYSIS (ADULT/NUTRITION AND METABOLISM)

194. #3. Growth hormone secreted after the epiphyses have closed causes an increase in bone density, not height. Blindness commonly occurs, unless the hormone secretion is stopped. ANALYSIS (ADULT/NUTRITION AND METABOLISM)

195. #4. Prolactin is secreted by the pituitary gland in pregnant and nursing women to produce lactation. A pituitary tumor can produce an excess of this hormone, causing galactorrhea. ANALYSIS (ADULT/NUTRITION AND METABOLISM)

196. #4. A serum calcium will give no information about the type of tumor or size of the lesion, whereas the other studies will. ASSESSMENT (ADULT/NUTRITION AND METABOLISM)

197. #2. Diabetes insipidus is a frequent complication following a hypophysectomy. Large volumes of urine may be excreted, causing critical problems if not treated. PLAN (ADULT/NUTRITION AND METABOLISM)

198. #1. Hypopituitarism is a common problem with clients who have had hypophysectomies, since the anterior pituitary gland has been affected. Pituitary hormone replacements may have to be given. ANALYSIS (ADULT/NUTRITION AND METABOLISM)

199. #3. The gonadal-stimulating hormones from the pituitary that affect pregnancy may be deficient, but replacements can be administered. IMPLEMENTATION (ADULT/NUTRITION AND METABOLISM)

200. #2. Tingling of the toes, fingers, or around the mouth is the first sign of hypocalcemia, which can lead to tetany. Thyroid surgery clients are at high risk for this problem because of the possibility of removal of or damage to the parathyroid gland. ASSESSMENT (ADULT/NUTRITION AND METABOLISM)

201. #3. Assist Mrs. Schiller to the semi-Fowler's position with her neck supported for optimal ventilation and to avoid strain on the neck muscles. IMPLEMENTATION (ADULT/NUTRITION AND METABOLISM)

202. #4. Hypoparathyroidism leads to hypocalcemia, which causes increased neuromuscular irritability and laryngospasm. ASSESSMENT (ADULT/NUTRITION AND METABOLISM)

203. #3. Respiratory distress from edema or hemorrhage is a potential complication of a subtotal thyroidectomy, so a tracheostomy set is kept at Mrs. Schiller's bedside. IMPLEMENTATION (ADULT/NUTRITION AND METABOLISM)

204. **#2.** Hypocalcemia can result from the accidental removal of 1 or 2 parathyroid glands, so calcium gluconate must be kept on hand. Calcium gluconate is more readily used than calcium chloride if given IV. ANALYSIS (ADULT/NUTRITION AND METABOLISM)

205. **#2.** Flexing or hyperextending the neck puts excessive tension on the surgical site. The other options are all appropriate nursing actions. IMPLEMENTATION (ADULT/NUTRITION AND METABOLISM)

206. **#2.** Prior to instructing the client on self-care related to diabetes, the nurse must establish a baseline regarding the client's knowledge of diabetes. Assessment of client knowledge is the priority prior to teaching. ASSESSMENT (ADULT/NUTRITION AND METABOLISM)

207. **#3.** Diabetes is a chronic disorder of carbohydrate metabolism and is one of the leading causes of death in the United States. It is not a curable illness. ANALYSIS (ADULT/NUTRITION AND METABOLISM)

208. **#1.** In diabetes, insulin deficiency results in hyperglycemia. Glucose is excreted in the urine and, acting as an osmotic diuretic, carries water and electrolytes with it. ANALYSIS (ADULT/NUTRITION AND METABOLISM)

209. **#3.** In addition, more rapid absorption can occur in unaffected sites leading to hypoglycemia. ANALYSIS (ADULT/NUTRITION AND METABOLISM)

210. **#1.** Peak hours of action for regular insulin are 2 to 4 hours after administration. ANALYSIS (ADULT/NUTRITION AND METABOLISM)

211. **#4.** The other options are symptoms of hyperglycemia. ASSESSMENT (ADULT/NUTRITION AND METABOLISM)

212. **#2.** Exercise is important for diabetic clients and is planned according to age and interests, and in balance with the prescribed insulin and diet regimen. ANALYSIS (ADULT/NUTRITION AND METABOLISM)

213. **#4.** Hunger is characteristic; but because the glucose cannot be used, weight loss occurs. ASSESSMENT (ADULT/NUTRITION AND METABOLISM)

214. **#1.** These are indicators of dehydration. This is the major initial problem to be treated. ASSESSMENT (ADULT/NUTRITION AND METABOLISM)

215. **#3.** The client has a fluid deficit of 8 to 12 liters, and replacement should be carried out as rapidly as tolerated. PLAN (ADULT/NUTRITION AND METABOLISM)

216. **#4.** This is the most therapeutic and most honest response. IMPLEMENTATION (ADULT/NUTRITION AND METABOLISM)

217. **#1.** Intermittent claudication is pain in the extremity with exercise, usually walking. When the energy demands exceed the oxygen supply, pain is experienced. ASSESSMENT (ADULT/NUTRITION AND METABOLISM)

218. **#2.** Keeping the feet covered with socks will keep the feet warm and not compromise circulation any further. Using external heat, such as hot water bottles, increases oxygen consumption and impairs arterial flow even more. IMPLEMENTATION (ADULT/NUTRITION AND METABOLISM)

219. **#3.** It is important for her to talk about her fears of body changes and loss, even if she will never need an amputation. IMPLEMENTATION (ADULT/NUTRITION AND METABOLISM)

220. **#4.** Even though Mrs. Carter is a type 2 diabetic, the stress of surgery may cause her blood sugar to rise for a short time; thus, it should be controlled with short-acting insulin administered according to her needs. IMPLEMENTATION (ADULT/NUTRITION AND METABOLISM)

221. **#1.** Irritability is often the first sign of hypoglycemia, particularly in the morning when the client has not had anything to eat for several hours. IMPLEMENTATION (ADULT/NUTRITION AND METABOLISM)

222. **#4.** Complex carbohydrates have much value in the diabetic diet as they are a good source of energy and keep the blood sugar more stable. IMPLEMENTATION (ADULT/NUTRITION AND METABOLISM)

223. **#3.** Elevating the legs is indicated for venous, not arterial, problems of the extremities. IMPLEMENTATION (ADULT/NUTRITION AND METABOLISM)

224. **#2.** Weakness and weight loss are symptoms of adrenocortical insufficiency. Increased skin pigmentation results as adrenal insufficiency allows melanocyte-stimulating hormone levels to increase. ASSESSMENT (ADULT/NUTRITION AND METABOLISM)

225. **#2.** Stress of any type increases the client's weakness. The client is vulnerable to stress, because she lacks the protection of the adrenal hormones. Exertion is a type of physiologic stress. PLAN (ADULT/NUTRITION AND METABOLISM)

226. **#4.** Addison's disease is characterized by inadequate amounts of cortisol, which results in hypotension. PLAN (ADULT/NUTRITION AND METABOLISM)

227. **#4.** Critical deficiency of glucocorticoids leads to vascular collapse. ASSESSMENT (ADULT/NUTRITION AND METABOLISM)

228. **#4.** The client with Addison's disease can live a normal life, provided the client takes the daily steroid medications without exception. IMPLEMENTATION (ADULT/NUTRITION AND METABOLISM)

229. **#1.** Clients at high risk for septic shock include the very young, the very old, those with genitourinary infections who undergo cystoscopy, and those with severe gastrointestinal blood loss. ASSESSMENT (ADULT/ELIMINATION)

230. **#4.** This answer gives Mr. Thomas an opportunity to express his concerns and fears. The other options do not acknowledge his concerns. IMPLEMENTATION (ADULT/ELIMINATION)

231. **#3.** Septic shock is insidious in onset, and slight changes in vital signs may be the only warning. Therefore, check the vital signs again in 15 minutes for any changes. IMPLEMENTATION (ADULT/ELIMINATION)

232. **#4.** Restlessness is an early sign of septic shock. Hypotension and cool, clammy skin are late signs. In early septic shock, urinary output is slightly decreased. ASSESSMENT (ADULT/ELIMINATION)

233. **#3.** Dried apricots are high in potassium and low in sodium; the other choices are high in sodium. EVALUATION (ADULT/ELIMINATION)

234. **#3.** It is important that the client with high blood pressure stop smoking. The other options are not correct statements. EVALUATION (ADULT/ELIMINATION)

235. **#1.** Forcing fluids serves as an internal irrigant, flushes the urinary tract, and decreases burning. Options #2 and #4 are important but focused more on prevention. Option #1 is most important for *treating* the infection. IMPLEMENTATION (ADULT/ELIMINATION)

236. **#4.** This is a sign of possible anaphylaxis. The client should be informed about the other reactions, which are normal. ASSESSMENT (ADULT/ELIMINATION)

237. **#2.** Activity aids in passage of the calculus. Even though she may need pain relief and will have to strain her urine, these do not aid in passage of stones. IMPLEMENTATION (ADULT/ELIMINATION)

238. **#1.** Calculi readily develop in immobile clients and especially in those with multiple myeloma, because the diseased bones release calcium, leading to the formation of calculi. ANALYSIS (ADULT/ELIMINATION)

239. **#1.** The etiology of bladder cancer is related to cigarette smoking and exposure to dyes used in rubber and cable industries. ASSESSMENT (ADULT/ELIMINATION)

240. **#2.** Painless, gross hematuria is the most common clinical finding and the first sign in 75% of clients with carcinoma of the bladder. ASSESSMENT (ADULT/ELIMINATION)

241. **#4.** Gentle acceptance of the client's anxiety and open-ended questioning allows the client the opportunity to express his feelings and concerns. IMPLEMENTATION (ADULT/ELIMINATION)

242. **#2.** Instruct the client to do range-of-motion exercises for his legs and teach him to keep his legs uncrossed. These activities decrease the risk of thrombophlebitis. IMPLEMENTATION (ADULT/ELIMINATION)

243. **#3.** A nasogastric tube may become obstructed with mucus, sediment, or old blood. It can be checked for patency by irrigating with 30 ml of normal saline. IMPLEMENTATION (ADULT/ELIMINATION)

244. **#3.** There is a risk of paralytic ileus when part of the bowel is removed. A nasogastric tube is used for 3 to 5 days or until bowel sounds return. ANALYSIS (ADULT/ELMINATION)

245. **#4.** The urinary stoma should be dark pink to red. A dark red color is indicative of inadequate circulation. ASSESSMENT (ADULT/ELIMINATION)

246. **#4.** Intramuscular or subcutaneous injections should not be administered because of the vasoconstriction in hypotension. Medications may not be absorbed and accumulate; then when perfusion improves, the client could experience an overdose. IMPLEMENTATION (ADULT/ELIMINATION)

247. **#2.** Normal potassium is 3.5 to 5.0 mEq/liter. Hyperkalemia can cause lethal cardiac dysrhythmias if not promptly treated. ASSESSMENT (ADULT/ELIMINATION)

248. **#1.** Fluid restriction is indicated during the oliguric phase of renal failure, when fluid overload is a problem. ANALYSIS (ADULT/ELIMINATION)

249. **#3.** Trousseau's sign is an indication of tetany, which results from the increased neuromuscular irritability caused by hypocalcemia. The method of eliciting this sign is to constrict the radial or brachial artery and observe the hand/fingers for spasm. The constriction can be done with a blood pressure cuff. ANALYSIS (ADULT/ELIMINATION)

250. **#1.** This is the only correct group of actions. In addition, bed rest should be maintained to reduce the buildup of lactic acid, which is released with muscle activity. Restrict fluids to reduce hypervolemia. IMPLEMENTATION (ADULT/ELIMINATION)

251. **#3.** The diuretic phase of acute renal failure causes loss of circulating volume, potassium, and sodium. This phase is exacerbated by the buildup of urea during the oliguric phase, which acts as a natural diuretic. ASSESSMENT (ADULT/ELIMINATION)

252. **#3.** The blood urea nitrogen becomes elevated because functioning nephrons are damaged and the body is unable to get rid of waste products through the kidneys. ANALYSIS (ADULT/ELIMINATION)

253. **#1.** A diet high in calories and low in protein is prescribed. The protein should be of high biologic value to prevent catabolism of body protein. IMPLEMENTATION (ADULT/ELIMINATION)

254. **#2.** Careful monitoring of the client's intake and output is important, as fluid replacement is often based on the output. PLAN (ADULT/ELIMINATION)

255. **#2.** These laboratory findings are consistent with renal failure. A decreased serum calcium results from both a decreased gastrointestinal absorption of calcium and an elevated serum phosphorus. The inability of the kidneys to excrete the potassium raises the potassium as well as the hydrogen ion level, and results in acidosis. ASSESSMENT (ADULT/ELIMINATION)

256. **#4.** Potassium shortens the repolarization phase of cardiac conduction, increasing cardiac irritability. This predisposes to irregularities, fibrillation, and eventual cardiac standstill. ANALYSIS (ADULT/ELIMINATION)

257. **#1.** The kidneys are unable to excrete the hydrogen ion or reabsorb the bicarbonate ion. The result is acidosis, for which the lungs attempt to compensate by blowing off excess hydrogen ion (carbon dioxide). ANALYSIS (ADULT/ELIMINATION)

258. **#4.** Phosphorus and calcium are inversely related. Potassium levels are usually inversely related to sodium. ANALYSIS (ADULT/ELIMINATION)

259. **#4.** Aluminum hydroxide antacids bind with the phosphate ion and are then excreted in the stool. ANALYSIS (ADULT/ELIMINATION)

260. **#3.** A client treated with peritoneal dialysis may need to be dialyzed 3 to 5 times per week for 8 to 12 hours each time. ANALYSIS (ADULT/ELIMINATION)

261. **#1.** Respiratory distress may indicate a fluid shift and pulmonary edema, requiring immediate attention. Hemorrhage is less likely once the catheter is in place; abdominal pain and peritonitis may also occur, but breathing is the first priority. ANALYSIS (ADULT/ELIMINATION)

262. **#2.** The life span of the shunt is 6 to 12 months. Major complications are clotting and infections, which are avoided by not using the arm for taking blood pressure or blood drawing. IMPLEMENTATION (ADULT/ELIMINATION)

263. **#1.** These are symptoms of the disequilibrium syndrome. It occurs when urea is removed more rapidly from the blood than the brain. The osmotic gradient caused by urea results in fluid passing to cerebral cells; thus, cerebral edema occurs. IMPLEMENTATION (ADULT/ELIMINATION)

264. **#2.** The Foley catheter is inserted to maintain urinary flow. Monitor intake and output throughout Mr. Rasmussen's pre- and post-op periods. PLAN (ADULT/ELIMINATION)

265. **#4.** A transurethral resection is the only type of prostatic surgery not requiring an incision through the skin. IMPLEMENTATION (ADULT/ELIMINATION)

266. **#1.** If increased blood is seen, first increase the speed of the irrigation. If this is not effective, notify the physician. Do not alter the traction on the Foley, as its purpose is to put pressure on the prostatic bed. Manual irrigation is done mainly for clots and requires a physician order. IMPLEMENTATION (ADULT/ELIMINATION)

267. #1. The large balloon on the Foley can stimulate spasms; therefore, administer narcotics plus anticholinergic drugs as ordered. IMPLEMENTATION (ADULT/ELIMINATION)

268. #4. Nursing strategies that can help prevent thrombophlebitis include helping with leg exercises and taking deep breaths, and obtaining an order for antiembolism stockings for the client. Nursing actions cannot prevent epididymitis, osteitis pubis, or urinary incontinence. ANALYSIS (ADULT/ELIMINATION)

269. #1. Mr. Rasmussen should refrain from sexual intercourse for approximately 6 weeks after surgery. In addition, he should avoid heavy lifting, straining at stool, and driving a car for approximately 6 weeks. IMPLEMENTATION (ADULT/ELIMINATION)

270. #2. Instruct Mr. Rasmussen to monitor his urine at home; it should be continually clear. EVALUATION (ADULT/ELIMINATION)

271. #1. A man with an enlarged prostate has difficulty emptying his bladder and has to strain to urinate. The stream lacks force and becomes weak, and dribbling occurs. Initiating a stream may also be a problem. ASSESSMENT (ADULT/ELIMINATION)

272. #2. Prostatic hypertrophy can be diagnosed by rectal digital exam. Gloves and lubricant are needed. ASSESSMENT (ADULT/ELIMINATION)

273. #3. The kidneys are located in the retroperitoneum, and the bowel must be cleared of any gas or fecal material that would obscure their visualization. Additional preparation for an intravenous pyelogram includes restricting food and fluids from midnight prior to the exam. IMPLEMENTATION (ADULT/ELIMINATION)

274. #2. Continuous bladder irrigation with saline or other solutions is done to remove clotted blood from the bladder. Blood and clots are normal in the first 24 to 48 hours post-TURP. PLAN (ADULT/ELIMINATION)

275. #4. A Foley catheter can irritate the bladder mucosa causing bladder spasms. The catheter must also be checked to ensure patency, but these sensations may be present with a patent catheter. ANALYSIS (ADULT/ELIMINATION)

276. #2. Temporary urinary frequency or incontinence, or both, can occur after removal of the catheter. ANALYSIS (ADULT/ELIMINATION)

277. #4. Race is not a factor in the client's ability to undergo surgery. It does have implications in the nursing care following surgery, especially in the assessment phase of the nursing process. ASSESSMENT (ADULT/ELIMINATION)

278. #4. There is post-op pain with this procedure but it can be managed with analgesics. IMPLEMENTATION (ADULT/ELIMINATION)

279. #2. The rectal area is less than 1 inch from the incision and prostatic bed; taking a rectal temp could cause trauma. An air ring can cause venous stasis and edema; a hard surface may increase pain. IMPLEMENTATION (ADULT/ELIMINATION)

280. #4. Sexual impotence is expected in suprapubic and retropubic prostatectomies, but not following transurethral resections. However, in the immediate post-op period it is too early to assess this activity. IMPLEMENTATION (ADULT/ELIMINATION)

281. #3. This requires a physician's order. In the early post-op period, active exercise is usually limited to leg dangling and brief ambulation. Passive exercise, however, is imperative for Mr. Lacona. PLAN (ADULT/ELIMINATION)

282. #1. Any invasive procedure on the urinary tract increases risk of urinary tract infections. ANALYSIS (ADULT/ELIMINATION)

283. #3. After removal of the catheter, incontinence is common in the older prostatectomy client because a Foley catheter decreases the contractility of the bladder muscle. PLAN (ADULT/ELIMINATION)

284. #1. The lower gastrointestinal tract must be clear for the exam. Cathartics are given at least 12 hours before the test, along with enemas till clear the morning of the exam. IMPLEMENTATION (ADULT/ELIMINATION)

285. #4. The knee-chest position provides maximum exposure for the proctosigmoidoscopy. IMPLEMENTATION (ADULT/ELIMINATION)

286. #2. No anesthetic is given and the client must relax, not bear down. The procedure is not painful, but it is uncomfortable. IMPLEMENTATION (ADULT/ELIMINATION)

287. #1. Stool samples for amoebae must be tested while they are warm and fresh, or the amoebae will die. IMPLEMENTATION (ADULT/ELIMINATION)

288. #1. Ulcerative colitis is characterized by very frequent diarrhea with mucus and blood, caused by inflammation of the colonic mucosa. ASSESSMENT (ADULT/ELIMINATION)

289. #1. Vitamin K, vital to the formation of prothrombin, is normally absorbed in the colon. ANALYSIS (ADULT/ELIMINATION)

290. #1. Sedation and decreased bladder tone may occur, but these drugs are given to decrease gastrointestinal motility. ANALYSIS (ADULT/ELIMINATION)

291. #2. An ileostomy involves removal of the whole colon and formation of an ileal stoma. ANALYSIS (ADULT/ELIMINATION)

292. #3. An ileostomy has liquid, almost continuous drainage. Weight gain may result from new found food tolerance. The drainage containing enzymes is irritating to the skin. ASSESSMENT (ADULT/ELIMINATION)

293. #1. Research indicates that virtually 100% of colon polyps are premalignant and can be expected to become cancerous if not excised. Colitis and amebiasis cause chronic irritation and therefore may predispose the client to colon cancer. ASSESSMENT (ADULT/ELIMINATION)

294. #3. Palpation is done last, because it can stimulate bowel sounds. Percussion usually does not stimulate bowel sounds as the technique is superficial to the bowel. ASSESSMENT (ADULT/ELIMINATION)

295. #4. Signs and symptoms of mechanical obstruction of the colon include decreased bowel sounds, abdominal distension, decreased flatus, and projectile vomiting. ASSESSMENT (ADULT/ELIMINATION)

296. #3. Fluid and electrolyte deficiency is the major problem, if the intestinal blood supply is not compromised. ANALYSIS (ADULT/ELIMINATION)

297. #2. The Miller-Abbott tube is an intestinal tube with an inflated bag designed to advance into the intestine. Taping it could traumatize nasal tissue as well as prevent further advance of the tube. IMPLEMENTATION (ADULT/ELIMINATION)

298. #1. Review deep breathing exercises. Mr. Hawkins's weight and a probable abdominal incision predispose him to post-op pulmonary complications. Preoperatively, a distended abdomen may prevent him from doing a return demonstration of deep-breathing exercises. IMPLEMENTATION (ADULT/ELIMINATION)

299. #2. Feces become increasingly firm as they progress through the colon because of water being reabsorbed back into the body. Stool in the transverse colon is mushy to semiformed, depending on the specific location. ASSESSMENT (ADULT/ELIMINATION)

300. #3. Colostomy irrigations should be done only once a day. IMPLEMENTATION (ADULT/ELIMINATION)

301. #3. The area around stoma must be kept dry and oil free in order for the colostomy appliance to adhere. IMPLEMENTATION (ADULT/ELIMINATION)

302. #1. Eating a balanced diet will provide proper stool consistency. A colostomy can be irrigated at any time that is convenient for the client. ANALYSIS (ADULT/ELIMINATION)

303. #4. Gradual involvement of the client in his ostomy care is more likely to increase acceptance. PLAN (ADULT/ELIMINATION)

304. #2. A nasogastric tube attached to suction keeps the stomach drained and decompressed. This prevents the risk of aspiration prior to, during, and after surgery. ANALYSIS (ADULT/ELIMINATION)

305. #3. Although the catheter can be used to check renal function, the proximity of the rectum and sigmoid colon to the bladder makes avoidance of injury a prime concern. ANALYSIS (ADULT/ELIMINATION)

306. #1. Colon tumors metastasize to other areas within the colon by direct extension. Enough colon needs to be removed so that the specimen margins are clear of any tumor cells. ANALYSIS (ADULT/ELIMINATION)

307. #3. Tube feedings circumvent swallowing, anorexia, and the gag reflex and can be administered regardless of appetite or level of consciousness; but the gastrointestinal tract distal to the feeding must be intact and functioning. ANALYSIS (ADULT/ELIMINATION)

308. #4. Talking to a person who has a colostomy and has it well under control can be very encouraging for the new ostomate. IMPLEMENTATION (ADULT/ELIMINATION)

309. #3. Warm tap water will cause the least irritation, while at the same time stimulating evacuation of the colon. IMPLEMENTATION (ADULT/ELIMINATION)

310. #4. The client must be relaxed for successful irrigation. ANALYSIS (ADULT/ELIMINATION)

311. #2. Excessive flatus is not symptomatic of colon cancer. A change in bowel habits is more common with left-sided lesions, while pain and obstructive symptoms are more common with right-sided lesions. ASSESSMENT (ADULT/ELIMINATION)

312. #3. While the carcinoembryonic antigen has been used in recent years to aid in diagnosing colon cancer, it is not as conclusive as a biopsy of the lesion. ANALYSIS (ADULT/ELIMINATION)

313. #2. Neomycin is given to achieve bowel sterilization. It destroys the normal flora of the bowel and will result in some loose stools. This enhances the bowel cleansing and is the desired outcome. IMPLEMENTATION (ADULT/ELIMINATION)

314. #1. The colostomy will be permanent as the cancerous rectum will be removed. Denial or lack of understanding may be the problem. In either case, further teaching is needed. EVALUATION (ADULT/ELIMINATION)

315. #2. Getting Mr. Simms to talk about his fears and concerns before he is discharged is the priority right now. IMPLEMENTATION (ADULT/ELIMINATION)

316. #2. Bone-marrow depression and stomatitis are the main side effects from this drug. A decreased white blood cell count can make him more prone to infection. PLAN (ADULT/ELIMINATION)

317. #3. Insulin shock must be ruled out as an etiology when dealing with a comatose client with no signs of injury. PLAN (ADULT/SAFETY AND SECURITY)

318. #1. Vital signs can reflect a client's increasing intracranial pressure. The other procedures are not indicated at this time. PLAN (ADULT/SAFETY AND SECURITY)

319. #1. All options except diabetic coma could cause unequal pupil reactions. ANALYSIS (ADULT/SAFETY AND SECURITY)

320. #3. Biot's respirations are totally irregular. ASSESSMENT (ADULT/SAFETY AND SECURITY)

321. #1. This describes decerebrate posturing, a sign of serious neurologic damage. ASSESSMENT (ADULT/SAFETY AND SECURITY)

322. #2. The most likely cause of Mrs. Swan's condition is an aneurysm; hypertension is a predisposing factor, and headaches may be a symptom. ANALYSIS (ADULT/SAFETY AND SECURITY)

323. #2. Unless a baseline is established, significant post-op changes could be overlooked. PLAN (ADULT/SAFETY AND SECURITY)

324. #1. The pupil and neurologic checks are important; however, maintaining respiratory status is the highest priority. PLAN (ADULT/SAFETY AND SECURITY)

325. #2. Pooling of secretions occurs when the client is in a side-lying position. These need to be suctioned before the client is repositioned. IMPLEMENTATION (ADULT/OXYGENATION)

326. #1. A tracheostomy is performed when an endotracheal tube is required for a long period of time in order to prevent tracheal necrosis. Postural drainage is done prior to or at least 2 hours after meals to prevent regurgitation. Options #2 and #3 are not correct. ANALYSIS (ADULT/OXYGENATION)

327. #4. The trachea is suctioned first using a sterile catheter. To suction the mouth first would contaminate the equipment. Remember the rule: clean to dirty. IMPLEMENTATION (ADULT/OXYGENATION)

328. #2. If the pharynx is not suctioned first, the secretions will be aspirated into the trachea when the cuff is deflated. IMPLEMENTATION (ADULT/OXYGENATION)

329. #2. Acidosis is not routinely treated with a respirator. ANALYSIS (ADULT/OXYGENATION)

330. #4. Restraints will likely increase client resistance. IMPLEMENTATION (ADULT/OXYGENATION)

331. #3. Of the options listed only anti-inflammatory drugs do not have respiratory depression as a side effect. ANALYSIS (ADULT/OXYGENATION)

332. #2. Diabetes insipidus occurs when there is suppression of antidiuretic hormone (ADH), leading to uncontrolled diuresis. ANALYSIS (ADULT/SAFETY AND SECURITY)

333. #3. ADH is stored and secreted by the posterior pituitary lobe. It is produced in the hypothalmus. ANALYSIS (ADULT/SAFETY AND SECURITY)

334. #2. The uncontrolled diuresis leads to loss of water and washout of most electrolytes. ANALYSIS (ADULT/SAFETY AND SECURITY)

335. #1. The urine will become very dilute, almost like water. ASSESSMENT (ADULT/SAFETY AND SECURITY)

336. **#3.** Tachycardia is a symptom of cardiac dysfunction. The options are related to the neurologic system. ASSESSMENT (ADULT/SAFETY AND SECURITY)

337. **#4.** Of the options listed, only a cerebral arteriogram is an invasive procedure. ANALYSIS (ADULT/SAFETY AND SECURITY)

338. **#2.** Control of emotions, personality, and higher level functioning is in the cortex of the frontal lobe. ANALYSIS (ADULT/SAFETY AND SECURITY)

339. **#4.** The client's safety and further assessment are paramount considerations. PLAN (ADULT/SAFETY AND SECURITY)

340. **#1.** All options are important to monitor; however, adequacy of respirations always has the priority. ASSESSMENT (ADULT/SAFETY AND SECURITY)

341. **#3.** The blood pressure is markedly abnormal, particularly the diastolic reading. The 3 other options are considered predisposing or risk factors, not direct etiologies. ANALYSIS (ADULT/SAFETY AND SECURITY)

342. **#2.** It is important to first assess functions necessary for maintenance of life. ASSESSMENT (ADULT/SAFETY AND SECURITY)

343. **#2.** A suction machine will allow the nurse to maintain a patent airway. Maintaining adequate oxygenation is a basic goal for all acutely ill clients. The second priority with a client whose mobility is impaired is correct positioning. PLAN (ADULT/SAFETY AND SECURITY)

344. **#2.** Mouth breathing commonly occurs during a coma. Even clients who are NPO can be properly hydrated and there is no evidence to suggest option #3. #4 is not correct. ANALYSIS (ADULT/SAFETY AND SECURITY)

345. **#4.** Although all options are appropriate, turning the client is the best way to prevent decubitus ulcers. IMPLEMENTATION (ADULT/SAFETY AND SECURITY)

346. **#1.** This is why contractures occur and why positioning is so vital in the stroke client. ANALYSIS (ADULT/SAFETY AND SECURITY)

347. **#2.** Although an increasing temperature may indicate an infectious or healing process, the changes in pulse and respirations indicate a more fundamental problem is occurring. ANALYSIS (ADULT/SAFETY AND SECURITY)

348. **#4.** Allowing her uppermost shoulder to fall out of alignment during the procedure could cause injury. Options #1 and #2 are advisable but are not critical to the procedure. IMPLEMENTATION (ADULT/SAFETY AND SECURITY)

349. **#3.** This is an abnormal finding. The red blood cell count in spinal fluid should be zero. ASSESSMENT (ADULT/SAFETY AND SECURITY)

350. **#1.** Emotional lability often follows this type of cerebral insult. This is the only correct option. IMPLEMENTATION (ADULT/SAFETY AND SECURITY)

351. **#4.** Movement of the head or neck is most likely to cause further trauma and must be avoided. PLAN (ADULT/SAFETY AND SECURITY)

352. **#2.** Spinal shock causes massive vasodilation, inconsistent with hypertension. ASSESSMENT (ADULT/SAFETY AND SECURITY)

353. **#3.** This is the top priority. With a C3-4 injury, paralysis of the diaphragm is likely. PLAN (ADULT/SAFETY AND SECURITY)

354. **#2.** In early stages of injury, no reflexes will be present and the client will have an atonic bladder. The bladder will become increasingly distended if the client is not catheterized. ANALYSIS (ADULT/SAFETY AND SECURITY)

355. **#3.** The sympathetic system controls the "flight or fight" response. The parasympathetic system is more concerned with normal body function. ANALYSIS (ADULT/SAFETY AND SECURITY)

356. **#4.** A reflex is a quick stimulus-response act such as a "hand-on-hot-stove" response. ANALYSIS (ADULT/SAFETY AND SECURITY)

357. **#3.** After a few months, automatic reflexes will return, even when there has been a complete cord transection. ANALYSIS (ADULT/SAFETY AND SECURITY)

358. **#2.** The person with spinal cord injury above T6 has sympathetic fibers that can be stimulated by ascending information entering the cord below level of lesion (i.e., sacral cord). The sympathetics are stimulated to fire, and since the cord is cut off from higher centers, firing is uncontrolled. The symptoms given are classic for autonomic hyperreflexia. ANALYSIS (ADULT/SAFETY AND SECURITY)

359. **#3.** The clamping of the Foley could have precipitated bladder distension. Fear does not stimulate autonomic hyperreflexia. There are no data to suggest that bowel distension may be present. ANALYSIS (ADULT/SAFETY AND SECURITY)

360. **#4.** Demineralization is a major problem with lack of stress on the long bones. Absorption is not changed. ANALYSIS (ADULT/SAFETY AND SECURITY)

361. **#3.** Erection can be stimulated by stroking the genitalia or other parts of the body, because it is a reflex action. Ejaculation may not be present with a complete injury, but may be possible with an incomplete injury. Orgasms may occur but will be different. IMPLEMENTATION (ADULT/SAFETY AND SECURITY)

362. **#3.** Face and neck (approximately) 4%; anterior chest (approximately) 9%; arms and hands 18% (9% each): total = 31%. ASSESSMENT (CHILD/SENSATION, PERCEPTION, PROTECTION)

363. **#3.** Options #1, #2, and #4 are characteristic of third-degree burns. ASSESSMENT (CHILD/SENSATION, PERCEPTION, PROTECTION)

364. **#3.** Persons with orofacial burns are at risk of developing upper airway edema. PLAN (CHILD/SENSATION, PERCEPTION, PROTECTION)

365. **#2.** Blood volume is reduced from the burn's fluid loss resulting in poor peripheral absorption. Burn clients need effective pain relief. ANALYSIS (CHILD/SENSATION, PERCEPTION, PROTECTION)

366. **#4.** More accurate measures are necessitated by the severity of the problem. EVALUATION (CHILD/SENSATION, PERCEPTION, PROTECTION)

367. **#1.** Sulfamylon is a carbonic anhydrase inhibitor and can lead to impairment of the renal buffering system. Options #2, #3, and #4 are side effects of silver nitrate. ASSESSMENT (CHILD/SENSATION, PERCEPTION, PROTECTION)

368. **#1.** Dressings on the donor site are never disturbed without a specific order. PLAN (CHILD/SENSATION, PERCEPTION, PROTECTION)

369. **#4.** A position of comfort often leads to a contracture, because clients tend to flex joints near the burn. Extension is a better position. PLAN (CHILD/SENSATION, PERCEPTION, PROTECTION)

370. **#3.** Since the major cause of death in burn clients is infection, this is the primary goal; however, all the options listed are important goals. PLAN (CHILD/SENSATION, PERCEPTION, PROTECTION)

371. **#3.** This is the area of the brain affected in Parkinson's disease. ANALYSIS (ADULT/SAFETY AND SECURITY)

372. **#3.** Tremors are characteristic of this disease, and the client cannot control them. ASSESSMENT (ADULT/SAFETY AND SECURITY)

373. **#3.** Motor function is tested by observing muscular movement, such as when the client walks. Options #1 and #4 test reflex function; #3 tests cognitive function. ASSESSMENT (ADULT/SAFETY AND SECURITY)

374. **#1.** There is no known cause for most cases of Parkinson's disease. Drugs and arteriosclerosis are implicated only in some cases. ANALYSIS (ADULT/SAFETY AND SECURITY)

375. **#4.** Tremors are the first symptom to appear and the last to be controlled. EVALUATION (ADULT/SAFETY AND SECURITY)

376. **#2.** Pain is the only option listed that is not commonly experienced by persons with multiple sclerosis. ASSESSMENT (ADULT/SAFETY AND SECURITY)

377. **#2.** There is no known benefit to long-term steroid therapy in treating multiple sclerosis. The other options given are all true. IMPLEMENTATION (ADULT/SAFETY AND SECURITY)

378. **#1.** This will prevent head injury. Once the seizure has begun, trying to place something in the mouth is dangerous. IMPLEMENTATION (ADULT/SAFETY AND SECURITY)

379. **#3.** Major seizures, also known as grand mal seizures, are characterized by a preceding aura. ANALYSIS (ADULT/SAFETY AND SECURITY)

380. **#2.** Most, but not all, cases of epilepsy can be controlled by medication. ANALYSIS (ADULT/SAFETY AND SECURITY)

381. **#2.** This test measures the electrical activity of the brain. Since epilepsy is caused by an abnormal discharge of the neurons, this test is the most specific. ASSESSMENT (ADULT/SAFETY AND SECURITY)

382. #4. Since seizures are controlled when clients take medication, they often begin to believe they are "cured" and stop taking the drugs at which time the seizures recur. While the other options may precipitate a seizure in an epileptic client, the effects are not consistent or common. ASSESSMENT (ADULT/SAFETY AND SECURITY)

383. #3. The definition of status epilepticus is continuous seizures. Consciousness is not regained until the seizures have been controlled. ANALYSIS (ADULT/SAFETY AND SECURITY)

384. #4. Respiratory failure is a potentially fatal sequela of myasthenia gravis. PLAN (ADULT/SAFETY AND SECURITY)

385. #3. Assessment of the hard palate in dark-skinned persons is done to observe early signs of jaundice. There is not enough vascular tissue in this area for cyanosis to be evident. ASSESSMENT (ADULT/SAFETY AND SECURITY)

386. #3. In myasthenia gravis, loss of voluntary breathing is a high risk. The other goals are important, but not priorities. PLAN (ADULT/SAFETY AND SECURITY)

387. #2. Color changes in the skin of dark-skinned persons are not easily assessed. All other parameters are used to assess a problem with an IV and are not dependent on skin color. ASSESSMENT (ADULT/SAFETY AND SECURITY)

388. #3. This is the only correct action for Solu-Cortef listed and describes the reason for administration. ANALYSIS (ADULT/SAFETY AND SECURITY)

389. #2. Cholinergic drugs act in the same way as acetylcholine. ANALYSIS (ADULT/SAFETY AND SECURITY)

390. #3. Cholinergic drugs cause vasodilation, not vasoconstriction. EVALUATION (ADULT/SAFETY AND SECURITY)

391. #1. The standard distance from an eye chart has been set at 20 feet. At this distance, letters of a certain size can be identified by a normal eye. Thus a person who reads the 20-feet line at a distance of 20 feet is said to have 20/20 vision. If a person can read only a line with larger letters (e.g., the 30-feet line), the visual acuity is 20/30, and so forth. ANALYSIS (ADULT/SAFETY AND SECURITY)

392. #3. The left occipital visual area contains fibers from the lateral half of the right retina. Thus, damage to the left occipital visual area produces the pattern of blindness described in option #3. The reverse pattern of blindness results from damage to the right occipital visual area. ASSESSMENT (ADULT/SAFETY AND SECURITY)

393. #3. This is the area defined as the anterior chamber. ANALYSIS (ADULT/SAFETY AND SECURITY)

394. #1. This is nearsightedness. Distant objects are not seen well. ANALYSIS (ADULT/SAFETY AND SECURITY)

395. #2. Presbyopia is a normal condition associated with aging. ANALYSIS (ADULT/SAFETY AND SECURITY)

396. #4. The best thing to do is cover the eye to decrease its movement and prevent possible damage until the client can be seen by a physician. IMPLEMENTATION (ADULT/SAFETY AND SECURITY)

397. #1. A blank spot or area in the field of vision is associated with retinal detachment. ANALYSIS (ADULT/SAFETY AND SECURITY)

398. #1. Bed rest is required, so that healing can occur. PLAN (ADULT/SAFETY AND SECURITY)

399. #3. This is an antiemetic but it is specific for motion sickness and acts on the inner ear. PLAN (ADULT/SAFETY AND SECURITY)

400. #3. The small incision to decrease pressure in the middle ear and prevent rupture of the eardrum heals quickly. ANALYSIS (ADULT/SAFETY AND SECURITY)

401. #3. Vertigo and nausea are classic signs of this syndrome. The remaining options are not characteristic of Ménière's. ASSESSMENT (ADULT/SAFETY AND SECURITY)

402. #3. The lens is the area of the eye affected by cataracts. ASSESSMENT (ADULT/SAFETY AND SECURITY)

403. #3. The opacity cannot be treated except by surgical removal of the lens. ANALYSIS (ADULT/SAFETY AND SECURITY)

404. #3. Paralytic ileus is not a complication that generally occurs following cataract extraction. How to use the call bell will be important because of post-op positioning and eye patches. Respiratory infections must be avoided as coughing and sneezing can increase intraocular pressure. PLAN (ADULT/SAFETY AND SECURITY)

405. #1. This option correctly describes the effects of cataract lenses. The client will need time to adjust to the distortion resulting with cataract lenses; new safety measures must be learned, as peripheral vision will be very distorted. ANALYSIS (ADULT/SAFETY AND SECURITY)

406. #1. Coughing increases intraocular pressure and is contraindicated for clients after eye surgery. PLAN (ADULT/SAFETY AND SECURITY)

407. #4. Prolapse of the iris can precipitate acute glaucoma. This is the most common post-op complication following lens extraction. ANALYSIS (ADULT/SAFETY AND SECURITY)

408. #3. Orient the client and observe her closely. Side rails are necessary, but applying restraints can increase anxiety and cause harm. IMPLEMENTATION (ADULT/SAFETY AND SECURITY)

409. #1. There is no reason to stay in a darkened room. In fact, this combined with impaired vision can lead to injury. PLAN (ADULT/SAFETY AND SECURITY)

410. #4. Weeding requires bending, which increases the intraocular pressure. The other options are all acceptable activities. PLAN (ADULT/SAFETY AND SECURITY)

411. #1. Mydriatics cause dilation of the pupil. A dilated pupil can block the outflow of aqueous humor and increase intraocular pressure. ANALYSIS (ADULT/SAFETY AND SECURITY)

412. #4. Normal intraocular pressure, measured by a tonometer, is 12 to 20 mm Hg. Glaucoma is a disease in which the intraocular pressure increases to pathologic levels, sometimes as high as 85 to 90 mm Hg. ASSESSMENT (ADULT/SAFETY AND SECURITY)

413. #2. The optic or second cranial nerve is responsible for vision. ANALYSIS (ADULT/SAFETY AND SECURITY)

414. #4. Lens opacity is characteristic of cataracts. In addition to options #1 through #3, optic nerve atrophy produces diminishing vision (first peripheral, then finally central vision). ASSESSMENT (ADULT/SAFETY AND SECURITY)

415. #4. Atropine sulfate is an anticholinergic drug that dilates the pupil secondary to inhibition of the parasympathetic nervous system. Neostigmine, pilocarpine, and physostigmine are all miotics and are used in the treatment of glaucoma. ANALYSIS (ADULT/SAFETY AND SECURITY)

416. #2. Routine care following eye surgery includes no coughing, no turning or turning only to the *unaffected* side, and adequate fluid intake. The client should not experience severe eye pain. PLAN (ADULT/SAFETY AND SECURITY)

417. #1. Usually the first symptom to be noted is decreasing peripheral vision. There may be some mild aching but generally no pain. Severe pain is characteristic of *acute* glaucoma. In the late stage, the client may see halos around lights. ASSESSMENT (ADULT/SAFETY AND SECURITY)

418. #2. Mr. James's vision in dark places may be decreased when using miotics to control the glaucoma; for safety reasons, more light is needed. Moderate exercise is indicated to promote better circulation, but excessive exercise would be contraindicated. PLAN (ADULT/SAFETY AND SECURITY)

419. #2. Pilocarpine is the miotic that is commonly used in the medical management of glaucoma. ANALYSIS (ADULT/SAFETY AND SECURITY)

420. #2. Miotics constrict the pupil and contract the ciliary muscles increasing the outflow of aqueous humor, thus decreasing intraocular pressure. Mydriatics (drugs that dilate the pupil) such as atropine can precipitate an acute episode of glaucoma. ANALYSIS (ADULT/SAFETY AND SECURITY)

421. #1. Putting pressure on the lacrimal duct at the inner canthus of the eyes is important to prevent systemic effects of miotics. IMPLEMENTATION (ADULT/SAFETY AND SECURITY)

422. #1. Reduction of aqueous humor is desirable. Acetazolamide (Diamox) is the drug commonly used to do this. ANALYSIS (ADULT/SAFETY AND SECURITY)

423. #1. Once vision has been lost, it cannot be restored. Treatment for glaucoma is aimed at preventing the loss of vision. PLAN (ADULT/SAFETY AND SECURITY)

424. #2. A tonometry exam measures the intraocular pressure and can reveal early glaucoma. Treatment can then be initiated. Surgical procedures are avoided if possible, as most of the filtering procedures can cause cataract formation. PLAN (ADULT/SAFETY AND SECURITY)

425. #4. Touching will provide stimulation and enhance the senses, one means to help prevent further regressive behaviors. IMPLEMENTATION (ADULT/SAFETY AND SECURITY)

426. **#4.** Nasal packing and splinting are utilized to prevent post-op edema and bleeding after a rhinoplasty. A HemoVac suction is never used. PLAN (ADULT/SAFETY AND SECURITY)

427. **#3.** Initial stools may be tarry due to swallowed blood. Since it may also indicate hemorrhage, further assessment is in order. IMPLEMENTATION (ADULT/SAFETY AND SECURITY)

428. **#1.** Blowing the nose is contraindicated, because it can cause bleeding. Increased pain and swelling are signs of infection and should be reported to the physician immediately. Rest, activity limitation, and adequate food and fluid intake help to prevent infection. Aspirin should be avoided if pain relief is necessary because of its effects on coagulation. IMPLEMENTATION (ADULT/SAFETY AND SECURITY)

429. **#4.** A history of hypertension is common with the occurrence of epistaxis. ASSESSMENT (ADULT/SAFETY AND SECURITY)

430. **#1.** Epinephrine is applied locally to create vasoconstriction and hemostasis. ANALYSIS (ADULT/SAFETY AND SECURITY)

431. **#2.** The sitting position will prevent the client from swallowing blood and secretions. PLAN (ADULT/SAFETY AND SECURITY)

432. **#3.** All the options are correct but keeping the airway open is the main priority. PLAN (ADULT/SAFETY AND SECURITY)

433. **#4.** The nose is a vascular area; thus, hemorrhage is the most common complication. Infection is possible but not a likely complication. Altered smell and inability to breathe through the nose are not complications. ANALYSIS (ADULT/SAFETY AND SECURITY)

434. **#1.** Vasoconstrictive nose drops stimulate the sympathetic nervous system. This is followed by relaxation of these vessels, accompanied by nasal stuffiness. Therefore, after obtaining temporary relief from nose drops, the nose becomes more stuffy than it was before. ANALYSIS (ADULT/SAFETY AND SECURITY)

435. **#4.** Vagal stimulation may produce dysrhythmias and bradycardia, not tachycardia. IMPLEMENTATION (ADULT/SAFETY AND SECURITY)

436. **#2.** The laryngectomy tube enters directly into the trachea and is considered sterile; it should be suctioned first. The nose can be suctioned last using the same suction catheter. IMPLEMENTATION (ADULT/SAFETY AND SECURITY)

437. **#2.** The nasogastric tube prevents food and fluid from contaminating the pharyngeal and esophageal suture line. PLAN (ADULT/SAFETY AND SECURITY)

438. **#1.** In addition to potassium and sodium loss, bicarbonate is also lost in diarrhea. The result is acidosis. ANALYSIS (ADULT/SAFETY AND SECURITY)

439. **#2.** Predisposing factors of cancer are known to be influenced by familial factors, sex differences, and environment, Long-term use of corticosteroids is associated with a higher incidence of cancer. ASSESSMENT (ADULT/CELLULAR ABERRATION)

440. **#2.** Speech rehabilitation can be started as soon as the esophageal suture line has healed. PLAN (ADULT/SAFETY AND SECURITY)

441. **#2.** Immediate first aid at the scene of the accident requires fractures to be immobilized in the position in which the fracture is found, in order to prevent further injury. Options #3 and #4 do not describe adequate splinting. IMPLEMENTATION (ADULT/ACTIVITY AND REST)

442. **#4.** Initial assessments of any injured client with a fracture would first rule out any life-threatening injuries, prior to dealing with the fracture. IMPLEMENTATION (ADULT/ACTIVITY AND REST)

443. **#3.** Increased blood pressure, confusion, and restlessness in a young adult are some of the first signs of fat emboli. Shock manifests with a decrease in blood pressure. A concussion presents signs of lethargy and possibly other signs of increased intracranial pressure. ANALYSIS (ADULT/ACTIVITY AND REST)

444. **#3.** Any malodor indicates a potential infection. A color other than white indicates drainage. ASSESSMENT (ADULT/ACTIVITY AND REST)

445. **#4.** The other options tend to dry the cast from the outside, leaving the inside damp and crumbly with potential irritation of the skin. Options #1 and #2 have risks of burning the client's exposed skin. IMPLEMENTATION (ADULT/ACTIVITY AND REST)

446. **#3.** Rubber makes the pillow hard, which can cause dents in the cast. The other options are correct. IMPLEMENTATION (ADULT/ACTIVITY AND REST)

447. **#2.** This is a good way of assessing the amount of bleeding. As described, the bleeding is not excessive, so the physician need not be notified. With internal fixation, some slight bleeding is normal. IMPLEMENTATION (ADULT/ACTIVITY AND REST)

448. **#1.** An infection would not be apparent on the first post-op day. Hemorrhage would not be painful. After the first post-op day, the cast would be almost dry, thus this pain could be from pressure. Casts are warm during the drying process but do not get hot enough to burn. ANALYSIS (ADULT/ACTIVITY AND REST)

449. **#2.** An unpleasant odor indicates infection. It need not include drainage. Temperature may not be elevated in local sites of infection. Option #3 is incorrect. ASSESSMENT (ADULT/ACTIVITY AND REST)

450. **#4.** Cyanosis is the result of poor circulation, not nerve damage. ASSESSMENT (ADULT/ACTIVITY AND REST)

451. **#4.** Shoe polish and alcohol might soften the cast. Shellac prevents evaporation of body moisture. Option #4 is correct. IMPLEMENTATION (ADULT/ACTIVITY AND REST)

452. **#4.** Pain unrelieved by analgesics is an early sign of compartment syndrome. Absence of the pulse and pallor are not reliable signs, because deep circulation may still be intact. Paralysis indicates nerve damage. ASSESSMENT (ADULT/ACTIVITY AND REST)

453. **#1.** Bivalving the cast will reduce the external constriction, which is the critical problem; the other options are inappropriate. IMPLEMENTATION (ADULT/ACTIVITY AND REST)

454. **#2.** Pressure on nerves and vessels entering and leaving the compartments of the arm cause paralysis and deformity of the arm and hand. Impaired circulation would be detected prior to development of gangrene. ANALYSIS (ADULT/ACTIVITY AND REST)

455. **#3.** Fat emboli cause petechiae. When they do occur, it is within 24 hours postfracture of a long bone. Frothy sputum indicates pulmonary embolus. Hypertension and coma indicate cerebral embolism. ASSESSMENT (ADULT/ACTIVITY AND REST)

456. **#4.** After menopause, osteoporosis becomes a problem for many women. Older women with this problem are at particular risk for fractures. ANALYSIS (ADULT/ACTIVITY AND REST)

457. **#3.** Buck's traction does not reduce the fracture; the pull is minimal. ANALYSIS (ADULT/ACTIVITY AND REST)

458. **#2.** The traction is applied directly to the skin, so it would irritate any existing ulcers. ANALYSIS (ADULT/ACTIVITY AND REST)

459. **#1.** The traction device can cause irritation and skin breakdown if the skin is not cared for. The bed acts as a splint when the client is turned on her affected side. Options #3 and #4 will cause the loss of countertraction and the effectiveness of the traction. PLAN (ADULT/ACTIVITY AND REST)

460. **#4.** High dietary fiber is a natural way to prevent constipation. Fluid intake should be encouraged. PLAN (ADULT/ACTIVITY AND REST)

461. **#1.** Total hip replacement is the treatment for avascular necrosis; it involves replacement of the femoral head. ANALYSIS (ADULT/ACTIVITY AND REST)

462. **#3.** Adequate blood supply is required for tissue to heal and survive; thus, the decision regarding the level of an amputation depends on the quality of vascularity of the tissue. This is best evaluated at the time of the surgery. ANALYSIS (ADULT/ACTIVITY AND REST)

463. **#2.** Firm application of an elastic bandage is necessary to prevent fluid accumulation and to continue to mold the limb if the rigid dressing comes off. Elevating the limb on the fifth day is contraindicated. Elevation of a lower extremity after amputation is only done for the first 24 hours postoperatively. After that, elevation promotes flexion contractures, the most common complication after amputation of lower extremities. IMPLEMENTATION (ADULT/ACTIVITY AND REST)

464. **#3.** A "shrinker" bandage is properly applied with tighter turns around the distal end of the affected limb to promote venous return and stump molding. IMPLEMENTATION (ADULT/ACTIVITY AND REST)

465. **#2.** The nurse should be direct and honest with the client concerning the accident and outcome of the surgery. IMPLEMENTATION (ADULT/ACTIVITY AND REST)

466. **#4.** The client needs to identify his new body boundary by touching and reorienting himself to his body. IMPLEMENTATION (ADULT/ACTIVITY AND REST)

467. **#4.** Inflammation and systemic symptoms are characteristic of rheumatoid arthritis. ASSESSMENT (ADULT/ACTIVITY AND REST)

468. **#4.** Clients with osteoarthritis should conserve energy when possible. IMPLEMENTATION (ADULT/ACTIVITY AND REST)

469. **#2.** Three to 5 grams/day for inflammation is the usual dose range. Regularly scheduled intake provides a constant plasma level and increases effects. Ringing in the ears is a first sign of overdose of aspirin. Enteric-coated tablets (e.g., Ecotrin) are helpful in preventing gastrointestinal distress. A hypersensitivity reaction can occur at any time. EVALUATION (ADULT/ACTIVITY AND REST)

470. **#1.** This is the only correct option. Gout occurs in the small joints and results when urate crystals are deposited in the joints. The age group is 30- to 40-year-old men. Option #4 is characteristic of osteoarthritis. ANALYSIS (ADULT/ACTIVITY AND REST)

471. **#4.** Fluid intake is increased to prevent the precipitation of urate in the kidneys. Clients often cannot tolerate the pressure of compresses on the affected areas. Salicylates antagonize the action of the uricosuric drugs. Deformities are rare in gout. PLAN (ADULT/ACTIVITY AND REST)

472. **#2.** Dietary restrictions of purine are not necessary after the acute attack, but the disease can be well controlled with medicines. The urine should be kept alkaline to prevent kidney damage. PLAN (ADULT/ACTIVITY AND REST)

473. **#4.** A thickening or lump noted in the breast is one of the signs of cancer cited by the American Cancer Society. A tumor itself does not cause pain; pain results from pressure exerted on surrounding tissue when the tumor enlarges and would be a later sign of cancer. ANALYSIS (ADULT/CELLULAR ABERRATION)

474. **#3.** Annual dental exams help to detect oral cancer. Breast exams should be done monthly. Prolonged exposure to sun is linked to skin cancer and should be avoided. Chest x-rays are no longer advocated for the general public on a yearly basis. EVALUATION (ADULT/CELLULAR ABERRATION)

475. **#1.** A Pap smear samples the cells from the cervix. ANALYSIS (ADULT/CELLULAR ABERRATION)

476. **#4.** Class I is a normal Pap smear and requires no follow-up until the next year. IMPLEMENTATION (ADULT/CELLULAR ABERRATION)

477. **#2.** The Hemoccult test is an excellent screening device for the general public; it can be done in the privacy of the home and has a low rate of false-negative results (i.e., if there is blood in the stool, this test will detect it most of the time). ASSESSMENT (ADULT/CELLULAR ABERRATION)

478. **#1.** Chest x-ray is the only practical screening method. ASSESSMENT (ADULT/CELLULAR ABERRATION)

479. **#3.** Only about 5% survive 5 years. The other options are true. ANALYSIS (ADULT/OXYGENATION)

480. **#2.** False reassurance that everything will be all right is inappropriate. The client should understand the extent of surgery as well as the type and care of the ostomy. PLAN (ADULT/CELLULAR ABERRATION)

481. **#1.** A margin of uninvolved tissue must be excised, but only as much tissue as necessary is removed. Wider or more radical excisions generally do not improve prognosis. ANALYSIS (ADULT/CELLULAR ABERRATION)

482. **#3.** Colon tumors tend to spread through the lymphatics and portal vein to the liver. While metastasis to the other sites listed is possible, the liver is most likely the first to be affected. ANALYSIS (ADULT/CELLULAR ABERRATION)

483. **#2.** Chemotherapy is a widely used systemic treatment that acts at the cellular level on both normal and cancer cells. Most chemotherapeutic agents cause some degree of side effects. ANALYSIS (ADULT/CELLULAR ABERRATION)

484. **#1.** Bland foods of moderate temperature and soft consistency facilitate food intake in the client with oral ulcers. The other options are all contraindicated. PLAN (ADULT/CELLULAR ABERRATION)

485. **#4.** Epithelial cells are extremely sensitive to chemotherapy because of their normally high rate of cell turnover. IMPLEMENTATION (ADULT/CELLULAR ABERRATION)

486. **#3.** It is important for the significant other to express anger, but allowing the client to know the diagnosis and treatment options cannot be delayed. IMPLEMENTATION (ADULT/CELLULAR ABERRATION)

487. #4. The other 3 options can prevent or assess potential bleeding. Eating a regular diet or whatever foods Mrs. Allen prefers will not cause bleeding. PLAN (ADULT/CELLULAR ABERRATION)

488. #2. When chemotherapy is initiated, there is a breakdown of many cancer cells. Uric acid is a cell metabolite. ANALYSIS (ADULT/CELLULAR ABERRATION)

489. #2. Allopurinol is very effective in inhibiting or decreasing uric acid formation. ANALYSIS (ADULT/CELLULAR ABERRATION)

490. #4. Thrombocytopenia is an abnormal decrease in the number of platelets, which results in bleeding tendencies. ASSESSMENT (ADULT/CELLULAR ABERRATION)

491. #3. A family history of cervical cancer is not considered a predisposing factor. ASSESSMENT (ADULT/CELLULAR ABERRATION)

492. #2. Many women with cervical cancer fear a loss of femininity. It is important to discuss the effects of treatment to enable the client to prepare for changes in sexual functioning. IMPLEMENTATION (ADULT/CELLULAR ABERRATION)

493. #1. Vital signs and the client's clinical status would be monitored every 2 hours to assess any systemic reactions such as those mentioned. IMPLEMENTATION (ADULT/CELLULAR ABERRATION)

494. #3. It is important to allow the client to express grief over the loss of her breast. False assurance will impede further communication. IMPLEMENTATION (ADULT/CELLULAR ABERRATION)

495. #1. Cancer of the breast can occur bilaterally. ANALYSIS (CHILDBEARING FAMILY/FEMALE REPRODUCTIVE ANATOMY)

496. #3. Mrs. Wu is expressing concern about her body image and how it will change after surgery. This option asks for clarification and gives Mrs. Wu an opportunity to tell the nurse more. IMPLEMENTATION (ADULT/CELLULAR ABERRATION)

497. #4. Raise the side rails after premedicating a client and leave the call light within easy reach. IMPLEMENTATION (ADULT/CELLULAR ABERRATION)

498. #1. Check under Mrs. Wu's back for drainage, as gravity will draw it toward the back. IMPLEMENTATION (ADULT/CELLULAR ABERRATION)

499. #1. Post-op goals for Mrs. Wu include preventing lymphedema and infection in her right arm. Only option #1 meets these criteria. IMPLEMENTATION (ADULT/CELLULAR ABERRATION)

500. #1. The other 3 options have been identified as influencing a couple's sexual adaptation to mastectomy, something that must be assessed in this case. ASSESSMENT (ADULT/CELLULAR ABERRATION)

501. #2. Denial is often the first response to a crisis or grief reaction. It is a defense against more anxiety than the client can cope with at the time. Mrs. Goldfarb may experience the other phenomena later, but her comments do not at present suggest them. ANALYSIS (ADULT/CELLULAR ABERRATION)

502. #2. This is the correct interpretation according to the International Tumor-Node-Metastasis (TNM) Classification System. ANALYSIS (ADULT/CELLULAR ABERRATION)

503. #3. Expressions of hopelessness or despair, or both, are defining characteristics of reactive (situational) depression. ASSESSMENT (PSYCHOSOCIAL, MENTAL HEALTH, PSYCHIATRIC PROBLEMS/ANXIOUS BEHAVIOR)

504. #1. This diagnosis reflects an actual change in the structure and function of a body. ANALYSIS (ADULT/CELLULAR ABERRATION)

505. #1. These safety measures must be instituted to promote adequate drainage and prevent infection in the affected arm. The other choices listed would actually contribute to tissue edema. PLAN (ADULT/CELLULAR ABERRATION)

506. #2. Cancer cells are generally the most rapidly dividing in the body. Healthy tissues such as bone marrow, gastrointestinal epithelium, and hair follicles are also rapidly proliferating and thus bear the brunt of the effects of many of the cytotoxic drugs. ANALYSIS (ADULT/CELLULAR ABERRATION)

507. #3. Some women have engorgement of the breasts premenstrually, which usually disappears a few days after the onset of menstruation. Because of this possible change, it is important that the breasts be examined at the same point in the menstrual cycle each month, ideally when the hormonal influences on the breast are the smallest. IMPLEMENTATION (CHILDBEARING FAMILY/FEMALE REPRODUCTIVE ANATOMY AND PHYSIOLOGY)

508. #3. A woman who is having a breast removed has many fears related to sexual and social acceptance, disfigurement, and death. Many women have been unable to discuss these feelings with significant others. The nurse can help the client verbalize her feelings and understand what the surgery means to her as a person. The client has a need to be understood and accepted by the nurse. The nurse can clarify any misconceptions and reduce the client's anxiety preoperatively. Sexual relations need not be altered as a result of the surgery, and a skin graft is not needed with a modified radical mastectomy. PLAN (ADULT/CELLULAR ABERRATION)

509. #3. Curling the tubing impedes free flow of the drainage and puts pressure on the skin. The skin will become irritated and could slough. In general, the wound exudate is a straw-colored fluid that is initially blood tinged. Obvious bleeding is bright red in color and should be immediately reported to the surgeon. To maintain suction, empty the HemoVac reservoir when it is half full and reestablish the negative pressure. IMPLEMENTATION (ADULT/CELLULAR ABERRATION)

510. #2. Because movement of the arm is painful, the nurse should support the arm the first few times the arm is exercised. Abduct and adduct it slowly; flex and extend the elbow, wrist, and fingers. Gentle exercises help reduce muscle dysfunction. The nurse's assistance helps to assure the client that movement of the arm will not cause any harm. Slings are to be avoided, and full range of motion cannot be achieved this early in the post-op period. IMPLEMENTATION (ADULT/CELLULAR ABERRATION)

511. #4. Clients should be encouraged to resume normal activities after returning home. The nursing care goals are to strengthen self-esteem, as well as contribute to the restoration of normal function with no activity restrictions after the wound is healed. IMPLEMENTATION (ADULT/CELLULAR ABERRATION)

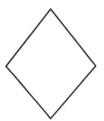

Reprints
Nursing Care of the Adult

A M E R I C A N   J O U R N A L   O F   N U [ ] N G

- pulmonary artery and right ventricular pressure rise at first
- depth and rate of respiration increase
- ratio of tidal volume to functional residual capacity increases
- elasticity of lungs and thorax is reduced
- cardiac output fluctuates

AFTER

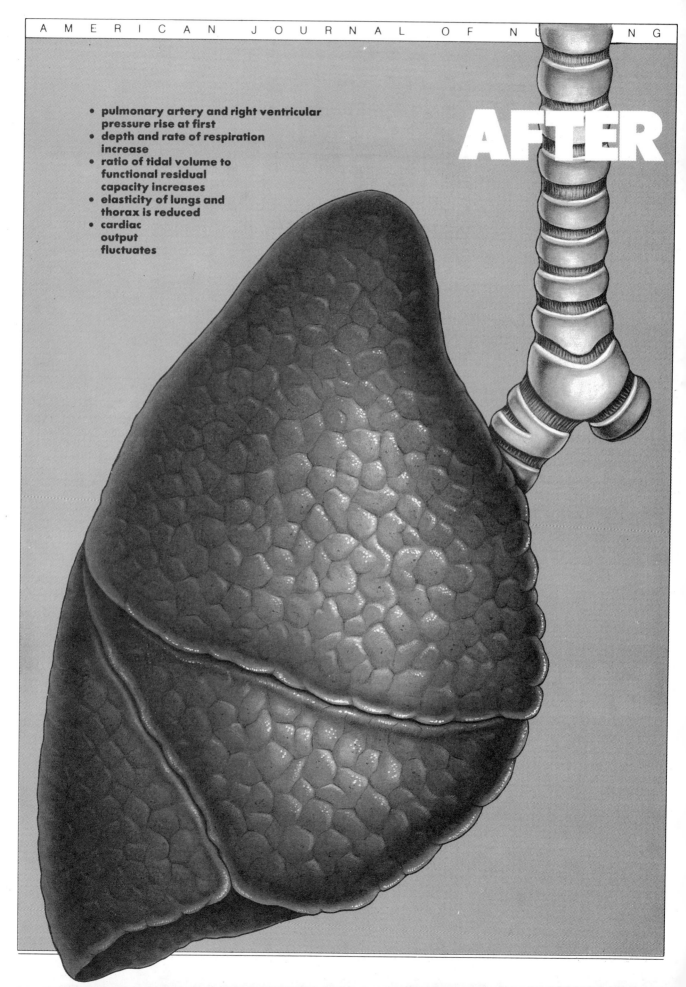

A M E R I C A N   J O U R N A L   O F   N U R S I N G

PNEUMONECTOMY

BY CAROL BURKHART

Reprinted from American Journal of Nursing, November 1983

Because of the great number of physiologic changes that follow pneumonectomy, postoperative care of pneumonectomy patients presents a particularly complex challenge.

Pneumonectomy is most often indicated for the treatment of bronchogenic carcinoma. If the disease is extensive—that is, if it has metastasized within the mediastinum—a radical pneumonectomy with *en bloc* mediastinal dissection including intrapericardial ligation of the hilar vessels may be indicated. Less frequent indications for this procedure are extensive unilateral tuberculosis, extensive unilateral bronchiectasis, multiple lung abscesses, and rare varieties of malignant lung tumors. Rarely, an inflammatory lesion, such as a fungal infection, cannot be eradicated except by pneumonectomy[1].

Some of physiological changes that follow this surgery relate to the anesthesia; others are a consequence of anatomical changes directly resulting from the procedure. While even short periods of anesthesia will adversely affect pulmonary function, such changes are especially marked following pneumonectomy and include the following:

• A temporary rise in pulmonary artery and right ventricular pressures with an eventual return to their preoperative level. This rise immediately follows surgery as the cardiopulmonary system attempts to compensate for loss of lung tissue (and, thus, alveolar surface area) for gas exchange. The rise in pressures may be permanent, although they will drop slightly. Nurses who are monitoring pulmonary artery (PA) pressures, therefore, expect an elevation above the normal.

Carol Burkhart, RN, BSN, is a surgical nurse clinician, at Michael Reese Hospital and Medical Center, Chicago, Ill. Ms. Burkhart cares primarily for thoracic and breast cancer patients. She is also the coordinator of the hospital's surgical nursing internship program.

• An increase in the depth and rate of respiration of the remaining lung. This state of hyperventilation leads to an increase in vital capacity and total lung capacity.

• An increase in the ratio of tidal volume to functional residual capacity, leading to improved functional residual capacity, leading to improved mixing of inspired gases. Diffusion of these gases, however, is decreased. This change reflects an attempt by the pulmonary system to compensate for the decreased alveolar surface. Even with compensatory mechanisms, however, the remaining pulmonary system is not able to equal the diffusion capacity of two lungs. Thus, the nurse must ensure that the patient's activities will be balanced with rest periods and that activities that markedly increase oxygen consumption are avoided.

• A reduction in compliance (elasticity of the lungs and thorax) with subsequent increases in the work of breathing, in oxygen consumption, and in energy expenditure.

• Reduced postoperative respiratory reserve in elderly patients and in patients with extensive chronic obstructive lung disease. (Children suffer less functional respiratory loss than adults. Diffusion capacity in children is normal if pneumonectomy is performed before puberty.)

• Fluctuations in cardiac output, with a moderate increase during exercise. Normally, cardiac output increases with moderate exercise. Now the remaining lung must accommodate the cardiac output for two lungs so that when cardiac output exceeds seven liters, the pulmonary artery pressure is noted to rise progressively. Thus, how much exercise a person can tolerate must be based individually. Onset of shortness of breath is one indication that the patient should stop at that point and rest. If PA pressures remain high, pulmonary hypertension can lead to cor pulmonale[2].

IMMEDIATELY POSTOP

Following removal of the lung, the chest is closed, without water seal drainage, and pressure in the pleural space is adjusted to minus 2 to 4 cm H_2O on inspiration and plus 2 to 4 cm H_2O on expiration, using a simple thoracentesis and manometer. Adjusting the pressure helps maintain the mediastinum midline. Mediastinal shift is most reliably determined by x-ray, but a shift in the position of the trachea or location of the apical impulse of the heart may also be determinants[3]. Normally, the pleural space is not drained. There are two reasons for this: First, progressive evacuation of the space could lead to overexpansion of the remaining lung, causing a shift of the mediastinum to the operative side. To prevent this shift, air and up to 3 liters of fluid are allowed to accumulate in the empty space. Second, if a chest tube were in place, the inevitable accumulation of fluid in the thoracic cavity could easily become contaminated from bacterial ingression along the chest tube tract, possibly resulting in an empyema[2].

The diaphragm on the operative side becomes elevated immediately following pneumonectomy, and the intercostal spaces narrow. Eventually, the fluid consolidates, a process that may take from three weeks to seven months to complete[2]. Because fluid collects in the pleural space, the patient must not be positioned with the remaining lung dependent. Such positioning could foster the development of a tension pneumothorax secondary to a mediastial shift or lead to drowning if the bronchial stump ruptures[4].

In general, because of the danger of inducing pulmonary edema in the remaining lung, close monitoring of fluid balance is especially important for the pneumonectomy patient. The patient must be kept hydrated, but not overhydrated. A central venous line and/or Swan Ganz catheter may be necessary in order to adjust fluid balance[5].

A M E R I C A N J O U R N A L O F N U R S I N G

Because of the potentially grave nature of the complications that can follow pneumonectomy, the patient's overall condition needs to be assessed frequently for emergent problems. Vital signs, for example, must be monitored frequently to note the presence of possible hypovolemia secondary to hemorrhage, infection, or respiratory insufficiency. The nurse must also continue to evaluate serial blood gas determinations, complete blood counts, and electrolyte reports, as well as serial chest x-ray results.

Maintenance of a patent airway is of prime importance. Pneumonectomy patients always receive supplemental oxygen therapy, usually in the form of a high humidity face mask. Vigorous nasotracheal suctioning is generally contraindicated to avoid the possible rupturing of the bronchial stump suture line from catheter trauma(6). It is imperative, therefore, to encourage the patient to use the incentive spirometer along with changing his position frequently.

Arm exercises and ambulation are initiated on the first or second postoperative day. Simple exercises include arm circles and lifting arms over the head and, on the affected side, out to the side(4,5).

POSSIBLE COMPLICATIONS

Respiratory insufficiency is the most frequently observed complication following pneumonectomy. If it is not corrected, it may progress to acute respiratory failure. Borderline preoperative pulmonary function is the clue to alert the nurse that postoperative respiratory insufficiency will most likely develop. Other possible causes include retention of secretions, mediastinal shift, gastric distention (from elevation of the left diaphragm after a right pneumonectomy), atelectasis in the remaining lung, and restriction of chest wall movement because of severe incisional pain(6,7).

Initially, respiratory insufficiency is clinically manifested by fever, tachycardia, tachypnea, and anxiety or mental confusion.

A patient who is likely to develop respiratory insufficiency will need to have his mental status, respirations, and arterial blood gases (ABGs) checked. We assess the patient's mental status preoperatively to obtain a baseline. Postoperatively, neuro checks are performed initially and then every one to two hours for the first 24 hours, and every four hours thereafter. Any change, especially confusion in an otherwise alert patient or extreme restlessness is reported to the appropriate physician as this may be an early warning symptom of hypoxia.

We check ABGs every four hours the first postoperative day by arterial catheter, once per shift (if acceptable) for the next 24 hours, and then as ordered according to the patient's clinical status. If the ABGs are within an acceptable range, no changes in oxygen therapy are made. ABGs may reveal a fall in both pO_2 and pCO_2 initially, followed by a rise in pCO_2 as compensatory hyper-

ventilation fails(7). If the pO_2 has dropped markedly, attempts are made to discover the cause and the fraction of inspired oxygen (FIO_2) is increased. If the ABGs and patient's clinical status continue to deteriorate to values associated with acute respiratory failure, the patient will be placed on assisted mechanical ventilation using synchronous intermittent mandatory ventilation (SIMV). The pressure is adjusted to suit the patient, and the endotracheal tube is positioned so that only the remaining lung is ventilated. We encourage the patient to use the incentive spirometer to prevent atelectasis of the remaining lung. Changing the patient's position will help mobilize secretions. The patient can only be positioned, however, on his back or on the operative side, with his head elevated. Ultrasonic nebulization is used if the patient is unable to mobilize secretions. To help the patient cough, we find it useful to splint the incision by placing our hands anteriorly and posteriorly over the chest wall on the operative side.

A posterolateral incision is the most painful thoracic incision; an anterolateral one is somewhat less painful(4). Using analgesics on a regular basis will help keep the pain in check and may encourage the patient to move, cough, and turn more readily. While narcotics can depress respiration, they must be given to the pneumonectomy patient as needed. Otherwise, the patient will breathe shallowly and ineffectively and will be unwilling to cough up accumulated secretions, all of which can lead to respiratory insufficiency(8).

We begin pain management in the

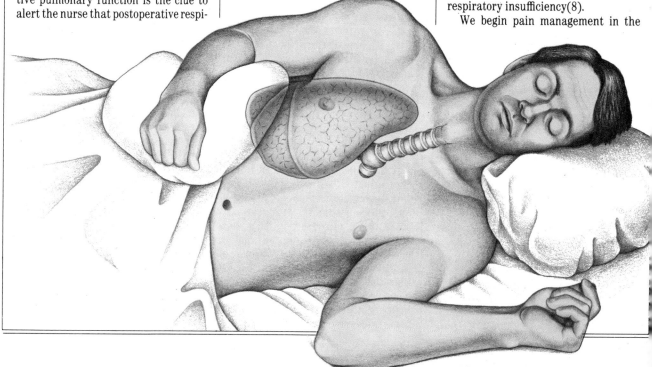

A M E R I C A N J O U R N A L O F N U R S I N G

Coughing up serosanguinous fluid may be a sign that the bronchial stump has ruptured.

recovery room with 75-100 mg meperidine (Demerol) IM q3h with the addition of IV-push morphine sulfate 2 mg per hour if the pain is not controlled. All pain medication is given with close analysis of the patient's clinical condition. All CNS depressors are withheld if the respiratory rate or level of consciousness is altered significantly. Naloxone HCl (Narcan), a narcotic antagonist, is always taped to the wall above the bed.

We find that giving 75-100 mg of Demerol every 3 hours (even if it is not requested) avoids peak periods of pain, making the patient more amenable to a pulmonary hygiene regimen. We have not found respiratory depression to be a common problem. In those rare instances when it has occurred, we use verbal and physical stimulation initially and have emergency oxygen and respiratory therapy equipment on close standby. We have had to administer Narcan to only one patient, who responded promptly.

After the second postop day, we discontinue the adjunctive IV morphine order and maintain the Demerol as described. Since true physical tolerance (even with q3-4h coverage) takes approximately two weeks to develop, we do not worry about making our patients addicts. After the first week, the dosage of Demerol is reduced to match patient need.

Cardiac Arrhythmias occur most often in patients over 60 years of age or in patients who have preexisting cardiac disease. The most common arrhythmia noted is sinus tachycardia (a heart rate over 110/minute), which generally is not treated. Pain, hypoxemia, hypovolemia, and acid-base imbalances can all contribute to its development. Atrial fibrillation or flutter, however, may appear in patients with known conges-

When the patient is lying on his side, keep the remaining lung uppermost to prevent mediastinal shift or drowning if the bronchial stump ruptures.

tive heart failure (CHF) or cardiac disease. Digitalis is commonly used to control atrial arrhythmias. Premature ventricular contractions are thought to result from hypoxemia, acid-base imbalance, and in those patients with a history of CHF or right bundle branch block (RBBB). Lidocaine therapy may be initiated for serious ventricular arrhythmias[6].

Fever during the first 24 hours is almost always due to atelectasis[7]. A wound infection or an infection elsewhere in the body is suspected when temperature rises within the fifth to tenth postoperative days. Aggressive pulmonary hygiene must be instituted if atelectasis is the cause. This approach includes suctioning, spirometry, turning, positioning, and ultrasonic treatment. Treatment of infection is aimed at identifying causative organisms and instituting appropriate antibiotic therapy[7].

Bronchopleural Fistulas occur in 3 to 5 percent of postpneumonectomy patients[1,2]. When it occurs on the first or second postop day, it could be a result of a slipped ligature. Symptoms include a massive air leak into the subcutaneous tissue (subcutaneous emphysema) and a mediastinal shift on x-ray. A bronchial air leak from the fifth to the tenth postoperative day generally indicates infection and lack of wound healing[2]. If a patient who is dyspneic and has a change in the mental status begins to cough up serosanguinous fluid, a ruptured ("blown") bronchial stump is immediately suspected. Fluid is evacuated by thoracentesis and the operative stump is resutured.

Hemorrhage, resulting in blood in the thoracic cavity (hemothorax), is another possible complication. A slipped ligature on an intercostal or bronchial artery is usually the cause. Fortunately, such an occurrence is relatively rare. This complication can be rapidly fatal. A mediastinal shift can be seen on x-ray, and cardiovascular collapse eventually occurs as shock progresses. Vital signs are monitored every five minutes.

Continuous invasive hemodynamic monitoring is instituted. Intake and output are also carefully monitored. The staff must be prepared to transfer the patient rapidly to the operating room.

Empyema is an infrequent complication and may or may not be associated with the development of a bronchopleural fistula[9]. The patient is usually febrile, has an elevated white count, and may be dyspneic. The empyema is drained, culture and sensitivity studies are obtained, and antibiotic therapy begun. To detect infection, the patient's temperature is monitored each shift every day.

Pneumonectomy is, thus, a major surgical procedure that carries the potential for the development of many serious and even life-threatening complications. Expert nursing care is crucial, therefore, for the smooth recovery of this patient, not only to recognize developing complications, but also to prevent them.

REFERENCES

1. Roe, Benson. *Perioperative Management in Cardiothoracic Surgery.* Boston, Little, Brown and Co., 1980, pp. 4-20.
2. Shields, Thomas, ed. *General Thoracic Surgery.* Philadelphia, Lea and Febiger, 1972, pp. 293-314.
3. Maier, H. C. Chest wall, pleura, lung, and mediastinum. IN *Principles of Surgery,* ed. by S. I. Schwartz and others. New York, McGraw-Hill Book Co., Vol. 1, 1969, p. 532.
4. Cameron, M. I. What patients need most before and after thoracotomy. *Nursing '78* 8:28-36, May 1978.
5. Beth Israel Hospital. *Respiratory Intensive Care Nursing.* 2nd ed. Boston, Little, Brown and Co., 1979, p. 218.
6. Dohi, S., and Gold, M. I. Comparison of two methods of postoperative respiratory care. *Chest* 73:592, 1980.
7. Condon, R., and Nyhus, L. *Manual of Surgical Therapeutics.* 4th ed. Boston, Little, Brown and Co., 1978, pp. 172-176.
8. McCaffery, Margo. *Nursing Management of the Patient with Pain.* 2nd ed. Philadelphia, J. B. Lippincott Co., 1979, p. 214.
9. Kinney, John, and others. *Manual of Surgical Intensive Care; Editorial Subcommittee.* (American College of Surgeons, Committee on Pre and Postoperative Care) Philadelphia, W. B. Saunders Co., 1977, pp. 300-305.

Glaucoma Update

Reprinted from American Journal of Nursing, May 1983

By Marion M. Resler
Gail Tumulty

To most people, glaucoma signifies vision loss and eventual blindness. Since one out of 10 cases of blindness is caused by this eye disease, such a perception is accurate(1). However, new developments in drugs and surgery, and now laser therapy, offer hope of reducing vision loss in the estimated 1.5 percent of people over 40 who develop glaucoma annually(2). The deciding factors in reducing blindness from this often asymptomatic disease are early detection, appropriate intervention, and long-term follow up.

Glaucoma is characterized by an increase in intraocular pressure that can lead to atrophy of the optic nerve and blindness. Normal intraocular pressure (13 to 22 mm Hg) is maintained by the aqueous fluid produced and secreted by the ciliary body. The fluid leaves through a channel from the anterior chamber through the iridocorneal angle, the trabecular meshwork, Schlemm's canal, and the aqueous veins (see diagram). Obstruction in any part of the outflow channel results in a backup of fluid and increased pressure within the eye.

Glaucoma may occur as a primary condition, or it can be secondary to other eye pathology. It may be acute, occurring abruptly with much pain, or it may be chronic, with an insidious onset, no pain, and silent progression.

Open-angle (wide-angle) or

MARION M. RESLER, RN, MSN is an assistant professor, School of Nursing, St. Louis University, St. Louis, Mo.

GAIL TUMULTY, RN, MSN, is assistant director of nursing and clinical supervisor, Bethesda General Hospital, and Eye Institute, St. Louis, Mo.

chronic glaucoma accounts for 90 precent of primary glaucoma. Usually caused by obstruction in the trabecular meshwork, this "silent thief" is often asymptomatic until considerable loss of vision has occurred. Treatment is aimed at facilitating aqueous outflow or decreasing aqueous production, or both. Pilocarpine is a parasympathomimetic agent that stretches the trabecular network, enlarging the outflow channel(3). However, miosis (constricted pupil), a side effect of pilocarpine, affects visual acuity and thus is troublesome for the patient who relies on clear vision for performance of tasks.

If pilocarpine is ineffective or not well tolerated by the patient, other parasympathomimetic drops can be used (see chart p. 755). Timolol (Timoptic), a beta-blocker that reduces the production of aqueous fluid, has recently replaced pilocarpine as the drug of choice. Its side effects are less severe than those of pilocarpine and it does not affect pupil size. Epinephrine drops are also used to increase outflow and, to some extent, to reduce aqueous secretion. However, because of the systemic effects of epinephrine, such as tachycardia and palpitations, its use must be carefully evaluated for each patient.

In addition to eye drops, an oral carbonic anhydrase inhibitor, such as acetazolamide (Diamox), may be prescribed to reduce the production of aqueous fluid. Other diuretics, such as chlorothiagide (Diuril), do not reduce intraocular pressure. Since acetazolamide acts as a diuretic, supplemental potassium may be needed. By assessing the patient's diet, the nurse can suggest adding such high-potassium foods as orange juice and bananas, if indicated.

All patients on a drug regimen for glaucoma must keep on their schedules even when hospitalized for other medical or surgical conditions. If other prescribed medications interfere with the glaucoma drugs, then substitutions should be made in the other drugs. Glaucoma control, like diabetes control, must be kept consistent in any treatment plan.

When the intraocular pressure is not adequately controlled by drugs, channels permitting outflow of the aqueous fluid must be created by surgery. In the past, trabeculectomy and trabeculotomy have been the procedures used. Both require hospitalization and often a general anesthetic. Now, laser therapy (discussed below) can in some cases accomplish the same goal more quickly and more easily.

The second (and less common) primary condition, called angle-closure or acute narrow-angle glaucoma, results from a narrowing or closing of the iridocorneal angle. Intraocular pressure rises abruptly, accompanied by pain in the eye, severe headache, and nausea and vomiting. The patient sees colored halos around lights and suffers a decrease in visual acuity in the affected eye. The pupil will be enlarged and fixed. Although accounting for only 5 percent of all primary cases, an attack of this type of glaucoma is an emergency because considerable loss of vision can occur in one attack(2). Aggressive treatment includes pilocarpine drops, which, by constricting the pupil, pull the iris away from the trabeculum. Strong miotic drops and mydriatics are contraindicated because they can worsen the condition. Patients are also cautioned not to take "over-the-counter" cold remedies such as decongestants. Os-

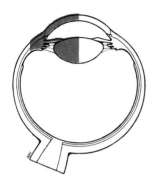

motic agents such as glycerol or mannitol are used to draw fluid from the eye, and an oral diuretic such as acetazolamide (Diamox) is given to inhibit aqueous production. The dosage of glycerol is 1.5 gm per kilogram of body weight, taken by mouth. The dosage of mannitol is 2 gm per kilogram of body weight, usually given IV(1). As soon as the intraocular pressure is under control, surgery is indicated to relieve the blockage. Peripheral iridectomy is usually the procedure of choice to reestablish the outflow of fluid. In some cases, laser iridotomy can accomplish the same purpose.

Some people may have a chronic form of angle-closure glaucoma, producing less dramatic episodes of elevated intraocular pressure, but causing considerable visual damage over time. Since these patients may eventually have acute attacks, surgery is recommended as soon as the condition is diagnosed.

Secondary glaucoma may result from ocular inflammatory processes, blood vessel changes, or tumors that obstruct the outflow of aqueous fluid. Trauma that causes hemorrhage into the eye or displacement of structures can also block aqueous drainage. Occasionally, glaucoma can develop after cataract extraction or other eye surgery, or as a complication of prolonged use of topical steroids. Treatment is directed at the cause as well as at lowering intraocular pressure.

Congenital or infantile glaucoma is rare, affecting 0.05 percent of all newborns(4). This type of glaucoma may be discovered at birth or during the first three years of life. The earliest signs are excessive lacrimation and photophobia. Later, enlargement of the eyeball may be noted. Early surgical intervention is necessary to prevent blindness.

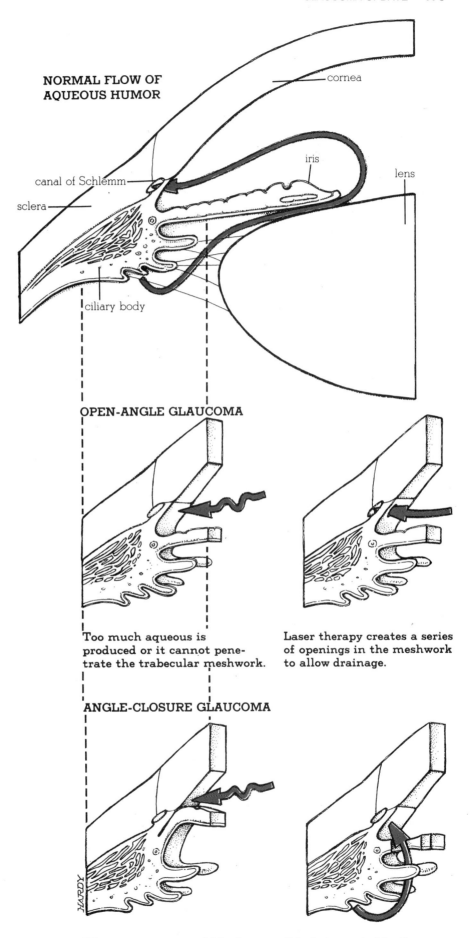

NORMAL FLOW OF AQUEOUS HUMOR

cornea

iris

lens

canal of Schlemm

sclera

ciliary body

OPEN-ANGLE GLAUCOMA

Too much aqueous is produced or it cannot penetrate the trabecular meshwork.

Laser therapy creates a series of openings in the meshwork to allow drainage.

ANGLE-CLOSURE GLAUCOMA

The iris tents up and blocks trabecular meshwork drainage to Schlemm's canal.

A hole is created in the base of the iris to permit drainage through the canal.

Three Patients' Experiences With Glaucoma

Ms. L, a 40-year-old legal secretary, suddenly developed pain, redness, edema, and vision loss in her right eye, which within hours sent her to her mother's ophthalmologist. Because her mother was being treated for glaucoma, Ms. L associated the disease with the aging process and assumed she was too young to develop it. The ophthalmologist diagnosed acute angle-closure glaucoma, and had the patient admitted to the hospital and immediately scheduled for a peripheral iridectomy. This traditional procedure is usually done in emergencies because it assures immediate relief. Since it was Ms. L's first hospitalization, the experience was terrifying for her. The surgery restored vision and lowered intraocular pressure in the right eye. Because of the threat of a similar attack in the left eye, a laser iridotomy was scheduled four weeks later.

Ms. B, a 60-year-old housewife, had been on a medical regimen for two years for chronic open-angle glaucoma in both eyes. Her medications included acetazolamide (Diamox) 125 mg BID, pilocarpine (Pilocar) 1 gtt TID, timolol (Timoptic) 1 gtt BID and 1% epinephrine (Epifrin) 1 gtt BID. Ms. B's intraocular pressure remained controlled between 20 to 25 on this regimen, but she experienced side effects from the medication. Her vision was blurred for two hours after the eye drops were instilled, making driving and reading impossible. Frontal headaches from the pilocarpine and generalized body tremors attributed to the acetazolamide were also problems. Ms. B had previous surgery for other conditions and was afraid to have

surgery on her eyes. Laser trabeculoplasty was presented as an alternative. It was decided, however, to do only half of one eye first. Good results were obtained and eventually she had further laser therapy. Her eye medications were resumed temporarily on the pretreatment schedule. Later, she was able to maintain safe intraocular pressure on a medication regimen that did not cause disturbing side effects.

Mr. F, a 44-year-old retail clerk, had been battling glaucoma for four years. Like all patients, he feared compromised visual acuity would affect his career, earning power, and life style. His eye medications were pilocarpine (Pilocar) 4% QID, timolol (Timoptic) 1/2% BID, and acetazolamide (Diamox Sequels) 500 mg TID. Even on this regimen, considered to be maximal medical therapy, his left intraocular pressure ranged between 27 and 36. The ophthalmologist decided to try argon laser trabeculoplasty. Mr. F's left eye was treated with 150 applications of .05 seconds duration, producing 50-micron spots around the 360° angle with 800 milliwatts of energy. Initially, pressure in his eye decreased to 14. Unfortunately, the pressure reduction was not permanent, and Mr. F subsequently underwent a trabeculectomy, or conventional surgical filtering procedure. (Traditional surgical correction is an option, since laser therapy does not rule out future surgery.) Naturally, the "failure" of laser therapy was disheartening to the patient, who required support and encouragement from the health care team to continue the grueling medical regimen.

Early Signs

One of the earliest findings indicative of open-angle glaucoma is the presence of increased introcular pressure, which is measured by a tonometer. For screening purposes, non-contact or air puff tonometers are most often used in community clinics and optometrists' and general physicans' offices. If glaucoma is not detected early by tonometry, the disease progresses and causes changes in the optic disk, such as deep cupping and displacement of the large vessels(2). The latter changes can be seen through an ophthalmoscope. Since some people may be genetically predisposed to the disease, patients should be asked about familial incidence of glaucoma as part of routine history-taking. Because the disease process affects the visual fields and the patient may be unaware of peripheral vision loss, those suspected of having glaucoma should have their visual fields measured by a tangent screen or perimeter. It is not sufficient to check vision on a standard E eye chart. A person may be able to read 20/20 yet have seriously diminished peripheral vision, almost to the point of legal blindness. Annual measurements of visual fields can monitor both the progress of the disease and the effectiveness of treatment.

Patients suspected of having glaucoma should be referred to the ophthalmologist for further evaluation. He will use the applanation tonometer, which is highly accurate, more sophisticated, and more expensive than other types of tonometers. Patients require topical anesthetic before being tested by this means. When glaucoma is suspected, an electronic tonometer may be rested on the eye for four minutes to measure and record the rate of aqueous outflow (tonography). The ophthalmologist examines the anterior chamber angle by gonioscopy, which involves use of special lenses, a light source, and a hand microscope or slit lamp. This method determines the structures of the angle and detects abnormalities that are present.

Many patients with glaucoma are managed effectively with a simple regimen of eye drops two to four times a day. Others require a number of types of drops at different times of the day, as well as an oral diuretic such as acetazolamide. All of these medications may produce some side effects that have an impact on the patient's sense of well being. They are costly as well. Because of the cost and, in many instances the absence of symptoms, some patients may stop using all or part of the drugs or fail to adhere strictly to the schedule.

When drug therapy is not successful, surgical intervention is needed—a frightening prospect for many patients. Laser treatment offers a noninvasive alternative. Laser therapy can be done as an outpatient procedure, making it both less risky and more cost effective

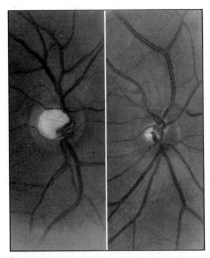

Deep cupping of the optic disk and displacement of large blood vessels occur (left) as glaucoma progresses. At right are normal disk and vessels.

than traditional surgery. Many patients may resume normal activities, including work, after 24 hours(5). The hazards of general anesthesia are avoided as are the complications of retrobulbar injection, which include infection, wound leak, and intraocular hemorrhage(6). The laser may also be more effective than lifelong multi-drug therapy, since poor adherence to medication regimens leads to advanced visual damage(7).

Laser Procedures

The traditional surgical correction for *angle-closure* glaucoma has been removal of a piece of the iris to facilitate aqueous flow from behind the iris into the anterior chamber, where the outflow chan-

MAJOR SIDE EFFECTS OF OCULAR DRUGS

Medication	Topical Side Effects	Systemic Side Effects
Parasympathomimetic pilocarpine hydrochloride (Pilocar) Dose: 1/4 – 10% 1-2 gtt up to 6 times daily	Blurred vision Cataract formation Miotic induced glaucoma Ocular pain	Bradycardia Exacerbation of asthma Diarrhea or vomiting Muscle tremors
Anticholinesterase Agent physostigmine salicylate (Eserine) Dose: 0.25 – 0.5% 1-2 gtt TID-QID	Blurred vision Cataract Frontal headache Iritis Ocular pain	Bradycardia Bronchial congestion Anoxeria Increased salivation Muscle twitching
Sympathetic Blocking Agents timolol (Timoptic) Dose: 0.25 – 0.5% 1 gtt daily or BID	Keratitis	Bradycardia Hypotension Exacerbation of asthma Lightheadedness, mental depression Fatigue, weakness Disorientation, memory loss
Sympathomimetic Agents epinephrine (Epifrin) Dose: 0.25 – 2% 1-2 gtt daily or BID	Hyperemia Conjunctival irritation Lacrimation Blurred vision Periorbital edema Ocular pain	Anxiety Headaches Tachycardia Palpitations Tremors
Carbonic Anhydrase Inhibitor acetazolamide (Diamox) Dose: 125 – 250 mg orally 1-2 QID or 500 mg sustained release capsule BID or may also be given IM or IV		Numbness & tingling in fingers & toes Irritability, muscle tremor Loss of appetite, nausea Dyspnea Fatigue, depression Hypokalemia Impotence

Adapted from K.W. Benjamin's Toxicity of ocular medications. *Int.Ophthalmo. Clin.* 19:199-255, Spring 1979.

nels lie. Now, in a procedure called iridotomy, the argon laser beam can penetrate the iris and create an opening for aqueous outflow.

A half-hour before the procedure, pilocarpine eye drops are instilled to prevent further contraction of the iris during treatment. A topical anesthetic, usually proparacaine hydrochloride (Ophthaine) 0.5% 1–2 gtt repeated as necessary, is used mainly to ease placement of the fundus contact lens. The lens serves to keep the lid open, enables visualization of the involved structures, and may also absorb some of the thermal energy that the laser might deliver to the corneal epithelium. Laser treatment usually begins with a delivery of 500 milliwatts for 0.2 seconds. In some instances, this level of power is enough to produce the desired penetration into the iris. If there is little effect at this level, the power may be increased to 1000 or even 1500 milliwatts, but no higher, because of the danger of damage to surrounding structures(8). The total number of laser deliveries is limited to approximately 50 per session; sessions are repeated at one-to-two week intervals if necessary. One or both eyes may be treated at one time.

Post-treatment discomfort is limited to headache and blurring of vision for the first 24 hours(8). Since a few patients experience moderate increases in intraocular pressure after the treatment, they are advised to continue their glaucoma medications until the pressure is rechecked, usually at one week or sooner. At that time their drops or oral medications are adjusted. To reduce inflammation from cellular debris, topical steroids are prescribed 4 times daily for 4 to 6 days for most patients.

Contraindications to laser iridotomy are few; however, it is not performed on eyes with hazy corneas. In some instances, additional treatments may be necessary. Long-term complications are not yet fully known, but no serious problems have been documented.

Laser trabeculoplasty is the procedure used in *open-angle* glaucoma. However, it is not clear exactly how the laser treatment works. The early intraocular pressure usually drops because the trabeculum has been opened, but it is doubtful that permanent openings remain(9). The desired effect is obtained by application of laser beam or spots (approximately 50 to 100) into and posterior to the pigmented band of the trabecular meshwork evenly spaced for 180° to 360° around the angle. Because the microburns scar rather than penetrate the trabecular meshwork, it is believed that a permanent increase in tension on the trabeculum results, opening the outflow channel (see diagram, p.753). Laser therapy applied in this manner is thought to act in much the same way that miotics do—by increasing radial trabecular tension(9). The post-laser care is the same as after iridotomy.

Involving the Patients

Prepare the patient and family member for laser treatment by carefully explaining the exact nature of the procedure, how to prepare for it, the equipment to be used, and what to expect afterward. The ramifications of the therapy are disclosed and informed consent is obtained.

Advise the patient to bring a friend or relative to accompany him on the day of the procedure, since blurred vision is common and would interfere with driving. Although there is no pain in the eye, some patients complain of headache afterward. Aspirin or acetaminophen can be given to reduce pain. There are usually no restrictions on fluids or food before or after therapy.

Before the procedure, seat the patient as comfortably as possible; adjust the chair height and chin support. Because he may be nervous, establish a calm atmosphere to make it easier for him to remain still during the treatment.

When instilling the anesthetic eye drops, reinforce correct instillation procedure by washing your hands. Ask the patient to look up before instilling the drops. Then gently pull down the lower lid and instill the drops into the conjunctival sac. Avoid placing the drop on the cornea or touching the bottle to the eye or skin. Offer a separate tissue to dry each eye.

After the laser procedure, an eye patch may be applied for a few hours to promote comfort by protecting the eye from light. Have the patient close the affected eye before applying the sterile 2" eye patch. Suggest that the patient sit a while before leaving. While he relaxes, review the physician's follow-up plans with him. The main points are the need to continue using the glaucoma eye drops until it is determined that the therapy has reduced the intraocular pressure; the need to use steroid drops (if prescribed) for 4 to 6 days to prevent inflammation; and, most importantly, the need to return for eye checkups both following the procedure and in the future. Some patients may be advised to continue with eye drops; frequent checkups will monitor the disease process and indicate adjustments in the drug regimen.

Since the possibility of loss of vision is frightening, each patient will respond differently to glaucoma. Some may display anxiety and overzealous attention to the condition and treatment regimen; others may react by denying the danger and appear to be indifferent. Still others may stop treatment, or, as they become older, become confused about their medication schedule. Therefore, patients need reinforced teaching, support, and encouragement.

References

1. Saunders, W., and others. *Nursing Care in Eye, Ear, Nose, and Throat Disorders.* 4th ed. St. Louis, the C.V. Mosby Co., 1979, pp. 112, 156.
2. Vaughn, D., and Asury, T. *General Ophthalmology.* 9th ed. Los Altos, Calif., Lange Medical Publications, 1980.
3. Jeglum, E. L. Ocular therapeutics. *Nurs.Clin.North Am.* 6(3):453-477, 1981.
4. Harley, R. D., and Manley, D. R. Glaucoma in infants and children. IN *Pediatric Ophthalmology,* ed. R. D. Harley. Philadelphia, W. B. Saunders Co., 1975, p. 391.
5. Schwartz, A. L., and others. Argon laser trabecular surgery in uncontrolled phakic open angle glaucoma. *Ophthalmology* 88:203-212, Mar. 1981.
6. Robin, A. L., and Pollack, I. P. Argon laser peripheral iridotomies in the treatment of primary angle closure glaucoma. *Arch.Ophthalmol.* 100:919-923, June 1982.
7. Wise, J. B. Long term control of adult open angle glaucoma by argon laser treatment. *Opthalmology* 88:197-202, Mar. 1981.
8. Quigley, H. Long-term follow-up of laser iridotomy. *Ophthalmology* 88:281-324, Mar. 1981.
9. Wise, J. B., and Witter, S. L. Argon laser therapy for open-angle glaucoma. A pilot study. *Arch. Ophthalmol.* 97:319-322, Feb. 1979.

Nursing Care of the Childbearing Family

Coordinator

B. Patricia Nix, MSN, RN

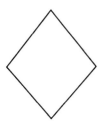

Questions

Juanita Romero has been married 1½ years. She stopped taking oral contraceptives several months ago and now suspects she is pregnant. She is being seen by her physician for the first time.

1. Mrs. Romero has numerous common signs and symptoms associated with pregnancy. Which of the following signs suggests she is probably pregnant?
   ○ 1. Amenorrhea
   ○ 2. Frequent micturation
   ○ 3. Enlarged and tender breasts
   ○ 4. Goodell's sign

2. Mrs. Romero's last menstrual period was from November 10 to November 15. She had intercourse on November 17. Her expected date of delivery is
   ○ 1. July 21.
   ○ 2. August 17.
   ○ 3. August 22.
   ○ 4. August 24.

3. Which of the following is true of pregnancy tests done on urine samples?
   ○ 1. A positive test is based on increased estrogen excretion in the urine.
   ○ 2. They are 100% accurate if done 10 to 14 days after fertilization.
   ○ 3. A positive test is based on the excretion of chorionic gonadotropin in the urine.
   ○ 4. Home pregnancy tests are not accurate, and clients should be cautioned not to use them.

4. Mrs. Romero is concerned about eating the proper foods during her pregnancy. Which of the following nursing actions is the most appropriate?
   ○ 1. Give her a list of foods to refer to in planning her meals.
   ○ 2. Emphasize the importance of limiting highly seasoned and salty foods.
   ○ 3. Ask Mrs. Romero to list her food intake for the last 3 days.
   ○ 4. Instruct her to continue her usual diet, as she appears to be nutritionally fit.

5. Mrs. Romero has a low hemoglobin. When counseling her to increase her iron intake, which of the following meals should the nurse recommend to her?
   ○ 1. Ham sandwich, corn pudding, tossed salad
   ○ 2. Hamburger, green beans, fruit cup
   ○ 3. Chicken livers, sliced tomatoes, dried apricots
   ○ 4. Omelet with mushrooms, spinach salad

6. The nurse should instruct Mrs. Romero to notify the physician immediately if which of the following symptoms occur?
   ○ 1. Swelling of the face
   ○ 2. Frequent urination
   ○ 3. Increased vaginal discharge
   ○ 4. The presence of chloasma

7. Which of the following changes is a pregnant woman most likely to notice in her breasts?
   ○ 1. Darkening of the areolae, tingling sensations, engorgement
   ○ 2. Lightening of the areolae, colostrum, increased size
   ○ 3. Colostrum, tingling sensations, darkening of the areolae
   ○ 4. Increased size, tenderness, flattening of the nipples

8. Mrs. Romero is treated for syphilis during the first trimester with intramuscular injections of penicillin. The baby's diagnosis at birth should most likely be
   ○ 1. congenital syphilis.
   ○ 2. stillborn.
   ○ 3. normal newborn.
   ○ 4. premature newborn.

9. Constipation during pregnancy is best treated by
   ○ 1. regular use of a mild laxative.
   ○ 2. increased bulk and fluid in the diet.
   ○ 3. limiting excessive weight gain.
   ○ 4. regular use of bisacodyl (Dulcolax) suppositories.

10. Which of the following symptoms would be considered normal if found while assessing Mrs. Romero?
    ○ 1. Vaginal bleeding and 1+ albuminuria
    ○ 2. Oliguria and glycosuria
    ○ 3. In the urine, 1+ sugar and urinary frequency
    ○ 4. Swelling of the face and increased vaginal discharge

Sharon Webb, aged 24, is delighted with confirmation of her first pregnancy, as she and her husband of 2 years hope to have a large family. Initial assessments indicate she is in good health and eager to learn about her needs during pregnancy. Richard Webb participates in the discussion, emphasizing their desire to adapt their life-styles to promote the health of the baby.

11. Mrs. Webb has a history of 28-day, regular menstrual cycles. At which point in Mrs. Webb's cycle was the mature ovum released from the ovarian follicle?
    ○ 1. On the 11th or 12th day
    ○ 2. On the 13th or 14th day
    ○ 3. On the 15th or 16th day
    ○ 4. On the 17th or 18th day

12. The young expectant father asks about leisure activities he can enjoy with his wife during pregnancy. Which response by the nurse best indicates an understanding of the needs of the couple during pregnancy?
    ○ 1. "Although she may tire easily, you can continue most activities you have been enjoying in the past."
    ○ 2. "You should explore more sedentary recreation now, as active exercise needs to be limited."
    ○ 3. "You may wish to continue with your hobbies, and allow your wife to enjoy leisure with her friends."
    ○ 4. "This is a time to prepare yourselves for the role of new parents, rather than thinking of yourselves."

13. The nurse determines that Mrs. Webb is in her tenth week of gestation. Which of the following signs of pregnancy would the nurse expect to observe?
    ○ 1. Breast tenderness
    ○ 2. Quickening
    ○ 3. Dyspnea
    ○ 4. Dependent edema

14. The nurse instructs Mrs. Webb what to do if vaginal bleeding occurs. Which of the following actions indicates that she understands prenatal instructions?
    ○ 1. She considers it normal, especially if bleeding occurs at the time of her usual period.
    ○ 2. She records the date and amount of bleeding and reports it on her next visit.
    ○ 3. She phones the physician to give duration and amount of bleeding.
    ○ 4. She remains on complete bed rest until the bleeding ceases.

15. After 2 clinic visits, Mrs. Webb seems discouraged. She tells you, "I guess I am pleased to be pregnant, but these visits are so routine. It's hard for me to take time from work to sit in the waiting room for just a urine check and weigh-in." What teaching should be most emphasized with this client?
    ○ 1. "Although pregnancy is normal, one must be prepared for any problems."
    ○ 2. "These routine visits are essential to the fetus and to your health."
    ○ 3. "Perhaps you might weigh yourself at home each week and call us."
    ○ 4. "Have you considered resigning from your job at this time?"

16. In Mrs. Webb's 4th lunar month of pregnancy, the physician advises her to adjust her daily routine as a typist. The nurse discusses her activities in the office and the nature of her work. Which of the following tasks needs to be modified for her to promote a healthy pregnancy?
    ○ 1. Sitting in 1 position for 6 hours without a break
    ○ 2. Delivering messages to several adjacent departments each day
    ○ 3. Answering phones as relief for the receptionist 1 hour each day
    ○ 4. Filing vouchers for sales personnel for 2 hours daily

17. Mrs. Webb calls the clinic to report that her younger sister has toxoplasmosis. In assessing the risk to Mrs. Webb, which factor is most critical?
    ○ 1. There has been no direct contact with her sister in 5 days.
    ○ 2. The client has a cat that recently gave birth to kittens.
    ○ 3. Both wife and husband are strict vegetarians.
    ○ 4. The client, at present, feels very well.

18. After a thorough assessment and lab work, it is determined that the client has no signs of toxoplasmosis. The physician is concerned about mild anemia, however, and asks the nurse to discuss dietary modifications with Mrs. Webb. Considering that she usually avoids meat and poultry, which foods should be included when planning a healthy daily diet?
    ○ 1. Egg yolks and dried fruit
    ○ 2. Cereal and yellow vegetables
    ○ 3. Leafy green vegetables and oranges
    ○ 4. Fish and dairy products

19. As the client approaches full term, the nurse discusses with Mr. and Mrs. Webb the antepartal classes they have attended. They tell the nurse of their participation in Lamaze classes with 10 other couples. Which statement by this couple best indicates understanding of key concepts?
    ○ 1. "Being well prepared will ensure delivery without anesthesia."
    ○ 2. "Self-hypnosis is the key to pain-free birth."
    ○ 3. "We will avoid all pain medication in labor."
    ○ 4. "We plan to continue using a wall hanging for a focal point."

20. Mrs. Webb calls the prenatal clinic and states that she thinks she is in labor. Which of the following signs would indicate that she is in true labor?
    ○ 1. Walking "eases" her contractions.
    ○ 2. She has urinary frequency and urgency.
    ○ 3. She thinks that the baby has dropped, as she can breathe better.
    ○ 4. Her contractions are increasing in frequency and duration.

One of the components of antepartal care is provision of childbirth education. The antepartal-care nurse is planning to conduct 8 weekly classes for women in their third trimester.

21. What is the main objective of this program according to modern concepts of childbirth education in the United States?
    ○ 1. A painless childbirth experience
    ○ 2. The participation of both parents in the birth process
    ○ 3. The elimination of medication in labor and delivery
    ○ 4. An emotionally satisfying birth experience

22. During the first childbirth class, one of the participants states, "I cannot relax! Just thinking of going through labor makes me tense all over." Which response is most appropriate?
    ○ 1. "Labor pains don't hurt as much as you have been led to believe. Childbirth can be a really enjoyable experience."
    ○ 2. "Once you understand the importance of natural childbirth, you will begin to relax and your fears will disappear."
    ○ 3. "It is quite common for women to be anxious about labor and delivery. Women can learn to relax through education and physical training."
    ○ 4. "Fear causes tension, which results in pain. When you learn about childbirth, your fear will be eliminated and pain will not occur."

Claire Ostrow, a primigravida, has encouraged her husband to attend prenatal classes with her. Although he has 2 children from a previous marriage, he did not participate in classes. Now he is eager to learn, and is enthusiastic when practicing breathing techniques. At the last class a film on childbirth is shown. Later the couple expresses concerns about the pain of labor and delivery.

23. It is recognized that the perception of pain during childbirth is influenced by many factors, including culture, education, and anxiety. How can the nurse best assess the level of pain experienced by the laboring client?
    ○ 1. Analyze objective and subjective data.
    ○ 2. Correlate dilatation and effacement with assessment.
    ○ 3. Consider gravity and parity as a variable.
    ○ 4. Use past experience as a guide to assessment of pain.

24. The Ostrow couple seem very frightened during the labor process. How should the nurse most effectively support the couple during early labor?
    ○ 1. Give a condensed course in childbirth education.
    ○ 2. Ask the couple what would help them at this time.
    ○ 3. Demonstrate comfort measures the father may use.
    ○ 4. Tell them it is normal to feel this way.

25. As the nurse teaches this couple about the birth process, which of the following is most appropriate?
    ○ 1. Assess present knowledge of couple.
    ○ 2. Teach at learners' level of understanding.
    ○ 3. Use a standard teaching plan.
    ○ 4. Reinforce key concepts as necessary.

26. When she reaches transition, Mrs. Ostrow tells her husband to leave her alone. What is the best nursing action at this time?
    ○ 1. Ask the father to leave the nurse and the client alone.
    ○ 2. Urge the client to remain quiet at this time.
    ○ 3. Explore their feelings for one another.
    ○ 4. Accept this behavior as normal in this situation.

27. Sibling visitation is arranged for Mrs. Ostrow's stepchildren. Upon visiting the infant, the 2-year-old sister seems uninterested and asks to go home. The nursing student asks the nurse if this is related to the family situation. What explanation to the student would be most appropriate?
    ○ 1. "The parents may not have prepared the child well."
    ○ 2. "The 2-year-old probably resents the stepmother."
    ○ 3. "The social worker should assess the family situation."
    ○ 4. "This behavior is common for this child's developmental level."

28. Later that evening, the client is informed that her stepdaughter has a fever and a tentative diagnosis of rubella. What statement made by the mother best indicates an understanding of the implications of this viral infection?
    ○ 1. "I'll remind my mother to give her aspirin for the fever."
    ○ 2. "My sister is 2 months pregnant; I'll ask her to stay away from our home."
    ○ 3. "If our infant catches the infection, she won't need a vaccination."
    ○ 4. "It's good that my husband and I both had German measles as children."

29. At the time of discharge, Mrs. Ostrow indicates a desire to learn about natural family planning or the ovulation method. The nurse refers her to classes held at the hospital and briefly discuss the method. Which information is essential to enable the client to successfully use this method?
    ○ 1. Observe temperature changes throughout the sexual cycle.
    ○ 2. Cervical mucus secretions are thicker and "stretchy" at ovulation.
    ○ 3. Keep a calendar recording of each menstrual period.
    ○ 4. Most couples find that intercourse is safe during menses.

30. When counseling Mrs. Ostrow about the signs of ovulation, which of the following points is most appropriate to include in your discussion?
    ○ 1. Ovulation comes predictably 14 days after the onset of menses.
    ○ 2. The cervical mucus becomes thin and watery after ovulation.
    ○ 3. A rise in temperature occurs before ovulation.
    ○ 4. Lower abdominal pain may be experienced at the time of rupture of the follicle.

31. Mrs. Ostrow confides that her husband wants her to have a tubal ligation in the future. Which statement most indicates a *lack* of understanding of this type of contraception?
    ○ 1. "I know it can be reversed later if I change my mind."
    ○ 2. "He tells me it involves just a few days of hospitalization."
    ○ 3. "My doctor says it is almost as safe as a vasectomy."
    ○ 4. "It will remove all worry about pregnancy from our marriage."

A telephone call is received in the antepartal clinic from 18-year-old Susan Winter, who has recently been diagnosed as being approximately 10 weeks pregnant. The nurse is told by a sobbing Mrs. Winter, "I am losing my baby! I am bleeding uncontrollably."

32. Which one of the following would be the most appropriate initial nursing response?
    ○ 1. "You must be quite upset right now. Why don't you come to the clinic immediately."
    ○ 2. "Go to bed immediately with your feet elevated. I will call for an ambulance."
    ○ 3. "It is very common for women to have some bleeding during early pregnancy."
    ○ 4. "Can you describe the bleeding to me and tell me when it first became apparent?"

33. When Mrs. Winter is seen by the physician in the emergency room, her cervix is found to be 2 cm dilated and she is having moderate, bright red vaginal bleeding. Which term best describes her condition?
    ○ 1. Incomplete abortion
    ○ 2. Inevitable abortion
    ○ 3. Threatened abortion
    ○ 4. Missed abortion

34. Mrs. Winter is admitted to the hospital. Her initial nursing management would include which of the following?
    ○ 1. Examine all perineal pads for tissues and clots.
    ○ 2. Place the bed in Trendelenburg's position.
    ○ 3. Prepare her for a Shirodkar procedure.
    ○ 4. Restrict all physical activity and fluid intake.

35. Mrs. Winter overhears the physician telling her roommate that she has had a "missed abortion". Mrs. Winter asks the nurse to explain what this means. Which response is most appropriate?
    ○ 1. "It's another name for a miscarriage."
    ○ 2. "The baby is deformed, resulting in an abortion."
    ○ 3. "The baby is no longer alive and growing, but the body hasn't expelled it yet."
    ○ 4. "There was no pregnancy; her body just responded as if there were."

James and Anne Collins have been trying to have a baby for 4 years. Mrs. Collins has been pregnant 3 times, but all 3 times she aborted between the third and fourth months. A medical diagnosis of incompetent cervical os was made.

36. Mrs. Collins is told that she will have a McDonald's procedure when she gets pregnant again. She asks the nurse about the procedure. Which of the following statements best explains the procedure?
    ○ 1. "It is a permanent suture that is put around the cervix around the fourteenth week of gestation."
    ○ 2. "The suture around the cervix means that a cesarean section will be performed at term."
    ○ 3. "The suture is temporary and will be removed at term. You may be able to have a vaginal delivery if all goes well."
    ○ 4. "You will have to spend most of the pregnancy in bed, but the suture will enable you to carry the baby to term."

37. Mrs. Collins has brought her temperature chart, and she discusses her fertile periods with you. She has a 30-day cycle. The chances of fertilization are greatest between which of the following days?
    ○ 1. Days 14 to 16
    ○ 2. Days 15 to 17
    ○ 3. Days 13 to 15
    ○ 4. Days 12 to 14

Sara Burns, in her first trimester of pregnancy, is seen in the antepartal clinic. An ectopic pregnancy is suspected.

38. Which of the following symptoms would the nurse most likely expect to be present in an ectopic pregnancy?
    ○ 1. Spotting, lower abdominal pain radiating to the shoulders
    ○ 2. Excruciating pelvic pain, an enlarged uterus
    ○ 3. Leukorrhea, an enlarged uterus
    ○ 4. Headache, profuse bleeding, lower abdominal pain

39. Which of the following factors is *not* considered a high-risk factor for ectopic pregnancy?
    ○ 1. History of infertility
    ○ 2. History of pelvic inflammatory disease
    ○ 3. History of gonorrhea
    ○ 4. History of 3 consecutive spontaneous abortions

40. The client with an ectopic pregnancy is a high-risk client. Which of the following reasons best accounts for this?
    ○ 1. Surgery is required to treat this complication.
    ○ 2. Hemorrhage is a major problem.
    ○ 3. Removal of the fallopian tube may result in sterility.
    ○ 4. The ovum may abort into the abdominal cavity.

Wi-Li Chin, who has completed 37 weeks of gestation, calls the clinic where she has been receiving antepartal care. She tells the nurse that there is a small amount of bright red blood coming from her vagina, but that she has no pain.

41. Based on the information given, what would the nurse best conclude?
    ○ 1. Lacerated vaginal mucosa
    ○ 2. Premature labor
    ○ 3. Abruptio placentae
    ○ 4. Placenta previa

42. Mrs. Chin is hospitalized. Which of the following nursing actions is most important at this time?
    ○ 1. Perform a vaginal examination.
    ○ 2. Estimate amount of blood loss.
    ○ 3. Take vital signs frequently.
    ○ 4. Assess fetal heart rate.

43. In caring for Mrs. Chin, the nurse should
    ○ 1. prepare for a vaginal examination.
    ○ 2. expect an emergency cesarean birth.
    ○ 3. keep her on bed rest.
    ○ 4. administer an enema.

44. Which of the following is most important for the nurse to teach Mrs. Chin?
○ **1.** Increase ambulation.
○ **2.** Decrease protein consumption.
○ **3.** Limit physical activity.
○ **4.** Avoid emotional upset.

45. Mrs. Chin tells the nurse that she was dancing the night before the bleeding began, and she feels responsible for her current condition. What would be the most appropriate response for the nurse?
○ **1.** "Don't feel guilty. It wasn't your fault."
○ **2.** "It's too late to change anything now."
○ **3.** "This was caused by an abnormal implantation of the placenta."
○ **4.** "No one knows why this happens."

Jayne Simmons, gravida 3, para 2, is admitted to the labor room in early labor. She has a history of precipitate deliveries and has had an elevated blood pressure since the 28th week of pregnancy. She is leaking amniotic fluid and currently has a blood pressure of 150/100 mm Hg.

46. Mrs. Simmons begins to have a vaginal discharge of bright red blood. The nurse recognizes this could be related to placenta previa or to abruptio placentae. Which of the following predisposing factors to abruptio placentae does Mrs. Simmons have?
○ **1.** Chronic hypertension
○ **2.** Pregnancy-induced hypertension
○ **3.** Multiple pregnancy
○ **4.** Rapid decrease in uterine volume

47. To further assess Mrs. Simmons, which of the following should be done?
○ **1.** Monitor urine output by inserting a Foley catheter.
○ **2.** Do a vaginal examination to evaluate progression of labor.
○ **3.** Check her vital signs every 30 minutes.
○ **4.** Conduct an abdominal examination for signs of tenderness or rigidity.

48. In providing care for Mrs. Simmons, which of the following measures would be most appropriate for the situation and be of most benefit to the fetus?
○ **1.** Turn Mrs. Simmons on her side.
○ **2.** Administer oxygen.
○ **3.** Estimate amount of blood loss.
○ **4.** Observe for changes in the pattern of uterine contractions.

49. The systemic effects of blood loss on both mother and fetus and the possibility of abruptio placentae are primary concerns when caring for Mrs. Simmons. What complication of abruptio placentae is of most concern?
○ **1.** Disseminated intravascular coagulation syndrome
○ **2.** Pulmonary embolus
○ **3.** Hypocalcemia
○ **4.** Urinary tract infection

50. The nurse notes Mrs. Simmons's vaginal discharge has changed from red to a watery brown. What does this change most probably indicate?
○ **1.** Cessation of bleeding
○ **2.** Old blood mixed with amniotic fluid
○ **3.** Meconium-stained fluid
○ **4.** Imminent danger to both mother and infant

51. In view of the change in the character of the vaginal discharge, what would be the most appropriate initial action?
○ **1.** Begin preparing Mrs. Simmons for an emergency cesarean birth.
○ **2.** Contact the physician immediately to report fetal distress.
○ **3.** Record a careful description of the vaginal discharge and of Mrs. Simmons's vital signs.
○ **4.** Check fetal heart tones and apply an external fetal monitor, if it has not already been applied.

Harriet Morton, aged 40, is hospitalized for severe pregnancy-induced hypertension (PIH). She is in her eighth month of pregnancy and has gained 66 lb.

52. Which nursing action should occur first after Mrs. Morton has been admitted?
○ **1.** Start an IV.
○ **2.** Record baseline vital signs.
○ **3.** Administer antihypertensive drugs.
○ **4.** Call the lab to draw blood.

53. Which of the following nursing actions would reduce the possibility of a convulsion?
○ **1.** Keep the side rails padded and up.
○ **2.** Place the client in the room closest to the nurse's station.
○ **3.** Keep the room dimly lit.
○ **4.** Stay with the client at all times.

54. The main purpose of bed rest as a treatment for PIH is to
- ○ **1.** reduce blood pressure by lowering body metabolism.
- ○ **2.** conserve energy in view of the impending labor.
- ○ **3.** lower the incidence of headaches.
- ○ **4.** limit contact with other clients.

55. The nurse administers magnesium sulfate to Mrs. Morton. What medication would the nurse have available to counteract toxicity?
- ○ **1.** Sodium chloride
- ○ **2.** Calcium gluconate
- ○ **3.** Adrenalin
- ○ **4.** Sodium bicarbonate

56. Mrs. Morton asks the nurse if the magnesium sulfate will affect her baby. What would be the best response?
- ○ **1.** "No, the placenta acts as a barrier to the medication."
- ○ **2.** "The doctor wouldn't order it if it would hurt the baby."
- ○ **3.** "It has a minor effect; however, the effects of a convulsion are much more severe."
- ○ **4.** "We don't know if this drug crosses the placental barrier."

Sally Dunsmore is a gravida 2, para 0, Class C diabetic. She is in her 34th week of pregnancy. At her weekly prenatal visit, her physician decides to hospitalize her because her fasting blood sugar is 325. Mrs. Dunsmore's previous fasting blood sugars have all been within normal limits.

57. Which of the following is true regarding insulin needs during pregnancy?
- ○ **1.** Insulin needs during pregnancy will be essentially the same as before pregnancy, as long as the client maintains a well-balanced diet.
- ○ **2.** Insulin needs will vary throughout the pregnancy and will need to be watched closely. It is not possible to predict when insulin needs will be greatest.
- ○ **3.** With a proper balance of nutrition and exercise, the client may not need insulin during pregnancy, as the baby will be producing insulin, which will be available for the mother's body to use.
- ○ **4.** Insulin needs will vary throughout the pregnancy. Need is likely to decrease during the first trimester and reach a peak at the end of the second trimester.

58. Mrs. Dunsmore inquires about how her baby will be delivered. Which of the following is the best response?
- ○ **1.** "You will probably have either a cesarean section or have labor induced about the 37th week of pregnancy."
- ○ **2.** "You will probably have a cesarean section to decrease the stress of delivery on the baby."
- ○ **3.** "Your insulin needs will be carefully monitored; and if they follow a normal pattern, your pregnancy will probably be allowed to progress to term with labor occurring naturally."
- ○ **4.** "Your pregnancy will be carefully monitored with the best time for delivery chosen on the basis of your status and tests of placental function and fetal maturity."

59. Baby Boy Dunsmore weighs 9 lb 6 oz at birth. Which of the following characteristics should the nurse expect to find in this infant?
- ○ **1.** Postmature
- ○ **2.** Active and alert
- ○ **3.** Neuromuscular irritability
- ○ **4.** Hypobilirubinemia

60. When caring for Baby Dunsmore in the delivery room, what is the nurse's first priority?
- ○ **1.** Ensure proper identification.
- ○ **2.** Establish a warm environment.
- ○ **3.** Maintain a patent airway.
- ○ **4.** Facilitate parental bonding.

61. Which of the following is of high priority when caring for Baby Dunsmore in the nursery?
- ○ **1.** Maintain hydration.
- ○ **2.** Assess gestational age.
- ○ **3.** Initiate early feeding.
- ○ **4.** Monitor blood sugar level.

62. Mrs. Dunsmore wants to breast-feed her baby. The nurse plans a response based on which of the following facts?
- ○ **1.** Insulin does not pass into breast milk.
- ○ **2.** Insulin does pass into breast milk.
- ○ **3.** The breast-feeding mother has a markedly decreased caloric demand.
- ○ **4.** The infant of the diabetic mother is often hypoactive.

63. In preparing Mrs. Dunsmore for discharge the nurse includes infant-care teaching. Which of the following is most important for this mother to know?
    ○ 1. Although the baby has a problem he is normal and should be treated like any infant.
    ○ 2. Give the child 24-calorie/oz formula to counteract hypoglycemia.
    ○ 3. See a pediatrician regularly throughout infancy and childhood.
    ○ 4. Feed the child skim milk to maintain weight in infancy.

Shelly and Mark Novak have been married for 5 years, and avoided pregnancy during that time on the advice of her physician. Mrs. Novak had corrective heart surgery as an infant, and there was fear that pregnancy might be unwise. After consultation with a cardiologist, the couple were advised that conception would be safe, and with regular care during the pregnancy, problems could be avoided. Mrs. Novak has visited the physician every 2 weeks, complies with dietary advice, and her blood pressure remains stable.

64. Which of the following would most likely indicate potential problems for a pregnant client with a history of heart disease?
    ○ 1. Reduced tolerance for activity
    ○ 2. Polyhydramnios
    ○ 3. Frequent urinary tract infections
    ○ 4. Frequent heartburn

65. Mrs. Novak delivers a healthy 7 lb son in a forceps-assisted delivery. Mother and infant remain in the recovery room for several hours for observation. The nurse notes that the mother's pulse rate is stable at 66. She received no medication other than oxytocin. What is the appropriate nursing action?
    ○ 1. Notify the physician immediately.
    ○ 2. Continue to assess vital signs routinely.
    ○ 3. Observe for toxicity to oxytoxic drugs.
    ○ 4. Monitor the level of consciousness.

66. In the immediate postpartal period, which physiologic adaptation would increase stress on this mother's heart?
    ○ 1. Moderate diaphoresis
    ○ 2. Release of prolactin
    ○ 3. Uterine contractions
    ○ 4. Increased blood volume

Juanita Lopez, a 15-year-old gravida 1 para 0, registers for antepartal care at 10 weeks gestation.

67. Which of the following is a priority for high-risk clients in a prenatal clinic?
    ○ 1. Encourage regular prenatal care.
    ○ 2. Encourage acceptance of the pregnancy.
    ○ 3. Arrange for financial support.
    ○ 4. Recommend genetic screening.

68. Juanita is facing the psychologic task of "accepting her pregnancy and incorporating the fetus into her body image," as identified by Rubin. Which of the following behaviors best characterizes this?
    ○ 1. Acknowledging the "surprise" she experiences at being in the pregnant state
    ○ 2. Planning for a "Lamaze" childbirth experience
    ○ 3. Arranging a baby nursery in the home
    ○ 4. Talking about the responsibilities of motherhood

69. During the initial antepartal appointment, which of the following nursing actions would most contribute to Juanita's positive reaction to her new physical status?
    ○ 1. Discuss patients' rights and explain informed consent.
    ○ 2. Provide a description of the scope of available services.
    ○ 3. Stay with the client and listen to her concerns.
    ○ 4. Reassure the client that many teenagers experience a temporary uneasiness at this time.

70. Basic nutritional counseling is an important component of Juanita's nursing care. Guidance in diet planning for pregnant teenagers differs from that of pregnant adults because of which basic consideration?
    ○ 1. The nutritional needs of pregnant women decline with advancing age.
    ○ 2. Metabolic alterations increase nutrient catabolism in pregnant adolescents.
    ○ 3. Postpubescent women have an increase in protein deposition.
    ○ 4. There is a pubertal acceleration in growth of pregnant adolescents.

71. Based upon the clinical findings of Juanita's examination at 32 weeks gestation, it is determined that she has iron-deficiency anemia. Which one of these findings supports the diagnosis?
    ○ 1. A hemoglobin less than 10 gm
    ○ 2. A hematocrit of less than 40%
    ○ 3. A hemoglobin less than 14 gm
    ○ 4. A hematocrit of less than 36%

72. The increased demand for iron during pregnancy is most likely caused by
    ○ 1. a decrease in hematopoiesis occurring in the third trimester.
    ○ 2. the rise in hemoconcentration occurring between 24 and 32 weeks gestation.
    ○ 3. an expansion in total blood cell volume and hemoglobin mass by approximately 25% to 50% during pregnancy.
    ○ 4. a decreased efficiency of iron absorption during pregnancy, and fetal inability to absorb the mineral.

73. The nurse asks Juanita to select foods that best meet her dietary needs for increased iron. Juanita's knowledge of foods highest in iron would be accurate if she selected which of these meals for lunch?
    ○ 1. A peanut butter and jelly sandwich, ½ cup cooked carrots, 1 cup whole milk
    ○ 2. An 8-oz strawberry yogurt, 1 banana, 1 cup apple juice
    ○ 3. Enriched macaroni, broccoli, 1 cup orange juice
    ○ 4. One-half chicken breast, split peas, 1 cup prune juice

Donna Walsh, a 16-year-old primigravida, is in the 28th week of her pregnancy. She has received no prenatal education and began receiving prenatal care only 2 weeks ago.

74. Which of the following best describes obstetric hazards experienced by the pregnant adolescent?
    ○ 1. They have an increased mortality rate and an increased incidence of anemia, vaginitis, urinary tract infections, and pregnancy-induced hypertension.
    ○ 2. They have decreased cognitive development, have little emotional support available, and display child-like behaviors, which may cause conflict.
    ○ 3. They usually experience economic and social handicaps leading to an unsafe physical environment.
    ○ 4. They usually have low self-esteem; therefore they have a decreased ability to establish meaningful relationships.

75. Donna reaches 40 weeks gestation. She arrives at the hospital with complaints of uterine contractions crying, "It's time to have the baby." Which of the following nursing actions should be first?
    ○ 1. Assess her contractions.
    ○ 2. Take a nursing history.
    ○ 3. Call the physician.
    ○ 4. Start an IV.

76. Donna has received no childbirth preparation. When will she be most receptive to learning breathing techniques?
    ○ 1. Any time between contractions
    ○ 2. During the contractions for simultaneous theory and practice
    ○ 3. When her anxiety has been reduced
    ○ 4. Early, when she is most alert and comfortable

77. During a strong contraction, Donna's membranes rupture. What nursing assessment is most important at this time?
    ○ 1. Color of amniotic fluid
    ○ 2. Extent of cervical dilatation
    ○ 3. Change in baseline vital signs
    ○ 4. Psychologic response to event

78. Donna delivered a 5-lb daughter yesterday after a difficult labor. She was alone during labor. She had spoken to the social worker about adoption, but has not made a final decision. She asks few questions of the staff and sleeps most of the time. The labor room nurse visits to follow up on the care of the previous day. Donna seems eager to talk. Which of the following statements made by the nurse is most appropriate?
    ○ 1. "Adoption is really the best solution to your situation."
    ○ 2. "It must be difficult to be in this position."
    ○ 3. "Was this pregnancy planned or unplanned?"
    ○ 4. "What would your parents like you to do?"

79. The nursing student expresses concern that the client continues to care for and feed the infant, while remaining ambivalent about an adoption decision. On what knowledge should the nurse base a response to the student?
    ○ 1. Such behavior is typical of adolescence.
    ○ 2. This care giving indicates guilt feelings.
    ○ 3. Such actions are a healthy grieving response.
    ○ 4. Caring for the infant delays decision making.

80. Donna agrees to sign the papers for adoption. After Donna has been discharged, the adoptive parents and social worker visit the 5-day-old newborn in the nursery. Based upon an understanding of the process of attachment, what should the nurse teach the adoptive parents?
    ○ 1. "Hold the infant and talk to her often."
    ○ 2. "Sleep with the baby to enhance bonding."
    ○ 3. "Learn basic infant care skills quickly."
    ○ 4. "It is too late to attach, but you'll learn to care."

81. While dressing the infant, which observation by the adoptive father is the most positive sign of early parenting?
    ○ 1. "Look at her watch me as I talk to her!"
    ○ 2. "See how great this pink sweater looks on her!"
    ○ 3. "Her eyes don't look much like anyone in the family."
    ○ 4. "I read that hiccoughs are normal for a newborn."

Jan Rondinelli, a 26-year-old primigravida in her 40th week of pregnancy, is admitted to the labor area. She has had no antepartal care. She is accompanied by her husband. Her membranes ruptured in the car on the way to the hospital.

82. Which of the following initial nursing assessments would be *least* important during her admission?
    ○ 1. Type of anesthesia requested for delivery
    ○ 2. Location, rate, and rhythm of fetal heart tones
    ○ 3. Maternal vital signs
    ○ 4. Onset, duration, and frequency of contractions

83. The admitting vaginal exam reveals that Mrs. Rondinelli's cervix is 6 cm dilated and 100% effaced. The fetus is at 1 + station and left occiput anterior. She is having difficulty coping with her contractions, which are occurring every 3 minutes. Which of these nursing actions is appropriate during her next contraction?
    ○ 1. Encourage her to bear down with the contraction.
    ○ 2. Check the perineum for crowning.
    ○ 3. Provide direct coaching using chest-abdominal breathing techniques.
    ○ 4. Show her husband how to apply firm pressure to her sacral area.

84. The nurse knows that Mrs. Rondinelli is in the transition phase of labor when she
    ○ 1. begins accelerated breathing.
    ○ 2. requests pain medication.
    ○ 3. requests sacral pressure.
    ○ 4. becomes irritable and frightened.

85. Mrs. Rondinelli is in the transitional phase of labor. Her contractions are lasting 75 seconds and occurring every 2 minutes. She begins to grunt and says she has to push. Upon vaginal exam, the nurse finds her cervix is dilated 9 cm. What is the most appropriate immediate nursing action?
    ○ 1. Roll her on her side and tell her to breathe slowly.
    ○ 2. Tell her to blow out until the urge passes.
    ○ 3. Explain that pushing will cause the cervix to swell and delay dilatation.
    ○ 4. Tell her to push with each contraction.

86. Mrs. Rondinelli begins to show symptoms of hyperventilation with her rapid panting during contractions. The nurse instructs her to slow down her breathing and breathe into her cupped hands. Which of the following would best indicate effectiveness of this action?
    ○ 1. Dizziness and finger tingling subside.
    ○ 2. Nausea increases.
    ○ 3. Amnesia between contractions lessens.
    ○ 4. The urge to push subsides.

87. Mrs. Rondinelli has now progressed to full cervical dilatation and effacement without perineal bulging. The nurse should
    ○ 1. prep and drape her for delivery.
    ○ 2. coach her how to push effectively with contractions.
    ○ 3. provide privacy for her and her husband.
    ○ 4. administer a narcotic analgesic.

88. Mrs. Rondinelli has an uneventful vaginal delivery with a midline episiotomy done under local anesthesia. During the fourth stage of labor, the nurse should include which of the following in the nursing care plan?
    ○ 1. Massage the fundus constantly.
    ○ 2. Monitor temperature every 30 minutes.
    ○ 3. Palpate the uterus to check muscle tone every 15 minutes.
    ○ 4. Monitor blood pressure every 5 minutes.

89. Baby Girl Rondinelli weighed 6 lb at birth and received routine care. Her eyes were treated prophylactically with 1% silver nitrate. This treatment is done to prevent
    ○ **1.** chemical conjunctivitis.
    ○ **2.** neonatal syphilis.
    ○ **3.** herpes infection.
    ○ **4.** ophthalmia neonatorum.

The professional nurse assigned to the labor and delivery unit of a hospital is required to manage care for a group of clients. The application of the nursing process in such a setting involves setting priorities as a part of decision making. The use of electronic fetal monitoring has enhanced the assessment of fetal response to labor, yet the nurse must constantly apply knowledge to interpret the tracings.

90. The nurse is going to care for Mrs. Sanchez, a multigravida, in the labor room. During an assessment the nurse notes a change in fetal-heart-rate variability on the monitor. Previous variability was 10 to 15 beats; it is now 2 to 3 beats over several minutes. Contractions are mild. What is the best analysis of these data?
    ○ **1.** The change is within normal limits.
    ○ **2.** There is indication of potential hypoxia.
    ○ **3.** Such variability is common in the fetus of a multigravida.
    ○ **4.** Insufficent data are given to assess fetal status.

91. The nurse sees that there are many variable decelerations on Mrs. Roberts's fetal monitor strip. Variable decelerations most likely are due to
    ○ **1.** head compression.
    ○ **2.** cord compression.
    ○ **3.** uteroplacental insufficiency.
    ○ **4.** posterior presentation.

92. Which of the following readings would be considered a normal finding?
    ○ **1.** Late decelerations, good variability
    ○ **2.** Early decelerations, no variability
    ○ **3.** Early decelerations, good variability
    ○ **4.** Variable decelerations, no variability

93. After asking the physician to examine Mrs. Sanchez, the nurse is called to a second labor room. The expectant father has noticed that the fetal heart rate drops slightly just prior to his wife's contraction, then recovers at the end of the contraction. What is the most appropriate *initial* nursing action?
    ○ **1.** Assess maternal vital signs.
    ○ **2.** Administer oxygen.
    ○ **3.** Notify the physican.
    ○ **4.** Reassure him that this is normal.

94. The physician orders an internal electrode for Mrs. Sakolov. The nurse is asked to assist in placement of the scalp electrode. This technique
    ○ **1.** is an invasive procedure.
    ○ **2.** routinely follows amniotomy.
    ○ **3.** is an extraordinary assessment.
    ○ **4.** is risk free.

95. Mrs. Sakolov is in the second stage of labor. Which of the following patterns would necessitate immediate action?
    ○ **1.** Baseline fetal heart rate between 120 and 130
    ○ **2.** Fetal heart rate that drops to 100 during contractions and returns to baseline when the contraction ends
    ○ **3.** An increase in baseline fetal heart rate to 150 just prior to the contraction
    ○ **4.** Fetal heart rate that drops to 120 during the contraction and returns to baseline 1 minute after the contraction ends

96. The nursing student asks the nurse to check her client. The baseline fetal heart rate has gradually decreased from 140 to 120. "But I know that is within normal range," comments the student. What is the appropriate nursing action?
    ○ **1.** Confirm that this is within a normal heart rate range.
    ○ **2.** Notify the physician immediately.
    ○ **3.** Elevate the foot of the bed in Trendelenburg's position.
    ○ **4.** Take the client's blood pressure and temperature.

97. Late decelerations are observed, on the fetal heart rate monitor; what should the first nursing action be?
    ○ **1.** Turn off the oxytocin.
    ○ **2.** Change the client's position.
    ○ **3.** Administer oxygen.
    ○ **4.** Inform the physician.

Marianne Stoner, aged 41, is admitted to the labor and delivery unit at 4:00 P.M. While taking the history, the nurse notes the following: gravida 8, para 7; weeks of completed gestation 41; membranes ruptured at 10:00 A.M. that day; contractions occur every 3 minutes; strong intensity with a duration of 60 seconds.

98. What nursing action would take highest priority at this time?
    ○ **1.** Get blood and urine samples.
    ○ **2.** Do perineal prep and give enema.
    ○ **3.** Attach monitors to client.
    ○ **4.** Determine extent of cervical dilatation.

99. Mrs. Stoner has just been given epidural anesthesia. What is the most important assessment at this time?
    - ○ 1. Maternal blood pressure
    - ○ 2. Fetal heart rate
    - ○ 3. Maternal level of consciousness
    - ○ 4. Fetal position

100. Mrs. Stoner has a normal spontaneous delivery. Why would she be considered at risk for development of postpartal hemorrhage?
    - ○ 1. Grand multiparity
    - ○ 2. Premature rupture of membranes
    - ○ 3. Postterm delivery
    - ○ 4. Anesthesia

101. Mrs. Stoner asks to be discharged after 24 hours, and her physician agrees. What is most important for the nurse to include in the discharge instructions?
    - ○ 1. Family-planning information
    - ○ 2. Newborn-care information
    - ○ 3. Need to have infant tested for phenylketonuria
    - ○ 4. Referral to social service

A nurse is summoned to the home of a neighbor, a multigravida, during a severe snowstorm. She appears to be in active labor. Both she and her husband are very apprehensive.

102. The initial nursing action should be to
    - ○ 1. call the hospital for an ambulance.
    - ○ 2. calm both parents.
    - ○ 3. prepare a clean delivery field.
    - ○ 4. assess the mother's status.

103. The assessment reveals the infant in a vertex presentation, crowning. As the nurse assists in the delivery of the head, which would be the most appropriate instruction to the mother?
    - ○ 1. Push during the contraction to aid in delivery.
    - ○ 2. Pant during contractions to avoid forceful expulsion.
    - ○ 3. Bear down continuously to assist the abdominal muscles.
    - ○ 4. Breathe slowly and deeply to ensure proper oxygenation of the fetus.

104. Before help arrives it appears that the newly delivered mother is bleeding excessively. What nursing action is most appropriate at this time?
    - ○ 1. Put the infant to breast.
    - ○ 2. Place sandbags on the fundus.
    - ○ 3. Pack the vagina with a towel.
    - ○ 4. Apply vigorous pressure to the uterus.

Angela Lopez is a primipara admitted for an elective cesarean delivery. Mrs. Lopez crushed her pelvis in an automobile accident as a teenager. This pelvic damage led to an extremely narrow pelvic outlet resulting in dystocia. The pregnancy has been normal.

105. Which of the following would *not* be included in preparation for the elective cesarean delivery?
    - ○ 1. Insert a Foley catheter.
    - ○ 2. Do an abdominal prep.
    - ○ 3. Ensure that blood has been typed and cross-matched.
    - ○ 4. Insert an internal fetal monitor.

106. Mrs. Lopez asks what is the most common reason for a cesarean delivery. Which of the following is the best explanation?
    - ○ 1. Hemorrhage
    - ○ 2. Toxemia
    - ○ 3. Dysfunctional labor
    - ○ 4. Cephalopelvic disproportion

107. After the cesarean delivery, Mrs. Lopez will need the usual post-op care as well as the usual postpartum care. Which of the following is true in this regard?
    - ○ 1. Fundal height should not be checked because of the location of the abdominal incision.
    - ○ 2. Lochia flow will be checked less frequently, as the uterus is cleansed more thoroughly during a cesarean delivery.
    - ○ 3. Perineal checks are less important, as there should not have been any perineal trauma.
    - ○ 4. The surgical incision will not need to be checked frequently, as increased vascularity in the area will speed healing.

108. Mrs. Lopez indicates she wants to breast-feed her newborn, but is uncertain if she can. The nurse's response should include which of the following?
    - ○ 1. Following a cesarean delivery, the mother's limited oral intake during the first 2 days will inhibit the production of milk.
    - ○ 2. She is likely to stay in the hospital for more than a week, but the baby does not need to stay this long.
    - ○ 3. Breast-feeding is not contraindicated by a surgical delivery.
    - ○ 4. The abdominal incision will make it very uncomfortable for her to breast-feed.

Judy Harris, aged 31, gravida 2, para 1, delivered her first child by cesarean birth because of footling breech. She is admitted for a planned, repeat cesarean delivery under regional anesthesia. During the initial assessment, she comments on the thrill she anticipates in watching the birth. Reviewing the prenatal record, the nurse notes that she kept her prenatal appointments.

109. Each of the following is noted on the chart. Which should be reported to the anesthesiologist prior to delivery?
    ○ 1. Corrective surgery for scoliosis at age 14
    ○ 2. Trace of glucose in urine throughout pregnancy
    ○ 3. Hemoglobin 12 gm; hematocrit 39%
    ○ 4. Acute episode of herpes type 2 prior to pregnancy

110. The physician orders an IV of 5% dextrose in normal saline to be infused over 6 hours prior to surgery. The IV inadvertently infuses more rapidly than desired. What assessments are most essential when fluids are administered too rapidly?
    ○ 1. Pulse and temperature
    ○ 2. Blood pressure and fetal heart rate
    ○ 3. Respirations and pulse rate
    ○ 4. Level of consciousness and hematocrit

111. The cesarean delivery proceeds normally under general anesthesia, and a healthy 6 lb son is delivered. As Mrs. Harris recovers from surgery in the postanesthesia recovery unit, which of the following assessments is most significant?
    ○ 1. Blood pressure is stable at 100/72 mm Hg.
    ○ 2. Respirations are 32 and shallow.
    ○ 3. Temperature is constant at 99.8°F (37.6°C) orally.
    ○ 4. Pulse is 68 and regular.

112. On the second post-op day, Mrs. Harris asks to have the infant room-in with her. In planning for her comfort and for the safety of the newborn, which nursing action is most appropriate?
    ○ 1. Suggest she delay breast-feeding for several days.
    ○ 2. Ask the father to remain with mother and infant.
    ○ 3. Inform her that the nurse is available to assist her.
    ○ 4. Place the signal light near her chair.

113. One evening during visiting hours, Mrs. Harris tells the nurse that she is afraid her 3-year-old son will be jealous of the new baby. The nurse should suggest that the parents take which of the following actions?
    ○ 1. "Ignore him; he will outgrow his jealousy."
    ○ 2. "Tell your son that he will learn to love their new baby."
    ○ 3. "Leave your son with his grandparents until the new baby is settled at home."
    ○ 4. "Bring your son a baby doll or other toy at the time the baby is taken home."

114. The parents notice a dark pigmented area on their son's lower back and buttocks. Which notation on the chart will best explain this observation?
    ○ 1. Positive rubella titer
    ○ 2. AB blood type
    ○ 3. Ethnic background: black
    ○ 4. Genetic screening positive for sickle cell disease

115. Both Mr. and Mrs. Harris are sickle cell carriers. The mother asks the nurse about the probability of inheritance of sickle cell disease. What response would be most appropriate to give?
    ○ 1. "It is not possible to predict."
    ○ 2. "There is a 25% probability."
    ○ 3. "There is no risk with 2 carriers."
    ○ 4. "Fifty percent of your offspring will have the disease."

116. On the third day, the nurse observes Mrs. Harris and the infant during feeding. The nurse notices that the infant nurses at the breast for a few minutes, then falls asleep. What other assessments are indicated?
    ○ 1. Observe the sleep periods.
    ○ 2. Note the mother's apprehension.
    ○ 3. Record the intake and output.
    ○ 4. Assess infant satisfaction.

Anna Wolinski had a low-segment cesarean delivery last evening for failure to progress in labor. She is now 12 hours post-op. Mrs. Wolinski has an intravenous infusion with 1,000 ml of 5% dextrose in water running at 150 ml/hour.

117. What primary advantage does the low-segment cesarean delivery have, compared with the classic cesarean delivery?
    ○ 1. Easier delivery of a fetus in a transverse lie
    ○ 2. Greater safety for delivery with an anterior placenta previa
    ○ 3. Simpler procedure to perform operatively
    ○ 4. Lower incidence of post-op infection and a smaller amount of blood loss

118. Mrs. Wolinski had an intrathecal injection for anesthesia. To prevent the occurrence of a postspinal headache, what should the nurse do during the first 8 hours postoperatively?
    ○ 1. Maintain an indwelling catheter.
    ○ 2. Ambulate her progressively.
    ○ 3. Administer analgesics and antiemetics.
    ○ 4. Maintain bed rest in a recumbent position.

Inga Swenson, aged 32, is admitted for induction of labor. It is estimated by ultrasound that the fetus is of 42 weeks gestation. She is very impatient for the birth of this planned child. The physician elects to rupture the membranes artificially. Subsequently, fetal heart beat is stable at 144. Amniotic fluid is clear.

119. As the nurse continues to care for Mrs. Swenson, she experiences sudden onset of dyspnea, cyanosis, and severe apprehension. This is followed by severe chest pain. Which of the following conditions is suggested by these data?
    ○ 1. Acute myocardial infarction
    ○ 2. Pulmonary embolus
    ○ 3. Hysterical reaction
    ○ 4. Massive infection

120. As Mr. Swenson watches, his wife is transferred to the intensive care unit (ICU). He remains in the waiting room, stunned. He refuses to talk to the resident and insists he will wait there for the safe delivery of his child. How could the nurse best meet his needs at this time?
    ○ 1. Insist that he go to ICU.
    ○ 2. Remain with him for the next few minutes.
    ○ 3. Allow him privacy and leave him alone.
    ○ 4. Ask the attending physician to see him later.

121. After 30 minutes, the husband joins his wife in the ICU. She is unresponsive. There is evidence of massive internal hemorrhage associated with disseminated intravascular coagulation. The physician orders immediate transfusions, but the husband refuses on religious grounds. Which action by the nurse is *least* appropriate at this time?
    ○ 1. Call the clergyman to speak with the father.
    ○ 2. Emphasize that religious values are not as important as saving lives.
    ○ 3. Clarify the physician's explanation of the situation.
    ○ 4. Ask the father if he wishes to consult with his family.

122. While awaiting a decision on the use of blood transfusions, the client's status is best evaluated by which of the following?
    ○ 1. Level of consciousness
    ○ 2. Blood pressure and pulse
    ○ 3. Observation of bleeding
    ○ 4. Repeated hematocrit levels

123. After discussion with clergy and physicians, Mr. Swenson agrees to life-saving measures and transfusions. However, the client does not respond to therapy, and both mother and fetus die. Which statement made to the distraught father by the nurse is most appropriate?
    ○ 1. "I am so sorry."
    ○ 2. "Try not to feel guilty."
    ○ 3. "It must be very difficult for you."
    ○ 4. "At least you have other children at home."

Suzanne Phillips is a 14-year-old, newly delivered primipara. She has just been admitted to her postpartum room after having been in the recovery room for 8 hours because of fluctuating blood pressure. She had a saddle block for delivery.

124. Suzanne has an IV infusing to which 10 ml of oxytocin (Pitocin) has been added. The rationale for administering oxytocin after delivery of the placenta is to
    ○ 1. shorten the third stage of labor.
    ○ 2. control postpartal bleeding.
    ○ 3. stabilize the mother's blood pressure.
    ○ 4. inhibit lactation in the bottle-feeding mother.

125. Suzanne states that her bladder feels full and that she needs to void but cannot. The nurse should
    ○ 1. walk her to the bathroom and encourage her to try to void.
    ○ 2. insert a Foley catheter to prevent postpartum cystitis.
    ○ 3. administer egonovine maleate (Ergotrate) as ordered.
    ○ 4. place her on a bedpan, dabble her fingers in water, and run water in the bathroom loud enough for her to hear.

126. Suzanne begins to tremble and shake. She states she is cold and cannot control her shaking. Nursing actions should include which of the following?
    ○ 1. Cover her with a warm blanket.
    ○ 2. Notify the physician immediately.
    ○ 3. Administer a tranquilizer.
    ○ 4. Discontinue the IV Pitocin.

127. Two days postpartum, Suzanne complains of perineal pain. Observing her midline episiotomy, the nurse sees that it is edematous but healing. Which of the following might help her?
    ○ 1. Apply ice packs to the perineal area.
    ○ 2. Encourage sitz baths as desired.
    ○ 3. Administer chlorotrianisene (TACE) as ordered.
    ○ 4. Encourage postpartal Kegel exercises.

Sally Noyamba is a primipara who is trying to breast-feed her infant for the first time.

128. Milk production after delivery is a direct result of
    ○ 1. a decrease in estrogen and progesterone.
    ○ 2. an increase in estrogen and progesterone.
    ○ 3. a decrease in oxytocin.
    ○ 4. an increase in prolactin.

129. Which of the following would be *least* helpful to Mrs. Noyamba?
    ○ 1. Stimulate the infant to suck by rubbing cheek on the side closest to the nipple.
    ○ 2. Use nipple rolling to get the nipple erect.
    ○ 3. Use a breast pump to bring the milk forward to the areola.
    ○ 4. Place most of the areola in the infant's mouth.

130. After 3 days, Mrs. Noyamba asks which type of contraceptive is acceptable to use before her first postpartal check. The nurse should advise which of the following?
    ○ 1. Birth control pills
    ○ 2. IUD
    ○ 3. Condoms
    ○ 4. Diaphragm and jelly

131. Which of the following statements by Mrs. Noyamba would indicate that she may need more teaching before her discharge?
    ○ 1. "I know how and when to bathe the infant."
    ○ 2. "I know that if my lochia becomes bright red I will need to rest and call my doctor."
    ○ 3. "I need to increase my calorie intake by 500 calories."
    ○ 4. "I plan on doing push-ups and sit-ups when I return home."

Sylvia Martino has just delivered a 10-lb girl.

132. In assessing Mrs. Martino immediately after delivery, which of the following would the nurse most likely find?
    ○ 1. Fundus located half way between the symphysis pubis and the umbilicus, lochia rubra
    ○ 2. Fundus displaced to the right and 3 cm above the umbilicus, lochia serosa
    ○ 3. Fundus located at the umbilicus, lochia rubra
    ○ 4. Fundus located halfway between the symphysis pubis and the umbilicus, lochia serosa

133. Mrs. Martino is having vaginal bleeding of bright red blood that is continuously trickling from the vagina. Her fundus is firm and in the midline. What is the most likely cause of this bleeding?
    ○ 1. Lacerations
    ○ 2. Subinvolution
    ○ 3. Uterine atony
    ○ 4. Retained placental fragments

134. Which of the following conditions predisposes a client to postpartal hemorrhage?
    ○ 1. Twin pregnancy
    ○ 2. Breech presentation
    ○ 3. Premature rupture of membranes
    ○ 4. Cesarean birth

135. Twenty-four hours later, Mrs. Martino has a temperature of 100°F (38.3°C), has voided 2,000 ml since delivery, and her skin is diaphoretic. Nursing actions should include which of the following?
    ○ 1. Notify the physician of the findings.
    ○ 2. Notify the nursery to feed the baby in the nursery, as the mother has a fever.
    ○ 3. Explain to Mrs. Martino that these symptoms are all very normal for a woman who has just delivered.
    ○ 4. Suspect a postpartal infection and isolate mother and newborn.

136. Mrs. Martino's sister warns her to expect afterpains. The nurse's teaching is based on the knowledge that the most likely candidate for afterpains is the
    ○ 1. primipara who is bottle-feeding.
    ○ 2. grand multipara who is breast-feeding twin boys.
    ○ 3. primipara who delivers prematurely and who is pumping her breasts.
    ○ 4. adolescent primipara who is breast-feeding.

137. Mrs. Martino is bottle-feeding her baby and asks when she should expect her first menses. The appropriate response would be
    ○ 1. "It usually takes at least 3 months before menstruation resumes after delivery."
    ○ 2. "As you aren't breast-feeding, it should occur in 4 to 6 weeks."
    ○ 3. "Two weeks is the average time for menses to return."
    ○ 4. "Ask your doctor. I'm sure that after doing a pelvic exam, she can tell you."

138. What modifications are made in formula to make it more comparable with breast milk?
    ○ 1. Water and simple carbohydrate are added.
    ○ 2. Simple carbohydrate is added.
    ○ 3. Water is added.
    ○ 4. Casein is added.

139. While attempting to diaper her baby for the second time, Mrs. Martino observes her infant crying. Her response is, "He can cry!" And with this, her eyes fill with tears. The tears shed by this mother are probably caused by
    ○ 1. relief that the child could function normally.
    ○ 2. fear that the child was sick.
    ○ 3. fear that she was not handling the child correctly.
    ○ 4. belief that the child did not like her.

Valerie Jackson, gravida 5 para 5, is in the fourth stage of labor after delivering a 9 lb 14 oz baby. The nurse has been checking her blood pressure, pulse, fundus, lochia, and perineum every 15 minutes for the past 45 minutes. The blood pressure has remained stable at 114/60 mm Hg, pulse 76, respirations 12. Her uterus tends to become boggy between checks, but firms readily with manual massage. Lochia is moderate, rubra. As the nurse approaches for the fourth check, she notices some large new blood stains on the top sheet. The nurse immediately removes the top sheet and blanket to discover Mrs. Jackson lying in a pool of blood that covers the Chux pad.

140. What should the nurse's first action be?
    ○ 1. Take her blood pressure.
    ○ 2. Start an IV.
    ○ 3. Give her oxygen per mask at 7 liters.
    ○ 4. Find and massage the uterus.

141. The most frequent cause of early postpartum hemorrhage and probably the cause of Mrs. Jackson's bleeding is uterine
    ○ 1. atony.
    ○ 2. inertia.
    ○ 3. lacerations.
    ○ 4. dystocia.

142. Mrs. Jackson has experienced a postpartal hemorrhage based upon her total blood loss in the first 24 hours. How much blood must be lost to be considered hemorrhage?
    ○ 1. 1,000 ml
    ○ 2. 800 ml
    ○ 3. 500 ml
    ○ 4. 300 ml

143. Mrs. Jackson's hemoglobin is 8.5 gm/100 ml and her hematocrit is 25%. She has a further diagnosis of anemia secondary to postpartum hemorrhage. Which of the following would *not* be included in discharge planning and teaching?
    ○ 1. Eat a diet high in protein and iron-rich foods.
    ○ 2. Take ferrous sulfate tablets as ordered by the physician.
    ○ 3. Stop breast-feeding the infant until the anemia is gone.
    ○ 4. Expect to feel tired for possibly 2 to 4 months.

Rosita Javier, a 1-day postpartum primipara, is Rh negative and has delivered an Rh-positive, 7-lb daughter.

144. Mrs. Javier is to receive Rh_0 (D) immune globulin (RhoGAM). Which action is essential prior to administration?
    ○ 1. Determine if Mrs. Javier has had a negative Coombs.
    ○ 2. Reverify the baby's blood type.
    ○ 3. Assess the paternal Rh factor.
    ○ 4. Assess maternal temperature.

145. Which of the following best describes how RhoGAM acts in the maternal system?
    ○ 1. RhoGAM attaches to maternal anti-Rh antibodies and directly destroys them.
    ○ 2. RhoGAM suppresses the immunologic production of maternal antibodies.
    ○ 3. RhoGAM destroys fetal Rh-positive red blood cells in the maternal circulation before sensitization occurs.
    ○ 4. RhoGAM prevents fetal-maternal bleeding episodes from occurring at the former placenta site.

146. Mrs. Javier asks if there is danger of this problem occurring in future pregnancies. Which of these understandings about Rh factor is most important for the nurse to communicate to Mrs. Javier?
- ○ **1.** This administration of RhoGAM will provide lifelong immunity against fetal Rh disease.
- ○ **2.** If Mrs. Javier delivers another Rh-positive infant, she will require a subsequent dose of RhoGAM.
- ○ **3.** The protective antibodies formed during this pregnancy increase the risk of hemolytic disease in future infants.
- ○ **4.** It is safe to assume that future infants have a 50% chance of being Rh negative.

Mindy Lowell, aged 21, is admitted in active labor. Prenatal history indicates she has taken heroin regularly during the past 3 years. Two months ago she attempted to change to methadone maintenance, but was not compliant in keeping appointments. Initial observations include jaundiced sclera and skin. Lab data confirms a diagnosis of type B hepatitis secondary to substance abuse.

147. A priority of nursing care for this client focuses on
- ○ **1.** maintaining strict enteric isolation.
- ○ **2.** using mask, gown, gloves during care.
- ○ **3.** disposing of syringes and needles separately.
- ○ **4.** taking no extraordinary precautions.

148. Following delivery of a 6 lb infant, the client is transferred to a medical unit and placed in isolation. Which of the following menus would meet Mrs. Lowell's needs as she recovers from hepatitis and adapts to the postpartal period?
- ○ **1.** Orange juice, eggs, wheat toast, tea with sugar
- ○ **2.** Grapefruit juice, prunes, eggs, tea with honey
- ○ **3.** Pineapple slices, sweet roll, bacon, tea with cream
- ○ **4.** Applesauce, pancakes, sausage, tea with milk

149. Which of the following signs observed in a newborn nursery would be indicative of withdrawal if the newborn is drug-addicted?
- ○ **1.** Dyspnea, bradycardia, restlessness
- ○ **2.** Hyperactivity, irritability, tremors
- ○ **3.** Pallor, subnormal temperature, weak cry
- ○ **4.** Petechiae, limpness, high-pitched cry

150. Baby Boy Lowell is placed in the isolation nursery for observation for several days. The pediatrician administers hyperimmune gamma globulin to the infant and plans to discharge him to his grandmother. What assessment of the family system is most important at this time?
- ○ **1.** Does the grandmother express an interest in the client and infant?
- ○ **2.** Has the cause of substance abuse been identified for this client?
- ○ **3.** Is the infant's father involved in plans for care?
- ○ **4.** Does the home situation appear to be adequate and safe for the infant?

151. What is the most serious potential problem for this neonate?
- ○ **1.** Developmental delays
- ○ **2.** Child abuse
- ○ **3.** Liver damage
- ○ **4.** Insufficient affection

Amy Williams is a gravida 1 para 1, 3 weeks postpartum. She calls the postpartum unit with questions about breast-feeding while she has the "flu." During the conversation, she tells the nurse her temperature is 103°F, and that she has a persistent headache and feels exhausted.

152. Which of the following topics would the nurse want to elicit more information about first?
- ○ **1.** Breast tenderness
- ○ **2.** Quality of sleep pattern at night
- ○ **3.** Character and amount of lochia
- ○ **4.** Status of the baby

153. Which of the following statements would *not* be included when counseling Mrs. Williams about her problem?
- ○ **1.** Take antibiotics and analgesics as ordered by the physician.
- ○ **2.** Wash the hands well before and after handling the breasts.
- ○ **3.** Breast-feeding will need to be discontinued indefinitely.
- ○ **4.** Apply heat locally and wear a supportive brassiere to decrease discomfort.

154. Which of the following nursing actions would most likely prevent the problem?
- ○ **1.** Administration of prophylactic antibiotics
- ○ **2.** Decreasing the frequency of nursing
- ○ **3.** Encouraging abrupt weaning
- ○ **4.** Limiting nursing time

Baby Speier is 3 days old. As the nurse bathes the newborn, she conducts a physical assessment.

155. In assessing Baby Speier's skin, which of the following observations would most likely require special attention?
    ○ 1. Cyanosis of the hands and feet
    ○ 2. Jaundice after 72 hours
    ○ 3. Harlequin sign
    ○ 4. Generalized cyanosis

156. In comparing Baby Speier's head and chest measurements, which of the following observations would the nurse expect to find?
    ○ 1. The chest circumference is approximately 1 inch smaller than the head circumference.
    ○ 2. The chest circumference is approximately 1 inch larger than the head circumference.
    ○ 3. The head and chest circumference are equal.
    ○ 4. The chest circumference is approximately 3 inches smaller than the head circumference.

157. If one of the following were found on Baby Speier, which one would require special attention?
    ○ 1. Erythema toxicum neonatorum
    ○ 2. "Stork-bite" marks
    ○ 3. Impetigo
    ○ 4. Mongolian spots

158. The nurse assesses Baby Speier's eyes. Which condition, if found, would most likely require special attention?
    ○ 1. Transient strabismus
    ○ 2. Subconjunctival hemorrhage
    ○ 3. Swelling and a watery discharge following administration of silver nitrate
    ○ 4. Opacity of a pupil

159. The nurse assessing Baby Speier's trunk at birth makes the following observations. Which one would alert the nurse to carry out further assessment?
    ○ 1. Breast engorgement
    ○ 2. Audible bowel sounds
    ○ 3. Palpable liver and kidneys
    ○ 4. Umbilical cord with one artery and one vein

160. Which of the following assessments would the nurse report to the physician concerning Baby Speier's ears?
    ○ 1. The upper part of the ears is on a plane with the angle of the eyes.
    ○ 2. The ears are set low on the head.
    ○ 3. Incurving of the pinna and instant recoil
    ○ 4. Responds to sound with a startle or blink

Juan and Conchita Hernandez are proud parents of 3-day-old Feliz. They have planned to have this first child for the past several years. The nurse on the postpartum unit notices that they are very careful with Feliz and tend to handle him with much anxiety, but they are interested in getting acquainted with their son and initiating play activities.

161. Mrs. Hernandez asks the nurse when she can "play" with Feliz. Which reply represents an understanding of developmental needs in infancy?
    ○ 1. "When do you think it would be appropriate?"
    ○ 2. "After he receives his first immunizations from the physician."
    ○ 3. "As soon as you feel comfortable with him, he is ready."
    ○ 4. "Babies should be allowed to sleep uninterrupted during the first month of life."

162. What is the newborn's visual capacity at birth?
    ○ 1. Long-distance vision
    ○ 2. Short-distance fixation
    ○ 3. Convergence of the eyes
    ○ 4. Coordinated peripheral vision

163. What are the most appropriate stimuli for the nurse to recommend for the first parent-child play activity?
    ○ 1. Rattles and small stuffed toys
    ○ 2. Books and pictures
    ○ 3. Swings and cradles
    ○ 4. Human faces and black-and-white objects

164. It would be most appropriate for the nurse to suggest the parents play with Feliz by which method?
    ○ 1. Turning him on his abdomen
    ○ 2. Propping him on a pillow in his crib
    ○ 3. Stroking him gently from head to toe
    ○ 4. Continuously rocking him during the day

165. To check the palmar grasp reflex in the newborn, the nurse would implement which of the following actions?
    ○ 1. Stroke either corner of the mouth.
    ○ 2. Apply pressure to the ball of the foot at the base of the toes.
    ○ 3. Rotate the head to one side and then the other.
    ○ 4. Exert pressure on the palm at the base of the digits.

166. To elicit Moro's reflex, the nurse would implement which of the following actions?
    ○ 1. Shake the infant rapidly from head to toe.
    ○ 2. Hold the infant in both hands and lower both hands rapidly about an inch.
    ○ 3. Place the infant in the prone position and observe posture.
    ○ 4. Stroke the lateral plantar surface of the infant.

Baby Girl Young is a 10 lb 2 oz, 38-week-gestation infant of a diabetic mother. The Apgar scores were 7 and at 1 minute and 9 at 5 minutes. After spending some time with her mother in the recovery room, she is transferred to the nursery.

167. Which of the following problems would the nurse be most alert for in this infant?
    ○ 1. Hypoglycemia
    ○ 2. Hyperglycemia
    ○ 3. Meconium aspiration
    ○ 4. Generalized sepsis

168. Which of the following orders would be included when planning care for an infant of a diabetic mother?
    ○ 1. Provide extra stimulation.
    ○ 2. Use oil on the body after bathing.
    ○ 3. Give early feeding of glucose water.
    ○ 4. Start early infusion of insulin.

169. How would the nurse record information about this infant's gestational age?
    ○ 1. Premature, large for gestational age
    ○ 2. Term, appropriate for gestational age
    ○ 3. Premature, appropriate for gestational age
    ○ 4. Term, large for gestational age

170. Mrs. Young asks the nurse if her baby has diabetes. What would be the nurse's best response?
    ○ 1. ''No, we are giving your baby medication to prevent that from occurring.''
    ○ 2. ''No, however, she will probably become diabetic sometime in childhood.''
    ○ 3. ''No, there is no connection between your diabetes and your baby.''
    ○ 4. ''No, however, you need to make regular visits to your pediatrician.''

171. On the third day of life, Baby Girl Young acquires hyperbilirubinemia and is placed under phototherapy. Which of the following would *not* be included in the nurse's plan of care?
    ○ 1. Cover her eyes with soft material.
    ○ 2. Keep the infant covered and warm.
    ○ 3. Give additional fluids.
    ○ 4. Record the type and amount of stools.

Following morning report, the head nurse and the nursing instructor take a group of students on rounds to orient them to the newborn nursery.

172. Which of the following infants would be at *lowest* risk for hypoglycemia?
    ○ 1. A 2-hour-old neonate at gestational age whose mother's blood-glucose level was 350 mg/100 ml during labor
    ○ 2. A large-for-gestational-age neonate 10 hours after birth whose Dextrostix test shows a reading of 60 mg/100 ml
    ○ 3. A 32-week-gestation neonate 5 hours after birth
    ○ 4. An small-for-gestational-age neonate 12 hours after birth who is NPO because of respiratory distress

173. Which of the following best indicates that a neonate with an infection is *not* fully recovered?
    ○ 1. Respiratory rate of 65 at rest
    ○ 2. Weight increase of 3 oz on 2 successive days
    ○ 3. Axillary temperature of 98.6°F (37°C)
    ○ 4. Hemoglobin of 20 gm/100 ml of blood

174. The mother of a boy born 2 days ago is refusing to care for her infant. Which of the following is the most appropriate action for the nurse to take?
    ○ 1. Care for the infant in the mother's room without making any demands on the mother.
    ○ 2. Encourage the mother to at least change the baby's diaper.
    ○ 3. Speak to the baby's father and encourage him to get the mother to care for the infant.
    ○ 4. Explain to the mother that corrective surgery will improve the infant's appearance.

175. A 34-week-gestation neonate in an incubator experiences sudden apnea. The nurse should first
    ○ 1. administer oxygen with positive pressure.
    ○ 2. call the pediatrician.
    ○ 3. increase the humidity in the incubator.
    ○ 4. gently shake the infant.

176. When examining the inside of a newborn's mouth, the nurse notices a small raised white bump on the palate; it does not come off nor does it bleed when touched. Which of the following is the most likely diagnosis?
    ○ 1. Milia
    ○ 2. Thrush
    ○ 3. Epstein's pearls
    ○ 4. Milk curd

177. Which of the following fetal circulatory structures are *not* needed for extrauterine life?
    ○ 1. Ductus arteriosus, foramen ovale, pulmonary artery, hypogastric arteries
    ○ 2. Ductus venosus, foramen ovale, portal vein, ductus arteriosus
    ○ 3. Foramen ovale, pulmonary artery, ductus venosus, umbilical vein
    ○ 4. Umbilical vein, foramen ovale, ductus venosus, ductus arteriosus

178. Neonates often "spit up" small quantities following feedings. Which of the following conditions offers the best explanation for this behavior?
    ○ 1. Immature cardiac sphincter
    ○ 2. Overfeeding by parents
    ○ 3. Activity of the infant during feeding
    ○ 4. Inadequate concentration of enzymes

179. Which of the following skull bones form the posterior fontanel?
    ○ 1. Frontal and parietal
    ○ 2. Parietal and occipital
    ○ 3. Temporal and frontal
    ○ 4. Frontal and occipital

180. How might the nurse best promote bonding while an infant is in an Isolette?
    ○ 1. Remind the mother that the staff is skillful.
    ○ 2. Allow the mother to touch the infant.
    ○ 3. Suggest the mother visit the intensive care unit occasionally.
    ○ 4. Inform the mother that the infant will be at home soon.

References

Jensen, M., Benson, R., & Bobak, I. (1981). *Maternity care—The nurse and the family*. St. Louis: Mosby.

Miller, M., & Brooten D. (1983). *The childbearing family: A nursing perspective*. Boston: Little, Brown.

Moore, M., & Strickland, O. (1983). *Realities in childbearing* (2nd ed.). Philadelphia: Saunders.

Olds, S., London, M., Ladewig, P., & Davidson, S. (1980). *Obstetric nursing*. Menlo Park, CA: Addison-Wesley.

Olds, S., London, M., & Ladewig P. (1984). *Maternal-newborn nursing*. Menlo Park, CA: Addison-Wesley.

Pillitteri, A. (1981). *Maternal-newborn nursing* (2nd ed.). Boston: Little, Brown.

Reeder, S., Mastrionni, L., & Martin L. (1983). *Maternity nursing*. Philadelphia: Lippincott.

Whaley, L., & Wong, D. (1986). *Nursing care of infants and children* (3rd ed.). St. Louis: Mosby.

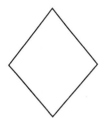

Section 4
Correct Answers

1. #4.	46. #2.	91. #2.	136. #2.
2. #2.	47. #4.	92. #3.	137. #2.
3. #3.	48. #2.	93. #4.	138. #1.
4. #3.	49. #1.	94. #1.	139. #1.
5. #3.	50. #3.	95. #4.	140. #4.
6. #1.	51. #4.	96. #2.	141. #1.
7. #3.	52. #2.	97. #1.	142. #3.
8. #3.	53. #3.	98. #4.	143. #3.
9. #2.	54. #1.	99. #1.	144. #1.
10. #3.	55. #2.	100. #1.	145. #3.
11. #3.	56. #3.	101. #3.	146. #2.
12. #1.	57. #4.	102. #4.	147. #3.
13. #1.	58. #4.	103. #2.	148. #2.
14. #3.	59. #3.	104. #1.	149. #2.
15. #2.	60. #3.	105. #4.	150. #4.
16. #1.	61. #4.	106. #4.	151. #2.
17. #2.	62. #1.	107. #3.	152. #1.
18. #1.	63. #3.	108. #3.	153. #3.
19. #4.	64. #1.	109. #1.	154. #4.
20. #4.	65. #2.	110. #3.	155. #4.
21. #4.	66. #4.	111. #2.	156. #1.
22. #3.	67. #1.	112. #3.	157. #3.
23. #1.	68. #1.	113. #4.	158. #4.
24. #3.	69. #3.	114. #3.	159. #4.
25. #1.	70. #4.	115. #2.	160. #2.
26. #4.	71. #1.	116. #4.	161. #3.
27. #4.	72. #3.	117. #4.	162. #2.
28. #2.	73. #4.	118. #4.	163. #4.
29. #2.	74. #1.	119. #2.	164. #3.
30. #4.	75. #1.	120. #2.	165. #4.
31. #1.	76. #4.	121. #2.	166. #2.
32. #4.	77. #1.	122. #4.	167. #1.
33. #2.	78. #2.	123. #1.	168. #3.
34. #1.	79. #3.	124. #2.	169. #4.
35. #3.	80. #1.	125. #4.	170. #4.
36. #3.	81. #1.	126. #1.	171. #2.
37. #2.	82. #1.	127. #2.	172. #2.
38. #1.	83. #3.	128. #4.	173. #1.
39. #4.	84. #4.	129. #3.	174. #1.
40. #2.	85. #2.	130. #3.	175. #4.
41. #4.	86. #1.	131. #4.	176. #3.
42. #2.	87. #2.	132. #1.	177. #4.
43. #3.	88. #3.	133. #1.	178. #1.
44. #3.	89. #4.	134. #1.	179. #2.
45. #3.	90. #2.	135. #3.	180. #2.

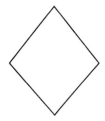

Correct Answers with Rationales

Editor's note:

Two pieces of information are supplied at the end of each rationale. First we tell you what part of the nursing process the question addresses. Second, in parentheses, you will find a reference to a section in the *AJN Nursing Boards Review* where a more complete discussion of the topic may be found should you desire more information.

1. **#4.** Goodell's sign is the only probable sign; the other choices are presumptive signs. ASSESSMENT (CHILDBEARING FAMILY/ANTEPARTAL CARE)

2. **#2.** Add 7 days, subtract 3 months, and add 1 year to the first day of the last menstrual period. This is Naegele's rule, which relates only to the first day of the menstrual cycle. There is no need to consider day of intercourse. ANALYSIS (CHILDBEARING FAMILY/ANTEPARTAL CARE)

3. **#3.** This is the only correct statement. HCG in the urine confirms the pregnancy. The urine test is 95% to 97% accurate. False positives and negatives are possible. Home tests are considered less accurate, most likely due to error in use. ANALYSIS (CHILDBEARING FAMILY/ANTEPARTAL CARE)

4. **#3.** The nurse must find out the eating habits of the client before she can teach or advise. A basic principle of the teaching-learning process is to access the learner by obtaining a diet history. If the learner is knowledgeable, she simply may require reinforcement. Providing a list of foods does not ensure that she will comply. Sodium is not restricted in pregnancy. IMPLEMENTATION (CHILDBEARING FAMILY/ANTEPARTAL CARE)

5. **#3.** Organ meats and dried fruits are high in iron. Spinach is also a good source, but option #3 lists 2 good sources. IMPLEMENTATION (CHILDBEARING FAMILY/ANTEPARTAL CARE)

6. **#1.** Swelling of the face is an indication of toxemia. The other symptoms are normal in pregnancy. Frequent urination is common in the first trimester because of pressure on the bladder from the uterus. Increased vaginal discharge is the result of an increase in glandular activity. Chloasma (also called the mask of pregnancy) results from an increased activity in the adrenal glands. IMPLEMENTATION (CHILDBEARING FAMILY/ANTEPARTAL CARE)

7. **#3.** Slight temporary enlargement of the breasts may cause sensations of weight and tingling. As pregnancy advances, the areolae become darker in color. Colostrum, a precursor of breast milk, may appear spontaneously in the second half of pregnancy. Engorgement occurs after delivery when the breasts begin to fill with milk. ASSESSMENT (CHILDBEARING FAMILY/ANTEPARTAL CARE)

8. **#3.** There is a placental barrier to syphilis until the 18th week of pregnancy. If the mother is treated prior to the 18th week, the baby will not be affected. However, titers will be positive at birth. ANALYSIS (CHILDBEARING FAMILY/ANTEPARTAL CARE)

9. **#2.** Bulk and fluid help increase peristalsis. Laxatives and suppositories should not be used in pregnancy. Prevention is more desirable than treatment. IMPLEMENTATION (CHILDBEARING FAMILY/ANTEPARTAL CARE)

10. **#3.** Urinary frequency and the spilling of sugar in the urine are normal conditions, because of the pressure of the growing uterus on the bladder (frequency) and the increase in glomerular filtration rate (sugar in urine). Vaginal bleeding may indicate the possibility of an abortion. Albuminuria and facial swelling are associated with toxemia. Oliguria would indicate renal failure. ASSESSMENT (CHILDBEARING FAMILY/ANTEPARTAL CARE)

11. **#3.** Ovulation occurs 14 days prior to the start of the next menstrual cycle. ANALYSIS (CHILDBEARING FAMILY/ANTEPARTAL CARE)

12. **#1.** The couple need to continue to enjoy recreation together, and most activities can be continued during pregnancy. New sports should not be introduced at this time. IMPLEMENTATION (CHILDBEARING FAMILY/ANTEPARTAL CARE)

13. **#1.** Breast changes are expected to appear during the first trimester. Quickening, the feeling of movement experienced by the mother, occurs at 18 to 20 weeks. Dyspnea, caused by pressure on the enlarging uterus on the diaphragm, and dependent edema, caused by the enlarging uterus impeding venous return, are expected in the third trimester. ASSESSMENT (CHILDBEARING FAMILY/ANTEPARTAL CARE)

14. **#3.** This may be a sign of threatened abortion. Remaining on bed rest is appropriate after the client's condition is assessed. EVALUATION (CHILDBEARING FAMILY/ANTEPARTAL CARE)

15. **#2.** Emphasis during antepartal care is on health promotion and early detection of problems. This response suggests a more positive approach than option #1. IMPLEMENTATION (CHILDBEARING FAMILY/ANTEPARTAL CARE)

16. **#1.** To promote comfort and enhance venous circulation, she must change position more frequently than once every 6 hours. The other activities described are not a problem. ASSESSMENT (CHILDBEARING FAMILY/ANTEPARTAL CARE)

17. **#2.** Toxoplasmosis is a protozoan infection transmitted via cat feces and undercooked meat. However, the risk to this client is lower because she is in her second trimester. ASSESSMENT (CHILDBEARING FAMILY/ANTEPARTAL CARE)

18. **#1.** Both of these foods are good sources of iron for the vegetarian. IMPLEMENTATION (CHILDBEARING FAMILY/ANTEPARTAL CARE)

19. **#4.** The chief concepts of Lamaze teaching include conditioned responses to stimuli through use of a focal point. An emotionally satisfying experience is promoted rather than discouraging use of analgesia and anesthesia. EVALUATION (CHILDBEARING FAMILY/ANTEPARTAL CARE)

20. **#4.** This is the only characteristic of true labor. Option #1 indicates false labor; options #2 and #3 are premonitory signs of labor. Walking has a tendency to increase true labor contractions. Urinary frequency is experienced after lightening or dropping of the fetus and is caused by uterine pressure on the bladder. Lightening occurs at approximately 38 weeks in the primipara. ASSESSMENT (CHILDBEARING FAMILY/INTRAPARTAL CARE)

21. **#4.** Education for childbirth classes is designed to increase the clients' understanding of pregnancy and birth, and to promote the optimum health of mother and baby. Through use of relaxation and other techniques, pregnant women are helped to cope better with labor and achieve an emotionally satisfying experience. PLAN (CHILDBEARING FAMILY/ANTEPARTAL CARE)

22. **#3.** Fear is a major pain-producing agent in labor. Through childbirth education, pregnant women learn techniques to assist in relaxing and preventing the fear-anxiety-pain syndrome. Pain is subjective. Understanding alone will not produce relaxation, nor will education alone eliminate pain. IMPLEMENTATION (CHILDBEARING FAMILY/ANTEPARTAL CARE)

23. **#1.** While there is validity to all responses, option #1 is the best because it includes all possible assessments (i.e., what the client describes and physical and psychologic changes). ASSESSMENT (CHILDBEARING FAMILY/INTRAPARTAL CARE)

24. **#3.** Involve the father as much as possible by demonstrating comfort measures he can provide. If the couple is frightened, an explanation would not be effective. The couple that is not coping because of fear would be unable to verbalize their needs. IMPLEMENTATION (CHILDBEARING FAMILY/INTRAPARTAL CARE)

25. **#1.** Assessment of the learner is the priority. Teaching can then be directed at the learner's level of understanding and key concepts reinforced. A standard teaching plan is not appropriate. IMPLEMENTATION (CHILDBEARING FAMILY/INTRAPARTAL CARE)

26. **#4.** As transitional labor approaches, such behavior is very common. It is not appropriate to ask the husband to leave or withdraw his support at this most crucial time. A woman in transition is not able to explore feelings. IMPLEMENTATION (CHILDBEARING FAMILY/INTRAPARTAL CARE)

27. **#4.** Sibling rivalry is normal. Grasp of the reality of a new sibling is difficult at this age. ANALYSIS (CHILDBEARING FAMILY/POSTPARTAL CARE)

28. **#2.** Any woman in the first trimester of pregnancy is at risk if exposed to rubella. Fetal defects often result from such an infection. EVALUATION (CHILDBEARING FAMILY/ANTEPARTAL CARE)

29. **#2.** The basis of the ovulation method is observation of changes in the character of mucus. Temperature variations and counting days of the cycle are elements of the rhythm method of planning. IMPLEMENTATION (CHILDBEARING FAMILY/ANTEPARTAL CARE)

30. **#4.** Mittelschmertz may be experienced at the time of ovulation. Ovulation occurs approximately 14 days prior to the onset of menstruation. The cervical mucus becomes thicker following ovulation. A temperature rise follows ovulation. IMPLEMENTATION (CHILDBEARING FAMILY/ANTEPARTAL CARE)

31. **#1.** While it is possible to reverse a tubal ligation in some cases (a 12% success rate), it is generally considered to be permanent sterilization. The other options are true. EVALUATION (CHILDBEARING FAMILY/ANTEPARTAL CARE)

32. **#4.** Bleeding during pregnancy is considered abnormal, but clients often overestimate the quantity of blood loss because of fear and lack of knowledge. As an initial response, the nurse should expand her data base by obtaining more specific information about the bleeding episode. Following complete assessment, a plan of care can be developed. IMPLEMENTATION (CHILDBEARING FAMILY/ANTEPARTAL CARE)

33. **#2.** In an incomplete abortion the fetus is expelled, but parts are retained. The term inevitable abortion is used to describe pregnancies complicated by bleeding, cramping, and cervical dilation (abortion is imminent). The term threatened abortion implies the pregnancy is jeopardized by bleeding and cramping, but the cervix is closed. In a missed abortion the fetus dies but is retained. ANALYSIS (CHILDBEARING FAMILY/ANTEPARTAL CARE)

34. **#1.** Because abortion is inevitable, all perineal pads must be inspected for the products of conception. Fluid replacement is necessary because of blood loss. There is no evidence of impending shock necessitating Trendelenberg's position. A Shirodkar procedure is done for an incompetent cervix, which is not the problem. IMPLEMENTATION (CHILDBEARING FAMILY/ANTEPARTAL CARE)

35. **#3.** This is the definition of a missed abortion. Findings in a missed abortion include spotting and a uterus that is smaller than expected for the length of pregnancy. If spontaneous evacuation of the uterus does not occur within 1 month, pregnancy will be terminated. IMPLEMENTATION (CHILDBEARING FAMILY/ANTEPARTAL CARE)

36. **#3.** McDonald's procedure is application of a temporary suture that is removed at term. Vaginal delivery may be possible if all else stays well. Shirodkar's procedure is the application of a permanent suture necessitating cesarean delivery. IMPLEMENTATION (CHILDBEARING FAMILY/ANTEPARTAL CARE)

37. **#2.** Day of ovulation is 14 days prior to menstruation; $30 - 14 = 16$. ANALYSIS (CHILDBEARING FAMILY/ANTEPARTAL CARE)

38. **#1.** These findings are consistent with an ectopic pregnancy. The referred pain is the result of bleeding into the peritoneal cavity and overstimulation of the vagus nerve. Vaginal bleeding is not evident nor is the uterus enlarged because the pregnancy is not implanted in the uterus. ASSESSMENT (CHILDBEARING FAMILY/ANTEPARTAL CARE)

39. **#4.** A history of repeated spontaneous abortions is consistent with a diagnosis of an incompetent cervix. A history of infection, producing tubal scarring, is a consistent finding in an ectopic pregnancy. ASSESSMENT (CHILDBEARING FAMILY/ANTEPARTAL CARE)

40. **#2.** Surgical intervention will be required; however, hemorrhage is the major life-threatening concern. If in ectopic pregnancy the tube ruptures, vascular collapse and hypovolemic shock may follow. The possibility of the ovum aborting into the abdominal cavity with a resulting abdominal pregnancy is rare. ANALYSIS (CHILDBEARING FAMILY/ANTEPARTAL CARE)

41. **#4.** Painless uterine bleeding occurring in the third trimester is a cardinal sign of placenta previa. ANALYSIS (CHILDBEARING FAMILY/ANTEPARTAL CARE)

42. **#2.** Persistent vaginal bleeding may seriously threaten the mother. Monitoring vital signs and fetal heart tones is important; however, significant changes may not occur until profound bleeding is present. IMPLEMENTATION (CHILDBEARING FAMILY/ANTEPARTAL CARE)

43. **#3.** Because symptoms suggest a possible placenta previa, bed rest might help prevent further separation. Options #1 and #2 will cause further bleeding. As she is in her eighth month and only bleeding a small amount, this client will most probably be kept under observation. IMPLEMENTATION (CHILDBEARING FAMILY/ANTE-PARTAL CARE)

44. **#3.** Physical activity may increase bleeding. Decreasing anxiety is advisable but bed rest is essential to limit the chances of her condition worsening. IMPLEMENTATION (CHILDBEARING FAMILY/ANTEPARTAL CARE)

45. **#3.** Location of the placenta and dilatation of the cervix are the causes of bleeding, and the condition cannot be prevented. Giving specifics is more useful than general reassurance. Options #2 and #4 imply that the client may have played a role. IMPLEMENTATION (CHILD-BEARING FAMILY/ANTEPARTAL CARE)

46. **#2.** While all the factors listed are predisposing factors associated with abruptio placentae, Mrs. Simmons' history supports only pregnancy-induced hypertension, which occurs after 24 weeks. Vasoconstriction in the placenta causes placental separation. ASSESSMENT (CHILDBEARING FAMILY/ANTEPARTAL CARE)

47. **#4.** Abdominal tenderness or rigidity or both are cardinal signs of abruptio placentae. A vaginal exam is definitely contraindicated. Options #1 and #3 are not specific for abruptio placentae. ASSESSMENT (CHILDBEARING FAMILY/ANTE-PARTAL CARE)

48. **#2.** The primary purpose of administering oxygen in this situation would be to increase the circulating oxygen in the mother to provide better oxygenation of the fetus. IMPLEMENTATION (CHILDBEARING FAMILY/INTRAPARTAL CARE)

49. **#1.** The hemorrhaging associated with abruptio placentae may deplete the woman's reserve of blood fibrinogen in the body's efforts to achieve clotting. Disseminated intravascular coagulation syndrome occurs when fibrinogen levels have been depleted. ANALYSIS (CHILD-BEARING FAMILY/ANTEPARTAL CARE)

50. **#3.** The bleeding has likely caused fetal stress. Fetal stress is associated with the release of meconium. As it has been established that Mrs. Simmons was leaking amniotic fluid, it is likely that this represents meconium-stained fluid. ANALYSIS (CHILDBEARING FAMILY/INTRA-PARTAL CARE)

51. **#4.** Meconium-stained fluid requires further assessment but is not necessarily an indication for emergency action. IMPLEMENTATION (CHILD-BEARING FAMILY/INTRAPARTAL CARE)

52. **#2.** Blood pressure should be monitored frequently in order to detect problems. Assessment of the client is a priority prior to designing a plan of care. IMPLEMENTATION (CHILDBEARING FAMILY/ANTEPARTAL CARE)

53. **#3.** A loud noise or bright light may be enough to precipitate a convulsion because of the hyperactive nervous system. Keeping the side rails padded and up will protect the client and careful monitoring of the client is in order; however, neither of these measures will reduce the possibility of convulsions. IMPLEMENTA-TION (CHILDBEARING FAMILY/ANTEPARTAL CARE)

54. **#1.** The client on bed rest has decreased physical activity and a reduced metabolic rate. There is also an increase in renal filtration rate. All of these physiologic adaptations may improve circulation to the uteroplacental unit. PLAN (CHILDBEARING FAMILY/ANTEPARTAL CARE)

55. **#2.** Keep an ampule of calcium gluconate available when magnesium sulfate is being administered. ANALYSIS (CHILDBEARING FAMILY/ANTEPARTAL CARE)

56. **#3.** Magnesium sulfate is an excellent anticonvulsant and vasodilator that lowers blood pressure. Therapeutic doses of this drug are generally well tolerated by the fetus, although some respiratory depression may result. Option #2 does not answer the client's question. IMPLEMENTATION (CHILDBEARING FAMILY/ANTE-PARTAL CARE)

57. **#4.** Insulin needs do vary throughout pregnancy. The greatest incidence of insulin coma during pregnancy occurs during the second and third months; the greatest incidence of diabetic coma during pregnancy occurs around the sixth month. ANALYSIS (CHILDBEARING FAMILY/ANTEPARTAL CARE)

58. **#4.** While a cesarean delivery at 37 weeks used to be common for diabetic mothers, current practice is to try and achieve delivery at the optimum time for mother and infant. Stress for the infant is greater during a cesarean birth than during a vaginal delivery. Tests of placental function and of fetal maturity help determine the prognosis of the fetus at any given time. IMPLEMENTATION (CHILDBEARING FAMILY/ ANTEPARTAL CARE)

59. **#3.** Newborn infants of diabetic mothers tend to be immature, lethargic, hyperbilirubinemic, and to have latent tetany or neuromuscular irritability. These problems can be attributed to early delivery, hypoglycemia, and hypocalcemia. ASSESSMENT (CHILDBEARING FAMILY/ HIGH-RISK NEWBORN)

60. **#3.** Although all are correct, the priority is establishing and maintaining a patent airway. PLAN (CHILDBEARING FAMILY/NORMAL NEWBORN)

61. **#4.** Excessive insulin may lead to hypoglycemia. Brain damage will result if not corrected. PLAN (CHILDBEARING FAMILY/HIGH-RISK NEWBORN)

62. **#1.** As insulin does not pass into the breast milk, breast-feeding is not contraindicated for the mother with diabetes. Breast-feeding is encouraged as it decreases the insulin requirements for insulin-dependent clients. ANALYSIS (CHILDBEARING FAMILY/HIGH-RISK NEWBORN)

63. **#3.** This infant has the usual risk related to heredity for diabetes and should be seen regularly during childhood. IMPLEMENTATION (CHILDBEARING FAMILY/HIGH-RISK NEWBORN)

64. **#1.** Reduced activity tolerance is differentiated from the normal fatigue of pregnancy; it may be an early sign of congestive heart failure, a condition to which the cardiac client is highly predisposed. ASSESSMENT (CHILDBEARING FAMILY/ANTEPARTAL CARE)

65. **#2.** This is a normal pulse rate for a newly delivered mother; continued routine assessments are all that is indicated. IMPLEMENTATION (CHILDBEARING FAMILY/POSTPARTAL CARE)

66. **#4.** A reduction in the pressure on the venous system allows fluid to move from the extravascular spaces into the blood stream. This increased blood volume requires increased cardiac output. This is a normal adaptation for all new mothers, but could pose a risk after delivery for the woman with a cardiac problem. ANALYSIS (CHILDBEARING FAMILY/POSTPARTAL CARE)

67. **#1.** Outcomes for the high-risk client and infant can be improved with regular prenatal care. PLAN (CHILDBEARING FAMILY/ANTEPARTAL CARE)

68. **#1.** During the first half of pregnancy, women question the reality of their condition and are often disbelieving. This may be expressed by ''Now?'' ''Who, me?'' or other statements of surprise. ASSESSMENT (CHILDBEARING FAMILY/ ANTEPARTAL CARE)

69. **#3.** It is most important for the nurse initially to establish rapport with the client by demonstrating a concerned and accepting attitude. IMPLEMENTATION (CHILDBEARING FAMILY/ ANTEPARTAL CARE)

70. **#4.** Adolescence is a time of great physical growth and development; to meet these needs as well as pregnancy needs, substantial nutritional intake is required. ANALYSIS (CHILDBEARING FAMILY/ANTEPARTAL CARE)

71. **#1.** The diagnosis of iron-deficiency anemia is made on the basis of a hemoglobin concentration value of 10 gm/100 ml blood or less, and a hematocrit value of 30% or less. ASSESSMENT (CHILDBEARING FAMILY/ANTEPARTAL CARE)

72. **#3.** To meet increased circulatory needs, especially to the mother, fetus, and placenta, the blood volume increases starting at about 3 months gestation. Beginning at about 6 months, the total red blood cell volume and hemoglobin mass increase. ANALYSIS (CHILDBEARING FAMILY/ANTEPARTAL CARE)

73. **#4.** The iron content of prune juice is 10.5 mg per cup and 4.2 mg per cup of split peas; ½ breast of chicken contains 1.3 mg of iron. EVALUATION (CHILDBEARING FAMILY/ANTEPARTAL CARE)

74. **#1.** The adolescent is prone to many complications during pregnancy. This can be attributed to lack of early prenatal care as well as to poor nutrition. The other options generally do not apply to the adolescent population. ASSESSMENT (CHILDBEARING FAMILY/ANTEPARTAL CARE)

75. #1. Assessment of the general situation is the first priority. What is important to know is how close is the delivery and how much time is available for preparation. Taking a nursing history, calling the physician, and starting an IV may follow assessment of contractions. IMPLEMENTATION (CHILDBEARING FAMILY/INTRAPARTAL CARE)

76. #4. In early labor, motivation is high and readiness to learn is enhanced. As labor progresses, concentration becomes more difficult to maintain. ANALYSIS (CHILDBEARING FAMILY/INTRAPARTAL CARE)

77. #1. Meconium-stained amniotic fluid frequently indicates fetal distress. ASSESSMENT (CHILDBEARING FAMILY/INTRAPARTAL CARE)

78. #2. This therapeutic communication fosters open expression of feelings. The nurse can only offer alternatives. The ultimate decision lies with the client. IMPLEMENTATION (CHILDBEARING FAMILY/POSTPARTAL CARE)

79. #3. Considering crisis theory and the knowledge of the grieving process, allowing the relinquishing mother to provide care is considered healthy adaptation. ANALYSIS (CHILDBEARING FAMILY/POSTPARTAL CARE)

80. #1. Adoptive parents, or any parent separated from the newborn in the period immediately following delivery, can still form a strong attachment to the infant. Encouragement and reinforcement of positive behaviors enhance such bonding. IMPLEMENTATION (CHILDBEARING FAMILY/NORMAL NEWBORN)

81. #1. This option indicates the father is alert to cues and responds to them. This is the only response that demonstrates interaction between infant and parent. EVALUATION (CHILDBEARING FAMILY/NORMAL NEWBORN)

82. #1. The other assessments have priority upon admission in determining her current clinical condition. ASSESSMENT (CHILDBEARING FAMILY/INTRAPARTAL CARE)

83. #3. Breathing techniques can help the laboring woman maintain control during contractions. The client should not bear down until she is completely dilated. Crowning will not occur until complete dilatation. Sacral pressure is a comfort measure used if the fetus is in a posterior position. IMPLEMENTATION (CHILDBEARING FAMILY/INTRAPARTAL CARE)

84. #4. This is the only assessment listed that is indicative of transition. The contractions are long and strong at this time resulting in heightened irritability and anxiety. Accelerated breathing and the need for medication and sacral pressure may occur at any time in active labor. ASSESSMENT (CHILDBEARING FAMILY/INTRAPARTAL CARE)

85. #2. If the client blows, she will not be able to push, which is contraindicated at this point. Option #3 is correct information, but it is not appropriate to explain things to a client in transition. She needs direction because of her pain and emotional status during that phase of labor. IMPLEMENTATION (CHILDBEARING FAMILY/INTRAPARTAL CARE)

86. #1. This action should reverse the initial symptoms of hyperventilation or carbon dioxide insufficiency (dizziness, tingling in the hands, or circumoral numbness) by enabling the client to rebreathe carbon dioxide and replace the bicarbonate ion. EVALUATION (CHILDBEARING FAMILY/INTRAPARTAL CARE)

87. #2. It is now safe to assist the client with effective pushing techniques to bring the baby down to the perineum. Prior to complete dilatation, pushing results in cervical edema and increases the danger of cervical lacerations and fetal head trauma. Narcotics should not be given after full dilatation. The client now requires constant monitoring by the nurse. IMPLEMENTATION (CHILDBEARING FAMILY/INTRAPARTAL CARE)

88. #3. The uterus must be assessed every 15 minutes to ensure that it is well contracted, thus preventing hemorrhage. The fundus should not be massaged unless it is relaxed. Constant massaging would tire the uterine muscle, contributing to hemorrhage. Blood pressure is monitored every 15 minutes and temperature every hour unless there are significant changes. IMPLEMENTATION (CHILDBEARING FAMILY/POSTPARTAL CARE)

89. #4. This treatment is to prevent gonorrheal ophthalmia neonatorum, which can lead to blindness. Chemical conjunctivitis may result from a reaction to the silver nitrate. Neonatal syphilis must be treated with penicillin. There is no cure for herpes. ANALYSIS (CHILDBEARING FAMILY/NORMAL NEWBORN)

90. #2. Absent variability is an ominous sign. Decreased or absent fluctuations indicate central nervous system depression. ANALYSIS (CHILDBEARING FAMILY/INTRAPARTAL CARE)

91. #2. Variable decelerations are the result of cord compression. Early decelerations result from head compression. Late decelerations result from uteroplacental insufficiency. Posterior positions should not affect fetal heart rate. ANALYSIS (CHILDBEARING FAMILY/INTRAPARTAL CARE)

92. #3. Early deceleration occurs in response to compression of the fetal head and does not indicate fetal distress. Lack of variability is considered a sign of possible fetal jeopardy. Fluctuations are caused by interplay of the parasympathetic and sympathetic components of the autonomic nervous system. When decreased variability is noted, the nurse must suspect compromise of these mechanisms. Variable decelerations result from cord compression and late decelerations result from uteroplacental insufficiency, both of which are abnormal. ASSESSMENT (CHILDBEARING FAMILY/INTRAPARTAL CARE)

93. #4. Early deceleration is often caused by head compression; no action is needed. IMPLEMENTATION (CHILDBEARING FAMILY/INTRAPARTAL CARE)

94. #1. This is an invasive technique requiring a written consent. Because internal monitoring is invasive, there is approximately a 17% chance of infection. ANALYSIS (CHILDBEARING FAMILY/INTRAPARTAL CARE)

95. #4. This signifies late decelerations, an ominous sign that indicates uteroplacental insufficiency. ASSESSMENT (CHILDBEARING FAMILY/INTRAPARTAL CARE)

96. #2. Even though the fetal heart rate is still within a normal range, the change is significant and must be investigated. IMPLEMENTATION (CHILDBEARING FAMILY/INTRAPARTAL CARE)

97. #1. Excessive oxytocin results in tetanic contractions that interfere with the fetal blood supply. It is necessary to stop the infusion to relax the uterine muscle. After turning off the oxytocin, changing the client's position and administering oxygen will help improve uteroplacental insufficiency. IMPLEMENTATION (CHILDBEARING FAMILY/INTRAPARTAL CARE)

98. #4. Contractions that are strong, last 50 to 70 seconds, and occur every 2 to 3 minutes usually signal the second stage of labor. In light of this client's pregnancy history, assessment is in order. IMPLEMENTATION (CHILDBEARING FAMILY/INTRAPARTAL CARE)

99. #1. Epidural anesthesia can cause maternal hypotension because of vasodilation. IMPLEMENTATION (CHILDBEARING FAMILY/INTRAPARTAL CARE)

100. #1. Uterine atony frequently occurs with older grand multiparas following spontaneous deliveries of full-term infants. Lack of muscle tone in the grand multipara predisposes to uterine relaxation. ANALYSIS (CHILDBEARING FAMILY/POSTPARTAL CARE)

101. #3. Phenylketonuria (PKU) tests are not performed within the first 24 hours. The infant must have ingested formula or breast milk before the test results can be considered accurate. PKU is an inborn error of metabolism caused by autosomal recessive genes. These infants have a deficiency in the liver enzyme phenylalanine hydroxylase, which is required to convert the amino acid phenylalanine to tyrosine. When the converting ability is lacking, phenylalanine accumulates leading to progressive mental retardation. IMPLEMENTATION (CHILDBEARING FAMILY/INTRAPARTAL CARE)

102. #4. Before taking any other action, assessment is a priority. The reaction of the mother is not necessarily reflective of the stage of labor she is in. IMPLEMENTATION (CHILDBEARING FAMILY/INTRAPARTAL CARE)

103. #2. The priority at this time is to prevent a precipitous delivery that may result in damage to the fetus as well as a perineal tear. The mother will experience the urge to push during the contraction, but panting will prevent her from doing so. It is important to deliver the baby in between contractions. IMPLEMENTATION (CHILDBEARING FAMILY/INTRAPARTAL CARE)

104. #1. The sucking of the infant triggers the release of oxytocin, which contracts the uterus. Fundal massage, not vigorous pressure, is also an important nursing action to stimulate contraction of the uterus. IMPLEMENTATION (CHILDBEARING FAMILY/POSTPARTAL CARE)

105. **#4.** There is no indication that Mrs. Lopez's membranes are ruptured or that her cervix is dilated, both of which are necessary conditions for internal monitoring. If fetal monitoring is desired, an external monitor will be employed. IMPLEMENTATION (CHILDBEARING FAMILY/INTRAPARTAL CARE)

106. **#4.** Cephalopelvic disproportion is the most common indication for a cesarean delivery. The other conditions are less commonly encountered indications. ASSESSMENT (CHILDBEARING FAMILY/INTRAPARTAL CARE)

107. **#3.** This is the only true statement. Checking fundal height, uterine massage as indicated, monitoring lochia, and assessing the incisional site are all important nursing actions following a cesarean delivery. ANALYSIS (CHILDBEARING FAMILY/POSTPARTAL CARE)

108. **#3.** A cesarean delivery is not a contraindication to breast-feeding. Certain adjustments in position may be necessary, but these should not limit breast-feeding. Intravenous fluids will be given until oral intake is established. The mother and baby are generally discharged together. IMPLEMENTATION (CHILDBEARING FAMILY/POSTPARTAL CARE)

109. **#1.** Regional anesthesia may be contraindicated based on this surgical history. Blood and urine findings are normal. Active herpes at the time of delivery necessitates a cesarean delivery. ASSESSMENT (CHILDBEARING FAMILY/INTRAPARTAL CARE)

110. **#3.** Rapid infusion of intravenous fluids may result in pulmonary edema if the heart is unable to adapt to the circulatory overload. ASSESSMENT (CHILDBEARING FAMILY/INTRAPARTAL CARE)

111. **#2.** The respiratory assessment indicates a potential problem following general anesthesia and should be reported immediately. Other findings are within normal limits. ASSESSMENT (CHILDBEARING FAMILY/POSTPARTAL CARE)

112. **#3.** While this may be quite early for rooming-in after a cesarean birth, with nursing assistance the client may be able to care safely for the infant. Asking the father to remain around the clock is not feasible. The signal light should be placed close to the client. IMPLEMENTATION (CHILDBEARING FAMILY/POSTPARTAL CARE)

113. **#4.** To help a 3-year-old adjust to a new sibling, a symbolic toy such as a baby doll may be provided. He may express his jealous feelings through symbolic play with this toy. IMPLEMENTATION (CHILDBEARING FAMILY/POSTPARTAL CARE)

114. **#3.** Parents of specific ethnic backgrounds (e.g., Afroamerican, Asian, Mediterranean) often note Mongolian spots on their newborn. These are clusters of pigment cells, of no consequence, that disappear at schoolage. ANALYSIS (CHILDBEARING FAMILY/NORMAL NEWBORN)

115. **#2.** Parents who are both carriers have a 1 in 4 chance of delivering a child with sickle cell disease; they should be made aware of the genetic implications. A carrier of sickle cell disease is heterozygous (Pp). A person with the disease is homozygous recessive (pp). Referral to a genetic counselor is appropriate. IMPLEMENTATION (CHILDBEARING FAMILY/HIGH-RISK NEWBORN)

116. **#4.** The infant weighed 6 lb at birth. This behavior is often normal for a smaller infant on the first days of life. If the infant seems satisfied after feeding, sufficient milk is probably being obtained with nursing. Weight of the infant is also a factor, but that response is not included among the listed options. IMPLEMENTATION (CHILDBEARING FAMILY/NORMAL NEWBORN)

117. **#4.** The incision is made in the lower segment of the uterus, the thinnest portion; thus there is minimal blood loss and repair is simplified. The procedure is associated with a lower incidence of post-op infection. ANALYSIS (CHILDBEARING FAMILY/INTRAPARTAL CARE)

118. **#4.** Postspinal headache is often attributed to the leakage of spinal fluid through the puncture site of the dura. Therefore, maintaining the client in a recumbent position while the puncture hole is healing may prevent this complication. Option #1 has no effect on spinal headache occurrence; #3 is appropriate treatment, not prevention. IMPLEMENTATION (CHILDBEARING FAMILY/POSTPARTAL CARE)

119. **#2.** After rupture of membranes, an amniotic fluid embolism may occur. In this case, the embolism apparently traveled to the lung. ANALYSIS (CHILDBEARING FAMILY/INTRAPARTAL CARE)

120. **#2.** The husband needs support during this time of crisis. He does not need to be left alone. A visit to the intensive care unit is probably not appropriate at this time. IMPLEMENTATION (CHILDBEARING FAMILY/INTRAPARTAL CARE)

121. **#2.** It is never appropriate to argue with the value system of an individual or family. The other options listed encourage more thoughtful consideration of the choice the husband is making. IMPLEMENTATION (CHILDBEARING FAMILY/INTRAPARTAL CARE)

122. **#4.** Hematocrit changes reflect blood loss most accurately and rapidly. Options #1 and #2 are important ongoing assessments, but option #4 is most specific. ASSESSMENT (CHILDBEARING FAMILY/INTRAPARTAL CARE)

123. **#1.** A therapeutic response at this time is one that reflects empathy. Option #3 might be appropriate at some later stage of the grieving process. IMPLEMENTATION (PSYCHOSOCIAL, MENTAL HEALTH, PSYCHIATRIC PROBLEMS/THERAPEUTIC USE OF SELF)

124. **#2.** Oxytocin is used to contract the uterus and minimize postpartal bleeding. ANALYSIS (CHILDBEARING FAMILY/POSTPARTAL CARE)

125. **#4.** The bedpan and running water should be tried first. Eventually, the nurse may need to insert a catheter but not as an initial action. Because of her fluctuating blood pressure and spinal anesthetic, it is not appropriate to get the client out of bed. IMPLEMENTATION (CHILDBEARING FAMILY/POSTPARTAL CARE)

126. **#1.** Postpartum chills are a common occurrence following delivery. Possible causes are reaction to the anesthesia, exhaustion, and a decrease in intra-abdominal pressure. Warming the client is the appropriate nursing action. IMPLEMENTATION (CHILDBEARING FAMILY/POSTPARTAL CARE)

127. **#2.** Ice is used during the first 24 hours; then switch to heat (sitz baths), which promotes vasodilatation and healing. TACE is a lactation suppressant. Kegel exercises will increase vaginal tone but will not relieve pain and swelling. IMPLEMENTATION (CHILDBEARING FAMILY/POSTPARTAL CARE)

128. **#4.** Prolactin is the direct cause of milk production. The decrease in estrogen and progesterone following delivery of the placenta stimulates prolactin production. ANALYSIS (CHILDBEARING FAMILY/POSTPARTAL CARE)

129. **#3.** Use of a breast pump is unnecessary when initiating feeding. The infant's sucking should stimulate the milk sufficiently. IMPLEMENTATION (CHILDBEARING FAMILY/POSTPARTAL CARE)

130. **#3.** The condom is the only safe, nonprescription contraceptive to use while a woman is lactating and before there is normal uterine involution. The intrauterine device is not inserted until healing takes place because of the increased risk of infection. Birth control pills are passed into breast milk. To be effective, a diaphragm must fit over the cervix, which has not undergone involution at this time. IMPLEMENTATION (CHILDBEARING FAMILY/POSTPARTAL CARE)

131. **#4.** These activities are considered too strenuous the first week after delivery. EVALUATION (CHILDBEARING FAMILY/POSTPARTAL CARE)

132. **#1.** Immediately after delivery, the fundus will be about halfway between the symphysis pubis and the umbilicus. Expect lochia rubra for about 3 days postdelivery. ASSESSMENT (CHILDBEARING FAMILY/POSTPARTAL CARE)

133. **#1.** Suspect lacerations if the client is bleeding and the fundus is firm. Subinvolution as well as uterine atony indicate that the uterus is not contracting properly; thus the fundus would not be firm. When placental fragments are retained, the uterus will not contract. ANALYSIS (CHILDBEARING FAMILY/POSTPARTAL CARE)

134. **#1.** Overdistension of the uterus causes poor uterine-muscle tone, which, in turn, causes poor uterine contractions postpartum leading to an increased risk of postpartum hemorrhage. ASSESSMENT (CHILDBEARING FAMILY/POSTPARTAL CARE)

135. **#3.** All these symptoms are expected for the first day postpartum. Maternal temperature during the first 24 hours following delivery may rise to 100.4°F as a result of dehydration. The nurse can reassure the new mother that these symptoms are normal. IMPLEMENTATION (CHILDBEARING FAMILY/POSTPARTAL CARE)

136. **#2.** Afterpains are more common in the multipara and the nursing mother. Multiparas have poorer muscle tone and the uterus has the tendency to contract and relax. Oxytocin is released during breast-feeding, causing the uterus to contract. ASSESSMENT (CHILDBEARING FAMILY/POSTPARTAL CARE)

137. #2. Menses return in 4 to 6 weeks in the non-nursing mother. IMPLEMENTATION (CHILDBEARING FAMILY/POSTPARTAL CARE)

138. #1. Ready-prepared infant formulas have additional water and carbohydrates, compared with breast milk. Commercial formulas are also fortified with essential nutrients. The higher casein content of formula makes it more difficult to digest than breast milk. ANALYSIS (CHILDBEARING FAMILY/POSTPARTAL CARE)

139. #1. As an essential part of the attachment process, the mother begins to "discover" her infant. This includes identification of physical characteristics and bodily processes. Identifying and relating to her infant as a separate and healthy human being may be accompanied by a sense of emotional relief in the mother. ANALYSIS (CHILDBEARING FAMILY/POSTPARTAL CARE)

140. #4. Of the options given, the only one that directly and immediately affects the bleeding is uterine massage. It would be important to start an IV with oxytocin at a rapid rate of flow and to give oxygen per mask at 6 to 7 liters/minute. However, the first action is to initiate uterine massage and compression. IMPLEMENTATION (CHILDBEARING FAMILY/POSTPARTAL CARE)

141. #1. The 3 causes of early postpartum hemorrhage in order of frequency are uterine atony, birth canal lacerations, and retained placental fragments. The client is a multipara who has given birth to a large baby, which results in decreased uterine tone. ANALYSIS (CHILDBEARING FAMILY/POSTPARTAL CARE)

142. #3. Postpartal hemorrhage is defined as blood loss equal to or in excess of 500 ml in the first 24 hours following delivery. ASSESSMENT (CHILDBEARING FAMILY/POSTPARTAL CARE)

143. #3. There is no documentation in the literature that breast-feeding is contraindicated following a postpartum hemorrhage and its resultant anemia. It is very important, though, to replace the lost iron stores. This is accomplished by diet and ferrous sulfate or ferrous gluconate tablets. Fatigue is a problem common in the postpartum period and is aggravated by the anemia in this case. Until the blood tests are within normal range, Mrs. Jackson would be expected to be fatigued on exertion, light-headed when arising too quickly, and pale in appearance. IMPLEMENTATION (CHILDBEARING FAMILY/POSTPARTAL CARE)

144. #1. The Rh-negative mother who has no titer (Coombs negative, nonsensitized) and who has delivered a Rh-positive fetus is given an intramuscular injection of anti-Rh_0 (D) (RhoGAM). IMPLEMENTATION (CHILDBEARING FAMILY/POSTPARTAL CARE)

145. #3. RhoGAM blocks antibody production by attaching to fetal Rh-negative blood cells in the maternal circulation before an immunologic response is initiated. ANALYSIS (CHILDBEARING FAMILY/POSTPARTAL CARE)

146. #2. RhoGAM must be administered to unsensitized postpartum women after the birth of each Rh-positive infant to prevent production of antibodies. If the father of future fetuses is Rh positive heterozygous, there is a 50% chance of an Rh-negative infant; if he is Rh positive homozygous, all infants will be Rh positive. IMPLEMENTATION (CHILDBEARING FAMILY/POSTPARTAL CARE)

147. #3. Serum hepatitis is transmitted through blood; thus needles and syringes must be disposed of properly. PLAN (ADULT/NUTRITION/METABOLISM)

148. #2. This menu meets the required amounts of vitamin C, iron, carbohydrates, and protein. As breast-feeding is contraindicated when the mother has hepatitis, milk does not need to be included in the meal. She can meet recommended daily allowances for milk without having a glass at every meal. IMPLEMENTATION (CHILDBEARING FAMILY/POSTPARTAL CARE)

149. #2. These are signs of withdrawal in an addicted newborn. The onset of withdrawal usually occurs within 24 hours of birth. The newborn may be jittery and hyperactive. The cry is often shrill and persistent with yawning and sneezing. Tendon reflexes are increased and the Moro reflex is decreased. ASSESSMENT (CHILDBEARING FAMILY/HIGH-RISK NEWBORN)

150. #4. A home visit is essential when preparing to discharge an infant into the care of others. Other factors will be considered but safety is the priority. ASSESSMENT (CHILDBEARING FAMILY/HIGH-RISK NEWBORN)

151. #2. The potential for abuse or neglect is significantly higher when the parent is a substance abuser. ANALYSIS (CHILDBEARING FAMILY/HIGH-RISK NEWBORN)

152. #1. Mastitis most frequently occurs at 2 to 4 weeks postpartum with the initial symptoms of fever, chills, headache, breast tenderness and/or a localized reddened area on the breast. The client may describe symptoms that are generally consistent with malaise. ASSESSMENT (CHILDBEARING FAMILY/POSTPARTAL CARE)

153. #3. There is controversy about whether a woman should temporarily stop breast-feeding or continue to breast-feed when mastitis is present. There is no scientific reason that, once the infection has passed the acute phase and the woman is no longer febrile, breast-feeding cannot be resumed. During the acute phase, it is important that counseling be given on how to manually massage or use a breast pump to empty the breasts to prevent stasis and further engorgement. IMPLEMENTATION (CHILDBEARING FAMILY/POSTPARTAL CARE)

154. #4. Limiting nursing time will prevent cracked nipples, a common cause of mastitis. Antibiotics are used to treat mastitis. Waiting too long between feedings and abrupt weaning may lead to clogged ducts, predisposing to mastitis. IMPLEMENTATION (CHILDBEARING FAMILY/POSTPARTAL CARE)

155. #4. Generalized cyanosis is a cause for concern that requires further assessment. Possible causes of cyanosis are hypothermia, infection, hypoglycemia, and cardiopulmonary disease. Acrocyanosis of the hands and feet is normal due to sluggish peripheral circulation. Jaundice after 72 hours is normal physiologic jaundice. Harlequin sign is a rare color change between the longitudinal halves of the infant (when the infant is on its side, the dependent half is noticeably pinker). ASSESSMENT (CHILDBEARING FAMILY/NORMAL NEWBORN)

156. #1. The head circumference is approximately 13 to 14 inches. The chest circumference is 1 inch smaller (12 to 13 inches). ASSESSMENT (CHILDBEARING FAMILY/NORMAL NEWBORN)

157. #3. Impetigo is a bacterial infection caused by staphylococci or streptococci, which can lead to a generalized infection, always serious in the newborn. Erythema toxicum is a normal newborn rash that disappears without treatment. Stork bites or telangiectases are clusters of small, red, localized areas of capillary dilation commonly found at the nape of the neck, upper eyelids, and bridge of the nose. They can be blanched with pressure of a finger and will disappear without treatment. Mongolian spots are bluish gray areas of pigmentation found over the lower back in black or Oriental infants. The spots fade within the first year or 2 of life. ASSESSMENT (CHILDBEARING FAMILY/NORMAL NEWBORN)

158. #4. An opaque pupil indicates a congenital cataract. Transient strabismus or nystagmus is present until the third or fourth month of life. Subconjunctival hemorrhage is due to the pressure sustained during birth and will resolve without treatment. The eyes may be irritated from the instillation of medication causing some discharge. ASSESSMENT (CHILDBEARING FAMILY/NORMAL NEWBORN)

159. #4. The single artery is associated with an increased incidence of various congenital anomalies and with higher perinatal mortality. Breast engorgement may be present as the result of maternal hormones. Bowel sounds are present within 1 to 2 hours after birth. The liver is large in proportion to the rest of the body and is easily felt. Kidneys are more difficult to feel. ASSESSMENT (CHILDBEARING FAMILY/NORMAL NEWBORN)

160. #2. Ears that are set lower than usual on the head may be associated with a congenital renal disorder or autosomal chromosomal abnormality. Incurving of the pinna and instant recoil are signs of maturity. The infant hears immediately following birth and hearing becomes acute as mucus from the middle ear is absorbed. ASSESSMENT (CHILDBEARING FAMILY/NORMAL NEWBORN)

161. #3. During periods of alert activity, play can be initiated with young infants. In the taking-hold period, the mother is particularly receptive to instruction and assistance in learning play and other parenting skills. IMPLEMENTATION (CHILDBEARING FAMILY/NORMAL NEWBORN)

162. **#2.** Fixation is present at birth. The newborn can see items with clarity that are within a visual field of 20 cm to 22 cm (9 inches). ANALYSIS (CHILDBEARING FAMILY/NORMAL NEWBORN)

163. **#4.** Young infants respond well to human faces and black-and-white objects, because of the visual contrast they provide. Newborns may fixate on visual stimuli for periods of 4 to 10 seconds. IMPLEMENTATION (CHILDBEARING FAMILY/NORMAL NEWBORN)

164. **#3.** Skin-to-skin touch provides a mild tactile stimulus appropriate for the infant. It can be accomplished by stroking the infant gently from head to toe. This procedure is very comforting and relaxing to the infant. IMPLEMENTATION (CHILDBEARING FAMILY/NORMAL NEWBORN)

165. **#4.** This reflex is also known as the grasping reflex and is elicited if the palm of the hand is stimulated by touch. The fingers close. ASSESSMENT (CHILDBEARING FAMILY/NORMAL NEWBORN)

166. **#2.** The infant experiences a sensation of falling when held in both hands and lowered rapidly about 1 inch. This will cause abduction and extension of arms and spreading of fingers bilaterally. ASSESSMENT (CHILDBEARING FAMILY/NORMAL NEWBORN)

167. **#1.** Maternal glucose crosses the placental barrier and stimulates the fetal pancreas to produce large amounts of insulin. At birth, the excess insulin causes the blood glucose level to fall rapidly. ANALYSIS (CHILDBEARING FAMILY/HIGH-RISK NEWBORN)

168. **#3.** Hypoglycemia may be prevented by the oral administration of glucose water. Oral feeding should be started as soon as the infant's condition permits. IMPLEMENTATION (CHILDBEARING FAMILY/HIGH-RISK NEWBORN)

169. **#4.** A term infant is one born between 38 and 42 weeks gestation; a weight of 10 lb is above the 90th percentile. ANALYSIS (CHILDBEARING FAMILY/NORMAL NEWBORN)

170. **#4.** There is an increased risk of development of diabetes later in life. IMPLEMENTATION (CHILDBEARING FAMILY/HIGH-RISK NEWBORN)

171. **#2.** Skin should be exposed to light to allow oxidation of bilirubin from the skin. The light may injure the delicate eye structures particularly the retina, so the eyes are patched. The infant requires additional fluids to compensate for the increased water loss through the skin and loose stools. Stools and urine are evaluated for green color and amount. IMPLEMENTATION (CHILDBEARING FAMILY/HIGH-RISK NEWBORN)

172. **#2.** Although large-for-gestational-age infants are often prone to hypoglycemia, the Dextrostix reading in this situation indicates an adequate blood-glucose level. All the other situations are at risk for hypoglycemia. The infant who is exposed to high blood-glucose levels in utero may experience rapid and profound hypoglycemia after birth because of the cessation of a high in-utero glucose load. The small-for-gestational-age infant has used up glycogen stores as a result of intrauterine malnutrition and has blunted hepatic enzymatic response with which to carry out gluconeogenesis. The preterm infants have not been in utero a sufficient period to store glycogen and fat. ASSESSMENT (CHILDBEARING FAMILY/HIGH-RISK NEWBORN)

173. **#1.** Increased respirations indicate a high metabolic rate. This happens with an infection. The other options are all within normal ranges. ASSESSMENT (CHILDBEARING FAMILY/HIGH-RISK NEWBORN)

174. **#1.** The mother's behavior indicates she is grieving over the infant's appearance. The nurse demonstrates acceptance of her feelings if she makes no demands on her, but allows infant contact. IMPLEMENTATION (CHILDBEARING FAMILY/HIGH-RISK NEWBORN)

175. **#4.** Periodic apnea is common in preterm infants. Usually, gentle stimulation is sufficent to get the infant to breathe. IMPLEMENTATION (CHILDBEARING FAMILY/HIGH-RISK NEWBORN)

176. **#3.** Epstein's pearls are small, white cysts on the hard palate or gums of the newborn. They are not abnormal and will disappear shortly after birth. Milia are blocked sebaceous glands located on the chin and nose of the infant. Thrush is a fungal infection characterized by white patches that appear to be milk curd on the oral mucosa. They have a tendency to bleed when removal is attempted. Thrush is caused by a monilial infection in the mother. ANALYSIS (CHILDBEARING FAMILY/NORMAL NEWBORN)

177. **#4.** The oxygenated blood flows up the cord through the umbilical vein; a fetal structure known as the ductus venosus shunts blood from the umbilical vein to the inferior vena cava. From the inferior vena cava, the blood flows into the right atrium and goes directly into the left atrium through the foramen ovale. It then flows into the left ventricle and out through the aorta. A fetal structure known as the ductus arteriosus provides a direct communication between the pulmonary artery and aorta. ANALYSIS (CHILDBEARING FAMILY/NORMAL NEWBORN)

178. **#1.** At birth, the newborn's cardiac sphincter is still immature, and the nervous control of the stomach is incomplete. As a result, some regurgitation may be observed, which may be minimized by small feedings and frequent bubbling. ANALYSIS (CHILDBEARING FAMILY/NORMAL NEWBORN)

179. **#2.** The posterior fontanel is located at the intersection of the sagittal and lambdoid sutures of the skull. The sagittal suture is the space between the parietal bones; the lambdoid suture separates the 2 parietal bones and the occipital bone. ANALYSIS (CHILDBEARING FAMILY/NORMAL NEWBORN)

180. **#2.** Parental contact promotes bonding and the parents' feeling that this is their infant. IMPLEMENTATION (CHILDBEARING FAMILY/NORMAL NEWBORN)

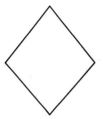

Reprints
Nursing Care of the Childbearing Family

A M E R I C A N   J O U R N A L   O F   N U R S I N G

VAGINAL DELIVERY AFTER C-SECTION

BY SHIRLEY L. BRENGMAN / MARGARET K. BURNS

With careful screening, many women can choose trial labor, regardless of their previous cesareans

Reprinted From MCN: American Journal of Maternal/Child Nursing, November 1983

DAVID KLEIN

A M E R I C A N   J O U R N A L   O F   N U R S I N G

Once a cesarean, always a cesarean." The dramatic rise in cesarean births in the past 10 years has led many consumers, providers, insurers, and government agencies to question the validity of that old dictum(1-4). Yet elective repeat sections continue, despite studies that show normal labor and vaginal delivery are possible and safe for the majority of carefully screened women who have had a previous C-section for a nonrecurrent problem(1-6).

The American College of Obstetricians and Gynecologists (ACOG) estimates that 25-30 percent of the annual 500,000 cesareans performed in this country are repeat sections(7). Many obstetricians fear uterine rupture or scar dehiscence if normal labor is permitted(1,2). But again, statistics show the risk is minimal, ranging from as little as 0.5 percent to 3.2 percent in studies of trials of labor(1,2,5). Most important, no maternal deaths have occurred in reported trials of labor(1,2,5).

What seems to be forgotten is that C-sections have risks too: Even under optimal conditions, abdominal delivery is associated with greater maternal mortality, morbidity, and blood loss than is a normal vaginal delivery(2). An elective repeat cesarean section also incurs greater medical costs, beginning with antepartal testing to determine fetal lung maturity, a usually routine procedure for repeat sections but only occasionally performed for vaginal deliveries, to increased delivery costs because of surgery and anesthesia, and a longer postpartum hospitalization for both mother and baby. At Ohio State University Hospitals, the average hospital cost for a vaginal delivery and postpartum stay is approximately 40 percent less than that for a cesarean and postop stay.

The overall rate of C-sections, as of January 1982, was 17 percent (of 3.5 million U.S. births annually), or 595,000 births(7). In some parts of the country C-sections have jumped by as much as

Shirley L. Brengman, RNC, and Margaret Burns, RNC, MS, were staff nurses in the labor and delivery unit during the Weekend Work Program, Ohio State University Hospitals, Columbus, Ohio. Ms. Brengman is head nurse in L and D at Mt. Carmel Medical Center, Columbus, Ohio, and Ms. Burns is assistant professor of nursing, Ohio Wesleyan University, Delaware, Ohio.

25 percent: OSU Hospitals' C-section rate, for instance, was 22 percent in 1982.

The introduction of electronic fetal monitors in the 1970s is believed to have contributed to the increase. By assessing fetal status moment by moment, these monitors can signal possible fetal compromise, which will be immediately evaluated and, in some cases, require emergency procedures.

A LAST RESORT

Prior to the 1900s, the occasional primary cesarean, performed as a last resort, usually resulted in a woman's sterility or death. Subsequent delivery was rarely a consideration(5). Cesareans consisted of vertical incisions into the thick, vascular, fundal portion of

---

WHO IS A CANDIDATE?

A woman who
- wants a normal labor and delivery
- has had a previous low transverse uterine incision
- has a nonrecurring problem (fetal distress, placenta previa)
- is in good health
- has had a normal pregnancy—vertex position, fetal weight less than 4,000 gm
- will be admitted to a hospital when labor begins, where fetal and uterine monitoring are available as well as surgical and pediatric services
- understands the risks and possibility of repeat section
- understands that analgesics may be limited during labor

---

the uterus. During a subsequent labor, such a scar might easily rupture from the force of contracting uterine muscles. Dehiscence from such scars is more likely to lead to maternal and fetal shock(6). The incidence of uterine rupture in a classical vertical scar is 4-5 times higher than rupture in a lower uterine segment scar—the operative procedure of choice today(7). The lower uterine segment is thinner and less vascular. And even if there is a dehiscence of this type of scar, there is usually minimal blood loss. No reported maternal deaths due to lower uterine segment scar rupture have been reported. However, deaths from unexpected uterine rupture have occurred in mothers who have not had a cesarean section(8). Should uterine rupture occur, hypovolemic shock may result from hemorrhage, and a hysterectomy may be necessary because of bleeding and tissue damage.

The risk of uterine rupture is believed to increase if the primary section is complicated by multiple cesarean births, additional vaginal deliveries following C-section, or placental implantation over the previous incisional site. There is, however, no statistical evidence to support these conclusions(8).

Febrile morbidity and endometritis increase significantly in patients delivered by repeat cesarean section following a trial of labor compared with those delivered by elective repeat cesarean section before labor begins. But there are no significant differences when the repeat section group is compared with those women delivered by primary cesarean section during labor(8).

Oxytocin (Pitocin) may be used in trial labor to induce or augment labor, just as it is in women with no history of section. However, use of the drug may increase the risk of scar dehiscence and reduce the likelihood of successful vaginal delivery(2,8). If Pitocin is used, ACOG recommends a dilute, controlled infusion, according to its guidelines(7).

Fetal mortality rates as high as 3.8 percent in vaginal deliveries following previous cesarean sections have been reported, but most of these statistics were compiled before electronic fetal monitoring became widely used(1,5). It is likely that current fetal mortality rates are much lower. In addition, the perinatal deaths reported in these studies were directly related to the vaginal delivery (prolapsed cord, birth asphyxia) or maternal complications (pregnancy-induced hypertension, diabetes), not uterine rupture(8).

SELECTING CANDIDATES

In 1982, ACOG developed guidelines for vaginal delivery after a cesarean. Highlights of these criteria, combined with those selected from the literature and our experiences. (See box, this page.)

Contraindications for such a trial include previous classical or unknown type of uterine incision; recurrent condition that resulted in previous cesarean; patient preference; inadequate birthing facilities; inadequate pelvis; patient refusal to accept blood or blood products; and other medical or obstetrical complications(5). A history of cephalopelvic disproportion is not necessarily a contraindication, reports Demianczuk, since 40 percent of women with this history in his study were safely delivered vaginally(2).

A M E R I C A N   J O U R N A L   O F   N U R S I N G

Parents need to know the risks involved; they must understand and accept that trial labor may again result in cesarean.

Most trials of labor are allowed to continue until vaginal delivery or indications for a cesarean section are clear(1). At our hospital forceps are only used at times to facilitate the birth. They are not used, as suggested in the literature, to shorten the second stage of labor and to reduce the chance of uterine rupture. Scar dehiscence is more likely in the second and third stages of labor, when the most stress occurs. Examples of trials of labor appear on page 1547.

UNDERSTANDING PARENTS' SPECIAL NEEDS

Women planning to undergo a trial labor have special needs. In most cases, the previous cesarean birth was not planned but was an emergency procedure because of fetal compromise or a long, nonprogressive labor. (Other indicators, besides fetal compromise, for primary cesareans are breech presentation, cephalopelvic disproportion, abruptio placentae, placenta previa, pregnancy-induced hypertension, and uterine dysfunction(5,6,8). In one study of 92 women, the most common causes of prior sections were cephalopelvic disproportion (33) and breech presentation (26)(2).

The cesarean undoubtedly caused the parents much anxiety concerning the physical well-being of mother and baby(10). The woman may have been greatly disappointed when she was not able to have a spontaneous vaginal birth. If general anesthesia was used, she may not have had a bonding period with the newborn immediately following the birth.

The father may have attended childbirth education classes as a labor coach, and expected to take an active part in the delivery. He, too, may have been disappointed over the loss of a natural birth experience, especially if he was not permitted in the delivery room for the cesarean birth. Every attempt should be made to involve the father in

the birthing experience, whether it is vaginal or abdominal.

During the antepartum period, both parents need to understand and accept that a trial of labor may again result in a cesarean birth. They need to know the risks and complications involved in a trial labor and vaginal delivery. The parents' possible unresolved grief at their loss of a normal delivery can lead to distrust of all providers; therefore, they need time to voice their concerns, as well as their expectations for the current pregnancy(10). Routine labor and delivery procedures and emergency cesarean procedures are explained, as is the necessity of limiting the use of analgesics and anesthetics during labor. The patient's record documents the teaching given.

The parents should be encouraged to attend classes in childbirth education and breathing techniques, to prepare for labor and its normal discomforts and pain. Finally, the patient is instructed to enter the hospital when contractions are regular and of increasing intensity (the nurse may have to describe labor signs if the woman has not experienced them), or if spontaneous rupture of amniotic membranes or vaginal bleeding occur.

INTRAPARTAL PERIOD

Upon arrival at the labor and delivery area of the hospital, the patient is immediately placed on external electronic monitoring to assess fetal well-being and uterine contractions. Appropriate anesthesia and nursery personnel are notified that a trial of labor is in progress (ACOG suggests 15 minutes as the maximum time to set up and begin a C-section.)(7). An intravenous infusion is begun with a large-bore intravenous catheter (at least 16-gauge, 2-in.). The woman is encouraged to restrict oral intake to small amounts of ice chips, since surgery and general anesthesia may be necessary. An antacid is given every 3-4 hours to neutral-

ize stomach acidity.

Supplies needed to ready the patient for an emergency cesarean, such as a Foley catheter, urinary drainage bag and abdominal prep kit, are stored in the patient's room. When the amniotic membranes rupture, an aseptic vaginal exam is done. A fetal scalp electrode is inserted and an intrauterine pressure catheter is passed into the uterus (both depicted in opening illustration) to better assess the fetal status and the strength of uterine contractions. Continuous assessment of maternal and fetal status by a professional nurse is mandatory. Abdominal pain may be an unreliable indicator because it can be due to peritoneal adhesions, a hypersensitive bladder, round ligament tension, scarring of the abdominal wall, or normal discomfort of labor. Some women do not experience any pain with uterine rupture(8).

Fetal distress (bradycardia and fetal heart rate decelerations) has been reported to be the only sign of uterine rupture in some cases(12). Fetal compromise appears secondary to placental separation, maternal hemorrhage, or, in rare cases, extrusion of the fetus into the abdominal cavity(9,11).

Minimal analgesics are offered during the trial of labor to avoid masking pain of uterine rupture. Epidural anesthesia is usually avoided for the same reason. A patient's experiencing more pain than would be expected from the strength of the uterine contractions could signal uterine rupture(9).

Maternal vital signs are recorded every 15-30 minutes, and temperature every two hours. The patient is encouraged to void often. Gross hematuria is reported to the physician immediately. Careful checking of the amount and character of vaginal discharge can help to distinguish normal bloody show from hemorrhagic bleeding. Observation of the suprapubic area before and after urination may reveal asymmetrical or abnormal contours; these could indicate

THREE WOMEN'S EXPERIENCES WITH TRIAL LABOR

The patient, a 25-year-old gravida 3, para 2, with a term pregnancy, wanted to deliver vaginally. Her first child was a spontaneous vaginal delivery. Her second pregnancy, complicated by twins in transverse lie, resulted in a low cervical transverse cesarean section.

After 10 hours of labor in the third pregnancy, she delivered a 4,200 gm (8 lb., 12 oz.) baby vaginally. She received meperidine (Demerol) and propiomazine (Largon) for analgesia during labor, and local anesthesia with a pudendal block for delivery. Although variable fetal heart rate decelerations were evident prior to delivery, the baby's Apgar scores were 9 and 9 at one and five minutes. The uterine scar was palpated after delivery and found to be intact.

A 22-year-old gravida 3, para 1, AB 1, with a pregnancy at term, desired a trial of labor. Her previous delivery had been by low cervical transverse cesarean section because of a footling breech presentation. She had and was treated for endometritis following her primary cesarean.

After 11 hours of labor, the patient experienced severe abdominal tenderness. Moderate fetal heart rate decelerations were observed. She had an immediate cesarean section under general anesthesia and delivered a 3,570 gm (7 lb., 7 oz.) baby with Apgar scores of 9 and 10 at one and five minutes. During surgery, a uterine rupture was found along the previous cesarean scar. Estimated blood loss during surgery was 700cc.

The patient, a 24-year-old gravida 3, para 1, AB 1, with a pregnancy at term, desired a trial of labor. She had not previously delivered a baby vaginally. Her first delivery was by low cervical transverse cesarean section because she was two weeks post-EDC and failed to progress in labor.

After 22½ hours of labor, she delivered a 5,040 gm (10 lb., 8 oz.) baby vaginally. She received no drugs for analgesia or anesthesia. No episiotomy was attempted (at the patient's request) and she received a second-degree perineal laceration, which was repaired. The baby's Apgar scores were 7 and 9 at one and five minutes. The uterine scar was found to be intact following delivery.

---

hematoma formation or fetal parts protruding from the uterus and should be reported immediately.

Encouraging the patient to use controlled breathing exercises: Those will relieve discomfort, as will backrubs, positioning, and cool cloths on the brow. If the patient is "up ad lib," ambulation with intermittent monitoring (10 min q1h) may stimulate labor. We encourage patients to change position often.

Should the trial of labor be terminated and a C-section scheduled, the nurse will prepare the woman and her husband by explaining what will be done, and offer support. The nurse will prep the woman's abdomen, insert a Foley catheter, and give any necessary medications. Following vaginal birth and removal of the placenta, the physician makes an internal exam of the uterus and palpates the old uterine scar to check if it is intact. The exam is uncomfortable, although it lasts less than 30 seconds.

POSTPARTUM CARE

The patient is moved to the recovery area where she is observed closely. An undetected uterine rupture may result in persistent heavy vaginal bleeding despite a firm fundus. With an empty bladder, the uterine fundus should remain in the midline, at or below the umbilicus. If the bladder is distended, encourage the patient to void. Record vital signs, fundal status (location, firmness), and description of vaginal drainage (color, amount, consistency) at least every 15 minutes for the first hour. Heavy vaginal bleeding, a dramatic change in vital signs, or fundus above the umbilicus (with an empty bladder) could indicate an undiagnosed uterine rupture[9].

If the patient remains stable during the recovery period, her postpartum care will be the same as that for any uncomplicated postpartum woman.

In our experience, many women who have had a previous section for a nonrecurring problem can experience a normal labor and delivery. Carefully explaining the risks and providing expert nursing can make the difference.

REFERENCES

1. Merrill, B. S., and Gibbs, C. E. Planned vaginal delivery following cesarean section. *Obstet.Gynecol.* 52:50-52, July 1978.
2. Demianczuk, N. N., and others. Trial of labor after previous cesarean section: prognostic indicators of outcome. *Am.J.Obstet.Gynecol.* 142:640-642, Mar. 15, 1982.
3. Marieskind, Helen I. *An evaluation of cesarean section in the United States.* Bethesda, Md., Department of Health & Human Services, 1979.
4. U. S. Department of Health and Human Services. *Draft Report of the task force on cesarean childbirth.* Bethesda, Md., National Institute of Child Health & Human Development, 1980.
5. Gibbs, C. E. Planned vaginal delivery following cesarean section. *Clin.Obstet.Gynecol.* 23:507-515, June 1980.
6. Hansen, G. F. A reevaluation of vaginal delivery after cesarean section. *Perinatol.Neonatol.* 3:46-48, July-Aug. 1979.
7. American College of Obstetricians and Gynecologists, Committee on Obstetrics Maternal and Fetal Medicine. *Guidelines for Vaginal Delivery after a Cesarean Childbirth.* Washington, D.C., The committee, Jan. 7, 1982.
8. Lavin, J. P., and others. Vaginal delivery in patients with a prior cesarean section. *Obstet.Gynecol.* 59:135-148, Feb. 1982.
9. O'Sullivan, M. J., and others. Vaginal delivery after cesarean section. *Clin.Perinatol.* 8:131-143, Feb. 1981.
10. Fawcett, J. Needs of cesarean birth parents. *JOGN* 10:372-376, Sept.-Oct. 1981.
11. Jensen, M. D., and others. *Maternity Care: the Nurse and the Family.* 2nd ed. St. Louis, C.V. Mosby Co., 1981.
12. Spaulding, L. B., and Gallup, D. G. Current concepts of management of the gravid uterus. *Obstet.Gynecol.* 54:437-441, Oct. 1979.

Are We Ignoring the Needs of the Woman With a Spontaneous Abortion?

Reprinted from MCN: American Journal of Maternal/Child Nursing, July/August 1982

The nurse plays an important role,
offering support and information,
when the woman aborts spontaneously.

SUZANNE KING WETZEL

A woman who has just had a spontaneous abortion may feel considerable shock and anger. The nurse caring for this woman requires an understanding of the processes of attachment and grief, along with a technical knowledge of spontaneous abortion. Since we know maternal-infant attachment starts as early as the planning stage in pregnancy, grief would be expected with a spontaneous abortion.

A spontaneous abortion is the natural termination of a pregnancy prior to twenty weeks of gestation. Spontaneous abortions are classified as threatened, inevitable, incomplete, complete, or missed abortions. The medical management of these classifications varies little; a dilatation and curettage (D&C) is generally performed as the bleeding or cramping increase (1). While the hospital stay for the woman is usually quite short, the contacts the woman and her mate have with the nurses are important.

Providing physical comfort is a nurse's primary concern immediately prior to and following the D & C. Frequent pad and Chux changes, along with perineal cleansing impart a sense of caring. Another vital provision is to teach simple relaxation and breathing techniques to help alleviate some of the stress. It takes only a short time to teach the slow, chest breathing exercises associated with prepared childbirth; and it is very beneficial, even following the abortion.

During the dilatation and curettage, itself, the woman is often without her usual support person

MS. WETZEL R.N., M.S.N., *at the time this article was written was the clinical nurse specialist in obstetrics and is now in the department of nursing education at the Medical College of Virginia, in Richmond.*

A woman having a spontaneous abortion

and upset and anxious. A nurse's simple act of holding the woman's hand during anesthesia provides a sense that others care and offer support. If the woman is awake during the procedure, it helps to use appropriate breathing techniques to aid in relaxation.

Another important consideration for the nurse is the careful use of medical terminology in front of the woman and her mate. Without an explanation, lay people may misunderstand a statement such as "This lady is aborting."

As the initial shock resolves and guilt ensues, the woman may have a dozen questions: What did she do (or not do) to cause the loss? Can she become pregnant again? What will happen to her ability to carry future pregnancies to term? And what has happened to her feminine identity?

Although a medical explanation of spontaneous abortion may have been inappropriate up to this time, now is the moment when it may help to explain these aspects. The woman needs to know that while many factors may enter into the etiology of spontaneous abortions, in 50 percent of the cases no cause for the loss can be determined (1). There is an approximately 20 percent occurrence rate for spontaneous abortions. They usually are not caused by working at a stressful job, having intercourse in early pregnancy, or by the previous use of contraception.

The woman probably will want to talk about her spontaneous abortion. This is similar to the need for a woman during postpartum to talk about her labor and delivery. A nurse with therapeutic listening skills can aid the grieving woman by allowing her the opportunity to discuss the entire experience.

If this was the woman's first pregnancy, she will require special support. She needs to talk with other women who have experienced a spontaneous abortion and later carried a baby to term. If available, the couple will benefit from a support group for bereaved parents, including those who had spontaneous abortions.

It is essential for the nurse to acknowledge the

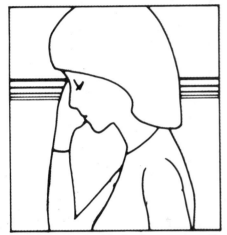

may feel considerable shock, anger, or guilt.

importance of the lost pregnancy. There is a great deal of emotional trauma caused by unthinking people who state, "It's for the best," "This is nature's way of getting rid of your defective children," or "Just get pregnant again." These comments only add to the woman's confusion, guilt, depression, and anger.

By understanding the attachment process, the nurse can offer support and empathy. A simple statement such as, "I know this hurt. That baby was special," can offer the woman an opportunity to grieve openly.

The Father's Part

Let us not forget that the abortion is experienced by the expectant father, as well as the mother-to-be. He too requires support. Often, at the time of the loss, the pregnancy is not a reality to him. His main concern may be only for the woman. If she has had physical discomfort or profuse bleeding, the man may fear for her safety. During hospitalization, he may need support and reassurance regarding the mother's condition.

The father may be ready for technical information much earlier than the woman (2). He also is just as

likely to experience feelings of guilt and fear regarding the woman's ability to carry a pregnancy to term. Providing accurate information to the father and encouraging him to discuss his fears will aid the couple toward a mutual resolution.

The father may need additional support once home. He may not understand that the woman may be emotionally labile for several weeks. The loss is resolved much more quickly in his mind. Often he becomes impatient when the woman is weeping several weeks after her loss. The differences in the return of libido may cause concern and stress if not understood. Just being told that this is a normal response can help resolve the feelings of marital discord. If tension does not ease, the couple should be referred to their obstetrician or other counseling resources in their area.

The Resolution Is Continuous

As the couple is overcoming the physical and emotional traumas, they may wish to learn more about their spontaneous abortion. The nurse can provide several references. (See * Bibliography and * References.) The nurse can also alert the couples that there will be occasional setbacks in the grieving process including at the time of the due date for the lost pregnancy and during the first few months of the next pregnancy (3).

The couple who has been fortunate enough to find a supportive and empathetic nurse in the community may continue to need her support for several months. Without the acknowledgment of her availability, they may fear intrusion on her privacy. Providing follow-up availability is as important here as any time such care is necessary.

The maternity nurse performs a greater service than just delivery care. She frequently is the salvation for a woman and her mate when they have had a spontaneous abortion.

REFERENCES

1. DANFORTH, D. N., ED. *Obstetrics and Gynecology.* 3rd ed. New York, Harper & Row, 1977.
*2. PIZER, HANK, AND PALINSKI, C. O. *Coping With A Miscarriage.* New York, Dial Press, 1980.
3. SEITZ, P. M., AND WARRICK, L. H. Perinatal death: the grieving mother. *Am.J.Nurs.* 74:2028-2033, Nov. 1974.

BIBLIOGRAPHY

*BORG, SUSAN, AND LASKER, JUDITH. *When Pregnancy Fails.* Boston, Beacon Press, 1981.
KOWALSKI, K., AND BOWES, W. A. Parents' response to a stillborn baby. *Contemp. OB/GYN* 8:53-57, Oct. 1976.
KUSHNER, LORRAINE. Infant death and the childbirth educator. *MCN* 4:231-233, July-Aug. 1979.
*PEPPERS, L. G., AND KNAPP, R. J. *Motherhood and Mourning: Perinatal Death.* New York, Praeger Publishers, 1980.
SAYLOR, D. E. Nursing response to mothers of stillborn infants. *JOGN Nurs.* 6:39-42, July-Aug. 1977.
ZAHOUREK, ROTHLYN, AND JENSEN, J. S. Grieving and the loss of the newborn. *Am.J.Nurs.*73:836-839, May 1973.

*Suggested reading for couples.

Emergency Delivery: How to Attend to One Safely

Reprinted from MCN: American Journal of Maternal/Child Nursing, May/June, 1979

While a qualified birth attendant is clearly the best person to assist a woman who is delivering a baby, at times one is simply not available. Often nurses who serve young families are the best, and only, second choice.

BETTY JENNINGS

The birth of a baby is imminent and the doctor or nurse-midwife has not arrived. Or a delivering woman is far from the hospital with a nurse the best qualified person to attend to her. Such situations are not uncommon. Nurses, especially those who practice in the area of labor and delivery, therefore need a basic working knowledge for providing a safe birth. The following review is not meant to minimize the knowledge, skill, and extensive preparation for a fully qualified birth attendant. On the other hand, in an emergency, labor and delivery nurses can ensure a safe birth as well as an emotionally satisfying experience for those involved.

In such a situation the nurse will most likely encounter a labor which has progressed unhindered and thus the likelihood of various problems are decreased. Furthermore, the woman usually has a relaxed, elastic perineum, reducing the chance of tissue injury, and the baby is unlikely to suffer the effects of cephalopelvic disproportion, so he usually fares well.

Various circumstances are likely in an emergency delivery. (See Common Circumstances Surrounding Emergency Deliveries on page 150.) Complications in the first three circumstances are unlikely. A precipitous labor, however, may cause maternal and

MS. JENNINGS, R.N., M.S.N., *is a certified nurse-midwife practicing at Colorado General Hospital in Denver. She is also assistant professor at the University of Colorado School of Nursing and a clinical instructor at the University of Colorado Medical School.*

fetal complications. The mother's tissue may be damaged as the presenting part descends too rapidly, and the fetus may experience distress as placental circulation is interrupted by uterine contractions which are more frequent and intense than normal. The premature baby, of course, has special needs depending on gestational age, but there are no physical complications specific to the mother.

What You Have to Know

The mechanisms and the average duration of each stage of labor are essential knowledge to the ordinary role of the labor and delivery nurse. Using the graph on page 152, the nurse may recognize when a woman is progressing more rapidly than usual and may even predict the time of delivery. Thus she will be better able to attend safely to a birth.

A woman's progress depends on the relationship of the fetal presenting part to the mother's pelvis and the quality of contractions. With a small presenting part and large maternal pelvis, labor progresses more rapidly. When the strength of labor is maximal and resistance to fetal descent through the pelvis is minimal, rapid labor can be anticipated. Most emergency labors are rapid ones.

If the woman in labor is not in the hospital, pelvic exams should be avoided, so determining dilatation and station will be difficult. There are, however, a number of other clues which warn the nurse that delivery is imminent. (See Physical and Behavioral Signs of Imminent Delivery on page 153.)

The mechanisms of normal labor (occiput anterior) are as follows[1]: Descent through the birth canal, which includes engagement, occurs continuously throughout a normal labor simultaneously with other mechanisms. In primigravidas significant descent should have occurred before the onset of labor. In multiparas engagement may not occur until labor is well established. Descent is accomplished by uterine contractions, the bearing down efforts of the second stage, and to some extent by gravity. Engagement refers to the point when the widest diameter of the baby's head (occipito frontal diameter) has passed the plane of the pelvic inlet. It usually occurs with the occiput transverse, the saggital suture being in the transverse diameter of the inlet. The baby is at zero station when the lowest portion of the head has reached the level of the ischial spines.

The baby's neck is flexed toward the chest throughout labor, reflecting the natural attitude of the fetus *in utero*. As descent progresses, the baby's chin more closely approximates the chest. This provides for the presentation of the smaller diameter of the fetal head (the suboccipitobregmatic diameter) through the maternal pelvis.

Internal rotation occurs as the baby's head twists on the shoulders, bringing the saggital suture in the anteroposterior diameter of the maternal pelvis. This allows the narrowest part of the fetal head (biparietal diameter) to pass the narrowest diameter of the maternal pelvis (the bispinous diameter) and aligns the fetus for the next step—birth of the head by extension. Internal rotation is usually complete by the time the head reaches the pelvic floor, having occurred mainly during the second stage of labor. Extension of the head occurs as the nape of the

What To Do

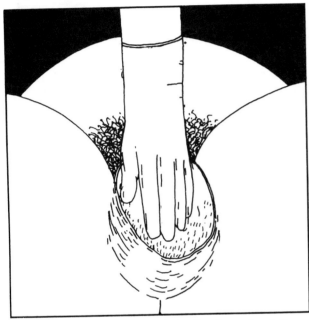

Apply gentle, even pressure with the flat of your hand, fingers and thumb close together, on the emerging head to slow the baby's progress and protect the mother's perineum.

Placing palms over baby's ears, apply gentle traction downward until the anterior shoulder appears fully at the introitus; then upward to lift out the other shoulder.

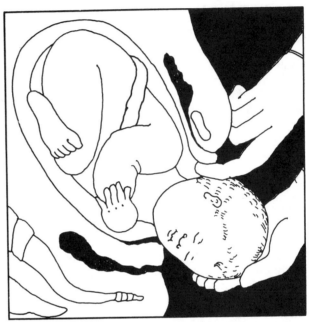

While gently supporting the head, during restitution and external rotation, feel around the neck for the umbilical cord, pulling gently to slacken it if necessary.

As the body emerges, slide your hand down the baby's back, cradling the buttocks in one hand, the head and the upper back in the other. Hold the head lower than the trunk.

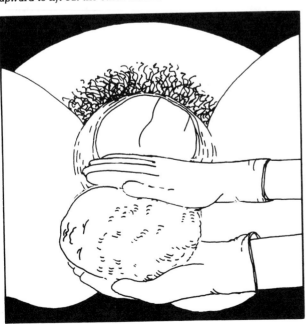

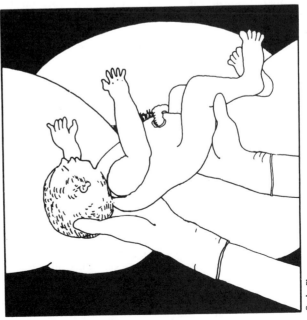

Creston Ely

baby's neck impinges under the *symphysis pubis* and the brow, nose, mouth, and chin emerge over the perineum. Restitution occurs as the baby's neck untwists on its shoulders, causing it to turn 45 degrees—that is, back to the position it was in prior to internal rotation.

External rotation is the visible result of the baby's *shoulders* rotating 45 degrees so that the bisacromial diameter is in the anteroposterior diameter of the mother's pelvis. The baby's head turns another 45 degrees so that the baby faces the mother's thigh. Then, as the anterior shoulder pivots under the *symphysis pubis*, the posterior shoulder is born over the perineum by a movement of lateral flexion(1).

Practical Hints for Delivery

WHERE? The woman may well be on the delivery table as you anticipate the immediate arrival of the birth attendant. A word to the wise: don't break the table. It takes practice to be able to handle a baby over a dropped table while accomplishing the following objectives:

- Holding the baby's head down to promote drainage of secretions
- Holding the baby close enough to the introitus so as not to pull on the cord
- Holding the baby at or above level of the introitus so as not to transfuse baby by gravity flow.

The labor bed or stretcher has certain advantages over the delivery table. First, if the mother is not already on the delivery table, the possibility of the baby's being born during the transfer from the bed to table is eliminated. The delivery of the baby's head cannot be controlled nor can the baby's overall safety be assured if birth occurs while the mother is being moved. Secondly, the labor bed or stretcher may well be more comfortable for the mother.

Disadvantages of the labor bed or stretcher include various factors. There may not be sufficient space to deliver the baby's shoulders, especially if the birth attendant is inexperienced. The perineum may not be clearly visible; the baby's nose and mouth may be inaccessible if you need to suction; or it may be difficult to keep the baby's face free from the amniotic fluid and blood pool. If necessary, the nurse may override these disadvantages by placing an upside-down, padded bedpan under the mother's hips. This provides as much as five inches of additional space between the perineum and the bed.

Another possibility is to ask the mother to raise her hips off the bed, which she can probably do rather easily with her feet planted firmly on the bed. Finally, one or two people may lift her a few inches off the bed with their hands under her buttocks.

MOTHER'S POSITION Elevate the head of the bed, table, or stretcher to at least 45 degrees. Lying flat is no way to give birth, primarily because the mother's *vena cava* and aorta are compressed and uteropla-

---

Common Circumstances Surrounding Emergency Deliveries

1. Multipara with history of rapid labors

2. Laboring woman who must travel a long distance to the hospital

3. Primipara with rapid labor (Adolescents seem to have labors at each extreme of the continuum—rapid or prolonged.)

4. Precipitous labor defined as less than three hours from onset to delivery

5. Unanticipated premature baby

---

cental blood flow is compromised in supine positions. A hypoxic baby is likely to be the result. An inexperienced birth attendant certainly wants to avoid a depressed baby at all costs. Maintaining good uteroplacental perfusion is the best way of assuring a well-oxygenated baby.

Elevating the head of the bed serves another purpose. The woman may well be frightened and need a great deal of support. Maintaining eye-to-eye contact, which is impossible if she is facing the ceiling, offers in itself more support and elicits more cooperation. The lateral Sims' position is probably the best choice, placing the least strain on the perineum and affording the best possible visualization of the birth. It also allows the necessary space for delivering the shoulders. Although few births in the U.S. are conducted using this position, some references do offer instruction about it(2).

STERILE TECHNIQUE Sterility is not a priority since surgery, vaginal intrusion, or the use of instruments is not involved in a normal vaginal delivery. It is important to bear several facts and principles in mind: The vagina intrinsically has a high bacterial count; few women have sterile uterine cavities during the postpartum period(3); vaginal examinations and cross-contamination are the primary causes of puerperal infection; and babies do not need to be in a sterile environment after birth.

The priorities relative to clean technique are: 1) cleansing one's hands, 2) cleansing mother's skin, 3) putting on gloves, 4) placing clean or sterile drapes under the mother, and 5) avoiding fecal contamination of the birth canal or baby.

PROTECTING THE PERINEUM Do not perform an episiotomy unless you are professionally and legally qualified to do so. The unexpecting birth attendant's greatest contribution will be fostering a slow birth of the baby's head. (See next paragraph.) Massaging and supporting the perineum may be helpful, but if you are inexperienced there are other priorities to consider. Trying to do too many things may cause you to forget the most important steps.

THE BIRTH Allow the woman to push during contractions until the perineum is thinning and distending and the infant's head is crowning. At this point coach her to blow through her contractions for the birth; the force of the uterine contractions will be sufficient to expel the baby.

As the head becomes progressively more visible, the attendant should gently place the flat of her hand, with fingers pointing toward the mother's rectum, on it. With this hand she can gently slow the baby's advance so that the maternal tissue gradually expands to accommodate it. Do not use great force. Do not apply uneven pressure with any part of your fingers or hand. Depending on the mother's tissue elasticity, she may go through one or several contractions with the head progressively more visible at the introitus. After the head is out to the forehead, it usually passes through smoothly and quickly.

Allow restitution and external rotation to occur, usually in a matter of seconds, gently supporting the head in your hand. With the other hand feel for the cord around the neck. It if is tight, pull gently to gain some slack so the shoulders may be born. Then place the palms of your hands on each side of the baby's head—over the ears. Apply gentle traction downward until you see the anterior shoulder appear fully at the vaginal opening, indicating that it has passed under the maternal *symphysis pubis*. Now apply upward traction to lift the posterior shoulder over the perineum.

As the body emerges, slide your hand down the baby's back, cradling the buttocks in one hand and the head and back in the other. Hold the head lower than the trunk. Place the baby on the mother's abdomen, steadying the baby as the mother takes the baby into her arms. Help her to keep the baby's head slightly lower than the rest of the body.

The following steps are then recommended:
1) Clear the airway and dry the baby with the baby at the level of the introitus.
2) Place the baby in the mother's arms or within her reach on her abdomen, attending to prevention of evaporative heat loss.
3) Clamp the cord when sterile equipment is available at about 60 seconds of age.

Caring for the Baby; Delivering the Placenta

Clearing the nose and mouth of mucus is important. A bulb syringe is useful for suctioning, but if you don't have one, passing your palm gently over the baby's face will wipe away much of the fluid and help decrease the possibility of aspiration.

The baby must be kept warm. This can be accomplished by placing mother, who should assume a semi-sitting position, and baby skin-to-skin and covering them with several layers of dry cloth, prefera-

bly warmed. The mother's body is a reliable heat source, and the layers of cloth will prevent evaporative loss of precious body heat(4). Don't forget to cover the baby's head, the largest portion of the baby's body.

With the baby cradled in this fashion, attend to the other priorities listed above, make essential observations, continue to clear the airway, and do the Apgar score. Meanwhile encourage the mother to put the baby to breast. Even if the baby nuzzles and licks but does not actually suck, oxytocin will be released from the pituitary, encouraging uterine contractions to help separate the placenta(4). After attending to all priorities, you can remove the wet inner layers from mother and baby and replace them with dry ones.

Writings conflict but most neonatologists advise against encouraging placental transfusion by milking the cord and awaiting the cessation of pulsation before clamping the cord. Placental transfusions can lead to hyperviscosity and significant problems for the baby. As a result, most experts recommend clamping at one minute of age to prevent hyperviscosity(5,6).

The rate of placental transfusion is dependent on time, gravity, and constriction of the umbilical vessels. Transfusion of the entire volume of placental blood can occur within three minutes, depending on the level of the baby at, above, or below the introitus. Minimal placental transfusion occurs with the baby at the level of the mother's breast when she is semi-

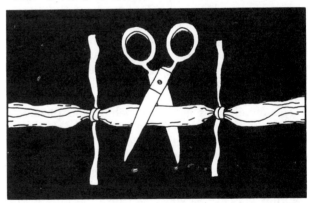

sitting. Significant and rapid transfusion occurs with the baby below the level of the introitus. The umbilical arteries effectively constrict by 45 to 60 seconds of age, while the umbilical vein is patent longer(6).

When clamping the cord, only sterile equipment (Kelly clamp, umbilical clamp, umbilical tape, boiled shoelaces) should be used. We know the disastrous results of clamping a cord with unsterile materials. Neonatal tetanus is a highly fatal, preventable disease.

Wait for the placenta to separate after clamping the cord. Signs of placental separation are: 1) a sudden gush of blood from the introitus, 2) lengthening of the cord, and 3) the fundus rising in the abdomen, becoming globular in shape, (previously dis-

Graphic Labor Record

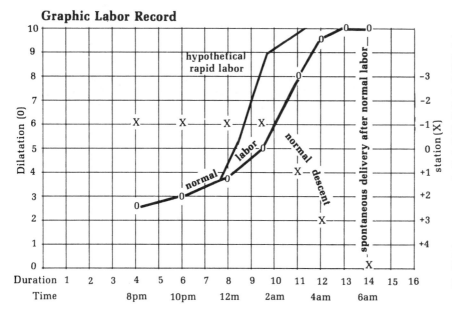

Normal labor is represented by the typical "S" curve for dilatation. The steeper curve indicates a hypothetical rapid labor. (Any curve which falls to the left of the S curve indicates a rapid labor.) If a woman progresses rapidly through the active phase of labor as shown by plotting her status on the graph, one may predict that all stages—including delivery—will progress rapidly. The mean durations of the active phase of labor are 4.6 hours for primiparas and 2.4 hours for multiparas.

Adapted from *Biological Principles and Modern Practice of Obstetrics* by J. P. Greenhill and Emanuel A. Friedman, Philadelphia, W. B. Saunders Co., 1974, p. 205. Used with permission.

coid, flatter, not quite as high in the abdomen). As the mother feels another urge to push, has a contraction, or feels pressure in the vagina, lift the placenta from the vagina by holding onto the umbilical cord. Guard against uterine inversion by placing your flat hand gently but firmly on the lower abdomen just above the *symphysis pubis*. Do not use much force as you guide the placenta along the curve of Carus (the curved angle from the cervix to the introitus which almost forms the lower fourth of a circle). Hold the umbilical cord near the introitus; the cord will be less likely to break or tear than it would be holding it farther back.

The membranes may trail behind the placenta. Take hold of them and with a gentle up, down, and out motion tease them out. After the delivery of the placenta and membranes, place one hand on the fundus and massage gently to firm the uterus, which occludes bleeding vessels at the placental site. Avoid vigorous massage as you may cause the muscles to fatigue and thus increase uterine bleeding. Another danger of vigorous fundal massage is prolapse or inversion of the uterus.

Some Problems You Might Encounter

MECONIUM PASSAGE   The infant is or has been stressed when this sign is present. Make additional effort to obtain assistance in case the baby needs to be resuscitated. With meconium in the amniotic fluid, clearing the oral and nasal passages before the onset of respiration becomes a top priority. This means suctioning the nose and mouth before the body of the baby is born if at all possible. A DeLee mucous trap is preferred for this purpose(7).

TIGHT NUCHAL CORD   If the cord is visible after the baby's head is born and seems to be stretched tautly, try to slide your finger under it and get some slack. If this isn't possible, clamping the cord twice and cutting between the clamps is in order. If no clamps are available, continue assisting with the baby's birth and unwind the cord as soon as the baby's body is born.

SHOULDER DYSTOCIA   In spite of efforts to recognize shoulder dystocia before a birth occurs and plan for a difficult delivery, such a potential disaster may still occur. The essential problem is one of the bisacromial diameter exceeding the anteroposterior or oblique diameter of the pelvic inlet. Several steps should be taken immediately:

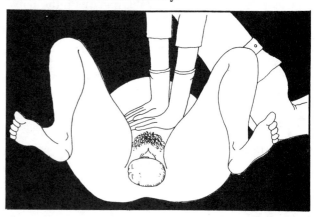

1) Have the mother flex her legs onto her abdomen as though she were squatting. This will increase the anteroposterior diameter of the outlet.
2) Don't apply fundal pressure.

3) Do apply suprapubic pressure. Have someone else apply straight arm pressure with two flat palms placed one over the other directly over the suprapubic area. Lean onto the mother's suprapubic area. This maneuver will serve to collapse the shoulders, allowing them to enter the pelvis. (This does not fracture the clavicles.) Proceed with steps for delivery of the shoulders(1).

DEPRESSED BABY The ABCs (airway, breathing, circulation) of infant resuscitation are essential knowledge and skill for anyone who is around newborns. Periodic review of the related theoretical information and supervised clinical practice in this technique will allow the nurse to provide this essential care for a newborn infant who requires it(8-10).

> **Physical and Behavioral Signs of Imminent Delivery**
>
> Involuntary catching of breath and pushing, even subtly, during a contraction
>
> Thrashing about in bed; absorption in self; change in breathing patterns; expressing the feeling, "I can't go on any longer." (These behaviors often indicate the transition phase of labor—which may be immediately followed by delivery.)
>
> Increasing bloody show
>
> Increased facial flushing and diaphoresis
>
> Increased sensation of pressure in pelvis
>
> Beginning of "blossoming" of the anus
>
> Appearance of fullness at perineum
>
> "Crowning"—appearance of head at introitus. (In multipara birth is very imminent. In primipara birth may be up to 30 minutes later. When head stays visible between contractions, birth is nearing.)

EXCESSIVE MATERNAL BLEEDING Postpartum hemorrhage can be life-threatening. Bleeding can arise from the uterus, cervix, or vagina.

Uterus. When excessive bleeding begins before the placenta is delivered, massage the fundus gently. This should stimulate the uterus to contract and facilitate placental separation. Putting the baby to breast will also promote this process. With the placenta delivered or retained, bimanual uterine compression done externally or internally may also help(3,11).

Cervical and Vaginal. Lacerations of the cervix and vagina are unlikely in a birth in which instruments and/or vigorous exams or manipulations are not used. They can happen, however, especially with a precipitous labor. Suturing will help control bleeding and, of course, approximate tissues. While awaiting the arrival of a physician, measures to prevent shock may be instituted. Using the Trendelenburg position and maintaining blood pressure with isotonic fluids are two important measures.

Perineal Lacerations. External lacerations may also bleed profusely. Direct pressure with sterile gauze or cloth compresses will probably control such bleeding. If such lacerations aren't bleeding excessively, nothing is required so long as they are sutured within a few hours so that closure by primary intention can occur(12).

Emotional Components

When a woman delivers her baby under unexpected circumstances, she will undoubtedly be anxious. Several simple measures will promote a positive birth experience and gain the cooperation of the woman in achieving a slow, gentle delivery. First, the nurse should speak calmly. Shouting for help and expressing your own fears will serve only to agitate the woman. As you proceed, explain what you are doing and give the mother clear, concise instructions, demonstrating and leading her breathing pattern whenever possible.

Finally, include any family members who are present or friends who are present. This will not only help put the woman at ease, but will ready people to assist you if necessary. While physical safety of mother and infant must clearly be the first concern, a birth is a very important emotional event as well. Making it as positive as possible from this standpoint will be gratifying for all concerned—mother, child, and nurse.

REFERENCES

1. OXORN, HARRY, AND FOOTE, WILLIAM. *Human Labor and Birth.* 3d ed. New York, Appleton-Century-Crofts, 1976.
2. TOWLER, JEAN, AND BUTLER-MANUEL, ROY. *Modern Obstetrics for Student Midwives.* Chicago, Year Book Medical Publishers, 1974, p. 360.
3. HELLMAN, L. M., AND OTHERS, EDS. *Williams' Obstetrics.* 14th ed. New York, Appleton-Century-Crofts, 1972.
4. KLAUS, M. H., AND KENNELL, JOHN. *Maternal-Infant Bonding: The Impact of Early Separation or Loss on Family Development.* St. Louis, C. V. Mosby Co., 1976.
5. KRAYBILL, ERNEST. Needs of the term infant. IN *Neonatology,* ed. by Gordon Avery. Philadelphia, J. B. Lippincott Co., 1975, p. 151.
6. YAO, A. C., AND LIND, JOHN. Cord clamping time—influence on the newborn. *Birth Fam.J.* 4:98, Fall 1977.
7. CARSON, B. S., AND OTHERS. Combined obstetric and pediatric approach to prevent meconium aspiration syndrome. *Am.J.Obstet.Gynecol.* 126:712-715, Nov. 15, 1976.
8. KLAUS, M. A., AND FANAROFF, A. A. *Care of the High Risk Neonate.* Philadelphia, W. B. Saunders Co., 1973, pp. 1-22.
9. TOOLEY, WILLIAM, AND PHIBBS, RODERIC. Delivery room management of the newborn. IN *Neonatology,* ed. by Gordon Avery. Philadelphia, J. B. Lippincott Co., 1975, pp. 111-125.
10. ABRAMSON, HAROLD, ED. *Resuscitation of the Newborn Infant.* 3d. ed. St. Louis, C. V. Mosby Co., 1973.
11. WHITE, GREGORY. *Emergency Childbirth, A Manual.* Franklin Park, Ill., Police Training Education, 1973, pp. 35-39. (3412 Ruby St., Franklin Park, Ill. 60131).
12. HARKINS, H. N. Wound Healing. IN *Surgery: Principles and Practice,* 3rd edition, edited by J. G. Allen and others. Philadelphia, J. P. Lippincott Co., 1965, p. 9.

Nursing Care of the Child

Coordinator

Mariann C. Lovell, MS, RN

Contributor to this Edition

Elizabeth J. Lipp, MS, RN

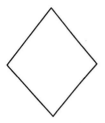

Questions

Toilet training is a problem for the mother of 18-month-old Susie. She states that "Grandma says Susie should be potty trained by now, but she's still wearing diapers because she's stubborn and won't use the potty."

1. What is the nurse's best response to Susie's mother?
   ○ 1. "Most children are not ready to be toilet trained until 18 months of age."
   ○ 2. "Susie should be potty trained by now, and needs to be evaluated for developmental delay."
   ○ 3. "Keep her in diapers and forget about toilet training; she'll train herself."
   ○ 4. "Susie is stubborn and must sit on the potty once every 2 hours during the day."

2. Which of the following is *not* a cue or sign of readiness for toilet training?
   ○ 1. Ability of child to walk confidently
   ○ 2. Capability of child to hold urine for 2 hours
   ○ 3. Child's awareness of soiled or wet diaper
   ○ 4. Child begins teething

Kelly Patrick is sitting with her 18-month-old daughter, Kathy, at the well-baby clinic. She tells the nurse that Kathy has been "driving her crazy" by saying "no" to everything, and she needs help in handling her.

3. The nurse explains to Mrs. Patrick that Kathy's negativism is normal for a toddler and that this helps her daughter meet which of the following needs?
   ○ 1. Discipline
   ○ 2. Independence
   ○ 3. Trust
   ○ 4. Consistency

4. Mrs. Patrick states, "This morning I gave Kathy her orange juice and she said 'No.' I'm worried and frustrated. She needs her fluids. What should I do?" What is the nurse's best response?
   ○ 1. Offer her a choice of 2 things to drink.
   ○ 2. Be firm and hand her the glass.
   ○ 3. Distract her with some food.
   ○ 4. Withhold fluids until she drinks the orange juice.

5. The nurse plans to talk with Mrs. Patrick about toilet training Kathy, knowing that the most important factor in toilet training is which of the following?
   ○ 1. Mother's willingness to work at it
   ○ 2. Starting early and being consistent
   ○ 3. Approach and attitude of mother
   ○ 4. Developmental readiness of child

6. Before Mrs. Patrick leaves the clinic, the nurse tells her she can best help Kathy learn to control her own behavior at this age by
   ○ 1. punishing her when she deserves it.
   ○ 2. setting limits and being consistent.
   ○ 3. allowing her to learn by her mistakes.
   ○ 4. letting her be a baby, because she is too young to control her behavior.

A nurse-consultant for a preschool nursery is asked to speak to the parents' group. They ask a number of questions. In each situation, what is the nurse's best response?

7. "My 4-year-old is a picky eater and only wants peanut butter sandwiches. What can I do to get him to eat a more balanced diet?"
   ○ 1. "Serve him a balanced diet and teach him to clean his plate."
   ○ 2. "Withhold all between-meal foods and serve him only at family mealtime."
   ○ 3. "Offer him a balanced diet and do not let him have dessert if he does not take at least 2 bites of each food."
   ○ 4. "Offer the child 1 small helping of each food at mealtime, and a protein or fruit snack at midmorning and midafternoon."

8. "I'm afraid my 4-year-old will get sick if he doesn't eat more; he used to be such a good eater. What can I do to increase his appetite?"
   ○ 1. "The fourth year is a slow-growth period, and the appetite will remain decreased until the growth spurt occurs in school-age years."
   ○ 2. "Four-year-olds should have an appetite increase to match normal rapid growth; take your child to the pediatrician for a checkup."
   ○ 3. "Withhold all between-meal foods and serve him only at family mealtime."
   ○ 4. "Gradually increase the size of servings on the child's plate and insist he remain at the table until the plate is clean."

9. "I can't believe how messy my 3-year-old is. How can I train her to have some table manners, so the rest of us can stand to eat with her?"
   ○ 1. "The 3-year-old can learn to hold a knife and fork and serve herself without spilling. Insist that she practice these behaviors."
   ○ 2. "The 3-year-old does not have the motor skills to sit quietly, hold a knife and fork perfectly, or serve herself without spilling. Establish a few rules and assist your child with cutting and serving."
   ○ 3. "Establish mealtime rules and insist that the 3-year-old learn the family table manners from the beginning."
   ○ 4. "Don't worry about table manners; just serve the child finger foods and let her eat by herself."

10. "My 4-year-old refuses to go to sleep without a light on. How can I get him to give up the night-light?"
   ○ 1. "Tell him that only babies have night-lights; he is too old for this behavior."
   ○ 2. "Let him go to sleep with the night-light, but then turn it off when he's asleep."
   ○ 3. "Give him a flashlight and tell him to use it to explore the dark room."
   ○ 4. "Lights help a child deal with fears; let him turn the light on and off as he wishes, and he will give it up when he does not need it any more."

11. "My 4-year-old is still wetting his bed almost every night. Is this abnormal, and what can I do to train him?"
   ○ 1. "Restrict all fluids after 5:00 P.M. and scold him; he is too old to wet the bed and must be trained to stay dry."
   ○ 2. "Get him up to urinate at midnight, and he will be able to stay dry until morning. He is too old to wet the bed."
   ○ 3. "Put him in diapers and tell him to get up if he has to urinate; 4-year-olds should learn to urinate in the potty."
   ○ 4. "Nighttime control is achieved between 3 and 5 years of age. Time and patience will lead to physical ability for nighttime control of urine."

12. "My 4-year-old tells lies all the time. What can I do about this?"
   ○ 1. "Confront the child with this behavior and let him know that lying is not acceptable."
   ○ 2. "The 4-year-old is old enough to tell the truth; ask him why he is not truthful."
   ○ 3. "The 4-year-old has a vivid imagination; ignore his lying and focus on reality."
   ○ 4. "The 4-year-old has a vivid imagination; acknowledge his stories or fantasies by saying, 'What a nice story,' or, 'That's a pretend story.'"

13. "How should I respond to my 3½-year-old when he touches his genitals or masturbates?"
   ○ 1. "Permit the child to explore his body and explain that masturbation is a private activity that is normal and acceptable in private."
   ○ 2. "Do not allow the child to masturbate; distract him with other interests."
   ○ 3. "Set firm limits and do not permit the child to indulge in this self-stimulation."
   ○ 4. "Masturbation is a sign of an emotional disorder and requires the assistance of a child-behavior specialist."

14. Two inquisitive parents want to know more about diphtheria and how it is diagnosed. The nurse begins the discussion by telling them which of the following tests is used in the diagnosis of diphtheria?
   ○ 1. Schick
   ○ 2. Dick
   ○ 3. Guthrie
   ○ 4. Heterophil antibody

15. The parents of a 2-year-old express concern about their daughter's temper tantrums. The nurse should include which piece of information about the child's behavior?
○ **1.** It indicates regression.
○ **2.** It should be controlled by parental discipline.
○ **3.** It is a normal expression of tension.
○ **4.** It suggests an interference with development.

Kimberly, aged 5, visits the pediatrician for her annual health visit. As an infant, she had the full recommended series of immunizations. Her last immunization was at 18 months of age.

16. Which of the following immunizations should Kimberly receive at this visit?
○ **1.** DTP and OPV boosters, Tine test
○ **2.** Tb and OPV vaccines
○ **3.** Measles and mumps vaccines, Tine test
○ **4.** No immunizations are indicated

17. As a 5-year-old in kindergarten, Kimberly would be expected to do all the following except one. Which of the following is *not* characteristic of this age?
○ **1.** Draw a person with 6 parts
○ **2.** Skip and hop
○ **3.** Use sentences of adult length
○ **4.** Tie her shoelaces

18. One day Kimberly's mother discovers Kimberly and her cousin, Will, aged 7, undressed and curiously looking at and touching each other's bodies. What is Kimberly's mother's best initial response?
○ **1.** "Will, it's time for you to go home."
○ **2.** "Kimberly, we're going to have a talk when your daddy gets home."
○ **3.** "Kimberly and Will, please put your clothes on. I'm going to wait in the kitchen for you."
○ **4.** "What are you children doing in here?"

19. Kimberly asks about her grandmother's death. Which statement is most characteristic of the child between 5 and 8 years of age regarding this topic?
○ **1.** The child conceptualizes death as a separate person such as the boogeyman or as a dead person.
○ **2.** The child is aware that death is permanent.
○ **3.** The child is aware that he himself will die.
○ **4.** The child is aware that death is inevitable.

Steve, aged 8, and his brother Charlie, aged 10, race to the breakfast table to see who gets a certain seat. This is usually followed by an argument.

20. Which of the following approaches is most effective in handling the above situation?
○ **1.** Tell the boys to eat at the counter.
○ **2.** Let Charlie choose his place, because he is older.
○ **3.** Assign the boys to places at the table.
○ **4.** Solicit the boys' ideas as to how to resolve the problem.

21. Which of the following guidelines is *least* appropriate for parents of school-age children?
○ **1.** Have the child eat most of the meal before offering second helpings or between-meal snacks.
○ **2.** Avoid forcing the child to eat or using desserts as rewards for eating disliked foods.
○ **3.** Deprive the child of a favorite food as punishment.
○ **4.** Maintain good nutrition by having only fruit, vegetables, cheese, and protein snacks available.

22. Which of the following is the *least* effective approach to teaching nutrition to school-age children?
○ **1.** Discuss nutrition without reference to "right" and "wrong."
○ **2.** Present consequences of eating a balanced versus an unbalanced diet.
○ **3.** Stress the importance of good table manners.
○ **4.** Encourage children to keep a journal for 3 days to monitor types of food consumed.

23. What is the major psychosocial task for both Steve and Charlie, according to Erikson's theory of development?
○ **1.** Trust versus mistrust
○ **2.** Autonomy versus shame and doubt
○ **3.** Industry versus inferiority
○ **4.** Identity versus role diffusion

24. Both boys are in the stage of cognitive development defined by Piaget as
○ **1.** concrete operations.
○ **2.** symbolism.
○ **3.** preoperational thinking.
○ **4.** formal operations.

Marian Taylor is a 6-year-old with recurrent infection of the tonsils.

25. Mrs. Taylor was told by the surgeon that the child would be scheduled for surgical removal of her tonsils and adenoids the following week. The nurse suggests that the mother can best prepare Marion by carrying out which of the following plans?
    ○ 1. Avoid talking about the surgery in Marian's presence because she will be frightened and uncooperative if she knows what is going to take place.
    ○ 2. Tell Marian that she is going on a "trip" to the hospital and it will be a very pleasant experience for her.
    ○ 3. Prepare Marian for the procedure by telling her that it will be very painful and unpleasant but there is nothing else to do but get it over with.
    ○ 4. Tell Marian about the proposed surgery 6 days before admission and emphasize that she will feel much better after her tonsils have been removed.

26. Marian will probably best accept her hospitalization if her mother does which one of the following?
    ○ 1. Tells her that she will be given medicine to make her sleep so she will not know what is going on while she is there
    ○ 2. Allows the child to help pack her own suitcase and choose the toys or books she wishes to take along
    ○ 3. Does not tell her about the hospital visit until just before the time to leave home
    ○ 4. Warns Marian that she must cooperate with the doctors and nurses or they will have to give her a "shot" to help her get well

27. Upon Marian's admission to the hospital, the laboratory technician visits Marian to obtain a sample of blood. Marian asks the nurse if the technician is going to hurt her. What is the best response?
    ○ 1. "Of course not. You won't feel a thing."
    ○ 2. "I don't know, but even if she does, you must not complain."
    ○ 3. "It will probably hurt a little bit, but we are doing this because we want to take very good care of you."
    ○ 4. "Yes, it will hurt, but we have to know your blood type if you need a blood transfusion after your tonsils are taken out."

28. Marian asks what they will do with her blood sample after it is taken. What is the best response to this question?
    ○ 1. "The technician will examine it carefully, so we will know exactly what we need to do to help you get well."
    ○ 2. "I can't explain that to you, because you are too little to understand."
    ○ 3. "They are going to take it to the laboratory and do experiments on it."
    ○ 4. "They will keep it in case something goes wrong while you are having your tonsils removed."

29. Before Marian goes to surgery it is very important that the nurse keep an accurate record of her vital signs. What is the reason for this?
    ○ 1. Any change in the vital signs would indicate the need for immediate surgery.
    ○ 2. An elevated temperature or change in vital signs may indicate an infection, which would prohibit surgery until the infection had subsided.
    ○ 3. Hemorrhage before surgery is quite common in cases of chronic tonsilitis.
    ○ 4. The child may need intravenous fluids or a blood transfusion before surgery if the vital signs are not within normal range.

30. Immediately after surgery, the nurse should place Marian in which of the following positions?
    ○ 1. Fowler's
    ○ 2. Semi-prone with pillow under chest, head lower than chest
    ○ 3. On her abdomen
    ○ 4. Lithotomy position

31. What is the most common complication in the post-op period?
    ○ 1. Loss of speech
    ○ 2. Hemorrhage
    ○ 3. Abdominal distension
    ○ 4. Loss of hearing

32. The evening of her operative day, Marian becomes restless and wants to get out of bed. What should the nurse do?
    ○ 1. Allow Marian's mother to hold the child in her lap and rock her for awhile.
    ○ 2. Tell Marian to sit quietly in bed so that she will get better faster.
    ○ 3. Permit Marian to walk in the halls, so she will sleep better at night.
    ○ 4. Restrain Marian to keep her from sitting up or getting out of bed.

33. The nurse should know that according to Piaget, Marian's level of cognitive development would most likely be
○ **1.** formal operational.
○ **2.** concrete operational.
○ **3.** preconceptual.
○ **4.** intuitive.

William Smith, 12 months old, has had an elevated temperature for 48 hours. There is evidence of nuchal rigidity, increasing lethargy, and nausea and vomiting. He is also dehydrated. Meningitis is suspected.

34. Which of the following observations would probably alert the nurse to William's dehydrated state?
○ **1.** Moist mucous membranes
○ **2.** Depressed anterior fontanel
○ **3.** Urine specific gravity of 1.007
○ **4.** 5% weight gain

35. William's physician will most likely need which of the following?
○ **1.** Thoracentesis tray
○ **2.** Lumbar puncture tray
○ **3.** Nasogastric tube
○ **4.** Foley catheter

36. William's physician has ordered 5% dextrose in 0.33% normal saline with 20 mEq of potassium chloride (KCl) to infuse at 32 ml/hour. Which of the following should be brought to the physician's attention immediately?
○ **1.** William has not voided in 4 hours.
○ **2.** William has had 3 liquid green stools.
○ **3.** William has vomited 50 ml mucus.
○ **4.** William is fussy and irritable when moved.

37. During the acute stages of Williams's illness, which of the following nursing actions should receive highest priority?
○ **1.** Give frequent tepid sponge baths.
○ **2.** Perform treatments as quickly as possible.
○ **3.** Reduce environmental stimuli.
○ **4.** Monitor vital signs every 5 to 10 minutes.

Eight-year-old Carlos comes to the physician's office with a sore throat, enlarged cervical lymph nodes, elevated temperature, and malaise. He has a history of frequent streptococcal throat infections.

38. Carlos has bacterial pharyngitis and is put on a regimen of oral penicillin. Which of the following instructions to Carlos's parents is most important at this time?
○ **1.** Have him gargle with a hot saline solution as needed.
○ **2.** Give Carlos the medicine for 10 days or until it is gone.
○ **3.** Feed him a soft diet until he feels better.
○ **4.** Ensure he gets a lot of vitamin C foods, such as orange juice.

39. Carlos returns in 2 months for a tonsillectomy. Preparation for hospitalization includes books for him to read. His mother should be advised to select a book with which of the following characteristics?
○ **1.** Small, paperback
○ **2.** Large-size print
○ **3.** Regular-size print
○ **4.** Large, with stiffened pages

40. After surgery, what assessment data may indicate that Carlos is hemorrhaging?
○ **1.** Tachycardia, hypertension, hemoptysis
○ **2.** Bradycardia, hypotension, increased swallowing
○ **3.** Tachycardia, hypotension, increased swallowing
○ **4.** Tachycardia, hypotension, decreased swallowing

41. Carlos's nurse prepares the family for his discharge. Which of the following instructions should be emphasized?
○ **1.** Return to school in 1 to 2 weeks
○ **2.** No vigorous activities for 3 to 4 weeks
○ **3.** Saline gargles as necessary for comfort
○ **4.** Delayed hemorrhage may occur on the third post-op day.

Four-year-old Judy is in a private room with "hand and linen precautions." She was admitted today for weight loss, anorexia, vaginitis, and insomnia. Lab tests include blood, urine, and stool tests. Results of lab tests are not on the chart yet. The nurse observes Judy scratching in the anal area at night.

42. Assessing the situation, the nurse suspects that Judy may have which one of the following problems?
○ **1.** Ulcerative colitis
○ **2.** Pinworm infestation
○ **3.** Diabetes
○ **4.** Ringworm

43. The nurse decides to assess further and writes which of the following nursing orders on Judy's care plan?
    ○ 1. Clinitest QID
    ○ 2. Scotch tape test in early morning before arising
    ○ 3. Scotch tape test after each bowel movement
    ○ 4. Bland diet, small frequent feedings

44. During nap time, Judy wet her bed. What action should the nurse take?
    ○ 1. Change Judy's clothes and bed and make no issue of it.
    ○ 2. Tell her big girls should call the nurse.
    ○ 3. Put her in diapers and note this in Kardex.
    ○ 4. Keep the bedpan in bed at nap time.

Carol Rauch yells for her nurse-neighbor to come and look at 2-year-old Kirsten Rauch. The nurse finds the child sitting in the middle of the bathroom floor with several open medicine bottles strewn around the room. She is chewing on something and has white powder around her mouth.

45. Mrs. Rauch says, "Do something!" What should be the nurse's first action?
    ○ 1. Call the poison control center.
    ○ 2. Determine what Kirsten ate or drank.
    ○ 3. Take Kirsten to the emergency room.
    ○ 4. Observe Kirsten closely to see if any symptoms develop.

46. The nurse determines that Kirsten ate only a few acetaminophen (Tylenol) tablets and a couple of her mother's arthritis capsules. The child is alert. The most appropriate nursing action would be which of the following?
    ○ 1. Give her milk to coat her stomach and delay absorption.
    ○ 2. Keep her NPO and observe her for symptoms.
    ○ 3. Give 15 ml of syrup of ipecac and lots of water.
    ○ 4. Give activated charcoal.

47. When Kirsten is out of immediate danger, the nurse explores with Mrs. Rauch how to prevent another episode such as this. The plan for prevention will *not* include which of the following?
    ○ 1. Label all containers.
    ○ 2. Place harmful substances out of Kirsten's reach.
    ○ 3. Teach Kirsten what is poisonous and what is not.
    ○ 4. Never refer to medicine as candy.

48. The best indicator that this teaching was successful is which of the following?
    ○ 1. Kirsten survives with no ill effects from the incident.
    ○ 2. Mrs. Rauch knows the correct first aid for poisoning.
    ○ 3. Kirsten returns to her normal activities.
    ○ 4. The Rauch home is modified to prevent a recurrence of this situation.

49. Which observation by the nurse best indicates that Kirsten is at her normal developmental level?
    ○ 1. Easily undresses herself, but needs help putting her clothes on
    ○ 2. Points to her body parts
    ○ 3. Puts objects into holes and smaller objects into larger ones
    ○ 4. Builds a tower out of 2 blocks

Three-year-old Sandy has cerebral palsy, spastic type, with a severe motor impairment. Her mother has brought her to the clinic because she is having difficulty feeding Sandy.

50. The nurse most likely observes which of the following manifestations in Sandy?
    ○ 1. Hypotonic muscles
    ○ 2. Mental retardation
    ○ 3. Scissoring of legs
    ○ 4. Absent deep tendon reflexes

51. To improve Sandy's eating abilities, the nurse should counsel her mother to do which of the following?
    ○ 1. Place Sandy in a semi-Fowler's position with her head to one side and allow her to suck liquids and pureed foods through a sturdy straw.
    ○ 2. Encourage Sandy to feed herself to increase her independence.
    ○ 3. Stand behind Sandy, support her jaw with one hand, and use the other hand to handle the cup or spoon to feed Sandy.
    ○ 4. Place Sandy in a sitting position, tilt her head slightly back, and use a Brecht feeder to give liquids and pureed foods.

52. Sandy's mother is pregnant and asks whether her second baby is likely to have cerebral palsy also. She states that the doctors do not know why Sandy has cerebral palsy. What is the nurse's best response?
    ○ **1.** "There is a strong possibility that your next baby may have cerebral palsy also."
    ○ **2.** "Perhaps you were exposed to some illness or took some harmful medication when you were pregnant with Sandy."
    ○ **3.** "You're concerned that your next baby may have cerebral palsy."
    ○ **4.** "Your attending prepared childbirth classes can lessen the possibility of birth trauma and decrease the risk of cerebral palsy."

Suzi Jones is a newborn with Down syndrome. Her parents have been told the diagnosis and are in the process of trying to adjust to this.

53. Which of the following is most appropriate to include when counseling Mr. and Mrs. Jones?
    ○ **1.** Suzi's developmental potential is greatest during infancy.
    ○ **2.** Suzi will be severely retarded.
    ○ **3.** Suzi will be spastic, so positioning should be discussed.
    ○ **4.** Suzi will be as susceptible to colds as her older brother.

54. Which of the following is an *incorrect* statement regarding Down syndrome?
    ○ **1.** It is associated with a higher incidence of congenital heart disease.
    ○ **2.** It is associated with a higher incidence of gastrointestinal defects.
    ○ **3.** It is associated with a higher incidence of leukemia.
    ○ **4.** It is inherited as an autosomal recessive trait.

55. Which of the following measures is of primary importance for parents with a young, mentally retarded child at home?
    ○ **1.** Limit the amount of environmental stimulation the child is exposed to.
    ○ **2.** Have the same parent teach the child new skills at all times.
    ○ **3.** Teach the child socially acceptable behaviors so s/he can join the family on outings.
    ○ **4.** Maintain a consistent routine for daily activities.

Baby Girl Carlton was born yesterday with a myelomeningocele, which is covered with a thin, fragile membrane. She is now in the special care nursery.

56. When her father visits her for the first time, he is most likely to exhibit behaviors that indicate which phase of the grief process?
    ○ **1.** Anger
    ○ **2.** Depression
    ○ **3.** Disbelief
    ○ **4.** Bargaining

57. Mr. Carlton is standing hesitantly beside the Isolette. What is the nurse's best initial action?
    ○ **1.** Show Mr. Carlton how to stroke and talk to his daughter.
    ○ **2.** Give him a detailed explanation of his daughter's defect.
    ○ **3.** Ask if he wants to hold his daughter.
    ○ **4.** Ask him how his wife is doing.

58. Preoperatively, what is the priority nursing goal for Baby Girl Carlton?
    ○ **1.** Prevent contractures of her lower extremities.
    ○ **2.** Protect the sac from injury.
    ○ **3.** Promote parent-infant bonding.
    ○ **4.** Maintain adequate hydration.

59. Which of the following measures would be most comforting for Baby Girl Carlton?
    ○ **1.** Decorate her crib with brightly colored mobiles.
    ○ **2.** Hold her closely and rock her.
    ○ **3.** Place a music box in her crib.
    ○ **4.** Sit at her cribside and talk to her.

60. Which nursing measure for Baby Girl Carlton would be most dangerous preoperatively?
    ○ **1.** Place her in a prone position.
    ○ **2.** Massage her skin periodically with lotion.
    ○ **3.** Apply dry sterile dressings on the sac.
    ○ **4.** Empty her bladder by applying downward pressure over the suprapubic area.

61. Baby Girl Carlton's defect is surgically closed. Postoperatively, it is imperative that the nurse assess her for
    ○ **1.** increased head circumference.
    ○ **2.** tachycardia.
    ○ **3.** lower extremity movement.
    ○ **4.** bladder function.

62. Postoperatively, Baby Girl Carlton's IV is prescribed to infuse at 8 ml/hour. How many drops per minute should the nurse regulate the microdrip to infuse?
    ○ **1.** 2 drops/minute
    ○ **2.** 4 drops/minute
    ○ **3.** 8 drops/minute
    ○ **4.** 12 drops/minute

63. Knowing the associated incidence of congenital hip dysplasia in infants with myelomeningocele, Baby Girl Carlton's hips should be maintained in which position?
    ○ **1.** Adduction
    ○ **2.** Abduction
    ○ **3.** Internal rotation
    ○ **4.** External rotation

64. Baby Girl Carlton's parents have named her Natalie. Three days postoperatively, while in her crib, Natalie begins to have a grand mal seizure with tonic and clonic movements. Which nursing measure should be implemented first?
    ○ **1.** Hold Natalie's arms close to her body.
    ○ **2.** Place a small padded tongue blade between her gums.
    ○ **3.** Administer oxygen by mask.
    ○ **4.** Put a blanket between Natalie and the crib rails.

65. Natalie is given phenytoin sodium (Dilantin) elixir. Children are generally given higher doses of phenytoin per kilogram of body weight than adults. What is the reason for this?
    ○ **1.** Children excrete anticonvulsants more readily from the body.
    ○ **2.** Children's seizures are usually more severe.
    ○ **3.** Children are less likely to develop toxic reactions to anticonvulsants.
    ○ **4.** Higher doses are necessary to prevent paradoxical effects from occurring.

66. Natalie will be discharged on a regimen of phenytoin. It is important to teach her parents to observe for all the side effects. Which of the following is *not* a side effect of this drug?
    ○ **1.** Gingival hypertrophy
    ○ **2.** Skin rash
    ○ **3.** Nausea and vomiting
    ○ **4.** Excessive sleepiness

67. After 1 month, Natalie is returned for an evaluation of her neurologic status. The physician decides to admit her because a CT scan shows developing hydrocephalus. When assessing Natalie for signs of increased intracranial pressure, the nurse observes which of the following signs that indicate her pressure is increasing?
    ○ **1.** High-pitched cry
    ○ **2.** Absence of neonatal reflexes
    ○ **3.** Sunken fontanel
    ○ **4.** Pinpoint pupils

68. A ventriculoperitoneal (VP) shunt is done, and a Holter valve is surgically inserted. Post-op nursing assessment and discharge teaching should be guided by the knowledge that which of the following are the most common complications of VP shunts?
    ○ **1.** Hemorrhage and subdural hematoma
    ○ **2.** Ascites and peritonitis
    ○ **3.** Obstruction and infection
    ○ **4.** Shunt or peritoneal catheter breakage

69. The physician has written an order to pump Natalie's shunt 4 times each shift. Natalie's parents ask why this needs to be done. The nurse explains that the primary purpose of pumping the shunt valve is to
    ○ **1.** maintain patency of the shunt.
    ○ **2.** prevent Natalie from having seizures.
    ○ **3.** minimize the possibility of the development of mental retardation.
    ○ **4.** prevent infection of the shunt.

70. What is the nursing priority for Natalie postoperatively?
    ○ **1.** Help Natalie's parents cope with having a disabled child.
    ○ **2.** Prevent skin breakdown of the scalp.
    ○ **3.** Prevent overhydration.
    ○ **4.** Promote adequate nutrition.

71. Which of the following is the best indicator of a successful outcome of Natalie's care?
    ○ **1.** The degree of attachment between Natalie and her parents
    ○ **2.** Natalie's physical growth
    ○ **3.** Natalie's cognitive and motor skills
    ○ **4.** Natalie's temperament and social skills

One morning, Doris and Carl Howard find their previously healthy 3-month-old daughter Hilary face down in her crib. She is not breathing and is limp. They rush her to the emergency room where Hilary is pronounced dead. The cause is attributed to sudden infant death syndrome (SIDS).

72. Three of the following nursing actions would be appropriate at this time? Which one would *not* be appropriate?
    ○ **1.** Provide the Howards with a fully detailed explanation of SIDS.
    ○ **2.** Allow the Howards to be alone with their daughter's body for a short time.
    ○ **3.** Call a relative or close friend to come to the hospital to be with them.
    ○ **4.** Place an arm around their shoulders and say, "I'm so sorry."

73. A short time later, Mr. Howard says, "She was so healthy. I just can't understand what would have caused this. What did we do wrong?" The nurse's response should be based on the knowledge that SIDS may be attributed to
○ **1.** an anaphylactic reaction to some allergenic substance.
○ **2.** suffocation by crib blankets.
○ **3.** previously undetected viral pneumonia.
○ **4.** an unknown cause.

74. While assessing the Howards during a follow-up home visit, what is the best indicator of their successful coping with the loss of their daughter?
○ **1.** Moving to a new residence
○ **2.** Involving themselves in a SIDS support group
○ **3.** Attending their church regularly
○ **4.** Returning to work

Six-month-old Jesus Sanchez is admitted to the pediatric unit with a diagnosis of bronchiolitis. He has a 2½-year-old sibling.

75. Which of the following manifestations is most suggestive of bronchiolitis?
○ **1.** Diminished breath sounds
○ **2.** Dry hacky cough
○ **3.** Serous nasal discharge
○ **4.** Shortened expiratory phase

76. Jesus is kept NPO. What is the best rationale for this?
○ **1.** Hypoxemia reduces gastrointestinal motility.
○ **2.** Oral fluids increase mucus production.
○ **3.** Tachypnea predisposes an infant to aspiration.
○ **4.** Hydration is not a concern with bronchiolitis.

77. Which of the following would *not* be included in a nursing care plan for Jesus?
○ **1.** Suction deeply.
○ **2.** Set up mist tent with oxygen.
○ **3.** Maintain adequate hydration.
○ **4.** Monitor for cor pulmonale.

78. Which position would be most appropriate for Jesus during the acute stages of his illness?
○ **1.** Modified Sims'
○ **2.** Semi-Fowler's
○ **3.** Supine
○ **4.** Prone

79. Chest physical therapy with postural drainage has been ordered for Jesus TID. When should these treatments be administered?
○ **1.** Before meals
○ **2.** After meals
○ **3.** Every 8 hours
○ **4.** When parents are present

80. Which of the following statements best describes Jesus's physical development? His weight should be
○ **1.** twice his birth weight.
○ **2.** 3 times his birth weight.
○ **3.** 4 times his birth weight.
○ **4.** 5 times his birth weight.

81. If Jesus's development is progressing normally, which of the following teeth should erupt first?
○ **1.** Upper lateral incisors
○ **2.** Upper central incisors
○ **3.** Lower central incisors
○ **4.** Lower lateral incisors

82. Once Jesus is able to tolerate feedings, which of the following foods would be most appropriate for the nurse to offer him?
○ **1.** Chopped egg white
○ **2.** Strained fruit
○ **3.** Crackers
○ **4.** Orange juice

83. If there is a history of food allergies in the Sanchez family, which of the following cereals would be most appropriate for Jesus?
○ **1.** Oatmeal
○ **2.** Rice
○ **3.** Mixed
○ **4.** Barley

84. At what age should Jesus begin drinking from a cup with assistance?
○ **1.** 4 to 6 months
○ **2.** 7 to 9 months
○ **3.** 10 to 12 months
○ **4.** 13 to 15 months

85. Mrs. Sanchez tells you that Jesus's immunizations are up-to-date. Which of the following should Jesus receive next?
○ **1.** Diphtheria and tetanus
○ **2.** Oral polio
○ **3.** Measles and mumps
○ **4.** Tuberculin test

Ten-year-old Pedro is admitted with airway obstruction.

86. A tracheostomy is performed; he requires frequent suctioning. The physician orders the instillation of 2 to 3 ml of sterile saline into the tracheostomy tube prior to suctioning. What is the best rationale for this order?
    ○ **1.** It will loosen secretions and stimulate coughing.
    ○ **2.** It will result in more normal sleeping patterns at night.
    ○ **3.** It replaces deep tracheal suctioning.
    ○ **4.** It provides humidity for the tracheal mucosa.

87. Prior to suctioning Pedro's tracheostomy, which of the following actions should the nurse perform?
    ○ **1.** Loosen the tracheostomy tube, to facilitate suctioning.
    ○ **2.** Ask him to hold his breath, to promote lung expansion.
    ○ **3.** Listen to his chest with a stethoscope.
    ○ **4.** Position him in a chair supported with pillows.

88. The nurse caring for Pedro should know that oxygenation prior to suctioning is essential for which of the following reasons?
    ○ **1.** It helps to loosen respiratory secretions.
    ○ **2.** Oxygenation will relax Pedro.
    ○ **3.** Suctioning removes oxygen from the lungs.
    ○ **4.** Oxygenation removes sodium ions from respiratory tissue.

89. Which of the following nursing actions would be most appropriate while providing tracheostomy care to Pedro?
    ○ **1.** Maintain sterile technique by using a sterile glove and catheter when suctioning.
    ○ **2.** Inject 5 ml air into cuff to prevent aspiration.
    ○ **3.** Cleanse the inner cannula with peroxide and sterile saline every day.
    ○ **4.** Remove the outer cannula at least every 8 hours for cleaning.

90. If suctioning was effective, an assessment of Pedro should reveal
    ○ **1.** increased breath sounds.
    ○ **2.** decreased breath sounds.
    ○ **3.** fine moist rales.
    ○ **4.** coarse rhonchi.

Pedro's recovery is uneventful. His tracheostomy has been plugged and he is able to perform daily activities with minimal assistance. He has been taking ampicillin 500 mg PO BID, cromolyn sodium (Intal) prn, and a regular diet.

91. The nurse should instruct Pedro's mother to include which of the following foods in his diet while he is taking ampicillin?
    ○ **1.** Honey
    ○ **2.** Yogurt
    ○ **3.** Bran
    ○ **4.** Oranges

92. Which of the following statements about cromolyn sodium (Intal) is most correct?
    ○ **1.** It enhances the release of histamine.
    ○ **2.** It is used during an acute asthmatic attack.
    ○ **3.** It is administered with milk PO QID.
    ○ **4.** It may cause irritation to the throat and trachea.

93. Which of the following developmental tasks are most descriptive of the child of elementary-school age?
    ○ **1.** Decreasing dependence upon family and satisfaction from peers and other adults increases
    ○ **2.** Developing the intellectual and work skills and social sensitivities of a competent citizen
    ○ **3.** Learning to handle the body using a variety of physical skills and to maintain good health
    ○ **4.** Settling into a healthful daily routine of adequately eating, exercising, and resting

Six-and-a-half-year-old Molly, a first-grader who has a history of asthma, is hospitalized with an acute episode.

94. Which of the following nursing actions is *contraindicated* during the acute phase of Molly's illness?
    ○ **1.** Encourage Molly to drink extra fluids.
    ○ **2.** Teach Molly to use her diaphragm for breathing.
    ○ **3.** Administer a cough suppressant to Molly.
    ○ **4.** Keep Molly's room quiet and darkened.

95. Molly's IV has infiltrated. When the nurse tries to apply a warm, moist washcloth to her swollen left forearm, she begins to whine and pull away. What should the nurse say to Molly to gain her cooperation?
    ○ **1.** "Molly, I'll come back in a few minutes after you calm down."
    ○ **2.** "Molly, the doctor says this washcloth will make your arm feel better."
    ○ **3.** "Molly, Susie didn't cry when I put one of these on her arm."
    ○ **4.** "Molly, this will feel warm. Let me show you what it feels like on your other arm first."

96. While hospitalized, Molly is especially at risk for developing feelings of
   ○ **1.** guilt.
   ○ **2.** mistrust.
   ○ **3.** inferiority.
   ○ **4.** shame.

97. While Molly is hospitalized, it is most important for the nurse to plan ways to
   ○ **1.** promote her sense of control.
   ○ **2.** maintain her gross motor skills.
   ○ **3.** maintain her school work.
   ○ **4.** promote attachment to her parents.

98. Molly is to be discharged tomorrow. Which of the following should be included in the discharge teaching plan for her parents?
   ○ **1.** Avoid dusting Molly's room at home too frequently.
   ○ **2.** Ensure Molly's immunizations and flu shots are current.
   ○ **3.** Have Molly sleep with her window open during cold weather.
   ○ **4.** Allow Molly to participate in quiet activities only.

Twelve-year-old LaTania is admitted to the adolescent unit with sickle cell disease. She is in vaso-occlusive crisis. Her right elbow is edematous, and she states that it is very painful.

99. In addition to pain, which of the following symptoms would LaTania most likely manifest?
   ○ **1.** Dactylitis
   ○ **2.** Chronic hemolytic anemia
   ○ **3.** Brushfield's spots
   ○ **4.** Jaundice followed by pallor after a sickling crisis

100. LaTania asks her nurse what she thinks caused this crisis episode. The nurse's reply is based on her knowledge of which of the following possible precipitating events?
   ○ **1.** Strenuous physical exertion
   ○ **2.** Developmental growth spurts
   ○ **3.** A recent spell of hot, humid weather
   ○ **4.** Overeating junk food at a pizza party

101. The nurse would do best to implement which of the following measures for LaTania?
   ○ **1.** Wrap a heating pad around her elbow.
   ○ **2.** Set up necessary equipment and fluid for a blood transfusion.
   ○ **3.** Limit her daily fluid intake to 900 ml.
   ○ **4.** Apply ice to her elbow to decrease the edema.

102. As the nurse prepares LaTania for discharge, what self-care principle is most important for her to know?
   ○ **1.** Hot weather presents a greater risk for crisis than cold.
   ○ **2.** Oxygen (per mask or cannula) will allay a sickling crisis.
   ○ **3.** Remain as physically active as possible.
   ○ **4.** Avoid high altitudes.

Fourteen-year-old Darryl has hemophilia. He is being seen in the clinic today for a periodic checkup.

103. When obtaining a history from Darryl and his father, which one of the following reported manifestations would be the greatest cause for concern?
   ○ **1.** Epistaxis
   ○ **2.** Pallor
   ○ **3.** Easy bruising
   ○ **4.** Hemarthrosis

104. Darryl's father tells the nurse privately that Darryl is "crazy about sports, especially football. He wants to try out for his junior high football team. My wife and I are having a hard time convincing him this is impossible."
   Which of the following alternatives is the best suggestion for Darryl?
   ○ **1.** Allow him to try out for the team as long as he wears a helmet and elbow and knee pads at all times.
   ○ **2.** Start a collection of football memorabilia.
   ○ **3.** Develop an interest in swimming or table tennis instead.
   ○ **4.** Try to become equipment manager for his junior high team.

105. Darryl is admitted to the hospital with an acute bleeding episode in his right elbow, which could not be controlled at home. Which of the following will *not* be used to control his bleeding?
   ○ **1.** Plasma
   ○ **2.** Plasma concentrate
   ○ **3.** Packed cells
   ○ **4.** Cryoprecipitate

106. During his bleeding episode, which one of the following nursing measures is indicated?
   ○ **1.** Apply a heating pad to the right elbow.
   ○ **2.** Keep the bedcovers off the right elbow.
   ○ **3.** Encourage Darryl to keep his right elbow as mobile as possible.
   ○ **4.** Administer aspirin 10 grains orally for pain relief.

107. Darryl is recovering and will be discharged tomorrow. His father expresses concern about Darryl's future as a ''family man.'' The nurse ascertains that Darryl's father is anxious to know if Darryl can have children who do not have hemophilia. Assuming that Darryl's future spouse is not a carrier of the disease, which explanation is most accurate?
    ○ **1.** All Darryl's children will be carriers.
    ○ **2.** Darryl's sons will have the disease and his daughters will be carriers.
    ○ **3.** There is a 50% chance that each of Darryl's children will have hemophilia.
    ○ **4.** Darryl's sons will be normal and his daughters will be carriers.

108. Which one of the following is the best indicator of a successful outcome of Darryl's long-term treatment?
    ○ **1.** Bleeding episodes are prevented or treated early to minimize sequelae.
    ○ **2.** Darryl is able to keep up with his peers academically.
    ○ **3.** Darryl's weight is maintained within age-appropriate ranges.
    ○ **4.** Darryl chooses a realistic career goal.

Angela Rodriguez brings her 1-year-old son, Miguel, in for a well-child examination.

109. Which of the following activities should Miguel be expected to do at this age?
    ○ **1.** Move around solid objects
    ○ **2.** Walk well, forward and backward
    ○ **3.** Have a vocabulary of 3 words
    ○ **4.** Feed himself with a spoon

110. Miguel receives a tuberculin skin test using purified protein derivative (PPD). The nurse instructs Mrs. Rodriguez to check the site in 48 hours and 72 hours. Which of the following most accurately describes a positive reaction?
    ○ **1.** A pruritic induration of 4 mm at the site
    ○ **2.** High fever and coughing
    ○ **3.** Induration of 10 mm at the site
    ○ **4.** Very erythematous site with 3 mm induration

111. A diminished reactivity to the Mantoux test may be expected in which of the following situations?
    ○ **1.** A child less than 6 months of age
    ○ **2.** A malnourished child
    ○ **3.** A child with a concurrent viral illness
    ○ **4.** All of the above cases will show diminished reactivity to the Mantoux test.

112. Miguel's condition is diagnosed as tuberculosis. Mrs. Rodriguez questions this since, ''Miguel doesn't act sick.'' The nurse explains that many children with tuberculosis may be asymptomatic. Which of the following would be an appropriate instruction for Mrs. Rodriguez?
    ○ **1.** Limit Miguel's activity.
    ○ **2.** Keep Miguel isolated from playmates.
    ○ **3.** Reinforce compliance with the medication regimen, as Miguel will probably be treated for at least a year.
    ○ **4.** Teach her how to obtain sputum specimens

Four-year-old Barbara Watson was admitted to the hospital for diagnostic studies and heart surgery for repair of aortic stenosis.

113. A cardiac catheterization is ordered for Barbara. Barbara's mother asks the nurse if the procedure will hurt. Which one of the following statements is the *best* nursing response?
    ○ **1.** ''A pushing sensation may be felt when the catheter goes into the vein.''
    ○ **2.** ''Momentary sharp pain will usually occur when the catheter enters the heart.''
    ○ **3.** ''It is usual for a 4-year-old to be aware of discomfort or pain during the procedure.''
    ○ **4.** ''It is a painless procedure although there is often a tingling sensation noted in the extremities.''

114. While doing morning care for Barbara, the nurse notes that the blanket that she brought from home is torn and tattered. What should the nurse do?
    ○ **1.** Keep it close to Barbara.
    ○ **2.** Ask her parents to take it and leave it at home.
    ○ **3.** Give her a new blanket.
    ○ **4.** Send the blanket to the laundry for a good washing.

115. After dinner, Mrs. Watson tells the nurse she has to leave. Barbara hears her and begins to cry loudly. Which action by the nurse would be best at this time?
    ○ **1.** Walk Mrs. Watson to the elevator.
    ○ **2.** Ask Mrs. Watson to stay until Barbara goes to sleep.
    ○ **3.** Stay with Barbara and try to comfort her.
    ○ **4.** Encourage Mrs. Watson not to visit for a while.

116. Mrs. Watson brings Barbara in for her checkup after discharge and her older brother, Eric, for his 5-year checkup. When taking Eric's vital signs, the nurse notices he has a sinus dysrhythmia. Which of the following nursing actions should be carried out?
   ○ 1. Notify the physician immediately.
   ○ 2. Obtain a 12-lead ECG.
   ○ 3. Ask Mrs. Watson if Eric has been taking digoxin.
   ○ 4. Have Eric hold his breath while listening to his apical pulse.

Ronald Fulton, 2 years old, was brought by his parents to the emergency room because of respiratory distress, an elevated temperature, and nasal congestion. A loud systolic murmur was noted over the left sternal border. His diagnosis was a large ventricular septal defect.

117. Which abnormal condition results from this defect?
   ○ 1. Peripheral hypoxia
   ○ 2. Elevated hemoglobin and hematocrit
   ○ 3. Volume overload in the lungs
   ○ 4. Decreased blood pressure

118. Children with congenital heart disease are extremely susceptible to which of the following problems?
   ○ 1. Gastrointestinal disorders
   ○ 2. Upper respiratory tract infections
   ○ 3. Urinary tract infections
   ○ 4. Allergic conditions

119. Children with congenital heart disease are often less able to adapt positively to frustrating situations. Which of the following provides the best explanation for their behavior?
   ○ 1. They have usually been spoiled by their parents.
   ○ 2. They have had fewer opportunities to learn to deal with frustrations
   ○ 3. They can manipulate others by their reactions.
   ○ 4. They are developmentally delayed in their socialization.

120. A cardiac catheterization confirms the diagnosis. Plans are made for Ronald to be followed up in an outpatient clinic and to return for corrective surgery when he is 3 years old. In discussing discharge plans with Ronald's parents, which of the following instructions would be most realistic?
   ○ 1. No restrictions or limits are needed.
   ○ 2. Diet should emphasize iron-rich meats and vitamins.
   ○ 3. Ronald's contacts should be limited to healthy adults.
   ○ 4. Ronald can set his own limits on exercise and activities.

When Ronald is 3 years old, he is readmitted to the hospital for repair of the ventricular septal defect. He is receiving a daily dose of digoxin and is admitted 3 days before the surgery is to be performed.

121. Ronald is placed in an oxygen tent for short periods of time before cardiac surgery for which primary reason?
   ○ 1. To accustom him to the experience
   ○ 2. To avoid contact with people who have upper respiratory infections
   ○ 3. To keep the body temperature low
   ○ 4. To reduce pre-op secretions from the respiratory tract

122. The nurse notes Ronald's apical pulse is 70. Which action by the nurse is *most* appropriate?
   ○ 1. Call an emergency alert because the child is in heart block.
   ○ 2. Give the digoxin because the pulse is within normal range.
   ○ 3. Take the radial pulse and compare it with the apical.
   ○ 4. Withhold the digoxin and notify the physician.

123. The nurse must administer 0.06 mg of digoxin, which comes in a solution of 1 ml = 0.05 mg. How many minims would the nurse give?
   ○ 1. 16
   ○ 2. 18
   ○ 3. 20
   ○ 4. 22

124. Therapeutic results of digoxin do *not* include which of the following?
   ○ 1. Slower heart rate
   ○ 2. Greater force in cardiac contraction
   ○ 3. Improved pulse rhythm
   ○ 4. Decreased urinary output

125. Hypothermia is used in open-heart surgery to
    ○ 1. lessen the dangers of post-op febrile episodes.
    ○ 2. stop cardiac activity.
    ○ 3. minimize respiratory action.
    ○ 4. reduce overall body metabolism.

126. Postoperatively, Ronald has a water-seal chest drainage system. This action helps drain air and fluid from
    ○ 1. the abdominal cavity.
    ○ 2. the alveoli.
    ○ 3. the myocardial sac.
    ○ 4. the pleural cavity.

127. For which of the following conditions would the nurse clamp off Ronald's thoracotomy tube?
    ○ 1. Obstruction of the drainage flow because of clots
    ○ 2. The appearance of large amounts of blood in the tubing
    ○ 3. Disconnection of the tubing
    ○ 4. Movement of the child from side to side

128. Which of the following nursing actions would best provide Ronald with physical support while encouraging him to cough?
    ○ 1. Sit him straight up in bed.
    ○ 2. Encircle the chest with both hands.
    ○ 3. Stimulate the cough reflex with a catheter.
    ○ 4. Clamp off the thoracotomy tube.

129. The nurse notices Ronald sucking his thumb. Which action would be most appropriate?
    ○ 1. Discuss with the parents how to break this habit.
    ○ 2. Gently remove the thumb from his mouth while diverting his attention.
    ○ 3. Recognize his behavior is expected regression and allow him to continue.
    ○ 4. Request permission to give him ice chips or sips of water by mouth.

130. Ronald's cardiac surgery has been successful. During the convalescent period, the Fulton family will probably need special counseling in
    ○ 1. becoming less protective.
    ○ 2. planning Ronald's educational goals.
    ○ 3. learning to avoid physical complications related to Ronald's childhood diseases.
    ○ 4. maintaining Ronald's restricted life-style.

131. Ronald's parents share their frustration with the nurse about his temper tantrums at home. Which parental response to the tantrums would best indicate that they are handling him appropriately?
    ○ 1. Ignoring the tantrums
    ○ 2. Reasoning with Ronald during the tantrum
    ○ 3. Restraining Ronald during the tantrum
    ○ 4. Placing Ronald alone after the tantrum

132. The nurse suggests that Ronald use which of the following activities to help him express his angry feelings?
    ○ 1. Reading a book
    ○ 2. Stacking blocks
    ○ 3. Throwing a ball
    ○ 4. Coloring in a coloring book

Twelve-month-old Marcus has been referred to the pediatric clinic by the public health nurse because of suspected failure-to-thrive syndrome. His mother is a 19-year-old single parent who lives alone with her son.

133. A first-year nursing student in the clinic asks what causes failure-to-thrive syndrome. The best reply would be that the most common cause is
    ○ 1. intestinal malabsorption.
    ○ 2. sensory overload.
    ○ 3. parent's lack of knowledge of correct feeding technique.
    ○ 4. disruption in parent-infant attachment.

134. Nursing assessment of Marcus is most likely to reveal
    ○ 1. intense eye-to-eye contact.
    ○ 2. extreme stranger anxiety.
    ○ 3. hyperresponsiveness to sensory stimuli.
    ○ 4. stiff posture when held.

135. During the assessment of Marcus, the nurse observes that he has good head control and can roll over, but cannot sit up without support or transfer an object from one hand to another. Based on this observation, the nurse concludes that Marcus is at what developmental age?
    ○ 1. 3 to 4 months
    ○ 2. 4 to 6 months
    ○ 3. 6 to 8 months
    ○ 4. 8 to 10 months

136. A plan of care to best meet the needs of this child would *not* include which of the following?
    ○ 1. A schedule of stimulation geared to the infant's present level of development
    ○ 2. A plan to teach the mother ways to provide stimulation during bathing and feeding
    ○ 3. A plan to have staff members pick him up and play with him whenever they can
    ○ 4. Consistent care with same primary care givers, as much as possible, each shift

137. Which nursing action would receive the highest priority in Marcus's nursing care plan?
    ○ 1. Suggest that Marcus and his mother move in with her parents.
    ○ 2. Provide Marcus's mother with anticipatory guidance concerning age-appropriate play activities for Marcus.
    ○ 3. Praise Marcus's mother's nurturing behaviors toward her son.
    ○ 4. Temporarily assume Marcus's mother's responsibilities for his care.

138. Which toys are *not* suited for Marcus, based on his present developmental age?
    ○ 1. Snap toys, large snap beads
    ○ 2. Soft, stuffed animals he can hold
    ○ 3. Brightly colored mobiles
    ○ 4. Squeeze toys

139. Mothers who neglect or abuse their children often
    ○ 1. were neglected or abused themselves as children.
    ○ 2. have knowledge of child growth and development.
    ○ 3. have knowledge of how to care for child and give affection.
    ○ 4. have low levels of stress.

140. There are several common characteristics of parents who abuse their children. Which of the following parental characteristics indicates a high risk for abusive behavior?
    ○ 1. Seldom touches or looks at the child
    ○ 2. Shows signs of guilt about the child's injury
    ○ 3. Is quick to inquire about the discharge date
    ○ 4. Is scrupulous in keeping the child's immunizations up-to-date

141. What is the best indicator that Marcus's failure to thrive is being resolved?
    ○ 1. His mother keeps scheduled clinic appointments.
    ○ 2. Marcus's physical growth is within normal limits.
    ○ 3. Marcus's sleeping, eating, and elimination patterns are predictable.
    ○ 4. Marcus's mother verbally expresses her fears and frustrations about being a parent.

Two-year-old Peter was admitted to the hospital for the second surgical repair of his cleft palate. His mother cannot stay overnight with her son or visit because of unexpected illness.

142. It is especially important to obtain which of the following pieces of information upon admission?
    ○ 1. Peter's sleeping habits
    ○ 2. Peter's feeding habits and ability to drink from a cup
    ○ 3. Peter's toilet training status
    ○ 4. Peter's favorite activities

143. On the morning after admission, Peter is standing in his crib crying. He refuses to be comforted and calls for his mother. The nurse approaches Peter to bathe him and he screams louder. She recognizes this behavior as which of the following stages of "settling in"?
    ○ 1. Protest
    ○ 2. Depression
    ○ 3. Denial
    ○ 4. Bargaining

144. What would be the most helpful nursing action at this time?
    ○ 1. Pick him up and walk him around the room.
    ○ 2. Be firm and begin with his bath.
    ○ 3. Sit at the bedside and spend time with Peter until his anxiety has decreased.
    ○ 4. Chart the behaviors and let the next shift bathe him.

145. Following surgical repair of his cleft palate, in which position should Peter be placed?
    ○ 1. On his abdomen
    ○ 2. On his back
    ○ 3. Fowler's position
    ○ 4. Any position that is comfortable for him

146. To prevent Peter from damaging the surgical repair, the nurse should apply
    ○ 1. a Logan bow to his mouth.
    ○ 2. elbow restraints.
    ○ 3. wrist restraints.
    ○ 4. gauze wrapping on Peter's hands.

147. Peter is 24 hours post-op. Which activity is most appropriate for him?
    ○ 1. Listen to a volunteer read a story
    ○ 2. Watch *Sesame Street* on television
    ○ 3. Play a toy piano
    ○ 4. Put together a puzzle with large pieces

148. On the third post-op day, Peter begins to regress and lies quietly in his crib with his blanket. The nurse recognizes that he is now in which stage of separation anxiety?
    ○ 1. Denial
    ○ 2. Despair
    ○ 3. Mistrust
    ○ 4. Shock and disbelief

149. By the end of the first week of hospitalization, Peter smiles easily, no longer cries when his father leaves after visiting hours, and goes to the nurses happily. He has not seen his mother since he was admitted to hospital. What should the nurse understand about Peter's present behavior?
    ○ 1. He feels better physically and so is behaving better.
    ○ 2. He has established a routine and likes the nurses.
    ○ 3. He is repressing feelings about his mother and has given up fighting separation.
    ○ 4. He is becoming more mature.

150. Peter's mother and father come to pick him up for discharge. This is the first time Peter has seen his mother since admission and he hides his face and clings to the nurse's leg. What is the best response the nurse can make?
    ○ 1. "Take Peter home immediately before he starts to cry."
    ○ 2. "Come to the playroom with Peter and me; let Peter come to you when he is ready."
    ○ 3. "Leave Peter in the hospital a few more days, because he's not ready to go home."
    ○ 4. Speak to Peter firmly and explain it is time to go home.

151. The nurse explains the meaning of Peter's behavior to the parents and tells them that after he goes home they should expect that
    ○ 1. it will take some time before the mother-child relationship becomes completely reestablished.
    ○ 2. Peter will miss the hospital routine and nurses.
    ○ 3. Peter will be happy and obedient at home.
    ○ 4. Peter will forget the whole experience right away.

Kristie, 8 hours old, has been diagnosed with tracheo-esophageal fistula (TEF). She is scheduled for surgery in 24 hours.

152. Preoperatively, the nurse will note which symptoms of TEF in Kristie?·
    ○ 1. Severe cyanosis and coughing
    ○ 2. Excessive drooling and abdominal distension
    ○ 3. Projectile vomiting and flatulence
    ○ 4. Bile-stained vomiting and choking

153. Which of the following nursing actions is most important for Kristie's care?
    ○ 1. Keep her as quiet as possible.
    ○ 2. Prevent infection.
    ○ 3. Provide normal sensorimotor stimulation.
    ○ 4. Prevent aspiration.

154. Preoperatively, Kristie should be placed in which position?
    ○ 1. On her abdomen
    ○ 2. Trendelenburg's position
    ○ 3. Semi-Fowler's position
    ○ 4. On her left side

155. Kristie has an IV of 5% dextrose in 0.25% saline solution prescribed to infuse at 12 ml/hour. The microdrip should be regulated to infuse at how many drops per minute?
    ○ 1. 6 drops/minute
    ○ 2. 12 drops/minute
    ○ 3. 24 drops/minute
    ○ 4. 30 drops/minute

156. Postoperatively, Kristie returns to the special care nursery following ligation of the fistula and an end-to-end anastomosis of the esophageal segments. She is to be given 15 ml of formula via gastrostomy tube every 2 hours. Which of the following nursing actions is not appropriate?
    ○ 1. Administer the feeding by gravity.
    ○ 2. Rinse the gastrostomy tube with a small amount of sterile water after each feeding.
    ○ 3. Clamp the gastrostomy tube after each feeding.
    ○ 4. Give Kristie a pacifier during each feeding.

157. Kristie is being discharged and will return in 1 month for removal of her gastrostomy tube. In the meantime, she will be fed by gastrostomy tube. Her parents should be advised to report immediately which one of the following symptoms?
    ○ 1. Difficulty swallowing
    ○ 2. Reddened skin around the gastrostomy tube
    ○ 3. Diarrhea
    ○ 4. Regurgitation of formula

Brooke White, aged 4, has cystic fibrosis. She is admitted to the pediatrics unit with bronchopneumonia, and dehydration secondary to diarrhea.

158. Brooke is put into a croup tent to relieve her respiratory distress. Which toy would be most suitable for her at this time?
○ **1.** Her favorite storybook
○ **2.** Her favorite doll
○ **3.** Her favorite puzzle
○ **4.** Her favorite stuffed animal

159. Which of the following would be an *inappropriate* nursing action based on Brooke's need for the croup tent?
○ **1.** Monitor temperature and oxygen concentration in the croup tent.
○ **2.** Change Brooke's linens and clothing as they become wet.
○ **3.** Leave the edges of the tent on top of the sheets.
○ **4.** Take Brooke out of the croup tent to use the bathroom.

160. Brooke is to receive 250 ml of IV fluid over 8 hours. Using a pediatric microdrip (1 ml = 60 drops), what is the desired rate of drops per minute?
○ **1.** 5 drops/minute
○ **2.** 31 drops/minute
○ **3.** 60 drops/minute
○ **4.** 83 drops/minute

161. Prior to administering the next dose of ampicillin, Brooke's mother informs the nurse that Brooke has begun to have diarrhea. Of the following, what is the best response?
○ **1.** Institute isolation precautions until an infectious disease is ruled out and administer the ampicillin.
○ **2.** Discontinue the ampicillin.
○ **3.** Do not withhold the dose unless you consult with the physician.
○ **4.** Institute isolation precautions and withhold the dosage.

162. Brooke has been running a fever and is still having frequent stools. The physician orders Brooke's temperature to be monitored q2h. The nurse should take
○ **1.** oral temperatures.
○ **2.** rectal temperatures.
○ **3.** axillary temperatures.
○ **4.** either oral or rectal temperature.

163. Gentamicin sulfate (Garamycin) 65 mg was ordered for IM injection. The multidose vial is labeled 40 mg/ml. How many ml of the medication should Brooke receive?
○ **1.** 0.61 ml
○ **2.** 1.22 ml
○ **3.** 1.60 ml
○ **4.** 3.20 ml

164. Discharge teaching for Brooke's parents should include which of the following factors to ensure optimal absorption of the oral form of ampicillin?
○ **1.** Administer on an empty stomach.
○ **2.** Give only with meals to prevent upset stomach.
○ **3.** Take care not to shake the container.
○ **4.** Always store and administer at room temperature.

Eight-year-old Matt received a diagnosis of cystic fibrosis at 9 months of age. He has been hospitalized several times since then but is now at home.

165. Which behavioral assessment is most age appropriate for Matt?
○ **1.** He has an imaginary friend named Germaine.
○ **2.** His favorite activity is riding his bicycle.
○ **3.** He overidentifies with his peers (clothes, etc.)
○ **4.** He is afraid of monsters.

166. Which of the following clinical signs of cystic fibrosis is most likely to be present in Matt?
○ **1.** Frequent urinary tract infections
○ **2.** Large, bulky stools
○ **3.** Ribbon stools
○ **4.** Poor appetite

167. The physician prescribes pancreatic enzymes (Pancrease) for Matt. Which of the following instructions is most essential regarding this medication?
○ **1.** Mix it with hot food or milk.
○ **2.** Give it q6h around the clock.
○ **3.** If Matt skips a meal, do not give the enzyme.
○ **4.** He will need more enzymes in very hot weather.

168. Which principle of care is most important for Matt and his family to know prior to discharge?
○ **1.** Restrict his fluids to reduce excessive sweating.
○ **2.** Encourage quiet activities.
○ **3.** Offer high-salt foods such as pickles and pretzels.
○ **4.** His diet should be higher than usual in fat content.

169. Matt's long-term nursing care plan is aimed primarily at which of the following?
  ○ **1.** Thoroughly educating his parents about cystic fibrosis
  ○ **2.** Preventing respiratory infections related to cystic fibrosis
  ○ **3.** Following his medical regimen
  ○ **4.** Teaching him how to live with cystic fibrosis

Fifteen-year-old Angela has recently been diagnosed with diabetes.

170. Which of the following situations would indicate that Angela is at greatest risk for a hypoglycemic reaction?
  ○ **1.** She has not taken her insulin for 3 days.
  ○ **2.** Her urine test is 4+ for sugar and positive for acetone.
  ○ **3.** Her urine test is negative for sugar.
  ○ **4.** She had an injection of NPH insulin one-half hour ago.

171. Angela is invited to a pajama party. Which option indicates the most appropriate action to meet her developmental needs?
  ○ **1.** Keep Angela at home until she knows her diet restrictions.
  ○ **2.** Have Angela explain to her friends that she is diabetic and will bring her own sugar-free drinks.
  ○ **3.** Adjust her diet and insulin before going to the party, so she does not need to eat.
  ○ **4.** Have Angela's mother call her friend's mother to explain her condition.

Bob Lee, aged 7, was admitted yesterday with acute glomerulonephritis and hematuria. He has orders for bed rest, intake and output, blood pressure q2h, a sodium-restricted diet, and daily weights. Bob is an only child, and his parents are almost always present, feeding him and caring for him. Bob seems embarrassed but complies.

172. In acute glomerulonephritis, changes in the glomeruli of the kidneys are *not* the result of which of the following?
  ○ **1.** Altered membrane permeability
  ○ **2.** Inflammation
  ○ **3.** Congenital causes
  ○ **4.** Antigen-antibody response caused by beta hemolytic streptococcus group A

173. What is the prognosis for acute glomerulonephritis?
  ○ **1.** Guarded
  ○ **2.** Impossible to predict
  ○ **3.** Favorable, 85% to 90% recover.
  ○ **4.** This is a terminal illness.

174. A potential problem for Bob is alteration in body image. Which age group is most concerned with body image and loss of body function?
  ○ **1.** Preschool
  ○ **2.** Kindergarten
  ○ **3.** Elementary-school age
  ○ **4.** Adolescent

175. Choose the primary nursing action to use when working with Bob's mother.
  ○ **1.** Inform her that her son needs more independence and encourage her to let him take care of himself.
  ○ **2.** Spend time at Bob's bedside to explain hospital rules or procedures or answer any questions that the family may have.
  ○ **3.** Encourage Mrs. Lee to attend the classes in family health education.
  ○ **4.** Teach her the basic functions of the kidneys.

176. Mrs. Lee tells the nurse, ''Bob was always a healthy boy until he started school. Now he gets colds and strep throat all the time. I'm afraid he has weak kidneys too.'' What is the nurse's best response?
  ○ **1.** ''A common factor in the history of children with glomerulonephritis is a strep infection 1 to 3 weeks preceding the present illness.''
  ○ **2.** ''Bob's kidneys are weakened and the damage is irreversible.''
  ○ **3.** ''Bob should be kept out of school to prevent infections.''
  ○ **4.** ''Bob's kidney condition has nothing to do with his colds and strep throat.''

Cindy, aged 12, reluctantly comes into the emergency room, brought by her mother. Cindy states, ''I'm OK now, my stomach doesn't hurt as much.'' Her mother says that Cindy has been complaining of abdominal pain, has been vomiting for 8 hours, is anorexic, and has been walking with a slight limp. As they got into the car to drive to the hospital, Cindy said that the pain was better.

177. Which of the following is *not* likely to be ordered for Cindy?
  ○ **1.** Admit for observation.
  ○ **2.** Give a clear-liquid diet.
  ○ **3.** Get a complete blood count.
  ○ **4.** Get an abdominal x-ray.

178. Cindy is 1 day post-op repair of a ruptured appendix. She has a Penrose drain in her incision site and is NPO. Nursing care for Cindy should *not* include which of the following?
   ○ **1.** Maintain her in semi-Fowler's position.
   ○ **2.** Position her on her right side.
   ○ **3.** Administer broad-spectrum antibiotics as ordered.
   ○ **4.** Change the dressing q24h.

179. Three days post-op, Cindy is observed lying on her back with her knees drawn up. Her respirations are irregular, temperature is normal, and her skin is warm and dry. Her abdomen is distended. When Cindy sees the nurse, she cries, "I'm so miserable, the pain is terrible." What is the best assessment of Cindy's pain reaction?
   ○ **1.** Marked psychic, autonomic, and skeletal muscle response
   ○ **2.** Marked psychic, moderate autonomic and skeletal muscle response
   ○ **3.** Moderate psychic, marked skeletal muscle response
   ○ **4.** Marked psychic response

180. Based on the assessment of Cindy's pain, what initial nursing action is most appropriate?
   ○ **1.** Call the physician immediately.
   ○ **2.** Calm Cindy down and reevaluate her pain in 1 hour.
   ○ **3.** Insert rectal tube, per physician's order.
   ○ **4.** Administer analgesic, per physician order.

181. In evaluating the effectiveness of the nursing action with Cindy, which of the following indicates relief?
   ○ **1.** Respirations regular
   ○ **2.** Pulse full and regular
   ○ **3.** Abdomen soft and flat
   ○ **4.** Normal perspiration

Hirschsprung's disease is a mechanical obstruction of the colon caused by a lack of colonic motility due to absence of innervation by the autonomic parasympathetic ganglion cells of the mesenteric and submucosal plexuses.

182. Which of the following is *not* characteristic of a newborn who has Hirschsprung's disease?
   ○ **1.** Failure to pass meconium within 24 to 48 hours after birth
   ○ **2.** Refusal to take liquids
   ○ **3.** Abdominal distension
   ○ **4.** Frequent, greenish stools

183. Which of the following is *not* characteristic of Hirschsprung's disease in the older infant?
   ○ **1.** Failure to thrive
   ○ **2.** Constipation
   ○ **3.** Diarrhea and vomiting
   ○ **4.** Steatorrhea

184. Pre-op care for the older child with Hirschsprung's disease should include which of the following diets?
   ○ **1.** Low residue, high calorie, high protein
   ○ **2.** High residue, high calorie
   ○ **3.** Clear liquids
   ○ **4.** High sodium, low potassium

185. When Hirschsprung's disease is not diagnosed in infancy, the nurse's role in later diagnostic workup should emphasize
   ○ **1.** bowel habits.
   ○ **2.** disposition.
   ○ **3.** feeding habits.
   ○ **4.** skin color.

186. Surgical treatment of Hirschsprung's disease is removal of the affected part of the colon with an accompanying colostomy. When explaining to the parents about the colostomy, the nurse should include which of the following?
   ○ **1.** The colostomy is usually temporary.
   ○ **2.** The colostomy is usually permanent.
   ○ **3.** The colostomy may not be necessary.
   ○ **4.** The child will have a colostomy until s/he reaches full growth.

187. The double-barrel type of colostomy is frequently performed on children following resection of the affected part of the colon. The nurse accurately evaluates the functioning of this type of colostomy in which of the following ways?
   ○ **1.** Both the proximal end and the distal end excrete feces.
   ○ **2.** Only the proximal end excretes feces.
   ○ **3.** The proximal end allows for excretion of feces; the distal end excretes mucus.
   ○ **4.** The proximal end allows for excretion of mucus; the distal end excretes feces.

188. Initial post-op care following colon resection does *not* include
   ○ **1.** a clear liquid diet.
   ○ **2.** nasogastric suction.
   ○ **3.** frequent abdominal dressing changes.
   ○ **4.** intravenous feedings to replace electrolytes.

189. A diet low in residue is encouraged postoperatively when full bowel function returns. A low-residue diet would *not* include which of the following foods?
    ○ 1. Jams, preserves
    ○ 2. White bread
    ○ 3. Vanilla ice cream
    ○ 4. Spaghetti with cream sauce

A school nurse is planning to screen a school population for scoliosis beginning with the high-risk group.

190. Which group of students would the nurse begin screening?
    ○ 1. Girls and boys, 8 to 11 years of age
    ○ 2. Girls, 10 to 15 years of age
    ○ 3. Girls, 15 to 19 years of age
    ○ 4. Boys, 12 to 16 years of age

191. Scoliosis can be most easily detected if the students are asked to assume which position?
    ○ 1. Bend at the waist, to the right, and then to the left
    ○ 2. Stand straight, face the nurse with arms raised overhead
    ○ 3. Bend forward at the waist with head and arms hanging freely
    ○ 4. Stand straight, with back to the nurse, and arms held out in front of the body

192. Tina Ford was found to have scoliosis during the initial school screening of high-risk groups. Tina states emphatically that it is a waste of time to get her back checked because she will never consider wearing a brace or having surgery. Tina's comment most likely indicates which of the following major fears associated with her age group?
    ○ 1. Intrusive procedures
    ○ 2. Body mutilation
    ○ 3. Change in body image
    ○ 4. Separation from her friends

193. Tina has wide mood swings: she acts like an adult one minute and behaves like a child the next. Which of the following best explains Tina's present behavior fluctuations?
    ○ 1. She has regressed because of her impending scoliosis treatment
    ○ 2. She is acting like a normal adolescent.
    ○ 3. She fears disruption in identity formation.
    ○ 4. She is reassessing her values.

194. Tina is fitted for a Milwaukee brace. Which suggestion would be best for the nurse to make when Tina asks how she can be comfortable in the brace?
    ○ 1. "Always wear a clean T-shirt under the brace."
    ○ 2. "Keep a back scratcher handy to scratch those itchy areas under the brace."
    ○ 3. "Rub baby oil on the parts of the brace that rub on the skin."
    ○ 4. "Leave the brace off at night only if you have a very firm mattress."

195. How does Tina's physical development probably compare to that of boys her age?
    ○ 1. She is probably 2 years behind them.
    ○ 2. She is developing at about the same rate.
    ○ 3. She is probably 2 years ahead of most boys her age.
    ○ 4. Since she has scoliosis, her physcial development can not be accurately assessed.

196. Denise Dean was also found to have a curvature of the spine. Which of the following observations would most likely alert the nurse to possible structural scoliosis?
    ○ 1. The shoulders are hunched excessively forward.
    ○ 2. Shoulder blades are equally prominent.
    ○ 3. One shoulder is higher or longer than the other.
    ○ 4. There is an increased angle between the lumbar spine and the sacrum.

197. Denise was found to have a curve of the spine in need of treatment. A Milwaukee brace was prescribed. The nurse in the scoliosis clinic explained the brace to Denise. It would be most important for the nurse to alert Denise to which of the following?
    ○ 1. Treatment of scoliosis is short term; the brace will be required for only a few months.
    ○ 2. Frequent adjustments of the brace will be needed, because of rapid growth rates during adolescence.
    ○ 3. Denise should wear the brace only at night.
    ○ 4. A tight fit is necessary, regardless of the discomfort.

198. The nurse is aware of the alteration in body image that Denise might experience as a result of the Milwaukee brace. Which of the following would be the most helpful action to foster a positive self-image for Denise?
- ○ **1.** Suggest that Denise limit her activities, especially outside school.
- ○ **2.** Suggest that Denise wear tight-fitting clothes or, when possible, wear clothing under the brace.
- ○ **3.** Encourage her to ask approval for wearing the brace from her family members.
- ○ **4.** Encourage Denise to maintain her personal hygiene and attractive hair style.

199. Denise's scoliosis continues to worsen, and she is admitted to the hospital for a spinal fusion. As part of the pre-op teaching, the nurse should include which of the following?
- ○ **1.** Demonstration of the Stryker frame to be used following surgery
- ○ **2.** Instructions not to move her head or extremities following surgery
- ○ **3.** A choice of food she desires to eat the first evening following surgery
- ○ **4.** The possible complications resulting from the surgery

Mary Anderson, 13 years old, is seen in the outpatient clinic. Her mother states that Mary has been complaining of knee and ankle pain. She also seems to bruise easily and upon examination, numerous petechiae and hematomas are noted. Mary has been anorexic, listless, and lethargic. A diagnosis of acute lymphocytic leukemia is made, and Mary is hospitalized.

200. Which of the following roommates would be most appropriate for Mary?
- ○ **1.** A 12-year-old with an elevated temperature
- ○ **2.** A 12-year-old with juvenile rheumatoid arthritis
- ○ **3.** A 12-year-old with sickle cell crisis
- ○ **4.** A 12-year-old with a fractured femur

201. Assuming Mary is a normal 13-year-old, which of the following areas will present the most problems for her?
- ○ **1.** Family roles
- ○ **2.** Limit setting
- ○ **3.** School work
- ○ **4.** Body image

202. Which of the following solutions would be most appropriate to use when flushing the IV tubing following Mary's blood transfusion?
- ○ **1.** Dextrose and water
- ○ **2.** Normal saline
- ○ **3.** Salt-poor albumin
- ○ **4.** Fresh frozen plasma

203. Epistaxis could be a serious problem for Mary. If this should develop, which of the following nursing actions would be most appropriate?
- ○ **1.** Place her in semi- or high-Fowler's position.
- ○ **2.** Place her in a supine position with a small pillow under her neck.
- ○ **3.** Administer oxygen per nasal cannula at 4 liter/minute.
- ○ **4.** Instruct her to gently blow her nose to dislodge the clot.

204. Mary spikes a temperature of 104°F (40°C) orally. Which of the following nursing actions would *not* be appropriate for Mary?
- ○ **1.** Encourage clear fluids as tolerated.
- ○ **2.** Monitor vital signs q1h to q2h.
- ○ **3.** Administer 2 adult-size aspirin tablets.
- ○ **4.** Sponge bathe her with tepid water.

205. While Mary is acutely ill, the nurse considers how she is likely to view death. Which statement is *inaccurate* about an adolescent's concept of death?
- ○ **1.** They believe that death will not happen to them.
- ○ **2.** They feel decreased anxiety about death.
- ○ **3.** They may attempt to exert their own power over mortality by tempting fate.
- ○ **4.** They may exhibit marked interest in religious beliefs concerning death.

206. Mary is receiving methotrexate. Which of the following is *contraindicated* with methotrexate administration?
- ○ **1.** Vitamins without folic aid
- ○ **2.** Anticholinergic medications
- ○ **3.** Vitamins with folic acid
- ○ **4.** Antihistamines

207. Mary is also receiving allopurinol. This drug is given to prevent
- ○ **1.** hypokalemia.
- ○ **2.** hyperkalemia.
- ○ **3.** hypouricemia.
- ○ **4.** hyperuricemia.

208. Which of the following nursing actions will be most appropriate for Mary while she is receiving allopurinol?
    ○ 1. Encourage oral fluids.
    ○ 2. Provide foods high in protein.
    ○ 3. Monitor diet for sucrose intake.
    ○ 4. Omit carbonated beverages.

209. Which of the following will be *contraindicated* for Mary until her disease is in remission?
    ○ 1. Antibiotics
    ○ 2. Immunizations
    ○ 3. Corticosteroids
    ○ 4. Bronchodilators

210. While Mary's bed is being changed, she cries out loudly and says, ''Don't touch me.'' Which of the following represents an accurate interpretation of this behavior?
    ○ 1. Children with leukemia have been overprotected by their parents.
    ○ 2. Children with leukemia are easily upset by disruptions in their routine.
    ○ 3. Children with leukemia are sensitive to touch and movement.
    ○ 4. Children with leukemia tend to employ manipulative techniques.

211. Mary responded well to treatment and was sent home. She has been seen in the outpatient clinic once a week for IV vincristine. Several weeks after discharge, Mrs. Anderson calls the clinic to say that Mary is complaining of weakness in her hands and feet, numbness, tingling, and jaw pain. What is the nurse's best approach?
    ○ 1. Tell her this is part of the disease process and it will disappear in 4 to 6 months.
    ○ 2. Recognize that Mary's mother will be very sensitive to any change in her condition.
    ○ 3. Suggest that Mrs. Anderson mention this at Mary's next checkup.
    ○ 4. Tell her to notify the physician, since these are manifestations of vincristine toxicity.

Wilms' tumor is the most frequent intra-abdominal tumor of childhood and the most common type of cancer of the kidney.

212. The highest occurrence of Wilms' tumor is at which age?
    ○ 1. Birth to 2 years
    ○ 2. 3 to 4 years
    ○ 3. 6 to 8 years
    ○ 4. 7 to 10 years

213. What is the most frequent sign of Wilms' tumor?
    ○ 1. Increasing abdominal girth
    ○ 2. Decreased urinary output
    ○ 3. Hypertension
    ○ 4. Weight loss

214. What is the best method of teaching the toddler about pre-op and post-op care?
    ○ 1. Mimicry using dolls
    ○ 2. Audiovisual devices
    ○ 3. Verbal explanations
    ○ 4. Peer play

215. Pre-op nursing care for the child with Wilms' tumor does *not* include
    ○ 1. preparing the child and family for pre-op tests.
    ○ 2. carefully monitoring blood pressure.
    ○ 3. palpating the abdomen to identify the tumor size.
    ○ 4. planning for post-op care.

216. Post-op care for the child following excision of Wilms' tumor does *not* include
    ○ 1. observing for signs of shock.
    ○ 2. monitoring gastrointestinal activity.
    ○ 3. monitoring intake and output.
    ○ 4. offering a diet high in sodium.

217. What is the overall goal in planning for discharge?
    ○ 1. Decreasing effects of chemotherapy
    ○ 2. Preventing nausea and vomiting.
    ○ 3. Planning for psychologic support
    ○ 4. Returning the child to normal pre-op lifestyle

218. Which of the following is most important in helping parents learn about home care needs for the post-op child?
    ○ 1. Include the parents in implementation of the care plans while the child is still in the hospital.
    ○ 2. Give the parents informative literature to read about home care.
    ○ 3. Save teaching until discharge is imminent.
    ○ 4. Allow the parents free time before teaching is begun.

References

Pillitteri, A. (1981). *Child health nursing: Care of the growing family* (2nd ed.). Boston: Little, Brown.

Smith, M., Goodman, J., Ramsay, N., & Pasternack, S. (1982). *Child and family: Concepts of nursing practice*. New York: McGraw-Hill.

Tackett, J., & Hunsberger, M. (1981). *Family-centered care of children and adolescents*. Philadelphia: Saunders.

Whaley, L. & Wong, D. (1986). *Nursing care of infants and children* (3rd ed.). St. Louis: Mosby.

Wieczorek, R. & Natapoff, J. (1981). *A conceptual approach to the nursing of children*. Philadelphia: Lippincott.

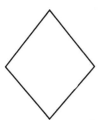

Section 5
Correct Answers

1. #1.	47. #3.	93. #1.	139. #1.
2. #4.	48. #4.	94. #3.	140. #1.
3. #2.	49. #1.	95. #4.	141. #2.
4. #1.	50. #3.	96. #3.	142. #2.
5. #4.	51. #3.	97. #1.	143. #1.
6. #2.	52. #3.	98. #2.	144. #3.
7. #4.	53. #1.	99. #2.	145. #1.
8. #1.	54. #4.	100. #1.	146. #2.
9. #2.	55. #4.	101. #1.	147. #1.
10. #4.	56. #3.	102. #4.	148. #2.
11. #4.	57. #1.	103. #4.	149. #3.
12. #4.	58. #2.	104. #4.	150. #2.
13. #1.	59. #2.	105. #3.	151. #1.
14. #1.	60. #3.	106. #2.	152. #2.
15. #3.	61. #1.	107. #4.	153. #4.
16. #1.	62. #3.	108. #1.	154. #3.
17. #4.	63. #2.	109. #1.	155. #2.
18. #3.	64. #4.	110. #3.	156. #3.
19. #1.	65. #1.	111. #4.	157. #1.
20. #4.	66. #4.	112. #3.	158. #2.
21. #3.	67. #1.	113. #1.	159. #3.
22. #3.	68. #3.	114. #1.	160. #2.
23. #3.	69. #1.	115. #3.	161. #3.
24. #1.	70. #3.	116. #4.	162. #3.
25. #4.	71. #3.	117. #3.	163. #3.
26. #2.	72. #1.	118. #2.	164. #1.
27. #3.	73. #4.	119. #2.	165. #2.
28. #1.	74. #2.	120. #4.	166. #2.
29. #2.	75. #1.	121. #1.	167. #3.
30. #2.	76. #3.	122. #4.	168. #3.
31. #2.	77. #1.	123. #2.	169. #4.
32. #1.	78. #2.	124. #4.	170. #3.
33. #4.	79. #1.	125. #4.	171. #2.
34. #2.	80. #1.	126. #4.	172. #3.
35. #2.	81. #3.	127. #3.	173. #3.
36. #1.	82. #3.	128. #2.	174. #4.
37. #3.	83. #2.	129. #3.	175. #2.
38. #2.	84. #2.	130. #1.	176. #1.
39. #3.	85. #4.	131. #1.	177. #2.
40. #3.	86. #1.	132. #3.	178. #4.
41. #1.	87. #3.	133. #4.	179. #2.
42. #2.	88. #3.	134. #4.	180. #3.
43. #2.	89. #1.	135. #3.	181. #3.
44. #1.	90. #1.	136. #3.	182. #4.
45. #2.	91. #2.	137. #3.	183. #4.
46. #3.	92. #4.	138. #1.	184. #1.

185. #1.	**194.** #1.	**203.** #1.	**212.** #2.
186. #1.	**195.** #3.	**204.** #3.	**213.** #1.
187. #3.	**196.** #3.	**205.** #2.	**214.** #1.
188. #1.	**197.** #2.	**206.** #3.	**215.** #3.
189. #1.	**198.** #4.	**207.** #4.	**216.** #4.
190. #2.	**199.** #1.	**208.** #1.	**217.** #4.
191. #3.	**200.** #4.	**209.** #2.	**218.** #1.
192. #3.	**201.** #4.	**210.** #3.	
193. #2.	**202.** #2.	**211.** #4.	

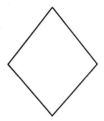

Correct Answers with Rationales

Editors note:

Two pieces of information are supplied at the end of each rationale. First we tell you what part of the nursing process the question addresses. Second, in parentheses, you will find a reference to a section in the *AJN Nursing Boards Review* where a more complete discussion of the topic may be found should you desire more information.

1. **#1.** Bowel control comes at about 18 months, depending on the developmental readiness of the child; daytime bladder training does not happen until 2 to 3 years of age. IMPLEMENTATION (CHILD/HEALTHY CHILD)

2. **#4.** Babies begin teething at 5 to 7 months; this is too early for bowel or bladder training. ASSESSMENT (CHILD/HEALTHY CHILD)

3. **#2.** Autonomy and independence are the tasks of this age. Option #3 is a task of infancy; options #1 and #4 are strategies for task achievement. ANALYSIS (CHILD/HEALTHY CHILD)

4. **#1.** This answer gives the child a limited choice and avoids a "no" answer, at least most of the time. Option #4 is unacceptable as it is unnecessarily punitive. IMPLEMENTATION (CHILD/HEALTHY CHILD)

5. **#4.** Unless the child is developmentally ready, toilet training only serves to train the parent and may produce frustration. ANALYSIS (CHILD/HEALTHY CHILD)

6. **#2.** Setting limits with consistency teaches the child habits that lead to self-control. It provides a sense of security for the child. PLAN (CHILD/HEALTHY CHILD)

7. **#4.** Four-year-olds have a decreased appetite, because their growth slows; they often pick a favorite food and need to choose the amount to eat. Small helpings at mealtime, plus nutritious snacks at midmorning and midafternoon, should be offered to them without bribes or threats. IMPLEMENTATION (CHILD/HEALTHY CHILD)

8. **#1.** This is the only correct option. The appropriate action is described in the above question. IMPLEMENTATION (CHILD/HEALTHY CHILD)

9. **#2.** Three-year-olds like finger foods and can feed themselves with a spoon; they do not have motor skills to sit quietly and eat with grown-up manners. They will learn family manners as they mature. IMPLEMENTATION (CHILD/HEALTHY CHILD)

10. **#4.** Allowing the child to explore the room with a flashlight would increase fears at this age. Options #1 and #2 do not allow the child to get used to the dark and deal with his overactive imagination. IMPLEMENTATION (CHILD/HEALTHY CHILD)

11. **#4.** This response is supportive and gently encouraging. Option #3 belittles the child and makes him feel bad about his lack of accomplishment. Options #1 and #2 are rigid and only emphasize his "failure." IMPLEMENTATION (CHILD/HEALTHY CHILD)

12. **#4.** It is important to acknowledge the child's imagination; this will be the source of creativity in later life. Options #1 and #2 are not true; the child is not lying. Option #3 is all right but does not have the positive aspect that #4 has. IMPLEMENTATION (CHILD/HEALTHY CHILD)

13. **#1.** Preschoolers need to explore their bodies and can begin to learn family and social limits on this behavior at this age. Option #4 is untrue. Options #2 and #3 falsely communicate to the child that masturbation is wrong. IMPLEMENTATION (CHILD/HEALTHY CHILD)

14. **#1.** The Dick test detects scarlet fever; the Guthrie test screens for phenylketonuria; heterophil antibody test determines the presence of mononucleosis. ASSESSMENT (CHILD/HEALTHY CHILD)

15. **#3.** Temper tantrums are the toddler's way of releasing tension and aggression and are used to gain control. It is a normal, age-appropriate behavior. IMPLEMENTATION (CHILD/HEALTHY CHILD)

16. **#1.** According to the American Academy of Pediatrics recommended schedule, Kimberly should receive DTP and OPV boosters (these should be given once between 4 and 6 years of age). An annual Tine test is also recommended. PLAN (CHILD/HEALTHY CHILD)

17. **#4.** The average child is unable to tie shoe-laces until 6 or 7 years of age. ASSESSMENT (CHILD/HEALTHY CHILD)

18. **#3.** This behavior is very normal at this age and should be handled matter-of-factly. However, Kimberly's mother should take the opportunity to explain to both children that there are other, more acceptable ways they can satisfy their curiosity, such as asking their parents questions or reading age-appropriate education materials. IMPLEMENTATION (CHILD/HEALTHY CHILD)

19. **#1.** Most children between 5 and 8 years of age are not aware that they themselves will die; this realization comes around age 9 to 10 years, along with the awareness that death is inevitable for everyone. ANALYSIS (CHILD/HEALTHY CHILD)

20. **#4.** School-age children are old enough to learn to problem solve, cooperate, bargain, and compromise; the family is the most important place to learn these skills. To motivate school-age children, listen to their ideas and facilitate a problem-solving attitude. IMPLEMENTATION (CHILD/HEALTHY CHILD)

21. **#3.** Depriving a child of food as punishment sets up a control struggle and is unnecessary; withholding other kinds of treats or utilizing methods relevant to causes of behavior is more effective in teaching healthy habits. PLAN (CHILD/HEALTHY CHILD)

22. **#3.** Stressing the importance of good table manners is not effective. It is more effective to give information or teach the child to increase his own awareness by keeping a journal. PLAN (CHILD/HEALTHY CHILD)

23. **#3.** According to Erikson, this is the task for the 6-to-12 age group. ANALYSIS (CHILD/HEALTHY CHILD)

24. **#1.** Concrete operations covers the ages from 7 to 11. Preoperational thinking occurs in the preschool age, and formal operations is the final stage. ANALYSIS (CHILD/HEALTHY CHILD)

25. **#4.** The child's age and stage of development as well as level of preparedness influence her reaction to the hospital. If the child has been told about the hospitalization and given a simple explanation of the need for it, she can adjust more easily than if not told ahead of time. PLAN (CHILD/ILL AND HOSPITALIZED CHILD)

26. **#2.** Allowing the child to take toys and books to the hospital helps to ease the transition from home to hospital. Scaring the child with threats or not telling the child ahead of time erodes trust and does not help the child accept hospitalization. PLAN (CHILD/ILL AND HOSPITALIZED CHILD)

27. **#3.** This option gives the child realistic information; lying or telling the child not to complain will not help the child adjust. Suggesting the child might get very sick and need a blood transfusion is unnecessary and frightening. Unloaded, simple explanations are best. IMPLEMENTATION (CHILD/ILL AND HOSPITALIZED CHILD)

28. **#1.** The nurse gives a truthful account of what will be done. The focus is positive and presented in terms of helping the child (child centered). The other options are threatening to the child because they are stated in negative terms or are belittling to her. IMPLEMENTATION (CHILD/ILL AND HOSPITALIZED CHILD)

29. **#2.** Infection is the greatest deterrent to surgery. There is no reason for hemorrhage before surgery because the tissues are still intact. Vital signs have little to do with indications for IV fluids (dehydration) or blood transfusions (low hemoglobin). ANALYSIS (CHILD/SENSATION, PERCEPTION, PROTECTION)

30. **#2.** This position prevents aspiration of any secretions or blood and helps to keep the airway clear. PLAN (CHILD/SENSATION, PERCEPTION, PROTECTION)

31. **#2.** Some bleeding is common, but hemorrhage is a serious and the most common complication. ANALYSIS (CHILD/SENSATION, PERCEPTION, PROTECTION)

32. **#1.** Children often regress in the hospital and need support from parents. Quiet holding and rocking prevent crying and facilitate healing. IMPLEMENTATION (CHILD/SENSATION, PERCEPTION, PROTECTION)

33. **#4.** Intuitive thought is Piaget's cognitive development phase for the 4- to 7-year-old child. ANALYSIS (CHILD/HEALTHY CHILD)

34. **#2.** Clinical signs of dehydration in infants include depressed anterior fontanels, dry mucous membranes, weight loss, poor tissue turgor, and increased specific gravity. ASSESSMENT (CHILD/SENSATION, PERCEPTION, PROTECTION)

35. **#2.** The definitive test for meningitis is a lumbar puncture. This is necessary to obtain a cerebrospinal fluid specimen for culture. ANALYSIS (CHILD/SENSATION, PERCEPTION, PROTECTION)

36. **#1.** Administration of potassium in the presence of diminished renal function may lead to hyperkalemia because potassium is excreted through the kidneys. ASSESSMENT (CHILD/SENSATION, PERCEPTION, PROTECTION)

37. **#3.** Children with meningitis are sensitive to noise, bright lights, and various other external stimuli. PLAN (CHILD/SENSATION, PERCEPTION, PROTECTION)

38. **#2.** Penicillin must be given for the entire course (usually about 10 days). Options #1 and #4 are contraindicated; option #3 is not as important as #2. IMPLEMENTATION (CHILD/SENSATION, PERCEPTION, PROTECTION)

39. **#3.** Vision is fully developed by age 7. Option #1 is more appropriate for an older child. Option #2 is fine from 3 to 7 years, #4 is appropriate for toddlers. IMPLEMENTATION (CHILD/SENSATION, PERCEPTION, PROTECTION)

40. **#3.** These are signs of post-tonsillectomy bleeding. ASSESSMENT (CHILD/SENSATION, PERCEPTION, PROTECTION)

41. **#1.** Recovery should be complete in 1 to 2 weeks. Gargling is contraindicated; delayed hemorrhage occurs after the fifth to the seventh day. IMPLEMENTATION (CHILD/SENSATION, PERCEPTION, PROTECTION)

42. **#2.** Scratching the anal area at night and insomnia are characteristic of pinworm infestation. ANALYSIS (CHILD/SENSATION, PERCEPTION, PROTECTION)

43. **#2.** The tape test is used to diagnose pinworms; the sticky surface of the tape over the anus can pick up ova in less than a minute in the early morning. PLAN (CHILD/SENSATION, PERCEPTION, PROTECTION)

44. **#1.** Children often regress to previous patterns when they are hospitalized; the child of 4 sleeps soundly and may sleep right through the urge to urinate. Putting a 4-year-old in diapers in the hospital is not appropriate, since this encourages regression and does not help the child move to the next developmental task. IMPLEMENTATION (CHILD/SENSATION, PERCEPTION, PROTECTION)

45. **#2.** Personnel at both the poison control center and the emergency room will need to know the substance consumed. Observing and waiting for symptoms to develop may use up too much valuable time. IMPLEMENTATION (CHILD/SENSATION, PERCEPTION, PROTECTION)

46. **#3.** This is the recommended dose for a child over 1 year of age. Option #1 is appropriate for hydrocarbon ingestion. By the time symptoms appear, the substance has been absorbed and time has been wasted. IMPLEMENTATION (CHILD/SENSATION, PERCEPTION, PROTECTION)

47. **#3.** She is too young to remember everything that is poisonous. It is the poorest of the 4 choices. The other options prevent access or condition her to respect medicine. PLAN (CHILD/SENSATION, PERCEPTION, PROTECTION)

48. **#4.** This is the only option that addresses prevention. She has actually followed through on what she learned and provided a safe environment for her toddler. The other options are short term or are aimed at intervention after poisoning has occurred. EVALUATION (CHILD/SENSATION, PERCEPTION, PROTECTION)

49. **#1.** This is characteristic of the 24-month-old child. All the other behaviors are characteristic of a younger child. ASSESSMENT (CHILD/SENSATION, PERCEPTION, PROTECTION)

50. **#3.** Spastic cerebral palsy results in hypertonicity of muscles and reflexes, leading to scissoring of legs. Mental retardation is not necessarily an associated problem. ASSESSMENT (CHILD/SENSATION, PERCEPTION, PROTECTION)

51. **#3.** Sandy needs assistance with feeding because of her motor impairment. This approach is the safest while providing motor stability to improve feeding. IMPLEMENTATION (CHILD/SENSATION, PERCEPTION, PROTECTION)

52. **#3.** Reflecting the mother's feelings opens communication for further exploration and expression of her specific concerns. IMPLEMENTATION (CHILD/SENSATION, PERCEPTION, PROTECTION)

53. **#1.** Children with Down syndrome are hypotonic, not spastic. This decreased muscle tone compromises respiratory excursion, making the child more prone to respiratory infections. Hypotonicity may also delay achievement of motor skills, but developmental potential is greatest during infancy. What to expect needs to be reinforced with parents, because they may see their child developing along a somewhat normal developmental curve and thus come to have unrealistic expectations of the final potential. IMPLEMENTATION (CHILD/SENSATION, PERCEPTION, PROTECTION)

54. **#4.** Trisomy 21, or Down syndrome, is caused by the presence of an extra chromosome 21. All other options are true. ANALYSIS (CHILD/SENSATION, PERCEPTION, PROTECTION)

55. **#4.** Limiting stimulation will not promote the mentally retarded child's optimal development. Having the same parent always work with the child to learn new skills is unrealistic. While teaching socially acceptable behaviors is important in "normalizing" the child, mentally retarded children really need consistency and structure in their daily routines to foster learning and promote security. PLAN (CHILD/SENSATION, PERCEPTION, PROTECTION)

56. **#3.** The initial phase of grief is shock and disbelief. ANALYSIS (CHILD/SENSATION, PERCEPTION, PROTECTION)

57. **#1.** It is very important for Mr. Carlton to have contact with his new baby so he can begin to develop an attachment to her, and to see her as a baby first, and then as a baby with a health problem. IMPLEMENTATION (CHILD/SENSATION, PERCEPTION, PROTECTION)

58. **#2.** Rupture of the sac can cause leakage of cerebrospinal fluid and lead to central nervous system infection with permanent brain damage. PLAN (CHILD/SENSATION, PERCEPTION, PROTECTION)

59. **#2.** Although the myelomeningocele requires taking special precautions, these infants can be held. Touch is the most comforting, highly developed sense in infants. The other measures would stimulate the visual and hearing senses, but would not be as comforting as touch. IMPLEMENTATION (CHILD/SENSATION, PERCEPTION, PROTECTION)

60. **#3.** If a dressing is ordered, it must be kept moist to prevent damage to the friable covering of the myelomeningocele. IMPLEMENTATION (CHILD/SENSATION, PERCEPTION, PROTECTION)

61. **#1.** The most common complication following surgical closure of a myelomeningocele is hydrocephalus. Daily measurement of the head circumference is essential for early detection and treatment of this complication. ASSESSMENT (CHILD/SENSATION, PERCEPTION, PROTECTION)

62. **#3.** The number of drops/minute is equal to the number of ml/hour when a microdrip is used. IMPLEMENTATION (CHILD/SENSATION, PERCEPTION, PROTECTION)

63. **#2.** Keeping her hips abducted encourages the hip joints to develop normally, decreasing the probability of congenital hip dysplasia. PLAN (CHILD/SENSATION, PERCEPTION, PROTECTION)

64. **#4.** The nurse should prevent Natalie from injuring herself on the crib rails during the seizure. IMPLEMENTATION (CHILD/SENSATION, PERCEPTION, PROTECTION)

65. **#1.** Children tend to eliminate anticonvulsants more readily and, therefore, are usually given higher doses to achieve desired blood levels of the drug. ANALYSIS (CHILD/SENSATION, PERCEPTION, PROTECTION)

66. **#4.** Although phenytoin may cause malaise, it does not cause excessive sleepiness in children (as phenobarbital may) and is often selected as the drug of choice for this reason. IMPLEMENTATION (CHILD/SENSATION, PERCEPTION, PROTECTION)

67. **#1.** A high-pitched cry is one of the key manifestations of increased intracranial pressure in infants. ASSESSMENT (CHILD/SENSATION, PERCEPTION, PROTECTION)

68. **#3.** The shunt may become obstructed with cells or tissue debris. Infection is also a common complication of shunt insertion. ANALYSIS (CHILD/SENSATION, PERCEPTION, PROTECTION)

69. **#1.** It is essential to maintain patency of the shunt by pumping the valve, in order to prevent any increase in intracranial pressure. PLAN (CHILD/SENSATION, PERCEPTION, PROTECTION)

70. **#3.** Overhydration can cause an increase in intracranial pressure and, thus, interfere with shunt functioning or cause damage to brain cells. PLAN (CHILD/SENSATION, PERCEPTION, PROTECTION)

71. **#3.** The major goal of treatment is to prevent neurologic damage. This is best evaluated by appraising the child's neurologic functioning using cognitive and motor development as indicators. EVALUATION (CHILD/SENSATION, PERCEPTION, PROTECTION)

72. **#1.** In their shock, numbness, and disbelief immediately after their daughter's death, the Howards will not be able to grasp a detailed explanation and may be overwhelmed by it. All the other options provide support and comfort, which are the priority goals. IMPLEMENTATION (CHILD/OXYGENATION)

73. **#4.** At this time, no clear etiology for sudden infant death syndrome (SIDS) has been identified. Research continues on SIDS, but options #1, #2, and #3 have been ruled out. ANALYSIS (CHILD/OXYGENATION)

74. **#2.** Involvement in a parents' support group indicates the Howards' willingness to face and deal openly with their daughter's death. EVALUATION (CHILD/OXYGENATION)

75. **#1.** Diminished breath sounds occur because of bronchiolitic obstruction. If a cough were present, it would be moist, not dry. Option #3 indicates upper respiratory problems. Expirations are long because air is trapped in lower field. ASSESSMENT (CHILD/OXYGENATION)

76. **#3.** An infant with very fast respirations barely has a chance to swallow before he must take another breath, thus making aspiration a real possibility. Hydration is a major concern because the infant loses fluid with easy respiration. Options #1 and #2 are false. ANALYSIS (CHILD/OXYGENATION)

77. **#1.** Accumulation of mucus occurs at the bronchiolar level; therefore, suctioning would not be effective. PLAN (CHILD/OXYGENATION)

78. **#2.** Semi-Fowler's facilitates expansion of the lungs. PLAN (CHILD/OXYGENATION)

79. **#1.** Performing chest physical therapy before meals minimizes the possibility of vomiting. Every 8 hours is too long an interval. PLAN (CHILD/OXYGENATION)

80. **#1.** An infant's birth weight should double by 5 to 6 months, and triple at 1 year. ASSESSMENT (CHILD/HEALTHY CHILD)

81. **#3.** Lower central incisors usually erupt around 5 to 6 months of age; drooling precedes this at approximately 4 months of age. Upper central incisors erupt next. ASSESSMENT (CHILD/HEALTHY CHILD)

82. **#3.** Voluntary grasping and improved eye-hand coordination enable the infant to begin picking up finger foods; also, the use of finger foods will foster increased independence. PLAN (CHILD/HEALTHY CHILD)

83. **#2.** Rice cereal is hypoallergenic and is easily digested. The other options have a higher propensity for causing allergy. PLAN (CHILD/HEALTHY CHILD)

84. **#2.** Seven to 9 months is the usual age for this activity. ASSESSMENT (CHILD/HEALTHY CHILD)

85. **#4.** Tuberculin testing provides systematic screening of the population; it is usually done before the measles, mumps, rubella vaccination. PLAN (CHILD/OXYGENATION)

86. **#1.** Instillation of several milliliters of sterile saline loosens thick secretions and mechanically stimulates the cough reflex. It has nothing to do with sleep patterns directly, nor does it replace deep suctioning. The saline instillation makes suctioning more effective. ANALYSIS (CHILD/OXYGENATION)

87. **#3.** This action provides baseline information regarding need for and effectiveness of suctioning. IMPLEMENTATION (CHILD/OXYGENATION)

88. **#3.** The act of suctioning mechanically removes oxygen directly from the airway. Presuction oxygenation replaces that oxygen so that the child does not become hypoxic. Oxygen will not directly relax Pedro, but the lack of oxygen will cause him to become agitated. ANALYSIS (CHILD/OXYGENATION)

89. **#1.** The outer cannula is never removed. The inner cannula is cleaned every shift and as needed. Pediatric trach tubes are not cuffed in order to prevent tracheal damage. IMPLEMENTATION (CHILD/OXYGENATION)

90. **#1.** Suctioning will improve respiratory exchange; therefore, breath sounds will be improved. Options #2, #3, and #4 are evidence of continued respiratory problems. ASSESSMENT (CHILD/OXYGENATION)

91. **#2.** Ampicillin destroys the normal flora of the gastrointestinal tract; yogurt will help promote its return. IMPLEMENTATION (CHILD/OXYGENATION)

92. **#4.** Cromolyn sodium is an inhalant that can irritate the throat and trachea. ANALYSIS (CHILD/OXYGENATION)

93. **#1.** Secure in relationships with the family, the elementary-school-age child explores the environment beyond the family and becomes more involved with peers and other adults. ASSESSMENT (CHILD/HEALTHY CHILD)

94. **#3.** Medications that interfere with the cough reflex are contraindicated. The priority concern during an acute asthma attack is to promote effective air exchange by loosening secretions, so they can be coughed up and expectorated. IMPLEMENTATION (CHILD/OXYGENATION)

95. **#4.** The 6-year-old is in a stage of concrete operations and needs to test new experiences firsthand. IMPLEMENTATION (CHILD/HEALTHY CHILD)

96. **#3.** The school-age child's psychosocial task is to develop a sense of industry. Hospitalization may interfere with mastery of this task, thus leading to feelings of inferiority. ANALYSIS (CHILD/ILL AND HOSPITALIZED CHILD)

97. **#1.** The school-age child's greatest fear is loss of control. This is especially accentuated by frightening experiences such as hospitalization and an acute asthma attack. PLAN (CHILD/OXYGENATION)

98. **#2.** The risk of having an asthma attack is lessened when the asthmatic child's immunizations are up-to-date and when she has received seasonal flu shots. Her room should be kept as dust free as possible. Option #3 is not safe and #4 is not necessary. IMPLEMENTATION (CHILD/OXYGENATION)

99. **#2.** Hemolytic anemia is present throughout the life of a child with sickle cell disease; option #1 is a condition seen in infants, and answer #3 is a clinical sign common in Down syndrome. Pallor precedes jaundice by several days. ASSESSMENT (CHILD/OXYGENATION)

100. **#1.** This is the most common cause of decreased circulation in the painful area. The other 3 options are not nearly as stressful to the body. ASSESSMENT (CHILD/OXYGENATION)

101. **#1.** Heat increases circulation (and oxygen) to the area that needs it most. Blood transfusions are not used unless the hemoglobin is 4 gm or less. Limiting fluids increases problems with sickling. IMPLEMENTATION (CHILD/OXYGENATION)

102. **#4.** High altitudes decrease available oxygen. Exogenous oxygen has little effect on the sickled red blood cells. Increased activity increases body demand for oxygen. IMPLEMENTATION (CHILD/OXYGENATION)

103. **#4.** Hemarthrosis (bleeding into a joint space) is the classic sign of hemophilia and the manifestation most likely to cause serious or permanent sequelae. ASSESSMENT (CHILD/OXYGENATION)

104. **#4.** This allows Darryl to be involved with his peers and also maintain his interest in football. PLAN (CHILD/OXYGENATION)

105. **#3.** Packed cells do not contain factor VIII, the needed coagulation factor. ANALYSIS (CHILD/OXYGENATION)

106. **#2.** The weight from the bedcovers may intensify the bleeding. Affected joints should be immobilized in a slightly flexed position during the bleeding episode. Aspirin and heat are contraindicated because they may exacerbate the bleeding. IMPLEMENTATION (CHILD/OXYGENATION)

107. **#4.** Hemophilia is a sex-linked recessive disorder transmitted to offspring by female carriers. Darryl's sons will receive a normal sex chromosome from each parent. His daughters will all receive the abnormal ''X^r'' chromosome from him and, thus, will be carriers. ANALYSIS (CHILD/OXYGENATION)

108. **#1.** Prevention and control of bleeding episodes is the priority concern. Therefore, the fewer the number of bleeding episodes the child has, the more successful the outcomes of treatment. EVALUATION (CHILD/OXYGENATION)

109. **#1.** A normally developing 1-year-old will be cruising and possibly walking. The other behaviors are accomplished in later months. ASSESSMENT (CHILD/HEALTHY CHILD)

110. **#3.** The PPD skin test is interpreted in terms of induration, not erythema. Induration of 10 mm or more is considered positive. A lesion with 5 to 9 mm of induration is considered doubtful, although it may indicate tuberculosis in a child less than 2 years old. ASSESSMENT (CHILD/SENSATION, PERCEPTION, PROTECTION)

111. **#4.** Infants under 6 months old, particularly those less than 3 months, may not be able to produce sufficient local inflammation for a positive skin test. Often there is a suppression of dermal sensitivity in children with viral diseases, who have received viral vaccines within the past 4 weeks, or who are malnourished. ASSESSMENT (CHILD/SENSATION, PERCEPTION, PROTECTION)

112. **#3.** Response to antituberculosis therapy is slow and requires prolonged treatment. Miguel's condition is not communicable. A sputum specimen is of little diagnostic value, since young children expectorate very small amounts and then promptly swallow the sputum. Gastric aspiration is usually of more diagnostic value. IMPLEMENTATION (CHILD/SENSATION, PERCEPTION, PROTECTION)

113. **#1.** In addition to addressing the mother's concerns, the nurse should give Barbara a simple, honest explanation of the basic steps in the cardiac catheterization. Because 4-year-old children are in the preoperational period of cognitive development, they are capable of prelogical reasoning about medical interventions. IMPLEMENTATION (CHILD/OXYGENATION)

114. **#1.** Barbara desperately needs her "security" object to give her a sense of constancy and comfort, especially during the stressful period of hospitalization. IMPLEMENTATION (CHILD/ILL AND HOSPITALIZED CHILD)

115. **#3.** The best course of action for dealing with a hospitalized toddler going through the protest phase of separation anxiety would be to stay with the child and offer support and comfort. IMPLEMENTATION (CHILD/ILL AND HOSPITALIZED CHILD)

116. **#4.** A sinus dysrhythmia is a normal physiologic phenomenon of childhood. The heart rate increases on inspiration and decreases on expiration. Breath holding causes the rate to remain steady, thus allowing assessment between breaths of any potentially pathologic dysrhythmia. ASSESSMENT (CHILD/OXYGENATION)

117. **#3.** The left-to-right shunt with a ventricular septal defect causes increased blood flow to the lungs because extra amounts of blood enter the right ventricle and are carried to the lungs via the pulmonary artery. ANALYSIS (CHILD/OXYGENATION)

118. **#2.** Children with cardiac problems are particularly susceptible to recurrent upper respiratory tract infections. This results from pulmonary vascular congestion, since large amounts of blood pool in the lungs. ANALYSIS (CHILD/OXYGENATION)

119. **#2.** Parents of children with congenital heart disease frequently attempt to overprotect their children, because of their fears of overexerting and exposing the child to environmental risks. The child may have had fewer opportunities for coping with frustrations or delayed gratification. ANALYSIS (CHILD/OXYGENATION)

120. **#4.** Most children with exercise intolerance rest when they need to do so. Option #2 is incorrect because a ventricular septal defect is an acyanotic problem that does not cause anemia. IMPLEMENTATION (CHILD/OXYGENATION)

121. **#1.** This is a part of pre-op teaching to decrease the child's fear of the tent after surgery. PLAN (CHILD/OXYGENATION)

122. **#4.** This is an abnormally slow pulse for a 3-year-old, and thus digoxin is contraindicated. IMPLEMENTATION (CHILD/OXYGENATION)

123. **#2.**

$$\frac{.05 \text{ mg}}{1 \text{ ml}} \times \frac{.06 \text{ mg}}{x \text{ ml}}$$
$$.05x = .06 \text{ ml}$$
$$x = 1.2 \text{ ml}$$
$$\frac{1 \text{ ml}}{15 \text{ min}} \times \frac{1.2}{x}$$
$$x = 18 \text{ minims}$$

IMPLEMENTATION (CHILD/OXYGENATION)

124. **#4.** Digoxin increases the force of myocardial contraction and produces a stronger systolic contraction of the heart; it also slows the heart rate. These actions result in increased cardiac output and venous pressure, which improve diuresis; pulse rhythm is also improved. ANALYSIS (CHILD/OXYGENATION)

125. **#4.** Hypothermia is used to reduce oxygen needs during surgery by decreasing overall body metabolism. ANALYSIS (CHILD/OXYGENATION)

126. **#4.** Two to 3 chest tubes are placed for drainage or suction, or both, to remove fluid and air that entered the pleural cavity and mediastinal space during surgery. ANALYSIS (CHILD/OXYGENATION)

127. #3. A chest drainage system will remove solids, such as fibrin or clotted blood; liquids, such as serous fluids; and gaseous materials. ''Milking'' the tubes prevents them from becoming plugged with clots or other material. The thoracotomy tube should be immediately clamped if it becomes disconnected to prevent air from entering the pleural cavity and causing a possible tension pneumothorax. IMPLEMENTATION (CHILD/OXYGENATION)

128. #2. Placement of the nurse's hands on either side of the operative site (encircling the chest) may reduce the pain associated with the coughing procedure by decreasing movement in the area. IMPLEMENTATION (CHILD/OXYGENATION)

129. #3. Hospitalization and stress cause regression in toddlers, and regression is best dealt with by accepting the behavior. IMPLEMENTATION (CHILD/OXYGENATION)

130. #1. During the convalescent period, it is most appropriate to focus upon management of the child in a manner that will promote a healthy life-style. The child's heart defect is likely to have been associated with parental anxiety and overprotective behavior. Parents must be told to treat a child like Ronald as they would any other child. PLAN (CHILD/OXYGENATION)

131. #1. Temper tantrums are best handled by ignoring them. Without the attention, toddlers will stop using this behavior. EVALUATION (CHILD/OXYGENATION)

132. #3. Use of large muscles, as in throwing, allows for a safe release of energy. IMPLEMENTATION (CHILD/OXYGENATION)

133. #4. Psychosocial failure to thrive is the result of an interference with parent-infant attachment during the critical period of infancy. ANALYSIS (CHILD/NUTRITION AND METABOLISM)

134. #4. The infant with failure to thrive avoids eye contact with others, has a flat affect, is withdrawn, and does not exhibit any stranger anxiety. When held, these infants often become very stiff and try to pull away. ASSESSMENT (CHILD/NUTRITION AND METABOLISM)

135. #3. Head control comes at 2 months; rolling over comes at 5 months; sitting without support and transferring objects from one hand to another come at 8 months. Marcus is around 6 to 7 months developmentally. ANALYSIS (CHILD/NUTRITION AND METABOLISM)

136. #3. The infant with failure to thrive needs to have one primary care giver per shift so that trust can be established; having many persons pick up the child ad lib does not help promote bonding. A schedule of stimulation geared to the infant's developmental level and given by the primary care giver would be more helpful. PLAN (CHILD/NUTRITION AND METABOLISM)

137. #3. Infant and mother must be cared for as a unit. Marcus can be helped most by promoting his mother's feelings of worth and confidence in her mothering role and behaviors. IMPLEMENTATION (CHILD/NUTRITION AND METABOLISM)

138. #1. Marcus would not be able to snap the snap toys, since he is unable to transfer objects. IMPLEMENTATION (CHILD/NUTRITION AND METABOLISM)

139. #1. According to research, mothers who neglect and abuse their children often were neglected and abused as children. They lack knowledge of growth and development as well as knowledge of child care and have high stress levels. ANALYSIS (CHILD/NUTRITION AND METABOLISM)

140. #1. The parents who abuse their children seldom touch or look at the children. The other responses are not characteristic of the abusive parent. ASSESSMENT (CHILD/NUTRITION AND METABOLISM)

141. #2. The ultimate concern in treating the infant with failure to thrive is restoring physical growth to normal limits for age. Weight gain especially is used as an indicator that the infant is responding to treatment. EVALUATION (CHILD/NUTRITION AND METABOLISM)

142. #2. Nutrition and feeding are key concerns pre- and postoperatively. This information is needed to plan for meeting Peter's nutritional and comfort needs postoperatively. ASSESSMENT (CHILD/NUTRITION AND METABOLISM)

143. #1. The child under 5 years of age is most vulnerable and at psychologic risk when separated from parents, especially the mother, if she is the primary care giver. Separation can interrupt emotional development and result in loss of trust in others. The child's initial reaction to separation anxiety is protest. ANALYSIS (CHILD/ILL AND HOSPITALIZED CHILD)

144. **#3.** Sitting at the bedside and spending time is a way to begin to build a trusting relationship, so that Peter will want to come to the nurse. IMPLEMENTATION (CHILD/NUTRITION AND METABOLISM)

145. **#1.** Prone position facilitates drainage of secretions, which may be copious following cleft palate surgery. PLAN (CHILD/NUTRITION AND METABOLISM)

146. **#2.** Elbow restraints will prevent Peter from getting his hands or fingers into his mouth. Exercise his arms one at a time at least q2h. IMPLEMENTATION (CHILD/NUTRITION AND METABOLISM)

147. **#1.** Listening to a story is appropriate in terms of Peter's energy level postoperatively, and promotes security through interaction with someone. Peter cannot use his arms because of the elbow restraints. IMPLEMENTATION (CHILD/NUTRITION AND METABOLISM)

148. **#2.** Regression and inactivity are behaviors of despair when the primary care giver, the mother, is lost. The child feels mother really is not coming back and begins to grieve. ANALYSIS (CHILD/ILL AND HOSPITALIZED CHILD)

149. **#3.** To survive, the child must repress feelings about the lost mother and bond to care givers who are present. ANALYSIS (CHILD/ILL AND HOSPITALIZED CHILD)

150. **#2.** This approach gives Peter time to make a transition from the nurse to the mother as primary care giver; he will need time to work out his feelings about the mother's having left him. Anger, fear, resentment, and mistrust are often present in this transition and need to be expressed in actions if the child is too young to express them with words. Then he can begin to bond to the mother again. IMPLEMENTATION (CHILD/ILL AND HOSPITALIZED CHILD)

151. **#1.** Peter needs time to reestablish trust and security in his mother. When he is home and involved in his usual routine for a while, the behavior will gradually dissipate. He will not miss the hospital because of the separation and procedures experienced there. Peter will not be happier or more obedient at home after hospitalization than he was prior to it. IMPLEMENTATION (CHILD/NUTRITION AND METABOLISM)

152. **#2.** In type III esophageal atresia, the upper esophageal segment ends in a blind pouch, and the lower segment communicates with the trachea. The former defect results in drooling and the latter in abdominal distension. ASSESSMENT (CHILD/NUTRITION AND METABOLISM)

153. **#4.** Maintaining a patent airway is the major problem in tracheoesophageal fistula. PLAN (CHILD/NUTRITION AND METABOLISM)

154. **#3.** This position prevents reflux of gastric contents into the trachea, which could result in aspiration pneumonia. PLAN (CHILD/NUTRITION AND METABOLISM)

155. **#2.** With a microdrip infusion, the number of ml/hour is equal to the number of drops/minute. IMPLEMENTATION (CHILD/NUTRITION AND METABOLISM)

156. **#3.** Clamping the gastrostomy tube prevents air from escaping from the stomach and can result in gastric distension, which can also cause tension on the esophageal anastomosis. IMPLEMENTATION (CHILD/NUTRITION AND METABOLISM)

157. **#1.** Difficulty swallowing usually indicates stricture at the site of anastomosis. Some reddening around the gastrostomy tube is normal. Diarrhea and regurgitation of the formula can be prevented with correct feeding technique. IMPLEMENTATION (CHILD/NUTRITION AND METABOLISM)

158. **#2.** A favorite toy will give her some sense of continuity with home. A doll can be dried off when it becomes wet yet does not pose a safety hazard in the croup tent. IMPLEMENTATION (CHILD/NUTRITION AND METABOLISM)

159. **#3.** The only inappropriate option listed is to leave the tent outside the sheets. Since oxygen is heavier than room air, it would settle to the bottom of the tent and leak out the edges. Tuck the edges into the sheets to prevent this. IMPLEMENTATION (CHILD/NUTRITION AND METABOLISM)

160. **#2.** When using the microdrip, drops/minute equals ml/hour. 250 ml ÷ 8 = 31.25. IMPLEMENTATION (CHILD/NUTRITION AND METABOLISM)

161. **#3.** Diarrhea is a side effect of ampicillin and is usually self-limiting. IMPLEMENTATION (CHILD/NUTRITION AND METABOLISM)

162. #3. Take axillary temperatures to avoid irritating the anal area or increasing her respiratory distress. PLAN (CHILD/NUTRITION AND METABOLISM)

163. #3. 40 mg/65 mg = 1 ml/x; 40x = 65; x = 1.62 ml. IMPLEMENTATION (CHILD/NUTRITION AND METABOLISM)

164. #1. For the most reliable absorption, ampicillin should be administered on an empty stomach. IMPLEMENTATION (CHILD/NUTRITION AND METABOLISM)

165. #2. Eight-year-olds can ride a bike; activities in options #1 and #4 occur at earlier ages; option #3 is characteristic of adolescence. ASSESSMENT (CHILD/HEALTHY CHILD)

166. #2. This type of stool results from the undigested fat in the gastrointestinal tract. ASSESSMENT (CHILD/NUTRITION AND METABOLISM)

167. #3. Enzymes must be given with every meal and snack to help digest the food. IMPLEMENTATION (CHILD/NUTRITION AND METABOLISM)

168. #3. Because of the particular exocrine glands involved, large amounts of salt are lost and must be replaced. IMPLEMENTATION (CHILD/NUTRITION AND METABOLISM)

169. #4. Cystic fibrosis is not curable and, at best, must be managed throughout life. PLAN (CHILD/NUTRITION AND METABOLISM)

170. #3. Children should never have completely sugar-negative urine because it does not allow correct assessment of the blood glucose level. ASSESSMENT (CHILD/NUTRITION AND METABOLISM)

171. #2. This is evidence that Angela can assume responsibility for her care and has accepted that she has the disease. PLAN (CHILD/NUTRITION AND METABOLISM)

172. #3. Acute glomerulonephritis is not a congenital condition. The other options are all possible etiologies. ASSESSMENT (CHILD/ELIMINATION)

173. #3. The prognosis is favorable if the condition is promptly treated. ANALYSIS (CHILD/ELIMINATION)

174. #4. The adolescent has many body changes and is establishing an identity; there is a heightened concern with body image and loss of function at this time. ANALYSIS (CHILD/ILL AND HOSPITALIZED CHILD)

175. #2. Initial actions should be designed to orient the client and family to the hospital, offer information about immediate procedures of care, and build a trusting relationship. IMPLEMENTATION (CHILD/ELIMINATION)

176. #1. Strep infection frequently precedes nephritis. Although there is some chance of chronic renal failure, at this stage it is too early to determine if the damage is permanent. After recovery from the acute episode, Bob should return to his normal life-style. IMPLEMENTATION (CHILD/ELIMINATION)

177. #2. Cindy's history is strongly suggestive of a ruptured appendix. Often there is sudden relief from pain after perforation, then a subsequent increase in pain when peritonitis occurs. If the appendix has perforated, Cindy will need surgery, so she should have nothing by mouth. The white blood cell count is often elevated with appendicitis, so a complete blood count would be a useful diagnostic tool. PLAN (CHILD/ELIMINATION)

178. #4. Frequent dressing changes are essential to prevent skin excoriation and infection from drainage and to permit inspection of the incision. A ruptured appendix releases many organisms into the peritoneal cavity, thus broad-spectrum antibiotics are needed in order to prevent infection. Positioning the child in semi-Fowler's or on the right side facilitates drainage and helps prevent formation of a subdiaphragmatic abscess. IMPLEMENTATION (CHILD/ELIMINATION)

179. #2. The client is experiencing pain and is demonstrating psychic (crying, etc.), autonomic (warm, dry skin; irregular respirations, etc.), and skeletal (knees drawn up) responses. ANALYSIS (CHILD/ELIMINATION)

180. #3. The use of a rectal tube is directed toward removal of the cause of her discomfort. IMPLEMENTATION (CHILD/ELIMINATION)

181. #3. A soft, flat abdomen indicates that flatus has been reduced. The other symptoms would indicate pain relief but that would be accomplished by relieving the distension. EVALUATION (CHILD/ELIMINATION)

182. #4. Due to the lack of distal colonic peristalsis, the infant is frequently unable to pass stool. When stool and flatus accumulate in the colon, the abdomen becomes distended and the infant refuses fluids. ASSESSMENT (CHILD/ELIMINATION)

183. #4. Steatorrhea (fat in the stool) indicates a problem with fat metabolism but is not a problem in Hirschsprung's disease. The infant may not want to eat due to the elimination problem. Constipation and vomiting are due to the "backup" of stool and flatus in the colon. Diarrhea may result when liquid stool seeps around the stationary hard stool. ASSESSMENT (CHILD/ELIMINATION)

184. #1. A high-residue diet would aggravate the problem by increasing the stool mass. Clear liquids would not provide adequate nutrition. This infant does not have a problem with sodium or potassium so option #4 has no purpose. PLAN (CHILD/ELIMINATION)

185. #1. While options #2, #3, and #4 are a part of the complete health history, the bowel habits pertain to this disease process. ASSESSMENT (CHILD/ELIMINATION)

186. #1. The colostomy is usually temporary and will be closed when the surgical repair of the colon is completely healed and the bowel functions normally. This usually takes from a few months to a year. IMPLEMENTATION (CHILD/ELIMINATION)

187. #3. Since the proximal end receives the stool, only mucus should be in the distal portion of the colon. EVALUATION (CHILD/ELIMINATION)

188. #1. As with any bowel surgery, the client is given nothing by mouth until bowel function returns. IMPLEMENTATION (CHILD/ELIMINATION)

189. #1. Jams and preserves contains portions of the fruit that provide residue (e.g., tiny seeds, skins). IMPLEMENTATION (CHILD/ELIMINATION)

190. #2. Preadolescent and young adolescent females are at highest risk for developing scoliosis. ASSESSMENT (CHILD/MOBILITY)

191. #3. The child's bending forward at the waist with head and arms hanging freely allows the nurse to most easily detect any flank asymmetry or rib hump. ASSESSMENT (CHILD/MOBILITY)

192. #3. Change in body image and loss of control are the major fears of adolescence. ANALYSIS (CHILD/MOBILITY)

193. #2. Mood swings are common in adolescence. ANALYSIS (CHILD/MOBILITY)

194. #1. A T-shirt protects the skin and absorbs perspiration. The other options are inappropriate advice. IMPLEMENTATION (CHILD/MOBILITY)

195. #3. During early adolescence, girls are about 2 years ahead of their male counterparts in physical development. ANALYSIS (CHILD/MOBILITY)

196. #3. This is the only physical finding listed that is indicative of scoliosis. ASSESSMENT (CHILD/MOBILITY)

197. #2. The other options are incorrect and would lead to inadequate bracing or skin breakdown. IMPLEMENTATION (CHILD/MOBILITY)

198. #4. Following the other options would result in a poor self-image. Denise must emphasize her positive qualities and present as attractive an appearance as possible. IMPLEMENTATION (CHILD/MOBILITY)

199. #1. It is important that she move her head and extremities after surgery to maintain range of motion. She will be on an NPO or clear-liquids regimen following surgery. The complications would already have been explained when the operative permit was signed prior to pre-op teaching. IMPLEMENTATION (CHILD/MOBILITY)

200. #4. Mary will be susceptible to infection, because of neutropenia. Clients in options #1, #2, and #3 have an infectious process associated with their conditions and are, therefore, not suitable roommates. PLAN (CHILD/CELLULAR ABERRATION)

201. #4. The developmental task of adolescence consists of developing a strong sense of identity; body image is an integral part of an adolescent's identity. This would be the same for any 13-year-old, and is not specific to her problem. ANALYSIS (CHILD/HEALTHY CHILD)

202. #2. Hemolysis will occur if dextrose is used; salt-poor albumin and fresh frozen plasma are never used to flush an IV line. IMPLEMENTATION (CHILD/OXYGENATION)

203. #1. Semi- or high-Fowler's position prevents choking or aspiration of blood. This position also lessens the pressure in the vessels to the head. Option #4 would increase bleeding; #3 would interfere with the flow of blood and clog the cannula. IMPLEMENTATION (CHILD/CELLULAR ABERRATION)

204. #3. Aspirin is contraindicated in clients with bleeding problems because it increases bleeding time. IMPLEMENTATION (CHILD/CELLULAR ABERRATION)

205. **#2.** Adolescents have increased anxiety about death and worry that they will die before they have a chance to live. ASSESSMENT (CHILD/ILL AND HOSPITALIZED CHILD)

206. **#3.** Vitamins with folic acid will interfere with the cytoxic action of methotrexate as it is a folic acid antagonist. ANALYSIS (CHILD/CELLULAR ABERRATION)

207. **#4.** Uric acid is released during cell destruction and can accumulate in the renal tubules, resulting in uremia. Allopurinol interferes with the metabolic breakdown of xanthine oxidase to uric acid; therefore, uric acid production is inhibited. ANALYSIS (CHILD/CELLULAR ABERRATION)

208. **#1.** Encouraging oral fluids ensures adequate excretion of the end products of metabolism. PLAN (CHILD/CELLULAR ABERRATION)

209. **#2.** Immunizations are contraindicated with clients receiving immunosuppressive drugs. ANALYSIS (CHILD/CELLULAR ABERRATION)

210. **#3.** Children with leukemia are sensitive to touch because of osseous invasion by leukemic cells. ANALYSIS (CHILD/CELLULAR ABERRATION)

211. **#4.** Vincristine can be neurotoxic; numbness, tingling, jaw pain, and ataxia are manifestations of vincristine toxicity. IMPLEMENTATION (CHILD/CELLULAR ABERRATION)

212. **#2.** The peak incidence for Wilms' tumor is 3 to 4 years. ANALYSIS (CHILD/CELLULAR ABERRATION)

213. **#1.** This is the most common sign. The child appears healthy except for increased abdominal size. Decreased output is seen only if the renal collecting system is involved in bilateral tumors. Hypertension is seen in children when there is pressure of the tumor on the renal artery (about 25% of the time). ASSESSMENT (CHILD/CELLULAR ABERRATION)

214. **#1.** Dolls, puppets, and such are familiar objects the young child can actively manipulate, and thus are good ways for the young child to learn. IMPLEMENTATION (CHILD/ILL AND HOSPITALIZED CHILD)

215. **#3.** The abdomen is not palpated unless absolutely necessary to prevent the spread of cancer cells into the surrounding abdominal areas. PLAN (CHILD/CELLULAR ABERRATION)

216. **#4.** A clear liquid diet is ordered when bowel function returns, and is advanced to regular diet. Additional sodium is not necessary. PLAN (CHILD/CELLULAR ABERRATION)

217. **#4.** While the other options may be objectives, the overall goal is to return the child to a normal life-style so that growth and development may continue along their normal course. PLAN (CHILD/CELLULAR ABERRATION)

218. **#1.** Including the parents in planning and implementation of care makes them feel useful, knowledgeable, and that they have an important role in the child's recovery. This increases compliance in the treatment regimen. Literature is a good teaching reinforcement but second in importance. Discharge planning begins with admission. Free time is important but not the sole factor for teaching objectives. IMPLEMENTATION (CHILD/CELLULAR ABERRATION)

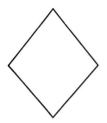

Reprints
Nursing Care of the Child

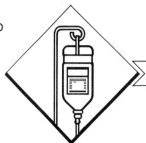

How To Administer
Blood Components To Children

Reprinted from MCN: American Journal of Maternal/Child Nursing, May/June 1985

By following these guidelines, nurses can help ensure that pediatric patients who need blood products will receive the right ones, and in the safest possible way.

WENDY C. LANDIER/MARGARET L. BARRELL
ELIZABETH J. STYFFE

When a young person needs blood or blood components, it is the pediatric nurse who must make the crucial decisions to ensure that they are administered safely. Whether the patient is a post-op infant who needs packed red bloods cells or an adolescent hemophiliac who needs cryoprecipitate, the nurse must be able to determine: How much? At what rate? What technique, observations, and interventions are needed? What tubing, filter, and needle size should be used? By keeping the following guidelines in mind, nurses can give blood products with confidence to the children in their care.

The basic principles of blood component therapy apply to children as well as to adults. However, a thorough understanding of these principles is even more necessary when working with chil-

WENDY C. LANDIER, R.N., B.S.N., *is an associate nurse in the medical-surgical units at Children's Hospital of Orange County in Orange, California.* MARGARET L. BARRELL, R.N., B.A., *is a staff nurse in the pediatric intensive care unit at Childrens Hospital of Los Angeles.* ELIZABETH J. STYFFE, R.N., B.S.N., *is charge nurse of the School Age/Adolescent Unit at Children's Hospital of Orange County.*

dren, because they differ so widely in age, size, weight, and health and medical condition.

First the nurse must identify which blood product the child should receive. Just as it is important to know which medication to administer, the nurse must understand the reason for giving a particular blood product in order to avoid errors and ensure that the child gets the most beneficial therapy. The chart Guidelines for Administering Blood Products to Children lists the various blood components and their indications as well as information on dosage and equipment.

Blood typing and crossmatching are both critical first steps in the transfusion process. Blood typing identifies the ABO and Rh groupings. Crossmatching determines the compatibility of donor and recipient cells. The chart indicates which products require typing and crossmatching and which do not; specific criteria for crossmatching will vary from one blood product to another. Blood for newborns is usually crossmatched against the mother's serum, which will contain equal or greater quantities of any antibodies present in the infant at birth. If the infant has already received a transfusion or is at least a week old, the crossmatch is done using a specimen of his own blood.

The nurse who obtains the blood for typing and crossmatching must be careful to identify the child properly and label the specimen accurately. By far the safest approach is to label the sample in the patient's presence immediately after it is drawn. If either the child or the blood specimen is incorrectly identified, a fatal transfusion reaction can result (1). The crossmatch must be repeated every 48 hours, as well, to ensure that any new antibodies that could cause a transfusion reaction

GIVING BLOOD PRODUCTS TO CHILDREN

are identified promptly (2).

ABO and Rh compatibility criteria are essentially the same as for adults (see chart). However, some centers are able to make multiple transfusions from a single unit (and thus save blood) by routinely administering O negative (universal donor) saline-washed red cells to infants under four months of age (3). This is because the young infant's immune system is not fully developed, so the risk of transfusion reaction is reduced.

Rh antigens are carried on red cells only, and no corresponding Rh antibodies occur naturally in the plasma. As a result, Rh compatibility criteria apply only to products that contain red cells. The nurse must never administer an Rh positive product to an Rh negative child, because one such transfusion may produce antibodies to the Rh(D) antigen and predispose the child to future transfusion reactions.

Furthermore, an Rh negative woman who was given Rh positive blood as a child may face serious consequences if she becomes pregnant. She has probably developed anti-Rh(D) antibodies, and if her fetus is Rh positive, it will be at risk for developing hemolytic disease of the newborn. If an Rh positive blood product that contains red cells or could be contaminated with red cells (including whole blood, packed cells, platelets, granulocytes, and cryoprecipitate) is incorrectly given to an Rh negative female who may someday bear a child, Rho(D) immune globulin (Rhogam) should be administered promptly (4). The chart shows which blood components require strict adherence to compatibility and which do not.

Determining the Dosage

The next step is deciding how much blood the child should receive. The primary difference between giving blood to adults and to children is that the dosage for children must be carefully calculated. Since pediatric patients can range from neonates to adolescents, the child's weight is the most important factor to consider, and dosage is often based on ml/kg as it is when administering other fluids and medications. The chart lists some standard dosages for a variety of components; a simple calculation will show whether the amount to be given is considered safe.

After the dose is confirmed, the physician may order the blood bank to prepare the blood in special pediatric units, called aliquots or pedipacks. A pedipack usually equals half a conventional unit, while an aliquot is a smaller fraction of a unit and can range from a few milliliters in a syringe to a bag containing a precisely measured amount.

Children are rarely given a full unit, but if nothing else is available, the nurse can measure the required dose and administer it safely using a burette and a volume control IV infusion pump. The remaining blood should be discarded once the transfusion has been completed.

Finally, the nurse must decide how much saline is required to flush between a maintenance IV solution and the blood product. Since fluid overload is a primary concern in pediatrics, it is important not to use any more than necessary; a one-ml barrier of normal saline is sufficient.

Once the blood product is ready for transfusion, two people in the blood bank should check all identifying data on the blood container and transfusion requisition. Then two professionals must confirm the match in the child's presence, verifying both the child's identity (by hospital armband) and the identity of the blood product by again comparing the transfusion requisition with the blood bag label. They must check the blood type, antibody screen, product name, amount, expiration date, the child's ID number, and the donor number. Any discrepancies must be resolved before the product is administered.

What Rate Is Best?

Any nurse who administers blood should consider the product's viability before choosing an infusion rate. Different rates are best for different components, and these are listed in the chart. The child's cardiorespiratory and hemodynamic status must also be considered. The nurse must periodically assess the child's vital signs, breath and heart sounds, and intake/output, and make any necessary rate adjustments indicated by the child's changing clinical condition. To determine both the initial rate and any rate changes, consultation with the physician is recommended.

For products that contain red cells, the initial infusion rate should be selected by calculating 5 percent of the total product to be given and infusing this amount over the first 15 minutes. This allows for early detection of a hemolytic reaction, and is comparable to the slowed infusion rate recommended when beginning a transfusion to an adult (5). If no signs of transfusion reaction occur within the first 15 minutes, the nurse may adjust the flow to match the ordered infusion rate.

Choosing the Right Equipment

Blood transfusions require a number of different pieces of equipment, and each one must be selected carefully to ensure the best results. The nurse

GUIDELINES FOR ADMINISTERING BLOOD PRODUCTS TO CHILDREN

COMPONENT	DESCRIPTION	INDICATIONS	DOSE
WHOLE BLOOD	Single donor anticoagulated blood	Massive hemorrhage (loss ≥ 10 percent to 15 percent of total blood volume)	20 ml/kg initially, followed by any volume required to stabilize child (correlate with clinical status and vital signs)
		Exchange transfusion (use blood ≤ 5 days old)	Two times child's blood volume (Note: must use blood warmer)
PACKED RED BLOOD CELLS	Concentrated red blood cells with most plasma, leukocytes, and platelets removed	Severe anemia Surgical blood loss Suppression of erythropoiesis (e.g., thalassemia or sickle cell anemia)	Usual dose is 10 ml/kg Dose should not exceed 15 ml/kg (1 ml/kg will increase hematocrit by approximately 1 percent)
SALINE-WASHED RED BLOOD CELLS	Red blood cells washed with normal saline, removing 93 percent of leukocytes	Children with history of repeated febrile transfusion reactions Immunocompromised children	SAME AS
FROZEN DEGLYCEROLYZED RED BLOOD CELLS	Specially processed red blood cells that can be stored for up to 3 years Most potential reaction-precipitating components are removed	Autotransfusion Rare blood types Pre- and post-transplant Children with history of repeated febrile transfusion reactions Children with anti-IgA antibodies (anaphylaxis prone children)	SAME AS
PLATELET CONCENTRATE	Platelets suspended in small amount of plasma	Severe thrombocytopenia (platelet count ≤ 20,000) Platelet count ≤ 50,000 in child who requires surgery or in child with hemorrhage or imminent bleeding Cardiac surgery with massive blood replacement	1 unit for every 7 to 10 kg body weight will increase platelet count by 50,000 per cu mm
GRANULOCYTES	Infection-fighting white blood cells	Sepsis in severe neutropenia (granulocyte count ≤ 500/cu mm) unresponsive to antibiotics for 48 hours Use with extreme caution in children receiving amphotericin B therapy	Dosage varies depending on child's blood counts and clinical condition Usual initial dose is 10 ml/kg/day
FRESH FROZEN PLASMA	Portion of blood that contains clotting factors and proteins	Massive hemorrhage Hypovolemic shock Multiple clotting deficiencies (e.g., liver disease, disseminated intravascular coagulation)	Acute hemorrhage: 15 to 30 ml/kg Clotting deficiency: 10 to 15 ml/kg May be repeated up to 3 times each 24 hours as necessary Monitor for congestive heart failure secondary to volume overload with increased use
CRYOPRECIPITATE	Concentrated Factor VIII and fibrinogen (approximately 100 units Factor VIII per unit)	Hemophilia A Von Willebrand's disease Hypofibrinogenemia Disseminated intravascular coagulation	One bag per 5 kg for mild bleed One bag per 2 kg for severe, life-threatening bleed Repeat every 12 to 24 hours as necessary
ALBUMIN	Blood protein	5 percent solution: Hypoproteinemia Volume expansion In neonates: to increase amount of bilirubin removed during exchange transfusion	1 gram/kg = 20 ml/kg
		25 percent solution: Severe burns Cerebral edema	1 gram/kg = 4 ml/kg
PLASMA PROTEIN FRACTION	Albumin plus some globulins	Volume expansion Hypoproteinemia	10 to 15 ml/kg/dose
FACTOR VIII CONCENTRATE	Concentrated, powdered blood clotting Factor VIII	Hemophilia A	Minor bleed: 20 units/kg Severe, life-threatening bleed: 40 units/kg
PROTHROMBIN COMPLEX	Concentrated, powdered blood clotting Factors II, VII, IX, and X	Hemophilia B Factor VIII deficiency with inhibitor to Factor VIII Liver disease Children on oral anticoagulants	Minor bleed: 10 units/kg Severe, life-threatening bleed: 40 units/kg

RATE	ABO/RH COMPATIBILITY	FILTER	TUBING
As rapidly as necessary to reestablish blood volume	Should be ABO/Rh identical. Exception: Rh positive child may receive Rh negative blood	Microaggregate	Standard IV mini or macrodrip tubing with burette, suitable for use with IV infusion pump
45 to 60 minutes (longer in hemodynamically unstable children)			
5 ml/kg/hour; 2 ml/kg/hour if child has incipient congestive heart failure. Note: If transfusion will take longer than 4 hours, unit should be divided into smaller aliquots and administered serially	Must be ABO/Rh compatibile (preferably identical). May use O Negative uncrossmatched blood for infants up to 4 months of age. RED CELL COMPATIBILITY — RECIPIENT / DONOR: A / A,O; B / B,O; AB / AB,A,B,O; O / O; Rh+ / Rh+ or −; Rh− / Rh−; undetermined / O−	Microaggregate	Standard IV mini or macrodrip tubing with burette, suitable for use with IV infusion pump
PACKED	RED	BLOOD	CELLS
PACKED	RED	BLOOD	CELLS
Administer each unit over 5 to 10 minutes via syringe or drip. If volume is a problem, administer total dose over 1 to 2 hours via pump	Must be Rh compatible; ABO plasma compatibility preferred (see Plasma Compatibility chart below). Type-specific platelets are commonly ordered for children receiving frequent platelet transfusions	Microaggregate. If platelet administration set is used, a platelet filter is incorporated into the set and additional filtering is not necessary	Standard IV mini or macrodrip tubing. May use burette. May use IV pump tubing. May use platelet administration set (adaptable for syringe or drip methods)
Slowly over 2 to 4 hours. Mild fever and chills are common reactions. Premedication with antihistamines, acetaminophen, steroids, and/or meperidine may be indicated. Must be transfused as soon as possible after collection, preferably within 6 hours, due to short lifespan of granulocytes	Should be ABO/Rh red cell compatible (see Red Cell Compatibility chart above). Crossmatch must be performed because granulocytes are contaminated with red cells. Granulocytes are often obtained from donors who are human lymphocyte antigen matched to the recipient	Standard blood filter or screen-type microaggregate filter (e.g., Pall Ultrapore). Do not use depth-type microaggregate filter (e.g., Bentley PFF-100) as it will trap granulocytes	Standard IV mini or macrodrip tubing with burette, suitable for use with IV infusion pump
Hemorrhage: As indicated by child's condition. Clotting deficiency: over 2 to 3 hours. Administer within 6 hours of thawing to preserve clotting factor activity	Donor's plasma should be ABO compatible with recipient's red cells. PLASMA COMPATIBILITY — RECIPIENT / DONOR: A / A,AB; B / B,AB; AB / AB; O / O,AB,A,B; undetermined / AB	Standard blood filter or microaggregate filter	Standard IV mini or macrodrip tubing with burette, suitable for use with IV infusion pump
Via syringe or drip as rapidly as solution will infuse. Administer within 6 hours of thawing	ABO plasma group compatible units preferred but not essential (see Plasma Compatibility chart above). Rh compatibility preferable	Standard blood filter or microaggregate filter	Standard IV mini or macrodrip tubing. May use burette or IV infusion pump
1 to 2 ml/minute (60 to 120 ml/hour)	No typing or crossmatching required	Filtered administration set packaged with the product	Use administration set provided with the product
0.2 to 0.4 ml/minute (12 to 24 ml/hour)			
4 to 10 ml/minute	No typing or crossmatching required	Filtered administration set packaged with the product	Use administration set provided with the product
2 ml/minute maximum via syringe	No typing or crossmatching required. Children on long-term therapy, if other than type O, should be monitored for hemolysis caused by isoagglutinins (anti-A and anti-B antibodies). Group specific concentrates are available if needed	Filter needle provided with product	Withdraw reconstituted solution from vial via filter needle, then administer via syringe
2 to 3 ml/minute	No typing or crossmatching required. Children on long-term therapy should have blood group determined, and if group other than O, should be monitored for hemolysis caused by infusion of iso-agglutinins (anti-A and anti-B antibodies)	Filter needle provided with product	Withdraw reconstituted solution from vial via filter needle, then administer via syringe

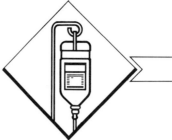

must be able to choose from a wide variety of needles, blood filters, tubing, pumps, and blood warmers, so here are some considerations to bear in mind.

First of all, it is not necessary to select large-gauge needles when administering blood products to children. The size of the needle or catheter depends on the child's venous access, not on the blood product. The nurse can safely employ a small-caliber needle without altering the integrity of the red cells. In vitro studies confirm that needles up to 27 gauge may be used to give whole blood at rates of up to 100 ml/hour and packed cells up to 50 ml/hour without significant hemolysis (6).

All blood products must be filtered, either before or during administration, because they contain debris ranging from large fibrin clots to tiny particles of fat, protein, clumped platelets, and leukocytes known as microaggregates. Standard blood filters (also known as gross-clot screen filters) are designed to remove particles larger than 170 microns and are generally built into commercial blood administration tubing sets. Microaggregate filters, on the other hand, are made to remove particles as small as 20 to 40 microns. Theoretically, these particles can cause microemboli in the pulmonary and cerebral blood vessels—which could be particularly dangerous for pediatric patients because of the relatively small size of these vessels. So as a precautionary measure microaggregate filters are used more often with children than with adults.

Microaggregate filters are generally available as separate units and can easily be added to any standard IV administration set. The two types currently available are the screen filter (such as the Pall Ultrapore), which traps microaggregate particles on a mesh-type surface, and the depth filter (such as the Bentley PFF-100), which holds the particles on a wetted surface by adhesion. The depth filter cannot be used, however, for the transfusion of granulocytes (7).

When microaggregate filters were first introduced, studies indicated that the smaller blood components, such as platelets, became trapped in them, but these initial studies were done with whole blood (8). More recent research suggests that microaggregate screen filters can be used to administer even the smallest components, including platelets and granulocytes, in concentrate form without trapping (7,9). The chart gives specific recommendations for these components.

Another factor for the nurse to consider when choosing a blood filter for the pediatric patient is the priming volume required. The manufacturer's guidelines should always be followed when using any blood filter, but it is also essential to prime the entire surface area with blood to ensure maximal filtration. Some filters require up to 80 ml of priming volume, which makes them impractical for pediatric transfusions. Most microaggregate filters can be used for several units of blood, but in pediatric transfusions they must be changed every two to four hours to reduce the risk of bacteria. One neonatal microaggregate filter has a 0.7 ml priming volume (Hemo-Nate) and can be attached directly to a syringe for small-volume transfusions. It must, however, be changed after processing every 20 ml of packed cells or 50 ml of whole blood.

Commercially available blood products, such as albumin and factor concentrates, are packaged with a filtered administration set or a filter needle. The manufacturer's instructions on filtration should always be followed when administering any of these products to children.

Some Tubing Pointers

Tubing is another important part of the transfusion equipment. All banked blood products can be administered through standard IV mini or macro-drip tubing, but some that are commercially prepared require specially filtered tubing, which is packaged by the manufacturer with the products. IV tubing that contains filters to remove air cannot be used for transfusions, since blood will become trapped in them. This is also the case with buretrols that have built-in air-eliminating filters.

The most common choice for adult transfusions is "Y" tubing primed with normal saline. But in pediatrics, where fluid volumes are most strictly controlled, only one ml of normal saline is necessary as a barrier between the IV maintenance solution and the blood product. Straight-line tubing may be primed with the blood product and attached directly to the IV catheter or extension set. During transfusions the IV tubing should be changed every time the filter is changed, and never used more than four hours. The chart summarizes what to consider when selecting tubing.

The use of an IV pump is strongly advised for all pediatric transfusions. Otherwise the rate of flow is hard to regulate when administering small volumes, and gravity flow puts the child at risk for receiving too much blood over a short period of

PROCEDURE	CONSIDERATIONS
1. Verify that the physician's order is appropriate: a) Component order is appropriate for child's clinical condition b) Dose ordered in ml/kg or units is within safe range for child's weight c) Rate of transfusion ordered is within safe range for blood component.	1. Refer to chart for blood product selection and dose calculation.
2. If specimen for typing and crossmatching is required, verify that ID of child matches lab requisition and carefully hand-label specimen in child's presence.	2. Refer to chart for products that require typing and crossmatching.
3. Order blood product from blood bank or pharmacy. If product is less than one standard unit, order amount to be given (in ml) and include the priming volume of the filter and blood administration set. Include any special instructions (e.g., "type specific" or "irradiated").	3. Certain banked blood products require extra time for processing (e.g., frozen products must be thawed). Check with blood bank to determine when product will be available.
4. Ensure adequate venous access. If current IV cannot be interrupted for transfusion, start another IV.	4. Products out of blood bank refrigerator for more than 30 minutes cannot be returned; infusion should be completed within 4 hours of obtaining product.
5. Obtain and assemble all necessary equipment for the transfusion.	5. Include IV pump, tubing, burette, filter, syringe with normal saline flush, and blood warmer if necessary.
6. Follow hospital procedure for obtaining blood product from blood bank (or pharmacy).	
7. Verify blood product and patient ID by comparing blood bag label, transfusion requisition, and child's ID band.	7. This should be done at the child's bedside by two licensed professionals.
8. Resolve any questions regarding compatibility before beginning the transfusion.	8. Refer to chart for compatibility information.
9. Prime filter, burette, and tubing with blood product.	9. Gloves can be worn to protect transfusionist from blood-borne infections, such as AIDS and hepatitis.

PROCEDURE	CONSIDERATIONS
10. Obtain baseline vital signs.	10. Include temperature, pulse, respiration, and blood pressure.
11. Disconnect maintenance solution, then flush IV extension set and/or IV catheter with normal saline.	11. Use at least 1 ml of normal saline as a barrier.
12. Connect blood-primed IV tubing to extension set or IV catheter.	
13. To begin transfusion, calculate 5 percent of total volume of product to be infused and set pump to deliver this amount over 15 minutes (e.g., if 50 ml of product is ordered, give 5 percent = 2.5 ml over 15 minutes = 10 ml/hour rate).	13. This step is necessary only if the blood product contains red cells. It allows for early detection of a hemolytic transfusion reaction and correlates with the slow flow rate recommended initially for adult transfusions.
14. Monitor child closely for first 15 minutes of transfusion. Obtain second set of vital signs after 15 minutes.	14. Observe for signs and symptoms of transfusion reaction (e.g., chills, vomiting, back pain, hematuria, fever, hypotension). It is not necessary to check vital signs throughout the entire transfusion unless child's condition warrants.
15. If reaction occurs or is suspected, stop transfusion immediately.	15. Disconnect tubing at IV catheter hub to avoid administering additional blood; flush IV catheter with normal saline and keep vein open while reaction is investigated.
16. If no signs or symptoms of a reaction occur, increase rate to ordered infusion rate.	
17. Evaluate child every 30 minutes during transfusion.	17. Observe for signs and symptoms of transfusion reaction; check IV site for infiltration.
18. When ordered amount is given, disconnect tubing and flush IV catheter/extension set with normal saline. Reconnect IV to maintenance solution or heparin lock, or discontinue IV as ordered.	18. Flushing the full length of tubing is not necessary unless an entire unit of product is being administered. In this case, normal saline should be used to flush product through the filter and tubing. This normal saline flush need not be administered to the patient; it will remain in the tubing once the product is cleared from the line.
19. Obtain post-transfusion vital signs.	19. Compare with baseline vital signs and report significant changes.
20. Complete hospital transfusion documentation as per hospital policy.	20. Include all vital signs, amount of product given, patient tolerance, amount of flush, and IV patency.
21. Dispose of tubing and blood container per hospital policy.	21. Should be considered contaminated waste.

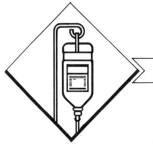

time. Most volumetric-type IV pumps are safe for administering blood products, but some may cause mechanical hemolysis of red cells (10). So select only pumps that the manufacturer recommends for giving transfusions.

Finally, commercial blood warmers should be available wherever children receive transfusions. The mechanism that regulates a child's body temperature is still immature, and cold stress is a danger. So when banked blood, which is stored at between 1°C and 6°C, is infused rapidly without warming, it can have serious negative effects on a pediatric patient. Therefore, blood that must be infused rapidly or in massive amounts should always be warmed, especially when it is given rapidly via a central line, since this may induce ventricular arrhythmias (11). Children with cold agglutinins in their blood and those getting exchange transfusions should also receive warmed blood.

Commercial blood warmers are designed to heat blood to a preset temperature between 32°C and 37°C, using either a water bath or an electric heating coil. However, the manufacturer's directions must be followed precisely. Heating blood under hot water faucets or in microwave ovens can cause hemolysis and is never acceptable.

Some Special Cases

While nurses must always make certain that their pediatric patients are receiving the appropriate blood products, in the correct dosage, at the correct rate, and with the proper equipment, some children may have health conditions that call for more specialized care. They may be at risk for transfusion reactions, or they may be immunocompromised. What can nurses do to ensure that these patients too receive blood safely?

Occasionally, children are premedicated with antipyretic, antihistamine, and/or anti-inflammatory medications to prevent allergic-type transfusion reactions. They are often treated before the administration of granulocytes, for example, because the incidence of reactions to this product is common. Pediatric patients are not routinely premedicated before receiving any specific blood product, however. Rather, the nurse should thoroughly review the medical history and then inform the physician if the child has had any documented reactions to blood products.

Many pediatric patients are also immunosuppressed. They include children with congenital or acquired immune deficiency syndrome, children

with malignancies, and some newborns. Each of these groups is at risk for developing graft versus host disease (GVHD) if they receive transfusions of blood products that contain lymphocytes (i.e., platelets, granulocytes, red blood cells, and whole blood) (12). GVHD is caused by donor lymphocytes that engraft in the recipient's marrow, and then attack the tissues and organs as if they were foreign. It is a serious complication that can result in a range of symptoms and may be fatal, but it can be prevented by inactivating donor lymphocytes via irradiation. Blood products can be safely irradiated using 1500 to 3000 rads before the transfusion is begun (13).

As we have seen, administering blood to young patients is more complex than administering blood to adults. Pediatric nurses must be prepared to give a wide variety of products to a population that ranges in age from newborns to adolescents and may have a number of very different health care needs. By following some specific guidelines, however, they can fulfill this responsibility both competently and confidently.

REFERENCES

1. AUSMAN, R. K. *Intravascular Infusion Systems: Principles and Practice.* Hingham, MA, Kluwer Academic, 1984, p. 148.
2. GILCHRIST, G. S., AND MOORE, S. B. Blood transfusion. IN *Practice of Pediatrics,* edited by V. C. Kelley, Philadelphia, F. B. Lippincott Co., 1985, Vol. 5, Chap. 60, p. 3.
3. OBERMAN, H. A., ED. *Standards for Blood Banks and Transfusion Services.* 10th ed. Washington, DC, American Association of Blood Banks, 1981, pp. 28–29.
4. HUESTIS, D. W., AND OTHERS. *Practical Blood Transfusion.* 3rd ed. Boston, Little, Brown and Co., 1981, p. 378.
5. KASPRISIN, C. A. Transfusion therapy for the pediatric patient. IN *Transfusion Therapy: Principles and Procedures,* 2nd ed. edited by R. C. Rutman and W. V. Miller. Rockville, MD, Aspen Systems Corporation, 1985, p. 183.
6. HERRERA, A. J., AND CORLESS, J. Blood transfusions: effect of speed of infusion and of needle gauge on hemolysis. *J.Pediatr.* 99:757–758, Nov. 1981.
7. SNYDER, E. L., AND OTHERS. Effect of microaggregate blood filtration on granulocyte concentrates in vitro. *Transfusion* 23:25–29, Jan.–Feb. 1983.
8. DUNBAR, R. W., AND OTHERS. Microaggreagate blood filters: effect on filtration time, plasma hemoglobin, and fresh blood platelet counts. *Anesth.Analg.* 53:577–583, July–Aug. 1974.
9. SNYDER, E. L., AND OTHERS. Effect of microaggregate blood filtration on platelet concentrates in vitro. *Transfusion* 21:427–434, July–Aug. 1981.
10. GIANINO, N. Equipment used for transfusion. IN *Transfusion Therapy: Principles and Procedures,* 2nd ed. edited by R. C. Rutman and W. V. Miller, Rockville, MD, Aspen Systems Corporation, 1985, pp. 161–165.
11. PAULEY, S. Y. Transfusion therapy for nurses. Part II. *NITA* 8:51–60, Jan.–Feb. 1985.
12. MALAVADE, V., AND OTHERS. Component transfusion therapy. IN *Critical Care Pediatrics: A Problem Oriented Approach,* edited by S. S. Zimmerman and J. M. Gildea. Philadelphia, W. B. Saunders Co., 1985, p. 123.
13. MILLER, D. R., AND OTHERS, EDS. *Blood Diseases of Infancy and Childhood.* 5th ed. St. Louis, The C. V. Mosby Co., 1984, p. 71.

Feeding Hospitalized Children With Developmental Disabilities

Reprinted from MCN: American Journal of Maternal/Child Nursing, May/June 1985

Making mealtimes more pleasant for children who have developmental disabilities only requires patience and sometimes a little creativity.

MARGARET MARY KOSOWSKI
DEBORAH LEE SOPCZYK

For millions of developmentally disabled children and adults, hospitalization is a common experience and frequently a difficult one. Mealtimes can be especially trying for all involved. Many disabled people who are eager and capable of participating during meals become distressed when they are forced into an unnatural role by frustrated hospital staff members who find feedings time-consuming and often unsuccessful.

The term *developmental disability* refers to intellectual and/or physical deviations that impair an individual's ability to meet age-specific standards. The intellectual and physical deviations can occur in any combination and with a wide range of severity. Authorities agree that normalcy is a goal to be strived for with all who have developmental disabilities. When individuals have seemingly overwhelming deficits, however, health care providers may forget that the basic principles of feeding still apply. These principles include appropriate positioning and using proper feeding utensils and feeding techniques.

MARGARET MARY KOSOWSKI, R.N., M.S.N., *is an assistant professor of nursing at Brenau College, School of Nursing in Gainesville, Georgia.* DEBORAH LEE SOPCZYK, R.N., M.S.N., *is a program associate at Regeants College Degrees Nursing Program in Albany, New York. The authors wish to thank Nina Herman-Blumlein, speech pathologist, United Cerebral Palsy Association of Western New York, Children's Center, for her technical assistance.*

The mealtime environment is equally important and must provide for a sensual and pleasant experience. In interviews with developmentally disabled people, Robert Perske and his associates found that nutrition and health were not given top priority by them. Instead, what happened at mealtimes was considered just as important, and sometimes more important, than the food itself. Those interviewed described the ideal mealtime as a time for feeling comradeship and belonging; for relaxing and being less defensive; for communicating in many ways—with voice, eyes, body, taste, smell, and touch; for laughing and feeling joyful; for being accepted and being happy with oneself; for making choices; for heightening all the senses; for feeling satisfied and relaxed; and for taking in nutrition for growth and good health (1).

Finding the Right Position

When feeding a disabled child, the initial step is to assist the child into a position that closely approximates the preferred sitting one. Eating in a sitting position promotes safe ingestion of food and enhances digestion of nutrients. However, in many instances developmental disabilities are accompanied by conditions that hinder the ability to sit upright. These conditions include abnormal muscle tone, persistent primitive reflexes, and orthopedic complications. Health care providers can compensate for the problems caused by these conditions by using adaptive equipment and individualizing feeding programs.

The sitting position can be strengthened by providing firm support for the child's feet and arms. Feet must be placed solidly on the floor or other firm surface. Adjustable bedside tables brought close to the child add support to the child's arms and trunk.

Since muscle tone strongly influences a child's ability to sit erect, health care providers must assess and compensate for an individual's limitations. The child who is hypotonic, for example, may have difficulty with head control. This child can be seated in a chair with a high back. In addition, a jacket or posey restraint can be used to stabilize the child's trunk and to support the child in an upright position.

On the other hand, a high-back chair is not essential for a hypertonic child unless arching is severe. For most hypertonic children, a wheelchair with foot supports is adequate. In order to diminish spastic responses, the child's hips and feet as well as the child's trunk may have to be restrained (see illustration below).

Since the spastic movements of a hypertonic child may impede the child's ability to assume and maintain a sitting position, simple relaxation techniques can be used prior to seating the child. For example, lying the child prone across the feeder's lap or a soft chair with the child's feet abducted helps diminish spasticity. To make the child feel more secure while in this postion, the feeder can place a hand on the child's back (see illustration below). Talking softly while gently rocking the child promotes further relaxation as does gently stretching the child's extremities.

Whenever possible, the child's head is placed in the usual position for swallowing (that is, head midline and bent slightly forward). This position becomes especially important when a child exhibits an asymetric tonic neck reflex (ATNR), a total body response that interferes with purposeful activity. The ATNR is a normal response in newborns and usually disappears by approximately six months of age. However, a child with a developmental disability may exhibit an ATNR throughout life.

The ATNR occurs when a child's head is turned. Thus, if the child does not have adaptive equipment designed to maintain the head in a midline position, the feeder must encourage this position by sitting directly in front of the child at eye level. Furthermore, all food and eating utensils must be placed directly in front of the child. Even when additional maneuvers to stabilize or manipulate the head or jaw are necessary, the child's head must remain in the midline position.

Although placing the child in an individually designed wheelchair generally permits the most advantageous position for feeding, one may not be available. If equipment on hand cannot be adapted adequately and if the child is small enough to fit comfortably on the feeder's lap, holding the child for feeding is a reasonable alternative. Care must be taken to support the child in a sitting rather than in a lying position.

Sometimes, sitting is compromised by spasticity of the abductor muscles of the hips and legs. Stimulation of these muscles during positioning may result in crossing of the legs (scissoring). Bending the child's knees helps to keep the child upright,

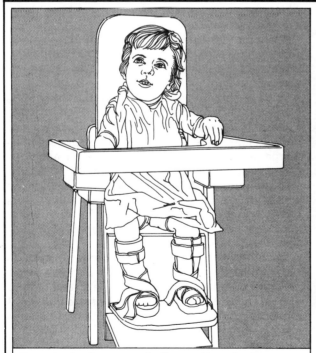

To maintain the proper feeding position, the hypertonic child's hips, feet, and trunk may have to be restrained.

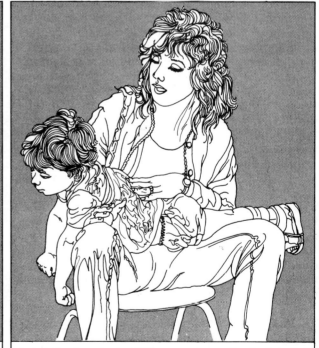

Lying the hypertonic child prone across the feeder's lap helps diminish the child's spasticity.

while putting an arm or pillow between the child's knees diminishes scissoring.

A major disadvantage of holding a child for feeding is fatigue. Feeding a child who is developmentally disabled usually is a lengthy process, and supporting the child's weight while compensating for abnormal muscle tone for an extended period of time can be exhausting for the feeder. A comfortable chair, pillows, and a footrest help to alleviate discomfort as well as to stabilize the child and feeder. Most authorities agree that bodily contact between child and feeder may overstimulate the child. This overstimulation is amplified when an uncomfortable feeder must make frequent changes in position during the meal.

In an acute care setting not equipped to meet the unique needs of the developmentally disabled child, health care providers must be creative in adapting available resources. Infant seats, umbrollers, lomax chairs, and lounge chairs can be used to provide a proper feeding position. Beanbag chairs are especially useful since they are inexpensive and can be molded to any desired shape. If it is necessary to use the child's bed, the child's head must be elevated and the child's knees must be gatched to most closely approximate a sitting position.

Rewriting the Menu

The physical impairments associated with developmental disabilities may interfere with a child's capacity to communicate preferences for food and eating untensils as well as impede the child's ability to consume food in a safe, effective manner. Nevertheless, promotion of normalcy must be the guiding principle when making decisions about food and eating utensils. Care must be taken not to compromise this principle for the sake of efficiency during meals. Although tube feedings or feeding by syringe are time-effective, these methods are abnormal and unnatural for people.

During the admission interview, the admitting nurse needs to obtain information about the child's typical eating and feeding routines. Specifically, the admitting nurse must document what kinds of food the child eats, how foods are eaten, and approximately how long the feeding process takes. If this information is not available, some general guidelines can be followed, although these guidelines may require modification according to the child's individual needs.

Food must be served at a moderate temperature (lukewarm rather than hot or cold). Since thin liquids usually are difficult for the developmentally disabled child to control, they have to be thickened. A number of commercially prepared products are available for this purpose. Alternately, formula can be thickened with pablum, apple juice with applesauce, and milk with yogurt. Wheatgerm can be used to thicken most foods.

Foods with a high sugar content increase salivation. Consequently, the child who has difficulty controlling secretions and swallowing can be given biscuits rather than cookies, fruit juice rather than soft drinks, and so forth. Moderately large pieces of food rather than very small ones may be easier for the child to control. For this reason, foods that crumble easily must be avoided. For example, moist tuna salad generally is easier for the developmentally disabled child to eat than is ground beef, which crumbles.

Proper utensils contribute significantly to the overall success of feedings. Each utensil selected must promote normalcy, efficiency, and most importantly safety.

The physical manifestations associated with developmental disabilities place the child at risk for injury. The mouth is especially vulnerable when a child has a bite reflex and spasticity causes excessive movement. Injury can be prevented by not placing anything in child's mouth that is brittle, breakable, or sharp. Metal or thin, disposable plastic utensils usually are not appropriate. Tefloncoated spoons are an inexpensive and safe substitute (see illustration on opposite page).

The same principle applies to the selection of drinking implements. Soft plastic or paper cups are safe, and their pliability allows them to be molded to the shape of the individual's mouth. When assisting a child with cup drinking, safety can be promoted by encouraging the normal head posture for swallowing (head held stable and bent slightly forward). A hand placed firmly on top of the child's head helps the child to maintain this position.

With a standard cup, the normal swallowing posture is very difficult to maintain since the feeder usually has to tilt the child's head backward in order to empty the cup. In this position, the child tends to gulp liquids and is at greater risk for aspiration. The problem can be avoided by using a cutout cup. It not only allows the feeder to empty the cup by tilting the cup rather than the child's head but also allows the feeder to observe the fluid in the cup and thereby control the flow of liquids (see illustration on opposite page).

Developmentally disabled children frequently have difficulty with hand control. Nevertheless, children who are capable of assisting with feeding are encouraged to do so through proper choice of food and utensils. For example, finger foods are always appropriate, but the most suitable finger foods are those that are large and sturdy enough to be handled with ease. Likewise, handles on utensils must be large enough for easy grasp. If a child's own utensils have not been sent to the hospital,

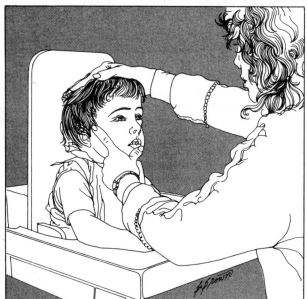

If jaw control is a problem, the feeder sits directly in front of the child and places hands to stabilize the child's head and to provide jaw control.

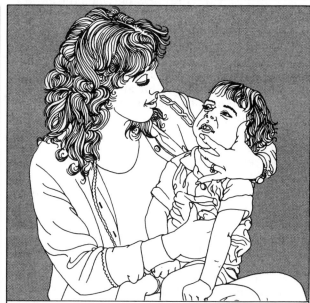

If the child with the problem of jaw control is sitting on the feeder's lap, the feeder adjusts placement of the fingers on the child's jaw as indicated in this illustration.

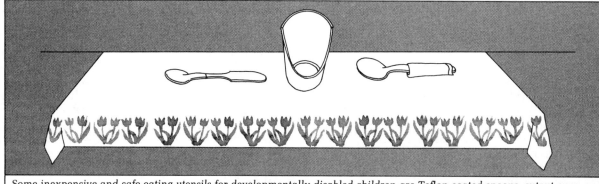

Some inexpensive and safe eating utensils for developmentally disabled children are Teflon-coated spoons, cutout cups, and utensils with handles built up with gauze and adhesive tape.

any utensil can be built up by taping the handle with gauze and adhesive tape (see illustration above).

Since poor hand control hinders the disabled child in carrying food from plate to mouth, foods that are thick enough to stay on the spoon must be provided. For greater stability, hand-over-hand feeding may be necessary. To do this, the feeder simply places a hand over the child's hand and provides the necessary support and guidance.

Some Techniques for Success

Neuromuscular abnormalities of the head and neck may impede the developmentally disabled child's ability to take in and swallow food. These abnormalities can create problems such as poor control of jaw and tongue or uncoordinated suck-

ing and swallowing patterns. Feeding techniques must be modified in order to compensate for these problems and to ensure safe ingestion of adequate amounts of food.

Control of the jaw implies the ability to open and close the mouth appropriately in response to stimuli. This process allows food to be taken into the mouth, kept in the mouth, and masticated. Abnormal muscle tone may impede the developmentally disabled child's ability to open or close the mouth at will. In addition, hypersensitivity may cause the child to open or close the mouth inappropriately in response to any stimuli.

The feeder can intervene by carefully supporting and directing the movement of the child's jaw and by identifying and minimizing offending stimuli. A simple and highly successful technique is to position the child in a chair with the feeder sitting directly in front of the child. The feeder places the fingers of one hand on the child's jaw. The child's jaw will open and close in response to the upward and downward pressure of the feeder's fingers (see illustration on previous page; also shown is the finger adjustment necessary when the child is sitting on the feeder's lap).

Control of the jaw is more complicated when the child has a bite reflex. This child clenches the teeth in response to stimulation. In addition to using the jaw-control technique, the feeder can stimulate the child's oral cavity to help minimize the bite reflex. Simple techniques such as rubbing the gums with a finger or brushing the teeth prior to feeding may prove successful. Care must be taken, however, to provide safety for the child and the feeder. Fingers must never be placed between the teeth, and a finger cot or a glove must always be used. For a more detailed, individualized program of oral stimulation, a speech and/or occupational therapist can be consulted.

A speech or occupational therapist also can be consulted when designing a program for children who have problems with lip closure. Lip closure can be encouraged during feedings by tilting the spoon upward and allowing the upper *lip*, not the teeth, to remove food from the spoon. Also, to promote lip closure and prevent lip retraction, the feeder can wipe the child's mouth with a patting rather than a rubbing motion.

Tongue thrust is an impediment to the feeding process. The child who has this problem pushes food out of the mouth instead of bringing food to the back of the mouth. Digital stimulation of the mouth may be used to reduce tongue thrust. It can be further diminished by using the jaw-control technique and firmly pressing the spoon downward on the first third of the child's tongue.

A hyperactive gag reflex is a common obstruction to feeding. Sometimes, a feeder may incorrectly interpret this reflex and inappropriately stop the meal. In children who have this problem, gagging is caused by stimulation of the oral cavity and does not usually indicate fullness or a need to vomit. The gag reflex can be diminished by consistently closing the child's mouth at the first sign of gagging and promoting the chewing response through jaw control.

Why Not Dim the Lights?

The overall feeding experience can be greatly enhanced by making the mealtime environment conducive to the comfort of both the child and the feeder. Initially, the child's ability to process stimuli must be assessed. Although public areas such as the nurses' station or the playroom often are used for feedings, some children find the noise, bright lights, and multitude of people in these areas overwhelming. Since a high level of stimulation may prevent a child from concentrating and relaxing, children who have difficulty processing stimuli may be more comfortable in their own rooms.

However, social interaction and appropriate stimulation are important mealtime activities. Meals should be uninterrupted and unhurried, with pleasant conversation and eye contact between feeder and child. For some children, as for some adults, quiet music and dim lights provide a pleasing mealtime atmosphere. When appropriate, the feeder can take advantage of mealtimes to identify and teach the child about food.

A Meal That Matters

Feeding the hospitalized developmentally disabled child does not have to be a frustrating experience. By properly positioning and supporting the child, offering appropriate foods, and using modified eating utensils and feeding techniques, the child can have an appealing, satisfying meal consumed in a safe, efficient manner. The extra touch of providing a pleasant mealtime environment can make feedings more than just a routine function for both the child and the caregiver.

REFERENCE

1. PERSKE, ROBERT. Introduction: a gentle call to revolution. IN *Mealtimes for Severely and Profoundly Handicapped Persons: New Concepts and Attitudes*, ed. by Robert Perske and others. Baltimore, University Park Press, 1977, p. XX.

BIBLIOGRAPHY

BLACKMAN, J. A. *Medical Aspects of Developmental Disabilities in Children, Birth to Three: A Resource for Special Service Providers.* rev. ed. Rockville, MD, Aspen Systems Corporation, 1984.

BLACKWELL, M. W. *Care of the Mentally Retarded.* Boston, Little, Brown & Co., 1979.

DARLING, R. B., AND DARLING, JON. *Children Who Are Different: Meeting the Challenges of Birth Defects in Society.* St. Louis, The C. V. Mosby Co., 1982.

FINNIE, N. R. *Handling the Young Cerebral Palsied Child at Home.* New York, E. P. Dutton, 1975.

GALLENDER, DEMOS. *Teaching Eating and Toileting Skills to the Multi-Handicapped in the School Setting.* Springflied, IL, Charles C Thomas, Publisher, 1980.

JOHNSTON, R. B., AND MAGRAB, P. R., EDS. *Development Disorders: Assessment, Treatment, Education.* Baltimore, University Park Press, 1976.

LEWIS, MICHAEL, AND TAFT, L. T., EDS. *Developmental Disabilities: Theory, Assessment, and Intervention.* New York, S. P. Medical and Scientific Books, 1982.

MORRIS, S. E. *Oral-Motor Function and Dysfunction in Children.* Paper presented at the Conference at the University of North Carolina at Chapel Hill, Division of Physical Therapy, held May 25-28, 1977.

MUELLER, H. A. Facilitating feeding and prespeech. IN *Physical Therapy Services in the Developmental Disabilities*, ed. by P. H. Pearson and C. E. Williams. Springfield, IL, Charles C Thomas, Publisher, 1972.

PIPES, P. L. *Nutrition in Infancy and Childhood.* 2nd ed. St. Louis, The C.V. Mosby Co., 1981, pp. 170-184.

SHEPPARD, J. J. *Treatment of Oral Motor Dysfunction in Infants and the Developmentally Disabled.* Paper presented at a meeting of the United Cerebral Palsy Association of Western New York, held June 30, 1983.

SPRINGER, N. S. *Nutrition Casebook on Developmental Disabilities.* Syracuse, NY, Syracuse University Press, 1982.

ZINKUS, C. Feeding skill training. IN *Feeding the Handicapped Child*, ed. by M. A. Smith. Memphis, TN, Child Development Center, 1971.

Sample Tests

The questions and answers in this section have been organized in such a way as to simulate 2 separate NCLEX-RN exams.

Each test has been divided into four books of 95 questions each. Each book tests your nursing knowledge in regard to care of the adult, the child, the childbearing family, and the client with psychosocial/psychiatric problems.

Instructions for Taking the Test

1. Review the information in Section One: Preparing for the NCLEX.
2. Time yourself, allowing one and one-half hours per book (6 hours per test).
3. Read each question carefully and select *one* best answer to each question.
4. Do not leave questions blank, as you will not be penalized for random answers on the NCLEX.
5. Score your exam using the answer key. Count any questions left unanswered as incorrect. A score of 75% (70 questions or more right answers per book) is roughly equivalent to a passing grade.
6. Review the questions you answered incorrectly and restudy that specific material.

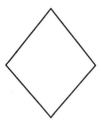

Test 1

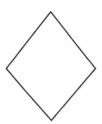

Test 1, Book I
Questions

Stella Garcia, aged 66, was brought to the hospital by ambulance after having suffered a fainting spell while shopping for the Christmas holidays. She was accompanied by her sister, who told the admitting physician that Mrs. Garcia recently learned she has diabetes mellitus. After a blood sample for sugar had been drawn, she was admitted for further evaluation with the diagnosis of hyperglycemia.

1. Before approaching Mrs. Garcia, what other information would be important to obtain from her sister?
   ○ 1. Is Mrs. Garcia a U.S. citizen?
   ○ 2. Does Mrs. Garcia speak or understand English?
   ○ 3. Was the sister present when Mrs. Garcia had her fainting spell?
   ○ 4. Does Mrs. Garcia have any medical insurance?

2. What information is most important to obtain during her admission process?
   ○ 1. Mental status
   ○ 2. Respiratory status
   ○ 3. Blood pressure
   ○ 4. Heart rate

3. Mrs. Garcia's understanding of the English language is limited. What would be the best means of communicating with her?
   ○ 1. Through a hospital interpreter
   ○ 2. Through a close family member
   ○ 3. Through a health practitioner fluent in both English and Spanish
   ○ 4. Through any one who is available who speaks both languages

4. Which of the following is an *inappropriate* goal in the care of Mrs. Garcia?
   ○ 1. Client will learn dietary principles and the role of diet.
   ○ 2. Client will be able to adapt her own cultural diet to meet diabetic requirements.
   ○ 3. Client will safely administer the prescribed hypoglycemia agents.
   ○ 4. Client will be able to adequately teach another newly diagnosed diabetic client in Spanish.

Ellen Evenson is a 20-year-old woman admitted to the psychiatric hospital after attempting to kill her 16-year-old sister, Tanya, by pushing her out of a second-story window. Her only explanation was, "She got in my way." She displays no remorse, nor any attachment to her family, and has a history of truancy and inability to retain employment. Both parents work full time and have been unable to provide close supervision.

5. Soon after Miss Evenson has been admitted to the unit, she shows interest in a young male nurse who is assigned to her. She is charming and cooperative and frequently says to him, "I'm so glad you're my nurse. You're the best nurse on the unit." Which of the following statements provides the best interpretation of Miss Evenson's behavior?
   ○ 1. She has finally found someone for whom she feels a real attachment.
   ○ 2. She recognizes the superior ability of this particular nurse.
   ○ 3. She is proficient at getting her way at the expense of others.
   ○ 4. She is demonstrating a willingness to change, so that a personal relationship with this nurse would be possible.

6. Which of the following statements most accurately describes factors that probably contributed to the character of Miss Evenson?
   ○ 1. There was ample opportunity for involvement with appropriate role models, but she chose to avoid close relationships.
   ○ 2. Early needs for security and love were met, but later associations with parents were distant.
   ○ 3. Impaired superego development occurred because she did not internalize parental values.
   ○ 4. Much of her lifelong pattern of difficulty is a result of below-average intelligence.

7. When working with Miss Evenson, the nurse should use which of the following strategies primarily?
   ○ 1. Allow the client to prepare as much of her own treatment plan as possible.
   ○ 2. Offer as many opportunities as possible for recreational and occupational therapies.
   ○ 3. Use interdisciplinary team planning to determine and enforce appropriate limits for behavior on the unit.
   ○ 4. Repeatedly provide sympathy and support for the client in her attempts to avoid anxiety.

8. One day Miss Evenson's sister comes to visit her. Miss Evenson says, "She can come in if she wants to. I really don't care." This best demonstrates what combination of responses common to the antisocial personality?
   ○ 1. Low self-esteem, poor impulse control
   ○ 2. Suspicion, aloofness
   ○ 3. Guilt, depression
   ○ 4. Self-centeredness, lack of consideration of others' feelings

9. Miss Evenson participates in family therapy with her parents. The parents frequently blame her for their difficulties and complain about the expense at the hospital. They also persist in requesting passes for her to go home and for an early discharge. Which of the following statements best describes the parents' beliefs or feelings?
   ○ 1. They believe she has improved enough to function efficiently outside the hospital.
   ○ 2. They believe she has been punished enough for her previous behavior.
   ○ 3. They have ambivalent feelings about her.
   ○ 4. They feel guilty about causing their daughter's antisocial behavior.

10. After having been in therapy several months, Miss Evenson shows signs of depression and feelings of guilt and remorse. What evaluation of her progress would be most appropriate?
    ○ 1. She has acquired a dysthymic disorder in addition to her antisocial personality.
    ○ 2. She has experienced a major depression in addition to her antisocial personality.
    ○ 3. She is gaining insight into the effect her behavior has had on others, and this resulted in depression.
    ○ 4. She is gaining insight into her problems, and this has made her realize that she has a poor prognosis.

11. One day in occupational therapy, Miss Evenson is observed briefly assisting a depressed client with a project. She is helpful but not superior in her attitude. Which of the following statements best describes her behavior?
    ○ 1. She is trying to impress the staff by her good behavior.
    ○ 2. She cares about the other client's completing the project.
    ○ 3. She is showing improvement by demonstrating more appropriate relationships with others.
    ○ 4. She is demonstrating apathy by doing no more than what she feels is expected of her.

Peggy Smythe excitedly shares with the nurse that she thinks she is pregnant. She wants to know how soon after she has missed her period she can expect laboratory test results to confirm her hopes.

12. Your response to Mrs. Smythe is based on knowledge of the hormonal changes of pregnancy. Which hormone is necessary for a positive pregnancy test?
    ○ 1. Estrogen
    ○ 2. Human chorionic gonadotropin
    ○ 3. Human placental lactogen
    ○ 4. Progesterone

13. Mrs. Smythe asks for information about how a fetus develops. In developing a teaching plan, the nurse identifies the terms used to denote the growth of the fetus. What are these terms in the correct chronologic order as they occur in pregnancy?
    ○ 1. Ovum, zygote, embryo, fetus, infant
    ○ 2. Zygote, ovum, fetus, embryo, infant
    ○ 3. Zygote, ovum, embryo, fetus, infant
    ○ 4. Ovum, embryo, zygote, fetus, infant

14. The nurse explains to Mrs. Smythe that a teratogen is any factor that has an adverse effect on the developing child in utero and that the timing of exposure to such a factor is significant. The greatest danger of teratogen exposure exists during the period
    ○ 1. from conception to the eighth week, during organogenesis.
    ○ 2. after 16 weeks, when the fetus begins swallowing amniotic fluid.
    ○ 3. beginning at 20 weeks, when the fetus is capable of producing antibodies.
    ○ 4. during the eighth to ninth month, which is a period of very rapid growth.

15. Fetal circulation differs from the circulatory pattern common after birth. Which major organ system is bypassed in fetal circulation, other than for purposes of nutrition?
   ○ **1.** Heart
   ○ **2.** Liver
   ○ **3.** Lungs
   ○ **4.** Spleen

16. Which of the following is a function of the placenta?
   ○ **1.** Prevents exchange between fetal and maternal blood
   ○ **2.** Allows exchange by osmosis across a semipermeable membrane
   ○ **3.** Protects the fetus from viral infections during the first 3 months
   ○ **4.** Allows exchange to occur only by the process of diffusion

Sam Weston, aged 21, was brought to the emergency unit for acute abdominal pain. His condition was diagnosed as acute appendicitis. He is currently in the emergency unit waiting to go to surgery.

17. In the limited time available, the nurse recognizes the need to include which of the following in the pre-op teaching?
   ○ **1.** Leg exercises to prevent venous stasis
   ○ **2.** Abdominal splinting for coughing and deep breathing
   ○ **3.** Explanation of the nasogastric tube he can expect postoperatively
   ○ **4.** Drainage he can expect on his dressing

18. Before administering Mr. Weston's pre-op medication, which of the following nursing actions is most essential?
   ○ **1.** Report to the physician the elevated white blood cell count.
   ○ **2.** Check to ensure the laboratory has completed the urinalysis.
   ○ **3.** Ensure the surgical consent form has been signed.
   ○ **4.** Provide a quiet environment.

19. Mr. Weston is taken to the operating room, and preparation for surgery begins. The circulating nurse's primary goal when positioning Mr. Weston on the operating room table is to achieve
   ○ **1.** a comfortable position for the client.
   ○ **2.** a position that is acceptable to the surgeon.
   ○ **3.** a position that prevents exposure and promotes privacy.
   ○ **4.** a position that avoids circulatory impairment and protects nerve function.

20. Mr. Weston receives a general anesthestic in the operating room. In order to suppress pain, general anesthesia must depress which part of the brain?
   ○ **1.** Medulla
   ○ **2.** Thalamus
   ○ **3.** Cerebellum
   ○ **4.** Cortex

21. Mr. Weston is admitted to the postanesthesia room. The nurse obtains admitting vital signs of blood pressure 90/60 mm Hg, pulse 100, respirations 18. Which of the following actions should the nurse take?
   ○ **1.** Recheck the vital signs in 5 minutes.
   ○ **2.** Increase the rate of the IV slightly.
   ○ **3.** Place him flat and elevate his feet.
   ○ **4.** Cover him with a warm blanket.

22. It is now 7 hours after Mr. Weston's surgery. He complains of being unable to void, even though he has the urge. Which nursing action is most appropriate?
   ○ **1.** Obtain an order to catheterize him.
   ○ **2.** Assist him to stand at the bedside to void.
   ○ **3.** Wait one more hour before taking any action.
   ○ **4.** Explain to him that this is a common sensation postoperatively.

23. Retained secretions in the lungs, especially postoperatively, most often result in
   ○ **1.** pulmonary edema.
   ○ **2.** fluid imbalance.
   ○ **3.** atelectasis and pneumonia.
   ○ **4.** CO_2 retention.

Five-year-old Marianne has varicella (chickenpox). Her fever is 102.5°F (39.2°C).

24. Marianne may be expected to have all the following manifestations *except* which one?
   ○ **1.** Pruritus
   ○ **2.** Lesions in 4 stages
   ○ **3.** Lymphadenopathy
   ○ **4.** Strawberry tongue

25. Marianne has 2 younger brothers. Marianne's mother should be advised to institute which type of isolation precautions at home?
   ○ **1.** Respiratory isolation
   ○ **2.** Strict isolation
   ○ **3.** Wound and skin isolation
   ○ **4.** Excretion precautions

26. It is also imperative to advise Marianne's mother to
    ○ 1. dim the light in Marianne's room.
    ○ 2. keep Marianne's fingernails short and clean.
    ○ 3. apply cool compresses to Marianne's lesions.
    ○ 4. avoid giving Marianne acidic foods or fluids.

27. Marianne's fever has subsided and she is very bored. Which activity is most appropriate for her as she convalesces?
    ○ 1. Watching cartoons on television
    ○ 2. Talking on the telephone with her friends
    ○ 3. Painting with watercolors
    ○ 4. Reading a book of riddles

28. Marianne's mother asks when Marianne can return to school. What would be the best response?
    ○ 1. "When she no longer has a fever."
    ○ 2. "In 2 weeks."
    ○ 3. "When all her lesions have dried."
    ○ 4. "When no new lesions have appeared for 24 hours."

Charles Arden, aged 25, the victim of an automobile accident, is admitted to the emergency room with a deep laceration on the right side of his head and a bleeding abrasion on his face. He is drowsy but able to respond to verbal stimuli. His vital signs are blood pressure 110/70 mm Hg, pulse 100, respirations 28. Dexamethasone (Decadron) is ordered, and he is admitted to the intensive care unit for further observation.

29. The nurse knows that injury to the right side of the brain will *not* include problems in which of the following?
    ○ 1. Speech
    ○ 2. Perception
    ○ 3. Coordination
    ○ 4. Personality

30. Which of the following would be *inappropriate* as an assessment priority for Mr. Arden?
    ○ 1. Level of consciousness
    ○ 2. Vital signs
    ○ 3. Bladder fullness
    ○ 4. Motor reflexes

31. Why is dexamethasone (Decadron) the corticosteroid of choice in this situation?
    ○ 1. It is an anti-inflammatory drug.
    ○ 2. It decreases the amount of spinal fluid secreted.
    ○ 3. It crosses the blood-brain barrier.
    ○ 4. It causes fewer side effects than any of the other corticosteroids.

Mr. Arden becomes confused during the night and falls quietly asleep. The nurse takes his vital signs and finds his blood pressure is 155/60 mm Hg, his pulse is 64, and his respirations are 18. The physician suspects increased intracranial pressure (ICP).

32. Which of the following nursing actions would be first?
    ○ 1. Institute seizure precautions.
    ○ 2. Start an IV infusion.
    ○ 3. Order a suction machine.
    ○ 4. Start oxygen by cannula at 6 liters.

33. Several hours later, Mr. Arden has a seizure. Which of the following nursing actions would be *inappropriate*?
    ○ 1. Protect his head.
    ○ 2. Restrain him.
    ○ 3. Turn his head or body to the side.
    ○ 4. Time the seizure.

34. After several diagnostic tests, it was determined that Mr. Arden's seizures were the result of increased ICP. Which of the following is the initial treatment?
    ○ 1. Craniectomy
    ○ 2. Induced barbiturate coma
    ○ 3. Osmotic diuretics, corticosteroids, hyperventilation
    ○ 4. Phenobarbital (Luminal) and phenytoin sodium (Dilantin)

35. Which drug is most likely to have a "rebound" effect in the treatment of cerebral edema?
    ○ 1. Dexamethasone (Decadron)
    ○ 2. Diazepam (Valium)
    ○ 3. Mannitol
    ○ 4. Prednisone

36. Two weeks later, Mr. Arden's condition has stabilized. He is restless, talks incessantly, and asks repetitive questions. These behaviors are most indicative of
    ○ 1. depression.
    ○ 2. anxiety.
    ○ 3. anger.
    ○ 4. denial.

37. Which of the following is probably not the underlying cause of his behavior?
    ○ 1. Powerlessness
    ○ 2. Fear of dying
    ○ 3. Decreased self-esteem
    ○ 4. Role acceptance

38. The most therapeutic independent nursing approach at this time is to
   - ○ 1. administer diazepam (Valium).
   - ○ 2. use active-listening skills.
   - ○ 3. obtain psychiatric consultation.
   - ○ 4. schedule a team conference.

Sixteen-year-old Scott Metzger is admitted to the hospital with severe injuries following a car accident in which his best friend had been driving. Both boys had been drinking, and his friend was driving at high speeds and in an erratic manner. When the police attempted to stop them, his friend tried to outrun the police. After speeds exceeding 80 mph, his friend lost control of the car and crashed into a telegraph pole. Scott suffered multiple fractures and a severely burned left foot. Extensive skin grafting and antibiotic therapy were instituted. Amputation of the foot remains a possibility. His friend suffered lacerations and bruises but was not hospitalized.

39. A week after admission, when his physical condition is well stabilized, Scott becomes extremely demanding of the nursing staff, putting on his call light constantly and yelling for the nurse if the light is not answered immediately. Scott's behavior is most likely related to which of the following?
   - ○ 1. Withdrawal from alcohol
   - ○ 2. Boredom
   - ○ 3. Psychotic depression
   - ○ 4. Reactive depression

40. What is the most therapeutic nursing approach to Scott's behavior?
   - ○ 1. Rotate the nurse assigned to his care on a daily basis.
   - ○ 2. Ignore his inappropriate demands.
   - ○ 3. Consider that he is frightened and angry and fulfill as many of his demands as possible.
   - ○ 4. Let him know that his inappropriate demands will be refused.

41. One morning Scott tells the nurse that he is feeling better because he has spent the night planning a way to ''get even'' with his friend. The nurse responds by saying, ''Sounds like you are feeling angry.'' This is an example of which of the following therapeutic communication techniques?
   - ○ 1. Accepting what the client says
   - ○ 2. Reflecting what the client says
   - ○ 3. Verbalizing inferred thoughts and feelings
   - ○ 4. Encouraging the client to express private thoughts

42. The physician writes an order that Scott may be out of bed on crutches only to use the bathroom in his room. The nurse finds Scott in another young client's room watching a football game. When the nurse confronts him about this, he responds, ''What does it matter? I'm going to lose my foot anyway.'' Which is the most therapeutically correct response?
   - ○ 1. ''Who told you that?''
   - ○ 2. ''You probably will if you keep up this behavior.''
   - ○ 3. ''You seem really worried about losing your foot.''
   - ○ 4. ''I'll get a wheelchair and take you back to your room.''

43. One evening as the nurse is helping Scott, he asks her for a date to go dancing after he is discharged. What explanation best fits his behavior?
   - ○ 1. He is acting out sexual feelings.
   - ○ 2. He wants to embarrass the nurse.
   - ○ 3. He wants to be reassured that his foot will heal normally.
   - ○ 4. His comments are normal, given the situation.

44. Which of the following would be the most therapeutic response from the nurse?
   - ○ 1. ''I don't go out with patients.''
   - ○ 2. ''Are you worried that you'll never be able to dance again?''
   - ○ 3. ''Don't you have a girlfriend?''
   - ○ 4. ''I'm your nurse, not your friend.''

Helen Jenkins, aged 8, is admitted to the pediatric unit with a diagnosis of acute bronchial asthma. She had a bad cold for several days before the attack and would awaken during the night with coughing and shortness of breath.

45. Which of the following is most characteristic of asthma?
   - ○ 1. Inspiratory stridor
   - ○ 2. Expiratory wheezing
   - ○ 3. Prolonged inspiration
   - ○ 4. Hoarse voice

46. Helen's physician has ordered epinephrine (Adrenalin) 0.03 ml stat, to be repeated in 20 minutes if no relief is obtained. What is the most common route of administration for epinephrine?
   - ○ 1. Intramuscular
   - ○ 2. Subcutaneous
   - ○ 3. Intravenous
   - ○ 4. Sublingual

47. Which of the following actions is expected of epinephrine?
○ **1.** Relax bronchial spasms
○ **2.** Liquefy respiratory secretions
○ **3.** Increase antibody formation
○ **4.** Reduce airway diameter

48. Following the administration of epinephrine, the nurse should monitor Helen for which sign of epinephrine toxicity?
○ **1.** Tinnitus
○ **2.** Coryza
○ **3.** Tachycardia
○ **4.** Dyspnea

49. Helen begins to show signs of increasing respiratory distress. These include all the following *except*
○ **1.** cyanosis and tachypnea.
○ **2.** intercostal retractions.
○ **3.** increased restlessness.
○ **4.** irregular respirations.

50. Helen is receiving a continuous IV drip of aminophylline. Which of the following is *not* an indicator of aminophylline toxicity?
○ **1.** Headache
○ **2.** Hypotension
○ **3.** Vomiting
○ **4.** Bradycardia

51. Which of the following nursing actions would be most appropriate for Helen?
○ **1.** Position Helen in a supine position.
○ **2.** Limit oral fluids in order to liquefy secretions.
○ **3.** Monitor intake and output and specific gravity.
○ **4.** Turn, cough, and deep breathe q2h.

52. Helen begins to receive hydrocortisone (Solu-Cortef) IV q12h. Prolonged use of steroids in children can lead to which of the following complications?
○ **1.** Laryngeal edema
○ **2.** Growth suppression
○ **3.** Grand mal seizures
○ **4.** Chronic osteoarthritis

53. What is the rationale for the administration of hydrocortisone (Solu-Cortef)?
○ **1.** It reduces anxiety.
○ **2.** It diminishes inflammation.
○ **3.** It mobilizes secretions.
○ **4.** It relieves bronchospasm.

54. Helen's mother asks if a pet would help her recovery after discharge. Which of the following pets would be most appropriate for Helen?
○ **1.** Parakeet
○ **2.** Dog
○ **3.** Cat
○ **4.** Fish

Armand and Julia Cirrone have been married 8 years. The first 2 pregnancies resulted in spontaneous abortions. This pregnancy has been healthy, and in the 7th month they decide upon delivery in a birthing center. The nurse conducts a tour of the suite and describes the adaptations common to such a birth.

55. As the nurse discusses the birth process with the couple, which statement best indicates they understand all options?
○ **1.** "We know that the midwife will call the physician if needed."
○ **2.** "If Julia needs pain medication, we know it is available."
○ **3.** "Armand and I will be together with our new baby for the first hours."
○ **4.** All the above statements indicate understanding.

56. Mrs. Cirrone's labor begins while her husband is on a business trip. She is very upset that he cannot be with her at this time, as they had prepared together for active participation in the birth. What approach can the nurse take to meet the client's needs at this time?
○ **1.** Ask if there is another individual she would like as support person.
○ **2.** Assign 1 nurse to remain with her.
○ **3.** Ask the operator to continue to try to locate her husband.
○ **4.** Reinforce the client's confidence in her own sense of control.

57. In assessing Mrs. Cirrone's progress during labor, which of the following observations best indicates imminent delivery?
○ **1.** Spontaneous rupture of membranes
○ **2.** 100% effacement
○ **3.** Bulging perineum
○ **4.** Contractions 50 seconds in duration

58. A healthy daughter is delivered just as Armand Cirone arrives at the birthing center. The happy couple hold the infant, and Mrs. Cirone initiates breast-feeding. In accordance with policies, she will be discharged in 8 hours, to be visited the following day by the nurse midwife. Which of the following aspects of postpartal teaching is of highest priority with an early discharge?
   ○ 1. Demonstrate correct breast-feeding techniques.
   ○ 2. Teach client palpation and massage of the fundus.
   ○ 3. Give a demonstration of infant bathing techniques.
   ○ 4. Answer all questions of both parents.

59. Which of the following is an appropriate goal for mother and infant for the first day?
   ○ 1. Promote health during perinatal period
   ○ 2. Teach developmental needs of first 12 months
   ○ 3. Prevent maternal and neonatal complications
   ○ 4. Promote attachment

Barbara Case's myasthenia gravis (MG) was diagnosed 4 years ago. The initial onset of symptoms occurred during a pregnancy. Her disease was well controlled with medication until she contracted an upper respiratory tract infection recently.

60. Mrs. Case asks why this had to happen to her when she is very careful to always take her pyridostigmine (Mestinon) on time, 3 times every day. What explanation would be most appropriate to give Mrs. Case?
   ○ 1. "You have become resistant to Mestinon, but there are other medications that work just as well."
   ○ 2. "Symptoms of MG are often exacerbated by any kind of stress such as infection."
   ○ 3. "You need to increase your medicine to 6 times a day."
   ○ 4. "Surgical excision of the thymus gland (thymectomy) often promotes better control of symptoms."

61. Which of the following would *not* be a typical finding in the physical assessment of Mrs. Case?
   ○ 1. Bilateral ptosis of the eyelids
   ○ 2. Difficulty swallowing and chewing
   ○ 3. Muscle rigidity and tremors at rest
   ○ 4. Inability to raise her arms over her head

62. To prevent aspiration, what should the nurse do before offering food or fluids to Mrs. Case?
   ○ 1. Check to see if she is NPO for a Tensilon test.
   ○ 2. Question her about muscarinic effects of the Mestinon (nausea, abdominal cramping, diarrhea).
   ○ 3. Assess cranial nerves III (oculomotor), IV (trochlear), and VI (abducens) for weakness.
   ○ 4. Assess cranial nerves IX (glossopharyngeal) and X (vagus) for weakness.

63. Mrs. Case is conscientiously taking her medication on time. What should the nurse teach her about her medication regimen at discharge?
   ○ 1. Never use atropine sulfate as an antidote for muscarinic effects.
   ○ 2. Edrophonium (Tensilon) will probably be given with the Mestinon until her infection is completely resolved.
   ○ 3. Take Mestinon on an empty stomach, 1 hour before meals.
   ○ 4. Take Mestinon with or immediately following meals.

64. To facilitate the management of MG, which is the most important information to discuss with Mrs. Case?
   ○ 1. No over-the-counter medications are known to affect the action of anticholinesterase medications used in the treatment of MG.
   ○ 2. Observe for symptoms of thyroid disease, because clients with MG also experience thyroid dysfunction.
   ○ 3. Planned rest periods throughout the day will maximize strength.
   ○ 4. Good body mechanics will prevent deformities.

65. Mrs. Case asks whether getting pregnant again will have any effect on her MG. What would be the nurse's best response?
   ○ 1. "Pregnancy has no effect on MG."
   ○ 2. "Pregnancy is considered to be a precipitating or aggravating event in MG."
   ○ 3. "What do you think?"
   ○ 4. "As long as you take your medication, you have nothing to worry about."

66. Mrs. Case asks, "Just what is MG?" What is the pathophysiologic principle upon which the nurse would base a response?
   ○ 1. It is an autoimmune process affecting nerves and muscles.
   ○ 2. It is an autoimmune process affecting the myoneural junction.
   ○ 3. It is a genetic defect that destroys myelin.
   ○ 4. It is a "slow" viral infection that attacks skeletal muscle.

67. The physician considers corticosteroid therapy for Mrs. Case. Which of the following can often result from long-term corticosteroid therapy?
   ○ 1. Adrenal gland hypertrophy
   ○ 2. Adrenal insufficiency in response to excess stress
   ○ 3. Elevated levels of corticotropin-releasing factor
   ○ 4. Atrophy of the posterior pituitary gland

68. Why must corticosteroid drugs always be stopped gradually?
   ○ 1. ACTH and corticotropin-releasing factor levels are diminished from the supplemental steroids, so no cortisol would be available with abrupt withdrawal.
   ○ 2. ACTH and melanocyte-stimulating hormone (MSH) levels are elevated, because the negative feedback loop has been lost.
   ○ 3. Ectopic ACTH syndrome could result with rapid withdrawal.
   ○ 4. Poor wound healing will occur with rapid withdrawal, along with sodium retention and edema.

Deborah Smolins, gravida 1, para 0, is 32 years old and classified as a class II cardiac client.

69. Careful assessments are particularly essential from weeks 28 to 32 because of the risk of
   ○ 1. premature delivery.
   ○ 2. cardiac decompression.
   ○ 3. fluid retention.
   ○ 4. fetal circulatory problems.

70. Teaching Mrs. Smolins the symptoms associated with congestive heart failure is very important. Which of the following statements best indicates that she understands what has been taught?
   ○ 1. "The doctor will be able to listen to my heart and lungs at my weekly visits and see how I am doing."
   ○ 2. "If there is swelling of my feet and hands, I should reduce the amount of salt that I take."
   ○ 3. "When I have inadequate rest, I will have palpitations."
   ○ 4. "If I have a cough or get tired more easily, I should see the doctor immediately."

71. Mrs. Smolins may need drugs during the antepartal period because of her cardiac status. Which one of the following is the most accurate statement about the use of drugs for cardiac conditions during pregnancy?
   ○ 1. Penicillin cannot be used prophylactically to prevent infections.
   ○ 2. Heparin is a safe anticoagulant, as it does not cross the placenta.
   ○ 3. Digitalis is safe, as it is not teratogenic.
   ○ 4. No drugs should be used, as they all cause damage to the fetus.

72. Mr. Smolins is concerned about the type of delivery that his wife might have. What is the nurse's most appropriate response in explaining the nature of the delivery?
   ○ 1. "A cesarean delivery would cause the least exertion, as she will not have to go through labor and delivery."
   ○ 2. "A forceps delivery will reduce the strain caused by pushing."
   ○ 3. "A normal delivery is possible, as she will be watched very carefully; and there will be no surgical intervention unless necessary."
   ○ 4. "What is important is that regional anesthesia is used. The type of delivery is not relevant."

73. What position will Mrs. Smolins need to assume in labor to allow for maximum functioning of her heart?
   ○ 1. Left lateral
   ○ 2. Sims's position
   ○ 3. Dorsal recumbent
   ○ 4. Semirecumbent

74. Which of the following statements would be most appropriate regarding Mrs. Smolins's interaction with the infant?
    ○ 1. If the labor, delivery, and postpartum were uneventful, it would be appropriate to breast-feed her baby.
    ○ 2. Rooming-in will be possible, and she will be able to care for herself and the baby.
    ○ 3. A regular schedule will have to be arranged for her to interact with the infant.
    ○ 4. Caring for the baby will be too great a strain on her for at least 6 weeks.

Vera Thompson, a 40-year-old woman, is brought to the emergency room by her sister. During the assessment, the nurse finds out that Mrs. Thompson's husband moved out that morning rather unexpectedly and into an apartment with his 24-year-old secretary. He has asked for a divorce. Mrs. Thompson has 2 girls, aged 12 and 14, a high school diploma, and has not worked outside her home in 18 years. The nurse noted a pulse of 120, blood pressure 130/70 mm Hg, tearfulness, narrowed perception, decreased attention span, and fidgeting.

75. Mrs. Thompson is most likely experiencing which of the following?
    ○ 1. Situational crisis
    ○ 2. Depression
    ○ 3. Psychosis
    ○ 4. Paranoid state

76. Which of the following is an important characteristic of crisis intervention?
    ○ 1. It is necessary to determine the cause before a solution to the problem can be found.
    ○ 2. It will not be of lasting value unless the client achieves insight and increased self-knowledge.
    ○ 3. The client is passive because of a decreased ability to function, so appropriate solutions are presented by the therapist.
    ○ 4. It deals only with helping an individual or family cope with the immediate presenting problem.

77. Factors that need to be assessed by the nurse when evaluating a client like Mrs. Thompson include which of the following?
    ○ 1. Precipitating events, coping styles, support systems
    ○ 2. Hallucinations, delusions, tensions
    ○ 3. Anxiety, suspicious behavior, irrational thoughts
    ○ 4. Eating habits, sleeping habits, affect, elimination difficulties

78. What is the nurse's first priority with Mrs. Thompson?
    ○ 1. Reassure her that all crises are time limited.
    ○ 2. Determine the extent of the immediate problems and how significant she perceives them to be.
    ○ 3. Advise her to contact an attorney and make an appointment for her to return the next day.
    ○ 4. Contact her husband and notify him of the situation.

79. Mrs. Thompson begins to cry. Select the correct nursing response.
    ○ 1. Provide her with privacy.
    ○ 2. "Everything will be all right in a day or so."
    ○ 3. Administer antianxiety medicine.
    ○ 4. "Tell me what's upsetting you, Mrs. Thompson."

80. Which setting would be the most appropriate referral for the emergency room nurse to make for Mrs. Thompson?
    ○ 1. Day treatment center
    ○ 2. Community mental health center
    ○ 3. Crisis center
    ○ 4. Inpatient psychiatric setting

81. In planning counseling sessions with Mrs. Thompson which of the following schedules should the nurse recommend?
    ○ 1. Every day for a week
    ○ 2. Two times a week for 2 weeks
    ○ 3. Three times a week for 3 weeks
    ○ 4. Once a week for 6 weeks

82. At the end of 6 weeks, Mrs. Thompson reports that she has begun working as a teachers' assistant at her daughters' school, has seen an attorney, and is receiving child support. Based on this information, at what level is Mrs. Thompson functioning?
    ○ 1. At the same level, since she has been unaffected by the crisis
    ○ 2. At a lower level, because of all the trauma she has experienced
    ○ 3. At a higher level, because of her personal growth
    ○ 4. At the same level. Despite the changes in her life, she is still the same person she was 6 weeks ago.

Tommy Miller is a 15-year-old with lymphosarcoma. During the terminal phase of his illness, he is hospitalized with nausea, edema, and pruritus. His mouth is ulcerated with some infected areas visible. His parents refuse to leave him. He is becoming very restless.

83. During the terminal stages of illness, the nurse needs to support Mr. and Mrs. Miller. Which of the following is *not* considered supportive nursing action?
   ○ 1. Call their religious advisor if they request.
   ○ 2. Arrange an opportunity for them to talk with the physician.
   ○ 3. Allow them to stay with Tommy and give them privacy with him.
   ○ 4. Limit conversations with Tommy and his parents.

84. When giving mouth care to Tommy, what should the nurse use?
   ○ 1. A toothbrush
   ○ 2. Peroxide solution
   ○ 3. A mild mouthwash solution
   ○ 4. Nothing; it will only annoy him.

85. Skin care for Tommy should include which one of the following?
   ○ 1. Keeping fingernails short
   ○ 2. Daily tub bath
   ○ 3. Shower as desired
   ○ 4. Scrub with pHisoHex

86. Mrs. Miller is overheard telling another visitor that Tommy will be going home soon and will be able to return to high school. Mrs. Miller is exhibiting behavior typical of which stage of loss?
   ○ 1. Denial
   ○ 2. Acceptance
   ○ 3. Restitution
   ○ 4. Guilt

87. Tommy has an order for meperidine (Demerol) 50 mg with hydroxyzine (Vistaril) 25 mg IM q3h to q4h prn for pain. Which of the following is *not* an action of hydroxyzine?
   ○ 1. Antiemetic
   ○ 2. Antihistaminic
   ○ 3. Central nervous system stimulant
   ○ 4. Opiate and barbiturate potentiator

88. Tommy requests that the radio be played at night, which is against hospital rules. What would be the best course of action for the nurse?
   ○ 1. Gently refuse and explain the rules.
   ○ 2. Let him play the radio but keep his door shut.
   ○ 3. Consider the possibility of obtaining earphones for the radio.
   ○ 4. Strictly enforce the rules and set limits.

89. Mr. Miller discussed Tommy's impending death with staff members. When the nurse who is working with the family of a dying child helps them to talk about the impending loss and what it means to them, s/he is doing all the following *except*
   ○ 1. overstepping her professional responsibilities.
   ○ 2. helping the family cope with the experience.
   ○ 3. practicing the principles of preventive medicine in mental health.
   ○ 4. indirectly assisting the client.

Sandra Gibson is admitted to the hospital with a diagnosis of acute bacterial pneumonia.

90. Miss Gibson's presenting symptoms are not likely to include
   ○ 1. cyanosis.
   ○ 2. dehydration.
   ○ 3. pleuritic pain.
   ○ 4. audible wheezing.

91. In caring for Miss Gibson, why must the nurse be careful to avoid overmedication with sedatives?
   ○ 1. They suppress bone-marrow function.
   ○ 2. They depress the cough reflex and cause accumulation of fluids in the lung.
   ○ 3. They increase the risk of superinfection.
   ○ 4. They cause hypersensitivity reactions.

92. Which of the following actions is *not* appropriate treatment for Miss Gibson's bacterial pneumonia?
   ○ 1. Auscultate the lungs q2h to q4h.
   ○ 2. Encourage fluids to 3 liters/day.
   ○ 3. Give ampicillin if the client is allergic to penicillin.
   ○ 4. Encourage the client to cough by splinting her chest.

93. What is the best reason for encouraging Miss Gibson to increase her fluid intake?
   ○ 1. To promote bronchial dilation
   ○ 2. To prevent the need for a nasogastric tube
   ○ 3. To improve antibiotic therapy
   ○ 4. To loosen and thin bronchial secretions

94. Why is aspiration pneumonia more common in the right lung?
   ○ 1. There is an increased amount of lung tissue available for infection on the right side.
   ○ 2. There is an absence of ciliated mucosal lining on the right.
   ○ 3. The right bronchus is shorter and wider.
   ○ 4. There is enhanced conduction through the airways on the right.

95. Which of the following statements best describes why a pleural effusion may be a complication of Miss Gibson's pneumonia?

○ **1.** Excess connective tissue accumulates in the lungs during healing and repair.

○ **2.** Increased hydrostatic pressure or decreased oncotic pressure occurs with movement of fluid out of the capillaries.

○ **3.** Thrombotic occlusion of the pulmonary arterial system occurs.

○ **4.** The pleurae become inflamed.

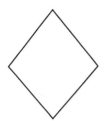

Test 1, Book I
Answers with Rationales

1. **#2.** Ability to communicate with the client is essential to the quality of care. ASSESSMENT (ADULT/NUTRITION AND METABOLISM)

2. **#1.** Because she fainted, cause unknown, the baseline mental status is most important. Vital signs are secondary in this situation. ASSESSMENT (ADULT/NUTRITION AND METABOLISM)

3. **#2.** During the admission process, a family member fluent in both languages is the best person to help gather the essential data. In Mrs. Garcia's culture, the family plays an important role in the care of the client and the success of treatment. IMPLEMENTATION (ADULT/NUTRITION AND METABOLISM)

4. **#4.** Adjusting to the life changes, especially for the older person, is a difficult process. Option #4 does not consider this problem of the difficulty of change. PLAN (ADULT/NUTRITION AND METABOLISM)

5. **#3.** Manipulation is a dominant characteristic of the client who exhibits antisocial behavior. Clients such as this have difficulty relating to others because of inner feelings of abandonment. Although it is possible that this particular nurse has superior abilities, it is likely that a number of other staff also have superior abilities. Clients such as Miss Evenson are rarely motivated to change. Any genuine changes that might occur will happen very slowly. ANALYSIS (PSYCHOSOCIAL, MENTAL HEALTH, PSYCHIATRIC PROBLEMS/SOCIALLY MALADAPTIVE BEHAVIOR)

6. **#3.** Lack of opportunity to associate with appropriate role models, such as parents, results in a poorly developed and unsocialized superego. It is not likely that Miss Evenson had appropriate role models. Clients like this often have developmental histories suggesting that early needs were not met adequately. There is no data suggesting below-average intelligence. ASSESSMENT (PSYCHOSOCIAL, MENTAL HEALTH, PSYCHIATRIC PROBLEMS/SOCIALLY MALADAPTIVE BEHAVIOR)

7. **#3.** The cooperation of all staff is necessary to achieve consistency in setting limits on behavior. Miss Evenson needs firm limits, not freedom of choice or independence. The client is not likely to do well in a group setting since she has not internalized self-control. The client needs a matter-of-fact attitude and firm limits. She will mistake sympathy for weakness and try to manipulate staff more. IMPLEMENTATION (PSYCHOSOCIAL, MENTAL HEALTH, PSYCHIATRIC PROBLEMS/SOCIALLY MALADAPTIVE BEHAVIOR)

8. **#4.** Clients demonstrating antisocial characteristics have no lasting attachments or sense of loyalty. They attempt to achieve pleasurable ends at the expense of others. Although these clients have low self-esteem and poor impulse control, this example does not demonstrate these traits. Although the client may be suspicious and aloof, her statement demonstrates option #4 is best. ANALYSIS (PSYCHOSOCIAL, MENTAL HEALTH, PSYCHIATRIC PROBLEMS/SOCIALLY MALADAPTIVE BEHAVIOR)

9. **#3.** Ambivalent feelings are exemplified by these opposing behaviors. Ambivalence is demonstrated in behaviors described in the question. Further information is necessary to determine whether guilt is present. Option #1 is unlikely. ANALYSIS (PSYCHOSOCIAL, MENTAL HEALTH, PSYCHIATRIC PROBLEMS/SOCIALLY MALADAPTIVE BEHAVIOR)

10. **#3.** After realizing how inappropriate past behavior was, the client often feels depressed. Depression occurs as a consequence of dealing with difficulties in therapy and an emerging awareness of how her behavior affects others. Dysthymic disorder refers to a neurotic depression. A major depressive episode has psychotic features including severe impairment of reality testing and physiologic disturbances. The client may begin to think her prognosis is not good, but such thoughts would not be as likely to occur at this time as option #3. EVALUATION (PSYCHOSOCIAL, MENTAL HEALTH, PSYCHIATRIC PROBLEMS/SOCIALLY MALADAPTIVE BEHAVIOR)

11. **#3.** More appropriate relationships with others demonstrates a decrease in antisocial behavior. Motivation for impressing the staff is difficult to discern. Her feelings for the other client are not known. The behavior described does not indicate apathy. EVALUATION (PSYCHOSOCIAL, MENTAL HEALTH, PSYCHIATRIC PROBLEMS/SOCIALLY MALADAPTIVE BEHAVIOR)

12. **#2.** Pregnancy tests are based on the presence of human chorionic gonadotropin (HCG) in the blood or urine of the woman. ASSESSMENT (CHILDBEARING FAMILY/ANTEPARTAL CARE)

13. **#1.** Before fertilization, the female cell is known as the ovum, after fertilization as the zygote, after implantation or nidation as the embryo, after organogenesis as the fetus, and after birth as the infant. ANALYSIS (CHILDBEARING FAMILY/ANTEPARTAL CARE)

14. **#1.** While teratogenic effects may be specific depending on the causative agent, the greatest danger exists during the formation of the organ systems, or organogenesis, which typically is completed by the end of the eighth week of pregnancy. IMPLEMENTATION (CHILDBEARING FAMILY/ANTEPARTAL CARE)

15. **#3.** Circulation to the lungs of the fetus is needed only for nutrition of the lungs, as oxygen exchange occurs across the placental barrier. ANALYSIS (CHILDBEARING FAMILY/ANTEPARTAL CARE)

16. **#2.** The placenta provides a semipermeable membrane across which exchange occurs by osmosis. In addition diffusion, facilitated diffusion, active transport, and pinocytosis occur. ANALYSIS (CHILDBEARING FAMILY/ANTEPARTAL CARE)

17. **#2.** The practice of abdominal splinting facilitates post-op performance of coughing and deep breathing. Practicing leg exercises is inappropriate, because they would increase abdominal pain preoperatively. A nasogastric tube is usually not required following a simple appendectomy. There is usually little wound drainage as a result of a simple appendectomy. PLAN (ADULT/SURGERY)

18. **#3.** After the client has received pre-op sedation, he is no longer considered competent to sign the operative permit. The other options are true but are unrelated to pre-op medication. IMPLEMENTATION (ADULT/SURGERY)

19. **#4.** The circulating nurse is responsible for ensuring the safety of the client and preventing any harm from positioning. PLAN (ADULT/SURGERY)

20. **#4.** The conscious interpretation of pain takes place in the cerebral cortex. ANALYSIS (ADULT/SURGERY)

21. **#1.** Movement of the client from the operating room table to the postanesthesia room may cause a transient drop in blood pressure. IMPLEMENTATION (ADULT/SURGERY)

22. **#2.** Standing a male client who is experiencing post-op urinary retention at the bedside to void may facilitate voiding. Waiting is not appropriate and explanations will not solve the problem. Catheterization may eventually be necessary but is not the first step. IMPLEMENTATION (ADULT/SURGERY)

23. **#3.** When secretions are retained, they block the small alveoli and cause them to collapse. The resultant inflammation often leads to pneumonia. ANALYSIS (ADULT/SURGERY)

24. **#4.** Strawberry tongue is characteristic of scarlet fever, an infection by beta hemolytic streptococci, group A. The other 3 options are characteristic of chickenpox. ASSESSMENT (CHILD/SENSATION, PERCEPTION, PROTECTION)

25. **#1.** Varicella is an airborne virus, and respiratory isolation procedures should be used to prevent its spread. IMPLEMENTATION (CHILD/SENSATION, PERCEPTION, PROTECTION)

26. **#2.** Keeping Marianne's fingernails short and clean decreases the chance of her acquiring a secondary infection of the pruritic lesions of chickenpox. IMPLEMENTATION (CHILD/SENSATION, PERCEPTION, PROTECTION)

27. **#3.** Painting with watercolors allows her to use her imagination for expression of feelings and ideas; it also promotes development of fine motor skills, which is important at this age. IMPLEMENTATION (CHILD/SENSATION, PERCEPTION, PROTECTION)

28. **#3.** Once the lesions have dried, chickenpox is no longer communicable and Marianne can return to school. A fever may be gone by the time the rash appears. Option #4 indicates she is still contagious. IMPLEMENTATION (CHILD/SENSATION, PERCEPTION, PROTECTION)

29. **#1.** The speech center is located in the left posterolateral side of the frontal lobe (Broca's center). ASSESSMENT (ADULT/SAFETY AND SECURITY)

30. **#3.** Bladder fullness is a priority assessment if the client has spinal cord injuries. There is loss of bladder reflex to empty during spinal shock that occurs within 30 minutes of injury. ASSESSMENT (ADULT/SAFETY AND SECURITY)

31. **#3.** Dexamethasone (Decadron) is the only corticosteroid that crosses the blood-brain barrier. It is the most commonly used steroid in neurologic clients because of its anti-inflammatory action. ANALYSIS (ADULT/SAFETY AND SECURITY)

32. **#1.** All the choices listed are important, but instituting seizure precautions is the priority. IMPLEMENTATION (ADULT/SAFETY AND SECURITY)

33. **#2.** During any seizure, restraining the client can create more trauma than the seizure itself. Other options listed are appropriate to protect client safety. IMPLEMENTATION (ADULT/SAFETY AND SECURITY)

34. **#3.** These are the appropriate measures to reduce the intracranial pressure. ANALYSIS (ADULT/SAFETY AND SECURITY)

35. **#3.** Mannitol is an osmotic diuretic. When it is discontinued, there is a temporary increase in fluid retention. ANALYSIS (ADULT/SAFETY AND SECURITY)

36. **#2.** These behaviors are signs of anxiety. Depression is usually manifested by withdrawal and lack of interest and energy. Yelling, threats, and demands would indicate anger. Someone in denial would not ask repetitive questions; rather would avoid the issues. ANALYSIS (PSYCHOSOCIAL, MENTAL HEALTH, PSYCHIATRIC PROBLEMS/ANXIOUS BEHAVIOR)

37. **#4.** It is too soon for role acceptance to be a major concern. Options #1, #2, and #3 are current issues that are inherent in the client's condition, given the suddenness of the accident, his age, and severity of injury. ANALYSIS (PSYCHOSOCIAL, MENTAL HEALTH, PSYCHIATRIC PROBLEMS/ANXIOUS BEHAVIOR)

38. **#2.** Active listening allows the gathering of more information and provides an opportunity for psychosocial intervention. Options #3 and #4 may be appropriate after further assessment. Option #1 is not an independent nursing action. IMPLEMENTATION (PSYCHOSOCIAL, MENTAL HEALTH, PSYCHIATRIC PROBLEMS/ANXIOUS BEHAVIOR)

39. **#4.** Reactive depression is related to precipitating stress and personal loss. In Scott's case, loss of freedom of movement and the possibility of the loss of his foot have caused a reactive depression. A common response is angry and demanding behavior. Withdrawal from alcohol probably would have occurred within 24 to 72 hours posthospitalization. Boredom usually manifests as complaining and restlessness, not yelling and demanding. The current behavioral presentation is not consistent with a psychotic depression; however, one would want to continue monitoring him for a possible delirium syndrome. ANALYSIS (PSYCHOSOCIAL, MENTAL HEALTH, PSYCHIATRIC PROBLEMS/ELATED-DEPRESSIVE BEHAVIOR)

40. **#4.** Firmness and consistency will make the client feel more secure and help to alleviate his fear. Minimizing the number of nurses who care for the client facilitates the implementation of a consistent approach. Ignoring or meeting the inappropriate demands only serves to escalate the behavior and does not solve the problem of his fear and insecurity. IMPLEMENTATION (PSYCHOSOCIAL, MENTAL HEALTH, PSYCHIATRIC PROBLEMS/ELATED-DEPRESSIVE BEHAVIOR)

41. **#3.** Anger is implied in his desire for revenge. Option #1 is not an acceptance of the retaliation theme but an inference of what the client may be feeling or thinking. A reflective statement uses part of what the client has already stated, i.e., "You are going to get even with your friend." #4 would hopefully be the outcome of using any one of the previously stated communication techniques. IMPLEMENTATION (PSYCHOSOCIAL, MENTAL HEALTH, PSYCHIATRIC PROBLEMS/ELATED-DEPRESSIVE BEHAVIOR)

42. **#3.** Reflecting is the proper therapeutic technique to use in this situation. It gives the client permission to express his feelings about the loss of his foot. Option #1 does not address his fears or concerns and will only provide the nurse with a factual option, not an exploration of feelings. #2 is a threat which, with an adolescent, will probably precipitate a power struggle. #4 will be perceived as a punishment and humiliating in front of a peer who could be beneficial in allowing and assisting the client to verbalize his fears. IMPLEMENTATION (PSYCHOSOCIAL, MENTAL HEALTH, PSYCHIATRIC PROBLEMS/ELATED-DEPRESSIVE BEHAVIOR)

43. **#3.** The fact that Scott asked the nurse for a date, to go dancing in particular, is the clue to his concern. Options #1 and #4 are possibilities; however, the specific activity for the date is dancing, which would require a healthy foot. He is taking a risk with this request, which could embarrass him, not the nurse. ANALYSIS (PSYCHOSOCIAL, MENTAL HEALTH, PSYCHIATRIC PROBLEMS/ELATED-DEPRESSIVE BEHAVIOR)

44. **#2.** This option both acknowledges the client's concern and allows him to discuss it if he wishes to do so. Options #1 and #4 establish a behavioral limit with the client; however, these responses also diminish the chance of the client sharing any feelings with this nurse. #3 completely misses and avoids the feeling tone of this client's request. IMPLEMENTATION (PSYCHOSOCIAL, MENTAL HEALTH, PSYCHIATRIC PROBLEMS/ELATED-DEPRESSIVE BEHAVIOR)

45. **#2.** Expiratory wheezing is the result of air attempting to pass through narrowed bronchial lumens. Option #1 characterizes croup and laryngotracheobronchitis; #4 relates to croup; expirations in asthma are prolonged. ASSESSMENT (CHILD/OXYGENATION)

46. **#2.** Subcutaneous is the preferred route. On occasion, it may be given IM, but the gluteal sites should be avoided. There is no adrenalin preparation suitable for sublingual use. The IV route may be used only if the drug is adequately diluted. IMPLEMENTATION (CHILD/OXYGENATION)

47. **#1.** Epinephrine relieves bronchospasm. It does not liquefy secretions (a subemetic dose of syrup of ipecac does this), nor does it increase antibody formation. The drug increases (not reduces) airway diameter. ANALYSIS (CHILD/OXYGENATION)

48. **#3.** Epinephrine is a beta-adrenergic agent that strengthens myocardial contractions and increases blood pressure, heart rate, and cardiac output. The vasoconstrictive effects predispose the child to tachycardia as well as elevated blood pressure, pallor, weakness, tremors, and nausea. ASSESSMENT (CHILD/OXYGENATION)

49. **#4.** Options #1, #2, and #3 are definite signs of respiratory distress. Irregular respirations may occur for many other reasons and are frequently normal in young children. ASSESSMENT (CHILD/OXYGENATION)

50. **#4.** Tachycardia, not bradycardia, is a manifestation of aminophylline toxicity as are the other 3 options. ASSESSMENT (CHILD/OXYGENATION)

51. **#3.** Intake and output and specific gravity are good indicators of hydration. Hydration is essential because it helps to liquefy secretions and enables the child to more easily expel the mucus. PLAN (CHILD/OXYGENATION)

52. **#2.** Adrenocortical steroids interrupt normal linear growth in children when used over a prolonged period of time. ANALYSIS (CHILD/OXYGENATION)

53. **#2.** Solu-Cortef's anti-inflammatory action relieves airway obstruction by reducing edema. It is administered IV when the usual drugs (e.g., epinephrine) are not effective. Solu-Cortef does not reduce anxiety, mobilize secretions, or relieve bronchospasm. The other asthma drugs achieve these actions. ANALYSIS (CHILD/OXYGENATION)

54. **#4.** The usual cause of asthma is an allergy or hypersensitivity to a foreign protein. A fish would be the most logical choice of pet for an asthmatic child. IMPLEMENTATION (CHILD/OXYGENATION)

55. **#4.** Couples preparing for delivery in a birthing center are well informed about these and other options, such as sibling participation. EVALUATION (CHILDBEARING FAMILY/INTRAPARTAL CARE)

56. **#1.** Allow the client to select another individual to take on the supporting role. If no one is available, it is helpful to assign 1 nurse. IMPLEMENTATION (CHILDBEARING FAMILY/INTRAPARTAL CARE)

57. **#3.** This indicates that the presenting part of the fetus is at the perineum; delivery will be very soon. ASSESSMENT (CHILDBEARING FAMILY/INTRAPARTAL CARE)

58. **#2.** Many clients are now discharged early from the hospital or birthing centers; it is essential to assess uterine firmness frequently and to massage as needed. The other options are important but can be addressed during follow-up visits. IMPLEMENTATION (CHILDBEARING FAMILY/POSTPARTAL CARE)

59. **#4.** While other goals are appropriate over a longer period, promoting attachment is the best short-term goal. PLAN (CHILDBEARING FAMILY/POSTPARTAL CARE)

60. **#2.** Myasthenia gravis is exacerbated by infection; emotional stress; menses; pregnancy; surgery; or accidental administration of curare, quinine, or quinidine. IMPLEMENTATION (ADULT/SAFETY AND SECURITY)

61. **#3.** Muscle rigidity and tremors at rest are symptoms of Parkinson's disease. ASSESSMENT (ADULT/SAFETY AND SECURITY)

62. **#4.** Myasthenia gravis frequently causes weakness in muscles innervated by cranial nerves IX and X, which is associated with difficult swallowing, regurgitation, and aspiration. ASSESSMENT (ADULT/SAFETY AND SECURITY)

63. **#4.** Mestinon is absorbed too quickly on an empty stomach. Exception: if the client is having symptoms, she may need to take the medication, or part of it, before a meal to aid chewing and swallowing. IMPLEMENTATION (ADULT/SAFETY AND SECURITY)

64. **#3.** Weakness becomes worse on exertion and at the end of the day (versus morning). Rest typically increases muscle strength. IMPLEMENTATION (ADULT/SAFETY AND SECURITY)

65. **#2.** Myasthenia gravis can be aggravated by pregnancy. Medication will need very careful management during pregnancy but may not be able to prevent problems. IMPLEMENTATION (ADULT/SAFETY AND SECURITY)

66. **#2.** Myasthenia gravis is caused by an autoimmune process that impairs receptor function at the myoneural junction. ANALYSIS (ADULT/SAFETY AND SECURITY)

67. **#2.** Exogenous steroids cause adrenal gland hypofunction. The body may not be able to respond in times of stress. ANALYSIS (ADULT/SAFETY AND SECURITY)

68. **#1.** Stopping steroids suddenly would mimic addisonian crisis, the major complication of which is cardiovascular collapse. ANALYSIS (ADULT/SAFETY AND SECURITY)

69. **#2.** This is a period of maximum cardiac output, and as a result, cardiac decompensation may occur. ANALYSIS (CHILDBEARING FAMILY/ANTEPARTAL CARE)

70. **#4.** These are the early symptoms of congestive cardiac failure and must be promptly recognized and treated. EVALUATION (CHILDBEARING FAMILY/ANTEPARTAL CARE)

71. **#2.** Heparin is the drug of choice when an anticoagulant is required because its large molecular weight prevents its crossing the placenta. Penicillin is used prophylactically to prevent subacute bacterial endocarditis. Digitalis may have teratogenic properties as it does cross the placenta. ANALYSIS (CHILDBEARING FAMILY/ANTEPARTAL CARE)

72. **#2.** Forceps application reduces the stress and exertion of pushing. Vaginal delivery is the preferred method of delivery for cardiac clients. IMPLEMENTATION (CHILDBEARING FAMILY/INTRAPARTAL CARE)

73. **#4.** The semirecumbent, or Fowler's, position allows for maximum functioning of her heart and respiratory system. IMPLEMENTATION (CHILDBEARING FAMILY/INTRAPARTAL CARE)

74. **#1.** Rooming-in is possible only with assistance and as she desires. A gradual increase in activity during the postpartum period is recommended. Breast-feeding is permissible if there were no cardiac problems during labor and delivery, and immediately postpartum. PLAN (CHILDBEARING FAMILY/POSTPARTAL CARE)

75. **#1.** Characteristics of a situational crisis are a precipitating event (divorce) and signs and symptoms of extreme discomfort, e.g., tearfulness, narrowed perception, loss of thinking ability, fidgeting, and increased values in vital signs. Any depressive symptoms would be related to the current situation and loss. Options #3 and #4 are diagnoses that are not consistent with the clinical situation. ANALYSIS (PSYCHOSOCIAL, MENTAL HEALTH, PSYCHIATRIC PROBLEMS/THERAPEUTIC USE OF SELF)

76. #4. The scope of crisis intervention is to deal with here-and-now problems and assist the client and family to find coping mechanisms effective in dealing with stress in the environment. New coping can be explored without knowing the cause of the problem. Insight and increased self-knowledge are valuable but may not always produce behavioral change. The client in crisis is facing the opportunity to change for the better or regress. The discomfort of the high anxiety provides leverage for the nurse to assist the client in learning how to problem solve and develop more effective coping. Giving advice reinforces the person's sense of helplessness. ANALYSIS (PSYCHOSOCIAL, MENTAL HEALTH, PSYCHIATRIC PROBLEMS/THERAPEUTIC USE OF SELF)

77. #1. Crisis intervention involves assessment of the client's support systems, coping mechanisms, and the precipitating event. Options #2, #3, and #4 can be behavioral manifestations of someone experiencing a crisis state; however, they are more indicative of chronic psychopathologic behavior. The crisis intervention framework focuses on the here and now and not chronic problems. ASSESSMENT (PSYCHOSOCIAL, MENTAL HEALTH, PSYCHIATRIC PROBLEMS/ THERAPEUTIC USE OF SELF)

78. #2. Initially, it is necessary to determine immediate problems and how they are viewed by the client. Reassurance at this time seldom lowers anxiety and tends to make the client feel misunderstood. Advice given before the problem is identified and feelings are explored is usually not taken because the client's anxiety is too high to make use of the suggestion. It is preferable to assist the client in coming up with her own solutions after the distorted perceptions have been corrected and her anxiety lowered. Rather than contacting the husband, explore with the client who her support system is, and encourage her to contact someone with whom she will feel comfortable. IMPLEMENTATION (PSYCHOSOCIAL, MENTAL HEALTH, PSYCHIATRIC PROBLEMS/THERAPEUTIC USE OF SELF)

79. #4. When dealing with Mrs. Thompson's crying, reflect the feeling and ask for more information. Some clients will want privacy, but this should be clarified with the client before the nurse automatically leaves a client alone to cry. False reassurance blocks communication. While antianxiety medications are commonly used to help clients be less nervous and gain control over themselves, crying is a healthy, emotional outlet and should be permitted and supported rather than circumvented with medication. IMPLEMENTATION (PSYCHOSOCIAL, MENTAL HEALTH, PSYCHIATRIC PROBLEMS/ THERAPEUTIC USE OF SELF)

80. #3. The emergency room nurse can refer clients like Mrs. Thompson to crisis centers for continued intervention. Mrs. Thompson's condition does not warrant inpatient psychiatric treatment or day care. Mental health centers are more focused on long-term therapy than crisis intervention. IMPLEMENTATION (PSYCHOSOCIAL, MENTAL HEALTH, PSYCHIATRIC PROBLEMS/THERAPEUTIC USE OF SELF)

81. #4. Crises are time-limited and are usually resolved within 6 weeks. Once a week is sufficient and allows time for the client to implement new coping behaviors and be supported during the entire time of the crisis. PLAN (PSYCHOSOCIAL, MENTAL HEALTH, PSYCHIATRIC PROBLEMS/THERAPEUTIC USE OF SELF)

82. #3. The information given suggests she has experienced personal growth. The goal of crisis intervention is to prevent hospitalization and regression to a permanently maladaptive state. This has been achieved. Even though the client has been traumatized and is the same person she was 6 weeks ago, her coping has become adaptive and enhances her life, so she is functioning at a higher level. EVALUATION (PSYCHOSOCIAL, MENTAL HEALTH, PSYCHIATRIC PROBLEMS/THERAPEUTIC USE OF SELF)

83. #4. Do not avoid Tommy and his parents; provide both privacy and emotional support. Tommy needs gentle physical care. PLAN (CHILD/MOBILITY)

84. #3. The toothbrush and peroxide solution might further damage Tommy's ulcerated and infected mouth. Doing nothing is not an appropriate measure, because discomfort will be increased. IMPLEMENTATION (CHILD/MOBILITY)

85. #1. Fingernails should be kept short to prevent scratching and injury to skin with pruritus. The other answers are inappropriate for a terminally ill client. IMPLEMENTATION (CHILD/MOBILITY)

86. #1. According to Kübler-Ross, Mrs. Miller is denying the consequences of the terminal phase of Tommy's illness. ANALYSIS (CHILD/MOBILITY)

87. #3. Hydroxyzine causes sedation and does not stimulate the central nervous system. ANALYSIS (CHILD/MOBILITY)

88. #3. This provides sound control for the other clients' benefit and allows Tommy to have his request. Music with earphones is also helpful for pain control and relaxation. IMPLEMENTATION (CHILD/MOBILITY)

89. #1. Working with the family of the child is an appropriate nursing action. ANALYSIS (CHILD/MOBILITY)

90. #4. Findings on physical examination of the chest may include dullness to percussion, diminished breath sounds, rales, and a pleural friction rub. Audible wheezing is a symptom of hyperinflated lungs such as are found with asthma. ASSESSMENT (ADULT/OXYGENATION)

91. #2. Sedatives can have this effect. Antineoplastic drugs usually suppress bone marrow. Antibiotics may increase the risk of superinfections. Penicillin-type drugs more commonly cause hypersensitivity reactions. ANALYSIS (ADULT/OXYGENATION)

92. #3. Ampicillin is in the penicillin family and should not be given to someone who is allergic to penicillin. IMPLEMENTATION (ADULT/OXYGENATION)

93. #4. Fluid intake of at least 3 liters/day facilitates the expectoration of bronchial secretions. PLAN (ADULT/OXYGENATION)

94. #3. The right and left mainstem bronchi are not symmetric; the right bronchus is shorter and wider, and continues from the trachea in a vertical course. This anatomic difference facilitates aspiration into the right lung. ANALYSIS (ADULT/OXYGENATION)

95. #2. Pleural effusions result from the movement of fluid out of the capillaries by an increased hydrostatic pressure or decreased oncotic pressure. ANALYSIS (ADULT/OXYGENATION)

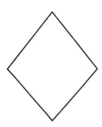

Test 1, Book II
Questions

Sheila Vogel is admitted to the labor room. Her gestation is estimated to be 35 weeks but she is having contractions. Attempts are made to stop labor.

1. Which of the following nursing actions is appropriate when caring for Mrs. Vogel?
- ○ **1.** Prepare for an oxytocin challenge test to determine fetal status.
- ○ **2.** Prepare for the application of an internal monitor.
- ○ **3.** Give frequent analgesia to relieve anxiety and promote comfort.
- ○ **4.** Discuss the potential problems and preparations being made for the infant.

2. Bed rest is prescribed for Mrs. Vogel primarily because it
- ○ **1.** will keep the pressure of the fetus off the cervix and enhance uterine perfusion.
- ○ **2.** may stop labor by decreasing uterine irritability.
- ○ **3.** will promote comfort and reduce anxiety.
- ○ **4.** will reduce fetal activity.

3. A tokolytic agent is administered to Mrs. Vogel to suppress her labor. Which of the following nursing actions would be most appropriate in preventing side effects from this type of medication?
- ○ **1.** Side-lying position, antiembolic stockings, adequate hydration
- ○ **2.** Reduction in extraneous stimuli, frequent assessment of fetal heart tones
- ○ **3.** Use of side rails, frequent monitoring of uterine contractions
- ○ **4.** Frequent monitoring of blood pressure and pulse

4. Which of the following drugs is considered a tokolytic agent?
- ○ **1.** Levallorphan tartrate (Lorfan)
- ○ **2.** Terbutaline sulfate (Brethine)
- ○ **3.** Phenobarbital
- ○ **4.** Betamethasone phosphate (Celestone)

5. Attempts to stop labor were unsuccessful, and Baby Boy Vogel is born weighing 4 lb 2 oz. Which of the following observations of Baby Vogel best suggest a gestational age of less than 40 weeks?
- ○ **1.** Small amounts of lanugo and vernix, testes descended, palmar and plantar creases
- ○ **2.** Parchmentlike skin, no lanugo, full areolae in breasts
- ○ **3.** Upper pinna of ear well curved with instant recoil, small amounts of lanugo, pink in color
- ○ **4.** Dark red skin, testes undescended with few rugations, abundant lanugo

6. The nurse carries out necessary precautions in the delivery room to meet the special needs of the premature infant. Which of the following is an important difference between a premature and term infant?
- ○ **1.** Owing to size, a premature infant will have a more efficient metabolic rate for heat production and maintenance.
- ○ **2.** In proportion to size, the premature infant will have more lanugo and more vernix than a full-term infant.
- ○ **3.** Gastrointestinal motility is decreased in the preterm infant. Stools may be infrequent resulting in abdominal distension.
- ○ **4.** Heat production is low in the premature infant because of the greater body surface related to weight and lack of subcutaneous fat.

7. Which of the following assessments would most likely indicate respiratory distress?
- ○ **1.** Abdominal breathing and acrocyanosis
- ○ **2.** Irregular shallow respirations
- ○ **3.** Respiratory rate of 30 to 60/minute
- ○ **4.** Nasal flaring

8. Baby Vogel's postdelivery hospital stay is uneventful. Which aspect of Baby Vogel's care will have the greatest permanent effect on emotional development?
   - ○ 1. The position in which he is placed in the crib
   - ○ 2. The way in which he is held and touched
   - ○ 3. The extent to which a quiet environment is provided for him
   - ○ 4. The number of caretakers who provide care for him

9. Provisions are made for Mrs. Vogel to spend time in the premature nursery. Which of the following is the most important reason for doing this?
   - ○ 1. To provide her with written instructions concerning feeding and bathing the infant
   - ○ 2. To provide a demonstration of feeding and bathing for her
   - ○ 3. To provide her with the opportunity to handle and care for the infant in a supportive atmosphere
   - ○ 4. To provide her with an opportunity to ask questions she may have concerning the infant's growth and development

Henry Nims, aged 58, is admitted with a diagnosis of chronic obstructive pulmonary disease (COPD). His orders include antibiotics and respiratory therapy, including intermittent positive pressure breathing (IPPB); chest physical therapy; and ultrasonic nebulizer.

10. Mr. Nims's tidal volume is 250 cc. This is commonly considered
    - ○ 1. high.
    - ○ 2. low.
    - ○ 3. normal.
    - ○ 4. high for his age group.

11. Mr. Nims's dead-space volume is most likely to be
    - ○ 1. 150 cc.
    - ○ 2. above 150 cc.
    - ○ 3. 100 to 150 cc.
    - ○ 4. below 100 cc.

12. Mr. Nims's vital capacity will be the greatest in which postion?
    - ○ 1. Supine
    - ○ 2. Prone
    - ○ 3. Fowler's
    - ○ 4. Sims'

13. Mr. Nims's arterial blood gases on admission were: pH 7.4, pO_2 60 mm Hg, pCO_2 60–80 mm Hg, HCO_3 30 mEq/liter. These values are most indicative of which of the following conditions?
    - ○ 1. Respiratory acidosis
    - ○ 2. Compensated respiratory acidosis
    - ○ 3. Respiratory alkalosis
    - ○ 4. Compensated respiratory alkalosis

14. Mr. Nims's blood gases could best be considered
    - ○ 1. normal.
    - ○ 2. normal for a COPD client.
    - ○ 3. abnormal.
    - ○ 4. abnormal for a COPD client.

15. Mr. Nims has most likely become adjusted to which of the following?
    - ○ 1. Elevated pCO_2 and pO_2 levels
    - ○ 2. Lowered pCO_2 and elevated pO_2 levels
    - ○ 3. Elevated pCO_2 and lowered pO_2 levels
    - ○ 4. Lowered pCO_2 and pO_2 levels

16. Mr. Nims has copious amounts of thick, tenacious yellow mucus, which he cannot manage. He requires suctioning, and the nurse becomes concerned that he might have an arrest during this procedure. Which of the following would not precipitate a cardiac arrest during suctioning?
    - ○ 1. Depletion of oxygen to the brain
    - ○ 2. Depletion of oxygen to the heart
    - ○ 3. Vagal nerve stimulation
    - ○ 4. Electrolyte imbalance

17. What is the primary purpose of the IPPB for this client?
    - ○ 1. Open clogged airways
    - ○ 2. Loosen accumulated secretions
    - ○ 3. Promote dilation of smooth muscle bands around airways
    - ○ 4. Provide adequate ventilation

18. Mr. Nims begins to exhibit restlessness, combativeness, and tachycardia, but he is not acyanotic. The nurse would expect to find his arterial pO_2 to be which of the following?
    - ○ 1. 48 to 52 mm Hg
    - ○ 2. 30 to 40 mm Hg
    - ○ 3. 60 to 70 mm Hg
    - ○ 4. Greater than 70 mm Hg

19. Which rate of oxygen flow per cannula would most likely be ordered for Mr. Nims?
    - ○ 1. Rate of 2 to 3 liters/minute
    - ○ 2. Rate of 4 to 6 liters/minute
    - ○ 3. Rate of 6 to 8 liters/minute
    - ○ 4. Rate of 8 to 10 liters/minute

20. Which is the *least* reliable sign of adequate ventilation?
    ○ **1.** Patent airway
    ○ **2.** Chest or abdominal movement with each respiration
    ○ **3.** Air flow at mouth or nose
    ○ **4.** Skin color

While riding his skateboard, 14-year-old Dennis falls and fractures his elbow.

21. Which of the following is a severe complication of this injury?
    ○ **1.** Fluid loss
    ○ **2.** Severe pain
    ○ **3.** Compartment syndrome
    ○ **4.** Infection

22. Which of the following is *not* a sign of this complication?
    ○ **1.** Increasing pain in the fascial compartment distal to the injury
    ○ **2.** Local heat, tenderness, and swelling
    ○ **3.** Painful passive motion of the fingers
    ○ **4.** Increasing pain in the fascial compartment proximal to the injury

23. Dennis's fracture is being treated with skeletal traction. Which of the following is *not* appropriate when caring for a child with skeletal traction?
    ○ **1.** Understand what the traction is supposed to accomplish.
    ○ **2.** Remove the traction weights if the child complains of excessive pain.
    ○ **3.** Check the pin sites frequently for bleeding, inflammation, or infection.
    ○ **4.** Check the bed position.

24. Dennis will be confined to his bed for several weeks. What type of play activity is *inappropriate* for Dennis during this time?
    ○ **1.** Reading
    ○ **2.** Playing board games with visitors
    ○ **3.** Building model airplanes
    ○ **4.** Viewing educational films

25. Pin care is important following skeletal surgery. Which of the following is *not* correct pin care?
    ○ **1.** Cover the pin ends to prevent injury.
    ○ **2.** Cleanse and dress the pin sites.
    ○ **3.** Make sure the pin moves freely through the bones.
    ○ **4.** Apply antibiotic ointments as ordered.

Calvin York is admitted to the coronary care unit with a diagnosis of myocardial infarction.

26. Two days later, Mr. York says to the nurse, "I don't know why they're keeping me here. I can rest at home. I have a lot of things I could be doing. I feel fine." Which of the following defense mechanisms is Mr. York utilizing?
    ○ **1.** Denial
    ○ **2.** Rationalization
    ○ **3.** Sublimation
    ○ **4.** Compensation

27. Mr. York has started eating a salt-restricted diet. When his tray is brought to him he shouts at the nurse, "Do you really expect me to eat this? It's not fit for human consumption. It has no taste." Which response by the nurse would be most therapeutic?
    ○ **1.** "Not fit for human consumption?"
    ○ **2.** "Mr. York, less salt will decrease the fluid in your body and make it easier for your heart to work."
    ○ **3.** "I'll arrange for you to see the dietitian."
    ○ **4.** "You're angry about the way things are going right now."

Karla Lu, a 25-year-old Chinese woman, is admitted to the hospital with a diagnosis of aplastic anemia.

28. Which of the following is a frequent cause of aplastic anemia?
    ○ **1.** Vitamin B_{12} malabsorption
    ○ **2.** Drugs
    ○ **3.** Folic acid deficiency
    ○ **4.** Genetic factors

29. Which diagnostic test will help the physician make the most conclusive diagnosis of aplastic anemia?
    ○ **1.** Bone-marrow aspiration
    ○ **2.** Schilling test
    ○ **3.** Hemogram
    ○ **4.** Differential blood count

30. When caring for Miss Lu, the most important nursing action is to
    ○ **1.** teach her about her diet.
    ○ **2.** help her conserve her energy.
    ○ **3.** encourage her to have some physical activity.
    ○ **4.** maintain her fluid and electrolyte balance.

During the assessment, the nursery nurse finds that newborn Steven Sims has a foot deformity. The deformity is diagnosed as bilateral talipes equinovarus (clubfoot).

31. Which of the following most likely alerted the nurse that Steven has an abnormality?
    ○ 1. The feet were in plantar flexion.
    ○ 2. The feet deviated from the midline when dorsiflexed.
    ○ 3. Manipulation of the feet seemed to induce pain.
    ○ 4. The feet were not in alignment with the knees.

32. Plaster casts are applied to both of Steven's feet to reestablish the correct alignment. Cast application is done as soon as possible after diagnosis for which of the following reasons?
    ○ 1. Developmental delays are prevented by early application of casts.
    ○ 2. The soft tissue of the infant's feet and ankles is pliable.
    ○ 3. Clubfoot abnormalities cannot be corrected after the age of 6 months.
    ○ 4. The skin of a newborn is less susceptible to breakdown.

33. Steven's parents take him home from the hospital with his new casts in place. It is most important that the nurse include which of the following in the instructions to the parents regarding cast care?
    ○ 1. Apply lotion to the skin under the cast edges.
    ○ 2. Sprinkle talcum powder into the cast to decrease odor.
    ○ 3. Watch for reddened areas on the skin around the cast edges.
    ○ 4. The infant can be bathed without concern about the casts.

34. Correction of Steven's foot abnormality was not achieved by casts alone. Steven was hospitalized at the age of 4 months for corrective surgery. Immediate post-op care would include
    ○ 1. elevation of the lower extremities to decrease edema.
    ○ 2. elevation of the head to prevent feeding difficulties.
    ○ 3. no turning until the casts are dry.
    ○ 4. positioning on the abdomen only.

35. Following several months of post-op cast-wearing, a brace is ordered to maintain the corrected position of Steven's feet. The nurse discusses important aspects about the brace and about Steven's care with his parents. To determine the parents' understanding of the information provided, the best question for the nurse to ask is which of the following?
    ○ 1. "Do you have any questions?"
    ○ 2. "Could you explain to me how to apply the brace?"
    ○ 3. "Could you show me how to apply the brace?"
    ○ 4. "How will you apply Steven's brace?"

Baby Girl Snow is beginning to show signs of respiratory distress.

36. What is one of the major symptoms that would lead the nurse to suspect a tracheoesophageal fistula in Baby Girl Snow?
    ○ 1. Stridor
    ○ 2. Apnea
    ○ 3. Refusal of food
    ○ 4. Persistent drooling

37. A diagnosis of tracheoesophageal fistula is made. The post-op nursing care of an infant with a repaired tracheoesophageal fistula would *not* include
    ○ 1. careful monitoring of IV solutions.
    ○ 2. vigorous nasotracheal suctioning.
    ○ 3. elevation of the head and thorax 30°.
    ○ 4. good skin care of gastrostomy site.

38. In collecting data about Baby Girl Snow, why should the nurse want to ask Mrs. Snow if she had a history of polyhydramnios during her pregnancy?
    ○ 1. In order to estimate how quickly Mrs. Snow will be able to care for her baby
    ○ 2. To determine if Mrs. Snow should be told to expect that her next child will be delivered by cesarean section
    ○ 3. A history of polyhydramnios is common in mothers of children with tracheoesophageal fistula
    ○ 4. To determine when Mrs. Snow will be able to begin breast-feeding

Ann Perry, a 45-year-old woman, was admitted to the nursing unit with the diagnosis of hyperthyroidism.

39. The initial assessment would include physical findings that support this diagnosis. What are they?
    ○ 1. Elevated vital signs, nervousness, weight gain
    ○ 2. Elevated vital signs, nervousness, weight loss
    ○ 3. Decreased vital signs, lethargy, weight gain
    ○ 4. Decreased vital signs, nervousness, weight loss

40. The nurse should monitor Mrs. Perry for which of the following signs and symptoms of complications?
    ○ 1. Cold intolerance
    ○ 2. Sensitivity to narcotics
    ○ 3. Increased tachycardia
    ○ 4. Increased lethargy

41. Mrs. Perry's nursing diagnosis of sleep pattern disturbance could be aided by
    ○ 1. restricting fluid intake.
    ○ 2. administering liotrix (Thyrolar).
    ○ 3. utilizing a private room.
    ○ 4. providing a warm environment.

42. Mrs. Perry will require which of the following dietary modifications?
    ○ 1. Six meals per day of a regular diet
    ○ 2. Low-fat, low-sodium, low-calorie diet
    ○ 3. High-protein, high-carbohydrate, high-calorie diet
    ○ 4. Low-carbohydrate, high-protein diet

43. Mrs. Perry was discharged on a levothyroxine (Synthroid) regimen following an uncomplicated, subtotal thyroidectomy. During her clinic visit several months later, Mrs. Perry complains of tiredness and of feeling cold. What content area would be most emphasized if the nursing diagnosis of knowledge deficit regarding self-management is made?
    ○ 1. The lack of thyroid hormones produced by the body requires daily intake of thyroid medication.
    ○ 2. Symptoms arise from taking too much thyroid-replacement medication, so the dose needs adjusting.
    ○ 3. The parathyroids will grow and will be able to meet the body's needs for the hormones.
    ○ 4. The parathyroids are overactive from having been disturbed during surgery, but symptoms should disappear soon.

Rachel Rosen has been given a diagnosis of cancer of the colon. Her physician has told her that the disease has progressed to the point that it cannot be treated and that her life expectancy is less than a year. Mrs. Rosen is 47 years old, married, and has 2 adult children.

44. After the physician and Mr. Rosen have left, the nurse enters the room to see how the client is feeling. Mrs. Rosen says, "That doctor must be crazy. He thinks I'm dying, but I'm not really that sick." What is the best interpretation of this remark?
    ○ 1. It indicates a normal response to what she has just been told.
    ○ 2. It implies she is unable to cope with her problem.
    ○ 3. It is an aberrant reaction.
    ○ 4. It requires further data for interpretation.

45. What is the most therapeutic response to Mrs. Rosen's remark?
    ○ 1. Remain silent and allow her to continue talking.
    ○ 2. Notify her physician and request appropriate orders.
    ○ 3. Ask her to say more about what she means.
    ○ 4. Reassure her.

46. What is the first goal in working with Mrs. Rosen?
    ○ 1. The client will begin to deal with impending death.
    ○ 2. The client will accept her impending death.
    ○ 3. The client will be able to say goodbye to relatives and friends.
    ○ 4. The client will verbalize an understanding of the disease process.

47. Which of the following would be included in planning for Mrs. Rosen's care?
    ○ 1. Help the client to identify the destructiveness of denial.
    ○ 2. Avoid questions about death and dying until later stages of the process.
    ○ 3. Stimulate expressions of anger and rage.
    ○ 4. Offer regular opportunities for the client to talk.

48. One day, Mrs. Rosen says, "I'll be so glad when this is all over and I can go back to work." How would the nurse respond?
    ○ 1. "Your work is really important to you."
    ○ 2. "I'm afraid you won't be going back to work."
    ○ 3. "It must be hard for you right now."
    ○ 4. "Tell me more about what you mean."

49. After about 3 weeks, Mrs. Rosen has not changed much in her responses to her diagnosis. One morning, she asks the nurse, "Do you think I'm going to die?" What is the best response for the nurse to make?
    ○ 1. "That is the diagnosis your doctor has given you."
    ○ 2. "Do you think you're going to die?"
    ○ 3. "What made you ask that question?"
    ○ 4. "This seems to be bothering you."

50. A few days later, the nurse enters the room to give Mrs. Rosen her bath. Mrs. Rosen says to the nurse, "Leave me alone. You're all like vultures hovering over me. Get out and don't come back!" What is the best nurse response?
    ○ 1. "Why are you so mad at me?"
    ○ 2. "You're pretty upset right now. Let's talk about it."
    ○ 3. "We may seem like vultures, but we're trying to help you."
    ○ 4. "I'll come back later when you've calmed down."

51. After Mrs. Rosen has spent more than 2 months in the hospital, Mr. and Mrs. Rosen express a desire to have Mrs. Rosen at home for the remaining time she has to live. What is the most appropriate nursing approach?
    ○ 1. Encourage them to reconsider this idea.
    ○ 2. Leave it up to them to work out with the physician.
    ○ 3. Help them to discuss the denial of the seriousness of Mrs. Rosen's illness.
    ○ 4. Assist them to make realistic arrangements.

52. Which statement indicates that the goal for Mrs. Rosen was met?
    ○ 1. Mrs. Rosen moves through the stages of the dying process and experiences a dignified death.
    ○ 2. Mrs. Rosen discontinues denial and expresses anger appropriately.
    ○ 3. Mrs. Rosen resumes a life-style comparable to that before her diagnosis.
    ○ 4. Mrs. Rosen becomes as independent as possible for her remaining life.

Four-and-a-half-year-old Erik is being prepared for correction of a mild pulmonary stenosis. He is not sure why he has to stay in the hospital.

53. Which assessment factor is most important in deciding how much information to give him?
    ○ 1. Developmental age
    ○ 2. Desire to learn
    ○ 3. Previous-hospitalization history
    ○ 4. Attitudes of his parents about hospitalization

54. Erik's parents ask about his cardiac problem. The nursing response is based on knowledge that pulmonary stenosis most often includes which of the following cardiac pathologic conditions?
    ○ 1. Left-to-right shunting of blood
    ○ 2. Left ventricular hypertrophy
    ○ 3. Right ventricular hypertrophy
    ○ 4. Aortic insufficiency

55. Preoperatively, which of the following nursing approaches is most important for Erik?
    ○ 1. Allow him to play with other children.
    ○ 2. Encourage him to express his feelings through play.
    ○ 3. Keep him isolated to prevent exposure to infection.
    ○ 4. Suggest vigorous exercise to build up his strength.

56. After surgery, the nurse prepares Erik and his parents for his return home. Which of the following suggestions by the nurse is most appropriate for the time when the recovery period is over?
    ○ 1. Limit his physical activity in the future.
    ○ 2. Provide for a tutor to decrease risk of infection from classmates.
    ○ 3. Help Erik understand that he will have special needs.
    ○ 4. Treat Erik like a normal child.

57. As a good-bye gift for the nurse, Erik draws a multicolor picture that has as its focus a figure consisting of 2 circles (head and body), 2 stick arms, and 1 stick leg. What is the best response for the nurse to make?
    ○ 1. "Oh, what a nice picture!"
    ○ 2. "Tell me about your drawing."
    ○ 3. "What is it?"
    ○ 4. "Is that your doctor?"

58. As Erik prepares to leave the hospital, which of the following motor skills would the nurse be *least* likely to see him perform?
    ○ 1. Lacing up his shoes
    ○ 2. Using scissors to cut out a favorite picture
    ○ 3. Tying a bow easily
    ○ 4. Climbing stairs like an adult

Steve Ray is admitted to the emergency room with a stiff neck and temperature of 102°F (38.8°C). He has had an earache for 1 week, but has not sought treatment for it.

59. Nuchal rigidity will *not* be seen in which of the following?
○ **1.** Meningitis
○ **2.** Intracranial mass with herniation
○ **3.** Intracranial hematoma
○ **4.** Cerebral concussion

60. Which of the following is a *contraindication* to lumbar puncture?
○ **1.** Unequal pupils
○ **2.** Lack of lateralization
○ **3.** Suspicion of meningitis
○ **4.** Nuchal rigidity

61. In addition to a brief explanation of the lumbar puncture procedure, which of the following is also the responsibility of the nurse?
○ **1.** Administer a narcotic to the client.
○ **2.** Position the client safely and properly in a lateral recumbent position with his knees flexed.
○ **3.** Administer procaine hydrochloride (Novocain).
○ **4.** Prepare a suture set, so it will be ready postprocedure.

62. Bacterial meningitis is confirmed by the cerebrospinal fluid culture. Mr. Ray has been transferred to a dimly lit private room. Why?
○ **1.** Increased stimulation such as bright lights may precipitate a seizure.
○ **2.** Inappropriate secretion of antidiuretic hormone (ADH) can be minimized.
○ **3.** It is easier to check his pupils in a darkened room.
○ **4.** Most clients with meningitis have photophobia.

63. Mr. Ray is placed on a hypothermia blanket. 20 minutes following the start of hypothermia treatments, what response would the nurse most likely expect to find?
○ **1.** Lowered vital signs
○ **2.** Elevated vital signs
○ **3.** Unchanged vital signs
○ **4.** Complaints of hot and cold flashes

64. The most desirable temperature for Mr. Ray while getting hypothermia treatment is
○ **1.** 98.6°F (37°C).
○ **2.** 95.6°F (35.3°C).
○ **3.** 91.6°F (33.1°C).
○ **4.** 89.6°F (32°C).

65. Hypothermia treatment will most likely put Mr. Ray at risk for the development of
○ **1.** emboli.
○ **2.** respiratory alkalosis.
○ **3.** metabolic alkalosis.
○ **4.** excess ADH secretion.

66. As Mr. Ray's temperature begins to drop, the nurse will most likely observe
○ **1.** loss of corneal response.
○ **2.** loss of gag reflex.
○ **3.** IM medications taking effect quickly.
○ **4.** fading of sensorium, including hearing.

67. Nursing measures for Mr. Ray should include
○ **1.** frequent turning.
○ **2.** thin coating of lotion to his skin followed by talcum powder, which is washed off and reapplied q8h.
○ **3.** passive range of motion.
○ **4.** all the above nursing measures.

68. The most desirable method of rewarming Mr. Ray is
○ **1.** surface rewarming.
○ **2.** natural rewarming.
○ **3.** bloodstream rewarming.
○ **4.** artificial rewarming.

69. A common complication to watch for during the rewarming process is
○ **1.** acidosis.
○ **2.** oliguria.
○ **3.** shock.
○ **4.** cardiac irregularity.

70. Mr. Ray continues on bed rest. During morning care, how should the nurse assist him with prevention of joint and muscle complications?
○ **1.** Active range of motion to all extremities
○ **2.** Passive range of motion to all extremities
○ **3.** Exercises to augment motor function as it returns
○ **4.** Nerve stimulation

Twenty-two-year-old Al Welch is admitted to the hospital with a diagnosis of manic-depressive illness, manic phase (bipolar disorder). He is bizarrely dressed with a colorful scarf tied around one arm and another tied around his leg. He wears a large gold earring in one ear and a beaded headband to hold back his long, flowing hair. He is obviously agitated and tells the nurse that he is Jesus Christ, and has come to save the world. He is accompanied by his parents, who report that Mr. Welch has not slept for at least 24 hours and only at 1- to 2-hour intervals for the past week.

71. Which of the following would *not* be an appropriate goal for Mr. Welch at this time?
  ○ 1. Client will participate in quiet activities.
  ○ 2. Client will remain free of injury.
  ○ 3. Client will experience increased sensory stimuli.
  ○ 4. Client will perform self-care and personal hygiene measures.

72. After admission procedures are completed, the most effective nursing measure would be which of the following?
  ○ 1. Take him on a tour of the unit to acquaint him with the other clients and staff.
  ○ 2. Suggest that he go to his room and get some sleep.
  ○ 3. Send him to the recreation room with several other young clients to develop his social skills.
  ○ 4. Accompany him to his room, sit, and talk quietly with him.

73. After assessing Mr. Welch, an additional action would be to
  ○ 1. treat physical problems that may result from hyperactive, manic state.
  ○ 2. promote increased physical activity.
  ○ 3. increase sensory stimuli.
  ○ 4. work with client regarding his low self-esteem.

74. Mr. Welch's physician orders lithium carbonate, 300 mg QID to control the symptoms. Why is lithium considered a potentially dangerous drug?
  ○ 1. The amount of the drug that is therapeutic is only slightly less than the amount that produces toxicity.
  ○ 2. The drug is potentially addicting.
  ○ 3. The drug has severe sedative effects.
  ○ 4. Lithium causes tardive dyskinesia with long-term use.

75. Lithium is often used in combination with an antipsychotic drug for initial treatment of acute manic episodes. Which of the following statements best explains the rationale for this?
  ○ 1. Antipsychotic drugs increase the beneficial effects of lithium.
  ○ 2. Manic-depressives are also usually schizophrenic.
  ○ 3. There is an initial lag period between administration of lithium and symptom reduction.
  ○ 4. Antipsychotic drugs reduce lithium toxicity.

76. Clients in the acute manic phase of manic-depressive illness often resist taking lithium. Which of the following is *not* likely to be the reason for their refusal?
  ○ 1. Lithium therapy produces temporary discomfort.
  ○ 2. The client often finds the manic periods to be pleasurable.
  ○ 3. Lithium therapy causes severe and permanent side effects.
  ○ 4. The client fears the mood change from elation to depression.

77. Mr. Welch loudly demands to be discharged so that he can go to South America. The nurse observes that he is agitated and is wearing bizarre clothing. Which of the following approaches would be most appropriate at this time?
  ○ 1. Call physician for a discharge order.
  ○ 2. Recognize that underneath his demands, the client is feeling dependent, unable to cope, and overwhelmed.
  ○ 3. Assess the client's abilities realistically.
  ○ 4. Involve the client in planning activities of daily living.

78. Mr. Welch has angry outbursts, calms down quickly, and is easily provoked a short time later. Which of the following actions would be most appropriate for this problem?
  ○ 1. Utilize measures to prevent overt aggression such as distraction and reduction of environmental stimuli.
  ○ 2. Encourage him to release his aggression by participating in competitive games.
  ○ 3. Set up a debate in the client-government group, so that he can practice stating his feelings.
  ○ 4. Distract him by taking him to the exercise yard whenever he appears angry.

79. Mr. Welch stays up all night, pacing the halls in his pajamas, and approaching male staff and clients in an aggressively sexual way. He states, "You are all frozen and impotent. You don't know how to live." Which of the following would be the *least* helpful approach?
  ○ 1. Avoid becoming defensive.
  ○ 2. Hold staff conferences to develop a plan for countering his aggressive sexual behavior.
  ○ 3. Confront him with his sexual behavior and inform him of his need to embarrass others.
  ○ 4. Involve the client in planning and participating in quiet, adaptive activities for nighttime.

80. Which of the following behaviors would *not* be an indication to anticipate client discharge?
   ○ 1. The client makes requests in a quiet voice.
   ○ 2. The client identifies and expresses feelings of depression.
   ○ 3. The client accepts limits on manipulative and acting out behaviors.
   ○ 4. The client is cheerful, is the life of the party, and denies depression.

Allan Miller, 4 years old, is admitted to the pediatric unit with a diagnosis of sickle cell crisis. Mrs. Miller is expecting her second child in 4 months.

81. Mrs. Miller is concerned that her next child will "have sickle cell." What is the nurse's best response to this concern?
   ○ 1. "Sickle cell affects every other child in a family."
   ○ 2. "The child will have either the trait or the disease."
   ○ 3. "There is a 25% chance the baby will have the disease."
   ○ 4. "There is no risk of developing sickle cell disease."

82. Mrs. Miller remarks that Allan never had any problems with sickle cell until about 1 year of age. Which of the following responses best addresses Mrs. Miller's concern?
   ○ 1. "Infections are not a problem until 1 year of age."
   ○ 2. "Fetal hemoglobin levels remain high during infancy."
   ○ 3. "Maternal antibodies protected Allan during the first year."
   ○ 4. "Breast-feeding provides passive immunity for the infant."

83. What is the most common cause of sickle cell crisis?
   ○ 1. Acute infections
   ○ 2. Emotional stress
   ○ 3. Strenuous activity
   ○ 4. Environmental change

84. Which of the following actions should receive the highest priority while caring for Allan?
   ○ 1. Hydration
   ○ 2. Elimination
   ○ 3. Mobility
   ○ 4. Oxygenation

85. Allan is to receive meperidine (Demerol) 20 mg IM q3h to q4h prn for pain. The vial reads "Demerol 50 mg/ml." How much will the nurse administer?
   ○ 1. 0.2 ml
   ○ 2. 0.3 ml
   ○ 3. 0.4 ml
   ○ 4. 0.5 ml

86. Which of the following behaviors indicate that the Demerol has been effective?
   ○ 1. Increased restlessness
   ○ 2. Respirations of 38
   ○ 3. Decreased attention span
   ○ 4. Apical heart rate of 96

87. A transfusion is ordered for Allan. Infusing the blood components too rapidly may lead to which of the following problems?
   ○ 1. Hypostatic pneumonia
   ○ 2. Cardiac failure
   ○ 3. Hemolytic anemia
   ○ 4. Stress ulcer

88. Thirty minutes after the transfusion begins, Allan's cheeks are flushed and he has hives on his abdomen and lower extremities. What should the nurse do first?
   ○ 1. Continue to monitor Allan for any increase in the symptoms.
   ○ 2. Stop the transfusion and begin an IV infusion of normal saline.
   ○ 3. Check Allan's vital signs and notify the physician immediately.
   ○ 4. Contact the blood bank to double check Allan's blood type.

Julie Warner is a 28-year-old, admitted on your shift with a fever of 102°F (38.9°C). Her complaints indicate dysuria, frequency, and malaise. Acute pyelonephritis is suspected.

89. Which of the following diagnostic findings would be *least* likely to be found in acute pyelonephritis?
   ○ 1. Cloudy, foul-smelling urine
   ○ 2. Bacteria and pus in the urine
   ○ 3. Low WBC count
   ○ 4. Hematuria

90. What is the most important nursing action when caring for Mrs. Warner?
   ○ 1. Encourage ambulation.
   ○ 2. Force fluids up to 3,000 ml/day.
   ○ 3. Restrict protein in the diet.
   ○ 4. Keep urine acid.

91. Phenazopyridine HCl (Pyridium) is ordered for Mrs. Warner. This drug has which of the following actions?
    ○ **1.** Antibiotic
    ○ **2.** Narcotic
    ○ **3.** Analgesic
    ○ **4.** Antipyretic

92. Long-term management for Mrs. Warner includes preventing reinfection. Which of the following nursing instructions should be included in teaching?
    ○ **1.** Void at least every 6 hours.
    ○ **2.** Use vaginal sprays to mask the odor.
    ○ **3.** Empty her bladder before and after intercourse.
    ○ **4.** Discontinue antibiotics when pain disappears.

93. Prior to administering the initial dose of Pyridium, what would the nurse tell Mrs. Warner about this drug?
    ○ **1.** This drug causes transient nausea.
    ○ **2.** Food interferes with absorption.
    ○ **3.** It colors the urine red or orange.
    ○ **4.** Bladder spasms are a side effect.

94. Sulfamethoxazole-trimethoprim (Bactrim DS) is a common antimicrobial agent ordered in combination with Pyridium. What does "DS" stand for?
    ○ **1.** "Dose specific"
    ○ **2.** "Decreased symptoms"
    ○ **3.** "Double strength"
    ○ **4.** "Deficient strain"

95. Methenamine mandelate (Mandelamine) is also prescribed for Mrs. Warner's urinary tract infection. Which of the following conditions is necessary to increase the effectiveness of this drug?
    ○ **1.** Crystalluria
    ○ **2.** Leukocytosis
    ○ **3.** Alkaline urine
    ○ **4.** Acid urine

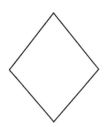

Test 1, Book II
Answers with Rationales

1. **#4.** Information should be given to the client. Oxytocin challenge testing would be contraindicated for a client experiencing the possibility of premature labor. An internal monitor cannot be applied unless membranes are ruptured. The client will receive little or no systemic analgesia if she goes into labor in order to prevent central nervous system damage to the fetus. IMPLEMENTATION (CHILDBEARING FAMILY/INTRAPARTAL CARE)

2. **#1.** This is the best description of the beneficial effects of bed rest for the client in premature labor. ANALYSIS (CHILDBEARING FAMILY/INTRAPARTAL CARE)

3. **#1.** Hypotension is among the expected side effects of tokolytic agents. These measures described in this option are employed to minimize hypotension. Assessment of blood pressure and pulse is important to detect hypotension but will not prevent its occurrence. IMPLEMENTATION (CHILDBEARING FAMILY/INTRAPARTAL CARE)

4. **#2.** Lorfan is a narcotic antagonist. Phenobarbital does not have tokolytic properties. Betamethasone is a glucocorticoid given to the mother to accelerate fetal lung maturity. ANALYSIS (CHILDBEARING FAMILY/INTRAPARTAL CARE)

5. **#4.** These signs are all indicative of a gestational age of less than 40 weeks. Lanugo and vernix wash away with maturity. Palmar and plantar creases increase with age. Development in the ears, breast tissue, and scrotum occur with age. Testes begin descent at approximately 36 weeks. Dark red skin in the premature infant is reflective of lack of subcutaneous fat. Parchmentlike skin is typical of the post-term infant. ASSESSMENT (CHILDBEARING FAMILY/HIGH-RISK NEWBORN)

6. **#4.** The premature infant is at greater risk for heat loss than the full-term infant. The nurse must keep this in mind while carrying out routine delivery-room procedures. Drying the infant is important to prevent heat loss by evaporation. ANALYSIS (CHILDBEARING FAMILY/HIGH-RISK NEWBORN)

7. **#4.** Nasal flaring is the only indication of respiratory distress listed. The nares flare to take in more oxygen to compensate for hypoxia. ASSESSMENT (CHILDBEARING FAMILY/HIGH-RISK NEWBORN)

8. **#2.** Research and observations of infants who have not been touched have shown that there are differences in the behavior of these babies when they are compared with babies who have received normal mothering. ANALYSIS (CHILDBEARING FAMILY/HIGH-RISK NEWBORN)

9. **#3.** It is desirable for parents to take an active role as care providers for their infants. This will promote attachment as well as help to develop their comfort and confidence in caring for the infant at home. PLAN (CHILDBEARING FAMILY/HIGH-RISK NEWBORN)

10. **#2.** Normal tidal volume is about 500 cc. ANALYSIS (ADULT/OXYGENATION)

11. **#2.** The amount of dead space in the lung increases with chronic obstructive pulmonary disease. Usual dead space is 100 to 150 cc. ASSESSMENT (ADULT/OXYGENATION)

12. **#3.** Fowler's position increases the expansibility of the lungs. IMPLEMENTATION (ADULT/OXYGENATION)

13. **#2.** The high pCO_2 is balanced by an increased bicarbonate, resulting in a pH of 7.4. The pH is within normal range (7.35–7.45); thus, he is compensated. If the pH is abnormal, then the client is said to be in a decompensated state. ANALYSIS (ADULT/OXYGENATION)

14. **#2.** The chronic obstructive pulmonary disease client's normal state is compensated respiratory acidosis. ANALYSIS (ADULT/OXYGENATION)

15. #3. A chronic obstructive pulmonary disease client adjusts to an increased pCO_2 and a decreased pO_2. ANALYSIS (ADULT/OXYGENATION)

16. #4. This client's electrolyte levels will not be affected by suctioning him. ANALYSIS (ADULT/OXYGENATION)

17. #2. Emphysema produces bronchiolar and alveolar changes that cannot be reversed. Treatment is aimed at relieving symptoms. ANALYSIS (ADULT/OXYGENATION)

18. #1. Mr. Nims is slightly hypoxic, but not cyanotic. This means his pO_2 is around 50 mm Hg. ASSESSMENT (ADULT/OXYGENATION)

19. #1. For chronic obstructive pulmonary disease clients, the breathing stimulus is based on their oxygen needs. Administration of more than 2 to 3 liters of oxygen impairs the respiratory drive. IMPLEMENTATION (ADULT/OXYGENATION)

20. #4. Skin color is affected by many things other than oxygenation, including circulation, hot or cold environment, and trauma. ASSESSMENT (ADULT/OXYGENATION)

21. #3. Compartment syndrome is possible because this type of fracture is frequently caused by substantial force that produces neurovascular disruption. Fluid loss is not a major problem. Infection (osteomyelitis) is a potential complication of any bone trauma and not specific to elbow fracture. Severe pain is associated with compartment syndrome but is a symptom of the complication and not a complication in itself. ANALYSIS (CHILD/MOBILITY)

22. #4. The pain is in the distal compartment due to the anatomy of the arm. ASSESSMENT (CHILD/MOBILITY)

23. #2. Skeletal traction adjustment is a medical function and is never altered by the nurse. IMPLEMENTATION (CHILD/MOBILITY)

24. #3. Model building usually requires fine motor skills and the use of both hands, and would be frustrating to Dennis. Reading and watching films are favorite activities of the young adolescent, and board games offer socializing opportunities. IMPLEMENTATION (CHILD/MOBILITY)

25. #3. The pin should be checked frequently to make sure it is secure and immobile in the bone. IMPLEMENTATION (CHILD/MOBILITY)

26. #1. The denial is evident. He is not yet able to consciously face the seriousness of his situation. Rationalization is an unconscious mechanism whereby a person creates a logical, socially acceptable explanation for a thought, feeling, or behavior. Sublimation is the conscious or unconscious channeling of ''unacceptable drives'' into acceptable activities. Compensation is a mechanism by which the individual attempts to make up for real or imagined deficiencies. ANALYSIS (PSYCHOSOCIAL, MENTAL HEALTH, PSYCHIATRIC PROBLEMS/LOSS, DEATH AND DYING)

27. #4. This response indicates to the client that the anger he is expressing was heard and offers the opportunity to deal with those feelings. Restating the most provocative part of his complaint will further escalate his anger. Option #2 is an excellent explanation of why he needs a low-sodium diet, but only after he has had an opportunity to verbalize his anger and feel understood will he be able to listen to it. #3 avoids the feeling tone of his complaint. He will only have numerous other complaints because the real issue has been circumvented. IMPLEMENTATION (PSYCHOSOCIAL, MENTAL HEALTH, PSYCHIATRIC PROBLEMS/LOSS, DEATH AND DYING)

28. #2. Many drugs can cause suppression of the bone marrow and aplastic anemia. ANALYSIS (ADULT/OXYGENATION)

29. #1. A sample of bone marrow will allow evaluation of the condition of the marrow and the number of erythrocytes, leukocytes, and thrombocytes. ANALYSIS (ADULT/OXYGENATION)

30. #2. When providing nursing care to a client who has a low hemoglobin, conserve the client's energy. With low hemoglobin, less oxygen will be carried and available to the cells. Maintenance of fluid and electrolyte balance is important for any client but is not specific to someone with a diagnosis of aplastic anemia. PLAN (ADULT/OXYGENATION)

31. #2. This is the physical finding that would indicate clubfoot. Pain is not associated with clubfoot. Newborns usually have bowed legs and frequently the foot is not aligned with the knee. ASSESSMENT (CHILD/MOBILITY)

32. #2. This is the only correct option. Temporary developmental delay may actually be caused by treatment. After the age of 6 months, clubfoot can be corrected but requires longer and more invasive treatment than if it were detected at birth. A newborn's skin is thin and fragile and has potential for breakdown. ANALYSIS (CHILD/MOBILITY)

33. #3. Reddened areas would alert one to skin breakdown. The other options are not appropriate because they could cause skin breakdown. IMPLEMENTATION (CHILD/MOBILITY)

34. #1. Elevation is critical to decrease edema and resulting circulatory compromise. Feeding difficulties have no relationship to the foot problem. Infant should be turned as usual and the foot casts supported on pillows or blankets. All positions can be used as long as the casted foot is supported. PLAN (CHILD/MOBILITY)

35. #3. This is the only question leading to a measurable outcome. The only true measurement of successful teaching is if the parents can apply the brace. EVALUATION (CHILD/MOBILITY)

36. #4. The most common form of tracheoesophageal fistula is one in which the proximal esophageal segment terminates in a blind pouch. When the child swallows saliva, water, or formula, it accumulates in the blind pouch resulting in excessive salivation or aspiration. Stridor, a crowing sound on inspiration, and apnea are conditions that may be caused by a number of factors. ASSESSMENT (CHILDBEARING FAMILY/HIGH-RISK NEWBORN)

37. #2. Vigorous nasotracheal suctioning may easily disrupt the integrity of the suture line, so it is contraindicated. Gentle oropharyngeal suctioning would be indicated if the infant cannot handle oral secretions. IV fluids will be necessary until the infant can be fed through a gastrostomy tube. Elevation of the head of the bed at 30° promotes pooling of secretions at the catheter tip if an indwelling nasal catheter is in use. Skin care will prevent skin breakdown and infection. IMPLEMENTATION (CHILDBEARING FAMILY/HIGH-RISK NEWBORN)

38. #3. Amniotic fluid is continually produced by the mother. A normal fetus swallows and excretes the amniotic fluid while in utero. If there is a gastrointestinal obstruction or neurologic problem that interferes with swallowing in the fetus, then the amniotic fluid accumulates and results in hydramnios. ASSESSMENT (CHILDBEARING FAMILY/HIGH-RISK NEWBORN)

39. #2. The thyroid (being the regulator for the metabolic rate) produces and releases more thyroid hormones in hyperthyroidism, which increases the metabolic rate. The increased metabolic rate leads to elevated vital signs, nervousness, and weight loss, because of increased activity in and demands on all body systems. ASSESSMENT (ADULT/NUTRITION AND METABOLISM)

40. #3. Tachycardia is usual in hyperthyroidism, and a further increase in cardiac rate indicates thyroid crisis, a more toxic state. ASSESSMENT (ADULT/NUTRITION AND METABOLISM)

41. #3. Assigning the client to a private room may promote rest by decreasing stimulation. PLAN (ADULT/NUTRITION AND METABOLISM)

42. #3. The client would have increased hunger as a result of the increased metabolic rate and requires a high-protein, high-calorie intake. PLAN (ADULT/NUTRITION AND METABOLISM)

43. #1. These symptoms are characteristic of hypothyroidism. The client will need lifelong daily replacement of thyroid hormones. ANALYSIS (ADULT/NUTRITION AND METABOLISM)

44. #1. The first stage in dealing with a terminal illness is denial, and the client's comment is a typical expression of denial. There is insufficient data to conclude that Mrs. Rosen may not be able to cope with her problem or that her behavior is unusual. ANALYSIS (PSYCHOSOCIAL, MENTAL HEALTH, PSYCHIATRIC PROBLEMS/LOSS, DEATH AND DYING)

45. #3. Respond to expressions of denial with statements that encourage exploration of feelings and thoughts, in order to help the client proceed through later stages. The client may interpret silence as agreement by the nurse and she may not continue talking. Reassurance would be false and nontherapeutic and suggests anxiety on nurse's part. IMPLEMENTATION (PSYCHOSOCIAL, MENTAL HEALTH, PSYCHIATRIC PROBLEMS/LOSS, DEATH AND DYING)

46. #1. Since the client is in the first stage of dealing with a loss, the first priority is to help her to begin dealing with her diagnosis. The client must begin to deal with impending death prior to initiating goals #2 and #3. Option #4 is not the first or more important goal, and it would not necessarily help her face death. PLAN (PSYCHOSOCIAL, MENTAL HEALTH, PSYCHIATRIC PROBLEMS/LOSS, DEATH AND DYING)

47. #4. The client needs opportunities to talk and to proceed at her own pace. She must not be abandoned or pushed into other stages. Deal with questions about death as they arise. Denial may be adaptive and normal up to a point. If client denies verbally the seriousness of the health threat but complies with treatment, denial can be adaptive. PLAN (PSYCHOSOCIAL, MENTAL HEALTH, PSYCHIATRIC PROBLEMS/LOSS, DEATH AND DYING)

48. #3. Respond to remarks indicating denial with realistic and empathic statements about the client's feelings. Do not encourage denial or try to interrupt it abruptly. Responding to client's work, rather than feelings, is an avoidance remark by the nurse. Option #2 is too confronting at this point and would cause a high anxiety level. #4 would encourage the client's denial. IMPLEMENTATION (PSYCHOSOCIAL, MENTAL HEALTH, PSYCHIATRIC PROBLEMS/LOSS, DEATH AND DYING)

49. #2. The client should be encouraged to express her own feelings about death. A willingness to talk about it should be met with encouragement to do so. Option #1 is unfeeling and cuts off further exploration of the client's concerns. Option #3 avoids the issue of death which the client is willing to talk about. #4 assumes the client is bothered, rather than exploring her feelings about accepting her prognosis. IMPLEMENTATION (PSYCHOSOCIAL, MENTAL HEALTH, PSYCHIATRIC PROBLEMS/LOSS, DEATH AND DYING)

50. #2. Anger is a normal stage in the dying process. Although it may be directed at nurses, it is usually displaced anger. The nurse should respond in a way that indicates acceptance of the client while encouraging her to talk about the underlying feelings. Option #1 indicates that the nurse has interpreted client's anger as personal. #3 is a defensive remark that avoids the client's feelings and may increase her guilt. Option #4 is a withdrawal reaction and may be helpful to the nurse, but it leaves the client with unresolved feelings. IMPLEMENTATION (PSYCHOSOCIAL, MENTAL HEALTH, PSYCHIATRIC PROBLEMS/LOSS, DEATH AND DYING)

51. #4. This is a reasonable request that should be pursued in order to determine whether or not it is possible. If so, the nurse can assist the client in making arrangements. Option #1 is not helpful because they need further information about this possibility. Discharge planning falls within purview of nursing and it is appropriate for the nurse to discuss this with the family. No data suggest denial of seriousness at this time. IMPLEMENTATION (PSYCHOSOCIAL, MENTAL HEALTH, PSYCHIATRIC PROBLEMS/LOSS, DEATH AND DYING)

52. #1. This indicates the realization of the most comprehensive and realistic goals for the client. Anger is not the end stage of the grief process; the expectation is for her to move beyond this phase. Option #3 is not realistic. Independence is an important achievement, but dealing with the emotional impact of impending death is more important. EVALUATION (PSYCHOSOCIAL, MENTAL HEALTH, PSYCHIATRIC PROBLEMS/LOSS, DEATH AND DYING)

53. #1. This determines a child's ability to handle information. Options #2, #3, and #4 are factors for consideration, but are not as important as #1. ASSESSMENT (CHILD/ILL AND HOSPITALIZED CHILD)

54. #3. This is the result of a backup of blood in the right ventricle, which enlarges to accommodate the extra volume. ANALYSIS (CHILD/OXYGENATION)

55. #2. It is most important to determine his understanding and allow him to express his feelings. Option #4 is contraindicated; option #3 is too severe a measure. PLAN (CHILD/OXYGENATION)

56. #4. Since his defect was mild, repair should be complete. He should not be encouraged to develop a chronically ill, dependent personality. PLAN (CHILD/OXYGENATION)

57. #2. Use an open-ended comment to encourage the child's own expressions. The other options are judgmental or discourage sharing of comments by child. IMPLEMENTATION (CHILD/ILL AND HOSPITALIZED CHILD)

58. #3. This skill comes at age 6. He should be able to do the other skills listed. ASSESSMENT (CHILD/OXYGENATION)

59. #4. Nuchal rigidity (the neck becomes rigid when flexion is attempted) results from meningeal irritation. This does not usually occur with concussions. ANALYSIS (ADULT/SAFETY AND SECURITY)

60. #1. Unequal pupils indicate possible increased intracranial pressure, which makes a lumbar puncture very dangerous. ASSESSMENT (ADULT/SAFETY AND SECURITY)

61. #2. Maintenance of proper positioning for a lumbar puncture is very important. Narcotics are avoided in clients with neurologic problems; they can mask symptoms and change pupil responses. Novocain is given as a local anesthetic, if used at all. IMPLEMENTATION (ADULT/SAFETY AND SECURITY)

62. #4. Meningitis is often accompanied by photophobia, a visual intolerance to light; therefore the client will be more comfortable in a dark room. ANALYSIS (ADULT/SAFETY AND SECURITY)

63. #2. The body will attempt to compensate for hypothermia, and the vital signs will initially become elevated; later they decrease. ASSESSMENT (ADULT/SAFETY AND SECURITY)

64. #4. The body's metabolic rate is reduced by almost 50% at this body temperature. PLAN (ADULT/SAFETY AND SECURITY)

65. #1. Circulation slows at low temperatures, predisposing the client to the formation of emboli. ANALYSIS (ADULT/SAFETY AND SECURITY)

66. #4. The gag and corneal reflexes are not lost until the client is completely comatose; an earlier sign is a fading of the senses. EVALUATION (ADULT/SAFETY AND SECURITY)

67. #4. All the options will help prevent vascular pooling without greatly increasing oxygen demand. IMPLEMENTATION (ADULT/SAFETY AND SECURITY)

68. #2. Natural rewarming is the least invasive and safest method of regaining the normal body temperature following induced hypothermia. PLAN (ADULT/SAFETY AND SECURITY)

69. #4. Cardiac irregularity is the most common complication of rewarming. ASSESSMENT (ADULT/SAFETY AND SECURITY)

70. #2. During the acute phase, complete bed rest and passive range of motion will help to conserve energy, yet maintain good joint mobility. PLAN (ADULT/SAFETY AND SECURITY)

71. #3. Mr. Welch needs decreased, not increased, sensory stimuli at this time. With sleep deprivation, the client may have impaired judgment so protecting this client from self-injury would be important. Although the client is delusional, he should be able to care for his personal hygiene. PLAN (PSYCHOSOCIAL, MENTAL HEALTH, PSYCHIATRIC PROBLEMS/ELATED-DEPRESSIVE BEHAVIOR)

72. #4. It is important to decrease environmental (sensory) stimulation for these clients and, at the same time, to keep them under close observation. Taking him on a tour of the unit may be too stimulating. He may not be able to sleep at this time due to being in a new environment. Developing social skills while in a delusional state is impossible and his bizarre dress might scare off others and not benefit the client. IMPLEMENTATION (PSYCHOSOCIAL, MENTAL HEALTH, PSYCHIATRIC PROBLEMS/ELATED-DEPRESSIVE BEHAVIOR)

73. #1. Initial actions with the hypermanic client would focus on physical problems such as poor nutrition, hygiene, and sleep and rest problems. Promoting increased physical activity would promote exhaustion. Increased sensory stimuli would overload him. Working on low self-esteem is not appropriate during a hypomanic state because he would not be able to pay attention. IMPLEMENTATION (PSYCHOSOCIAL, MENTAL HEALTH, PSYCHIATRIC PROBLEMS/ELATED-DEPRESSIVE BEHAVIOR)

74. #1. Lithium has a very narrow therapeutic index. Therefore, clients must be closely observed for signs of lithium toxicity. Lithium is not addicting, nor does it have sedative side effects. Lithium does not cause tardive dyskinesia, but is often given with antipsychotic agents, which do. ANALYSIS (PSYCHOSOCIAL, MENTAL HEALTH, PSYCHIATRIC PROBLEMS/ELATED-DEPRESSIVE BEHAVIOR)

75. #3. Once a therapeutic serum level is attained, it takes 7 to 10 days for a clinical response from lithium. Therefore, antipsychotic drugs that have a therapeutic-response time that can be measured in minutes are used to alleviate the acute symptoms of mania until lithium begins to take effect. Manic-depressives are not usually schizophrenics, but both have psychotic features. Antipsychotic drugs do not reduce lithium toxicity or increase the beneficial effects. ANALYSIS (PSYCHOSOCIAL, MENTAL HEALTH, PSYCHIATRIC PROBLEMS/ELATED-DEPRESSIVE BEHAVIOR)

76. **#3.** There is no evidence to date that lithium therapy causes irreversible side effects with long-term use. Lithium therapy does produce mild discomfort such as nausea, vomiting, dizziness, headache, impaired vision, and diarrhea, among other symptoms. Manic clients often report liking the euphoric feeling and once the lithium takes effect, clients fear having to face their underlying depression. ANALYSIS (PSYCHOSOCIAL, MENTAL HEALTH, PSYCHIATRIC PROBLEMS/ELATED-DEPRESSIVE BEHAVIOR)

77. **#2.** Manic-depressive clients cover their dependency needs and confusion by acting independent, controlling, and bossy. Calling the physician for discharge orders would not be appropriate when the client is agitated and shows bizarre grooming. Distraction only works temporarily and may only increase his irritation when the real issue is not addressed. IMPLEMENTATION (PSYCHOSOCIAL, MENTAL HEALTH, PSYCHIATRIC PROBLEMS/ELATED-DEPRESSIVE BEHAVIOR)

78. **#1.** Competitive games, group debates, and physical movement serve to escalate manic behavior and should be avoided. IMPLEMENTATION (PSYCHOSOCIAL, MENTAL HEALTH, PSYCHIATRIC PROBLEMS/ELATED-DEPRESSIVE BEHAVIOR)

79. **#3.** Confronting this client is not helpful and serves to escalate his manic, anxious behaviors. A staff conference would help to reduce defensiveness of the staff and define consistent, helpful strategies to promote adaptive activities for nighttime. IMPLEMENTATION (PSYCHOSOCIAL, MENTAL HEALTH, PSYCHIATRIC PROBLEMS/ELATED-DEPRESSIVE BEHAVIOR)

80. **#4.** This option describes hypermanic behavior and would not be an indication for discharge. Option #1 indicates the client is in good control of his feelings. Option #2 indicates the client has an awareness of his underlying feelings of depression. Option #3 indicates the client will not use his hostility to threaten others into doing what he wants. EVALUATION (PSYCHOSOCIAL, MENTAL HEALTH, PSYCHIATRIC PROBLEMS/ELATED-DEPRESSIVE BEHAVIOR)

81. **#3.** Sickle cell disease is an autosomal recessive disease. Both parents are carriers; therefore, with each pregnancy, Mrs. Miller has a 25% chance of having a child with the disease, a 50% chance of having a child with the trait, and a 25% chance of having a child without the disease or the trait. IMPLEMENTATION (CHILD/OXYGENATION)

82. **#2.** The presence of fetal hemoglobin prevents sickling; it begins to decrease around 4 to 6 months of age, and the child eventually develops symptoms of the disease. IMPLEMENTATION (CHILD/OXYGENATION)

83. **#1.** Children with sickle cell disease have an increased susceptibility to infections. The exact cause is unknown, but supporting data suggest that many organisms thrive in a state of diminished oxygen and that phagocytosis is reduced in a hypoxic state. ANALYSIS (CHILD/OXYGENATION)

84. **#1.** Hydration promotes hemodilution, which in turn decreases blood viscosity and prevents further sickling; hydration also interferes with the cycle of stasis, thrombosis, and ischemia. PLAN (CHILD/OXYGENATION)

85. **#3.**
$$\frac{50 \text{ mg}}{1 \text{ ml}} = \frac{20 \text{ mg}}{x \text{ ml}}$$
$$50x = 20 = \frac{20}{50} = 0.4 \text{ ml}$$

IMPLEMENTATION (CHILD/ILL AND HOSPITALIZED CHILD)

86. **#4.** The normal heart rate for a 4-year-old is approximately 100 beats/minute; a heart rate of 96 would indicate that the child is resting comfortably. EVALUATION (CHILD/ILL AND HOSPITALIZED CHILD)

87. **#2.** Infusion of blood too rapidly may lead to hypervolemia, which in turn may lead to heart failure. ANALYSIS (CHILD/OXYGENATION)

88. **#2.** The child is experiencing an allergic reaction. The transfusion should be stopped immediately, but the patency of the IV line is maintained as a route for emergency drugs, if they become necessary. IMPLEMENTATION (CHILD/OXYGENATION)

89. **#3.** Leukocytosis (an elevated white blood cell count) is present with a bacterial infection. ASSESSMENT (ADULT/ELIMINATION)

90. **#2.** Increased fluids will help treat the symptoms of infection (i.e., elevated temperature, dysuria). PLAN (ADULT/ELIMINATION)

91. **#3.** Pyridium is a urinary analgesic. ANALYSIS (ADULT/ELIMINATION)

92. **#3.** The female urethra is short, and its proximity to the vagina predisposes the client to infection. Bacterial contamination can result from sexual intercourse, and emptying the bladder before and after intercourse reduces this risk. IMPLEMENTATION (ADULT/ELIMINATION)

93. **#3.** The azo dye in Pyridium stains the urine reddish orange. It is important to inform the client, when the initial dose is given, so that she does not think something is wrong when she voids. IMPLEMENTATION (ADULT/ELIMINATION)

94. **#3.** The "DS" product denotes "double strength." ANALYSIS (ADULT/ELIMINATION)

95. **#4.** Methenamine decomposes to formaldehyde and ammonia. The urine should be maintained at a pH of 5.5 or less for effective treatment. ANALYSIS (ADULT/ELIMINATION)

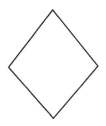

Test 1, Book III
Questions

Joan Plum, a 35-year-old physicist, tripped and fell while walking to work. The next day she found her lower extremities "very weak." She can stand only with assistance. She is admitted to the hospital with complaints of back pain. A motor assessment reveals flaccid paralysis in the lower extremities. She states her hands feel "numb." A brief health history reveals Miss Plum has been healthy, "never sick." She did have a slight upper respiratory infection 2 weeks ago. A diagnosis of polyneuritis (Guillain-Barré syndrome) is made after cerebrospinal fluid (CSF) reports have been returned showing a negative culture, increased protein, with normal pressure and cell count.

1. When planning care, why must respiratory-assistance equipment be kept immediately available?
   ○ 1. The pattern of the paralysis is ascending, and respiratory failure can occur if intercostal muscles are affected.
   ○ 2. Intracranial pressure can exert pressure on the medulla, causing respiratory arrest.
   ○ 3. High fever associated with this syndrome often disrupts the normal respiratory patterns.
   ○ 4. The particular bacteria or viruses or both in the cerebrospinal fluid have a special affinity for the nerves that control respiration.

2. Cranial nerves can be affected by Guillain-Barré syndrome. The facial nerve is most frequently involved. A baseline has been established and the cranial nerves are being assessed at frequent intervals. What would the nurse most likely observe if the motor nucleus of the facial nerve becomes dysfunctional?
   ○ 1. Decreased ability to distinguish tastes in the anterior ⅔ of the tongue
   ○ 2. Pain in the distribution of the affected nerve
   ○ 3. Inability to wrinkle the forehead and smile
   ○ 4. Inequality of pupils and sluggish response to light

3. What is the primary role of the nurse in caring for Miss Plum during this acute phase?
   ○ 1. To make accurate assessments and prevent complications
   ○ 2. To give medications on time and control blood pressure
   ○ 3. To provide nutrition and control of temperature
   ○ 4. To prevent contractures and suction the respiratory tract.

4. When Miss Plum asks whether or not she has a fatal disease, the nurse should reply
   ○ 1. "The great majority of people with Guillain-Barré syndrome recover completely, so your chances of recovery are good."
   ○ 2. "You never know what can happen when something goes wrong with your nervous system."
   ○ 3. "You should have checked with your doctor when you fell down yesterday."
   ○ 4. "Most clients have remissions, but eventually an exacerbation is apt to occur, because this disease has a long, progressive course."

5. As Miss Plum's recovery begins, the nurse notes that neurologic return is taking place in a descending order. However, she still retains some paresthesia in her right hand, even though she is ambulatory. During discharge planning, what should the nurse emphasize most to Miss Plum considering this sensory impairment?
   ○ 1. Maintain bed rest for several months to prevent fatigue and exacerbation of the disease.
   ○ 2. Test bath water with a bath thermometer as a safety precaution in order to avoid burns.
   ○ 3. Avoid contact with others until the first clinic visit, so she will not contract a viral infection.
   ○ 4. Surgery may be required to correct the paresthesia.

Daphne Runyon was admitted to the psychiatric hospital with a diagnosis of conversion disorder. She is a 21-year-old college student, who was functioning adequately until yesterday, when she suddenly lost the use of her right arm. She was taken to the emergency room, where no physical reason could be found for the paralysis. She was then transferred to the psychiatric unit.

6. What is most important for the nurse to know concerning Miss Runyon's symptoms?
○ **1.** They are caused by a demonstrable physical lesion.
○ **2.** They follow motor-nerve paths.
○ **3.** There is no primary gain as a result of the symptoms.
○ **4.** They represent symbolic dysfunction.

7. The cause of Miss Runyon's symptoms can best be explained as tension resulting from
○ **1.** a fixation at the anal stage of development producing feelings that are converted into the symptom.
○ **2.** repression of feelings converted into a symptom that has special meaning to the person.
○ **3.** suppression of feelings converted into the presenting symptom.
○ **4.** sublimation of feelings converted into the presenting symptom.

8. When meeting the rest of the clients on the unit, Miss Runyon laughs and smiles in an animated manner. Miss Runyon is demonstrating
○ **1.** ambivalence.
○ **2.** lability.
○ **3.** *la belle indifférence.*
○ **4.** narcissism.

9. When Miss Runyon's parents come to visit, they are very concerned about their daughter's condition. Which of the following will most likely apply to Miss Runyon?
○ **1.** She will receive secondary gain of increased attention from her family because of her symptoms.
○ **2.** She will have her dependency needs met and have no school responsibilities as long as she has symptoms.
○ **3.** She may assume a chronic illness role over a period of time as a result of symptoms.
○ **4.** All of the above are likely to apply.

10. One of the most important aspects of Miss Runyon's care will be which of the following?
○ **1.** Confrontation to help her become aware of her feelings
○ **2.** Supportive measures so she will have increased feelings of acceptance
○ **3.** Diversion from the sick role to other more productive behaviors
○ **4.** Antipsychotic medication to keep her comfortable until her symptoms are gone

Three-year-old Mark Elliot has just been admitted to the pediatric unit. Upon entering his room to begin the initial admission assessment, the nurse finds Mark sitting upright in bed, leaning forward with his mouth open. He is drooling and complaining of a sore throat.

11. The nurse should realize that Mark's problem most likely is
○ **1.** spasmodic croup.
○ **2.** infectious laryngitis.
○ **3.** laryngotracheobronchitis.
○ **4.** acute epiglottitis.

12. In developing a nursing care plan for Mark, which of the following should receive the highest priority?
○ **1.** Airway
○ **2.** Hydration
○ **3.** Mobility
○ **4.** Elimination

13. Which of the following manifestations would best indicate that Mark's respiratory distress is increasing?
○ **1.** Progressive hoarseness
○ **2.** Productive cough
○ **3.** Change in heart rate
○ **4.** Expiratory wheeze

14. Mark has been placed on a regimen of ampicillin 450 mg IV q6h. Which of the following nursing actions should receive the highest priority?
○ **1.** Check for hypersensitivity.
○ **2.** Monitor patency of the IV line.
○ **3.** Check client's name band.
○ **4.** Administer correct dose of medications.

15. Mark is placed in a Croupette with cool mist. What is the best rationale for this action?
○ **1.** To restrict his activity
○ **2.** To control his elevated fever
○ **3.** To stimulate the cough reflex
○ **4.** To reduce mucosal edema

16. While Mark is in the Croupette, 3 of the following nursing actions would be appropriate. Which one would *not* be appropriate?
○ **1.** Periodically change Mark's linen and pajamas.
○ **2.** Frequently monitor Mark's vital signs.
○ **3.** Loosely tuck the tent edges around the mattress.
○ **4.** Encourage Mark's mother to stay with him if possible.

17. Which one of the following lab reports would give the nurse the most information about Mark's hydration status?
    ○ **1.** White blood cell count of 12,500
    ○ **2.** Urine specific gravity of 1.005
    ○ **3.** Blood pO_2 of 85 mm Hg
    ○ **4.** Serum potassium of 3.8 mEq/liter

18. Mrs. Elliot states that Mark reports he has an imaginary friend who plays with him. She is obviously concerned. The nurse's response should include which of the following?
    ○ **1.** Suggest she discuss this with her pediatrician.
    ○ **2.** Tell her that imaginary friends are normal for this age group.
    ○ **3.** Encourage her to spend more time with Mark.
    ○ **4.** Discuss preschool or day care experience with her.

19. Developmentally, Mark would be expected to perform which of the following activities?
    ○ **1.** Tie his shoelaces
    ○ **2.** Hop in place
    ○ **3.** Jump rope
    ○ **4.** Walk backward

Earnest Washo has had diabetes mellitus for 20 years. He is admitted to the hospital with dry gangrene of the right great toe.

20. When assessing Mr. Washo's gangrenous condition, the nurse will *least* likely expect
    ○ **1.** intense pain in the affected area.
    ○ **2.** extension of the metatarsal-phalangeal joints.
    ○ **3.** changes in skin temperature of both feet.
    ○ **4.** tissue destruction.

21. When the nurse is working with Mr. Washo, what information is most important to ascertain?
    ○ **1.** His age when diabetes mellitus developed
    ○ **2.** His understanding of hygienic skin measures
    ○ **3.** His technique in administering insulin
    ○ **4.** His willingness to look at, touch, or talk about his gangrenous foot

22. Mr. Washo is placed on bed rest. Which nursing care measure would be *least* therapeutic for this client?
    ○ **1.** Heel protectors
    ○ **2.** Footboard
    ○ **3.** Foot cradle
    ○ **4.** Sheep skin or foam pad

23. To prevent complications of the bed rest imposed on Mr. Washo, which nursing action would be *contraindicated*?
    ○ **1.** Inspect Mr. Washo's feet.
    ○ **2.** Teach about appropriate foot care.
    ○ **3.** Restrict fluid intake.
    ○ **4.** Exercise joints and muscles.

24. The nurse should perform which of the following when providing care to the skin surrounding the lesion?
    ○ **1.** Apply an occlusive dressing.
    ○ **2.** Dry the skin thoroughly.
    ○ **3.** Put lotion on the healthy tissue.
    ○ **4.** Soak the foot.

25. The physician ordered sodium hypochlorite and boric acid (Dakin's solution) to the lesion and petroleum jelly to the adjoining healthy skin. Which of the following best describes their actions?
    ○ **1.** Dakin's solution is an anti-inflammatory agent; petroleum jelly is an anti-absorbent agent.
    ○ **2.** Dakin's solution debrides the wound; petroleum jelly protects the healthy tissue.
    ○ **3.** Dakin's solution drys out the lesion; petroleum jelly lubricates the surrounding tissue.
    ○ **4.** Dakin's solution cleanses the wound; petroleum jelly moisturizes the skin.

26. If an infection develops, which effect is this most likely to have on Mr. Washo's need for insulin?
    ○ **1.** Undeterminable
    ○ **2.** No effect
    ○ **3.** Increase the need
    ○ **4.** Decrease the need

27. Mr. Washo asks you if his toe will be amputated. Which of the following approaches is the most therapeutic?
    ○ **1.** Discuss the meaning this would have for him.
    ○ **2.** Explain the different types of medical management.
    ○ **3.** Help him value the importance of his health.
    ○ **4.** Refer the question to his physician.

Sean O'Connor has become increasingly depressed and is brought to the emergency room after slashing his wrists with a razor blade. He is conscious and crying uncontrollably.

28. Which of the following actions by the emergency room nurse should have the highest priority?
   ○ 1. Examine the extent of his wounds.
   ○ 2. Check his pulse, respiration, and blood pressure.
   ○ 3. Sit quietly with him until he is calmer.
   ○ 4. Talk with him about the problems he has been experiencing.

29. Mr. O'Connor's condition stabilizes and he is admitted to the psychiatric unit. He states dejectedly, ''I don't know why they saved me. As soon as I can, I will try it again. Nothing in my life is ever going to get better.'' What would be the best response by the nurse?
   ○ 1. ''You'll feel differently after you've been here awhile.''
   ○ 2. ''You're feeling things are pretty hopeless right now.''
   ○ 3. ''You're quite angry at the people who saved you.''
   ○ 4. ''It sounds as if you've already made up your mind.''

30. In assessing the suicide potential as reflected in Mr. O'Connor's statement, what other information would be the most useful for the nurse to have?
   ○ 1. Does he have a workable plan?
   ○ 2. Is there a family history of suicide?
   ○ 3. Have there been suicide attempts prior to this one?
   ○ 4. What precipitated this attack?

31. What would be the best placement for the client at this time?
   ○ 1. A single room on a locked psychiatric unit
   ○ 2. A single room on an open psychiatric unit
   ○ 3. A double room on either type of unit
   ○ 4. Any room where he can be closely observed

32. Mr. O'Connor has been taking amitriptyline (Elavil) for 7 days. He continues to appear depressed and expresses a desire to commit suicide. What is the most likely explanation for this?
   ○ 1. Amitriptyline is not effective for Mr. O'Connor.
   ○ 2. This is a side effect of amitriptyline.
   ○ 3. Tolerance to amitriptyline has developed.
   ○ 4. Amitriptyline may take 4 weeks to take effect.

Cheryl Fick is seen in the obstetric clinic in her third month of pregnancy. She complains of an intermittent brownish-red discharge and excessive nausea and vomiting. Abdominal palpation reveals the uterus to be at the level of the umbilicus. Fetal heart tones are absent.

33. The symptoms described above are characteristic of
   ○ 1. ectopic pregnancy.
   ○ 2. hyperemesis gravidarum.
   ○ 3. hydatidiform mole.
   ○ 4. threatened abortion.

34. In order to confirm the diagnosis, further assessment is carried out. Which of the following would best confirm the above diagnosis?
   ○ 1. Dilatation and curettage
   ○ 2. Ultrasound
   ○ 3. Laparoscopy
   ○ 4. Estriol levels

35. Which of the following will *not* be a treatment option for Mrs. Fick?
   ○ 1. Dilatation and curettage
   ○ 2. Induced abortion
   ○ 3. Hysterectomy
   ○ 4. Laser treatments

36. Following removal of the hydatidiform mole by dilatation and curettage, the nurse counsels Mrs. Fick. In her teaching, the nurse considers the prognosis of the client. Of the following complications, which would be of greatest concern?
   ○ 1. Ectopic pregnancy
   ○ 2. Choriocarcinoma
   ○ 3. Pelvic inflammatory disease
   ○ 4. Cancer of the cervix

37. Mrs. Fick indicates she is very disappointed that this pregnancy did not have a successful outcome. She wonders how soon she can plan to become pregnant again. The nurse will base an answer on the knowledge that there is an established preferred time frame for the next pregnancy after having a hydatidiform mole. What is this time period?
   ○ 1. As soon as possible
   ○ 2. After 6 months
   ○ 3. After 1 year
   ○ 4. After 2 years

38. Of the following responses, which would best indicate to the nurse that Mrs. Fick has understood discharge instructions?
   ○ 1. She maintains a diet high in iron.
   ○ 2. She avoids the use of tampons.
   ○ 3. She is taking oral contraceptives.
   ○ 4. She avoids heavy lifting for 6 weeks.

Ralph Damian is a 60-year-old client admitted to the surgical unit with complaints of left lumbosacral pain that occasionally radiates down to his groin. He reported that, a year ago, his physician told him that he had kidney stones. He also has a long history of recurrent gout. Medication for pain is listed on his admitting orders.

39. In Mr. Damian's case, the renal stones are most likely caused by
   ○ 1. urinary stasis.
   ○ 2. increased excretion of calcium.
   ○ 3. increased uric acid in the urine.
   ○ 4. urinary infection and large intake of milk.

40. Untreated kidney stones can dislodge, obstructing the ureter. In turn, this obstruction is the primary cause of
   ○ 1. kidney abscess.
   ○ 2. hydronephrosis.
   ○ 3. glomerulonephritis.
   ○ 4. nephrosis.

41. One evening while in bed, Mr. Damian complains of severe pain in the left, posterior, lumbar region radiating down to his groin. The first nursing responsibility would be to do which of the following?
   ○ 1. Strain his urine.
   ○ 2. Give an analgesic (e.g., morphine) as ordered.
   ○ 3. Encourage movement about to facilitate excretion of the stone.
   ○ 4. Encourage large fluid intake.

42. A urea-splitting organism such as streptococcus favors the growth of inorganic renal calculi by causing the urine to become
   ○ 1. alkaline.
   ○ 2. acidic.
   ○ 3. neutral.
   ○ 4. concentrated with sediments.

43. If the client's urine has a pH of 7.8, which of the following would most likely be given?
   ○ 1. Methenamine mandelate (Mandelamine)
   ○ 2. Vitamin C
   ○ 3. Sodium bicarbonate
   ○ 4. Sodium phosphate

44. The use of bethanechol (Urecholine) in the treatment of temporary post-op urinary retention is suggested because of its action as
   ○ 1. an anticholinergic.
   ○ 2. a cholinergic.
   ○ 3. an anesthetic.
   ○ 4. a urinary antispasmodic.

45. Decompression drainage of the bladder is used specifically
   ○ 1. to alleviate discomfort by providing continuous drainage.
   ○ 2. to prevent increased intra-abdominal pressure by avoiding bladder distension.
   ○ 3. to provide a means of constant irrigation of the bladder.
   ○ 4. to aid the muscles of the bladder to maintain their tone.

Three-and-a-half-year-old Courtney has been hospitalized with nephrosis.

46. Which of the following manifestations would most likely be observed?
   ○ 1. Ascites
   ○ 2. Elevated blood pressure
   ○ 3. Low urine specific gravity
   ○ 4. Hematuria

47. Because of their work commitments, Courtney's parents are not able to stay with him in the hospital. In addition to the stress created by his separation from his parents, Courtney will most likely be fearful of
   ○ 1. intrusive procedures.
   ○ 2. unfamiliar caretakers.
   ○ 3. dying.
   ○ 4. monsters.

48. When planning Courtney's nursing care, the nurse should include activities that promote a sense of
   ○ 1. trust.
   ○ 2. industry.
   ○ 3. esteem.
   ○ 4. initiative.

49. Courtney is receiving prednisone by mouth. Which of the following actions is *not* indicated?
   ○ 1. Give the prednisone with an antacid.
   ○ 2. Withhold the prednisone if Courtney's blood pressure becomes elevated.
   ○ 3. Observe Courtney closely for signs of infection.
   ○ 4. Provide foods high in potassium in Courtney's diet.

50. During the acute phase of his illness, which position is best for Courtney to be placed in?
   ○ 1. On his left side
   ○ 2. On his back
   ○ 3. On his abdomen
   ○ 4. Semi-Fowler's

51. Which of the following snacks would be the best choice for Courtney?
    ○ 1. 1 oz processed cheese spread, celery sticks, Kool-Aid
    ○ 2. ½ cup vanilla pudding, grape juice
    ○ 3. ½ peanut butter sandwich, apple slices, ½ cup hot cocoa
    ○ 4. ½ cup corn flakes, milk, raisins

52. Which activity would be most appropriate for Courtney while he is hospitalized?
    ○ 1. Playing with other children in the playroom
    ○ 2. Riding a push-pull toy in the hall
    ○ 3. Having a volunteer read him a story about a child in the hospital
    ○ 4. Playing with housekeeping toys in his room

James Lee is a 23-year-old graduate student, who has just been admitted to the unit with behaviors of withdrawal, flat affect, disregard of hygiene and grooming, and associative looseness. His diagnosis is paranoid schizophrenia.

53. Which of the following is *not* characteristic of the client with paranoid schizophrenia?
    ○ 1. Delusions
    ○ 2. Hallucinations
    ○ 3. Decreased sensitivity
    ○ 4. Ideas of reference

54. Which defense mechanism is most characteristic of the client with paranoid schizophrenia?
    ○ 1. Denial
    ○ 2. Projection
    ○ 3. Rationalization
    ○ 4. Suppression

55. Which of the following would *not* be an appropriate goal when working with a client with paranoid hallucinations?
    ○ 1. The client will learn to define and test reality.
    ○ 2. The client will devalue internal voices and hallucinations.
    ○ 3. The client will discuss feelings with primary nurse.
    ○ 4. The client will act out his fantasies in group therapy.

56. Which of the following would *not* be appropriate if the goal was, "Client will develop a relationship with a staff member"?
    ○ 1. Allow client to set the pace of the relationship.
    ○ 2. Suggest solitary activities for the suspicious client.
    ○ 3. Allow ample time for response if the client is very regressed.
    ○ 4. If the client withdraws from social interactions, allow the client to be alone.

57. Which of the following actions would *not* be helpful when dealing with paranoid hallucinations?
    ○ 1. Assist the client to relate with real persons.
    ○ 2. Avoid giving attention to the content of hallucinations or delusions, after initial investigation of these.
    ○ 3. Relate to the client to discover the meaning and purpose of the hallucination, focusing on immediate situation.
    ○ 4. Listen carefully to the content of hallucinations and delusions and encourage the client to describe them.

58. Which of the following would be most helpful to meet the goal, "Client will demonstrate improved hygiene and grooming"?
    ○ 1. Identify specific client needs for assistance.
    ○ 2. Ignore messy clothes and lack of hygiene.
    ○ 3. Insist that the client participate in a good-grooming group.
    ○ 4. Encourage the client by doing hygiene and grooming for him.

59. Mr. Lee approaches a staff member with hostile comments about another client who is "out to get me." In responding to Mr. Lee, which of the following would *not* be appropriate?
    ○ 1. Assist Mr. Lee to acknowledge and name feelings.
    ○ 2. Explore appropriate outlets for hostility such as physical activities, exercise, sports.
    ○ 3. Confront Mr. Lee with his hostility.
    ○ 4. Explore the source of the hostility with Mr. Lee.

60. Thioridazine (Mellaril), an antipsychotic, is usually effective in treating all the following symptoms of schizophrenia. Which symptom will not be affected by this drug?
    ○ 1. Agitation
    ○ 2. Hallucinations
    ○ 3. Delusions
    ○ 4. Ambivalence

61. Which of the following is *not* a common side effect of thioridazine (Mellaril) therapy?
    ○ 1. Dry mouth
    ○ 2. Constipation
    ○ 3. Urinary hesitancy
    ○ 4. Addiction

Ten-year-old Jackie is admitted to the hospital with a medical diagnosis of rheumatic fever. She relates a history of a sore throat "about a month ago." She is placed on bed rest with bathroom privileges.

62. Which of the following nursing assessments should be given highest priority when assessing Jackie?
   ○ **1.** Jackie's response to being hospitalized
   ○ **2.** The presence of a macular rash on her trunk
   ○ **3.** Her sleeping or resting apical pulse
   ○ **4.** The presence of polyarthritis and pain in her joints

63. Jackie exhibits manifestations of Sydenham's chorea. Which of the following is *not* a manifestation of this condition?
   ○ **1.** Intellectual impairment
   ○ **2.** Muscle weakness
   ○ **3.** Purposeless tremors
   ○ **4.** Emotional lability

64. Which of the following nursing plans should receive the highest priority during Jackie's hospitalization?
   ○ **1.** Minimize cardiac damage by keeping Jackie on bed rest.
   ○ **2.** Relieve pain by administering prescribed analgesics.
   ○ **3.** Help Jackie cope with hospitalization by providing age-appropriate activities.
   ○ **4.** Prevent injury by padding the bed side rails.

65. Which activity is most appropriate for Jackie during the acute phase of her illness?
   ○ **1.** Playing Nerf basketball
   ○ **2.** Visiting other children on the unit
   ○ **3.** Keeping a written diary
   ○ **4.** Listening to records of her favorite singing groups

66. Three of the following laboratory results are crucial indicators of Jackie's progress. Which one is *not*?
   ○ **1.** Antistreptolysin-O titer
   ○ **2.** C-reactive protein
   ○ **3.** Urine protein
   ○ **4.** Erythrocyte sedimentation rate

67. Jackie is discharged after 3 weeks of hospitalization. Which of the following statements best indicates that Jackie's parents have understood discharge teaching?
   ○ **1.** ''Jackie should lead a sedentary life-style for at least a year.''
   ○ **2.** ''Jackie must take daily antibiotics for an extended period of time to prevent a recurrence of rheumatic fever.''
   ○ **3.** ''Jackie should not return to her fifth-grade classroom but should have a home teacher the rest of the year.''
   ○ **4.** ''Jackie may have permanent neurologic sequelae as a result of the Sydenham's chorea.''

Aurelio Juarez is admitted to the emergency room with an abdominal gunshot wound.

68. Which of the following descriptions of the bleeding is best for the nurse's notes?
   ○ **1.** A moderate to large amount of sanguinous drainage noted from abdominal wound
   ○ **2.** Severe bleeding from wound
   ○ **3.** Copious amounts of blood coming from abdomen
   ○ **4.** Sanguinous drainage from abdominal wound soaked 2 towels and 6 abdominal pads in 10 minutes

69. Towels can be used to pack the gunshot wound because
   ○ **1.** the injury is usually fatal.
   ○ **2.** the wound is already grossly contaminated.
   ○ **3.** towels absorb more than ABD pads.
   ○ **4.** the client is probably bleeding minimally.

70. Mr. Juarez also has a knife protruding from his chest. The best nursing action is to
   ○ **1.** immediately remove the knife.
   ○ **2.** leave the knife in, until an operative setup is arranged.
   ○ **3.** clean the exposed knife blade with povidone-iodine solution.
   ○ **4.** cover area with a sterile towel soaked in saline.

71. Select the most correct statement about subcutaneous emphysema.
   ○ **1.** It is caused by air sucked into the chest wall from a superficial wound.
   ○ **2.** It is caused by internal injury.
   ○ **3.** It can always be noted easily.
   ○ **4.** It is not exacerbated by coughing.

72. Mr. Juarez is unable to void. A catheterization yields a small amount of bloody urine. This is most likely an indication of
   ○ **1.** urethral tear.
   ○ **2.** urethritis.
   ○ **3.** ruptured bladder.
   ○ **4.** prostatitis.

73. Several blood transfusions were ordered. When administering a blood transfusion, what is a mandatory nursing function requiring 2 nurses?
    ○ 1. Check the type and crossmatch data, numbers on the lab slips, and the information on the blood with that on the client's blood band.
    ○ 2. Check the type and crossmatch data, numbers on the lab slips, and the information on the blood with that on the client's chart.
    ○ 3. Check for the best possible vein to ensure correct infusion.
    ○ 4. Ensure Mr. Juarez is rational in order to establish a baseline of behavior.

74. Mr. Juarez's girlfriend volunteered to donate blood for him. What information is necessary to ascertain if she can be a donor?
    ○ 1. History of gonorrhea within the last year
    ○ 2. History of bacterial endocarditis within the last 4 years
    ○ 3. History of hepatitis within the last 5 years
    ○ 4. History of upper respiratory tract infection within the last 6 months

75. When assembling the equipment to start the blood transfusion, which of the following solutions is used to start the IV?
    ○ 1. Sterile water
    ○ 2. Normal saline
    ○ 3. 10% dextrose in water
    ○ 4. Lactated Ringer's

76. The nurse must remain at the bedside for 15 minutes after the blood is started to assess for any transfusion reaction. Which one of the following is *not* a sign or symptom of such a reaction?
    ○ 1. Chills, fever, dyspnea
    ○ 2. Decreased blood pressure, increased pulse rate
    ○ 3. Bleeding under the skin at the IV site
    ○ 4. Hives, itching

77. Which one of the following nursing actions must be taken immediately if a transfusion reaction occurs?
    ○ 1. Notify the physician.
    ○ 2. Check the vital signs and take a urine sample.
    ○ 3. Stop the blood transfusion and infuse normal saline.
    ○ 4. Slow down the rate of blood flow and continue the assessment.

Aretha Benson is admitted to the labor room for induction. She is 20 days past her estimated date of delivery. Her cervix is 50% effaced and fingertip dilated.

78. Prior to the induction, Mrs. Benson has an oxytocin challenge test. What does this test demonstrate?
    ○ 1. Lung maturity of the fetus
    ○ 2. The response of the fetal heart rate to fetal activity
    ○ 3. The degree of well-being of the feto-placental-maternal unit
    ○ 4. The ability of the fetus to tolerate the stress of uterine contractions

79. An infusion of oxytocin (Pitocin) is administered to Mrs. Benson, and labor is initiated. Which of the following observations would be most critical at this time?
    ○ 1. Fetal heart rate and uterine contractions
    ○ 2. Vaginal discharge and vital signs
    ○ 3. Fetal heart rate and maternal blood pressure
    ○ 4. Uterine contractions and maternal responses

80. In evaluating the action of the oxytocin, which of the following would be most indicative of an adverse effect?
    ○ 1. A contraction lasting over 120 seconds
    ○ 2. A decrease in blood pressure
    ○ 3. Urinary output of 100 ml per hour
    ○ 4. Increasing intensity of contractions

81. Mrs. Benson, now in active labor, expresses concern about her ability to continue to behave as she would wish during the remainder of labor. Which of these nursing actions would be most supportive?
    ○ 1. Reassure her of your competency.
    ○ 2. Reassure her that medication is available.
    ○ 3. Instruct her in relaxation and breathing exercises.
    ○ 4. Reassure her that she will be accepted regardless of her behavior.

82. An external monitor has been applied to Mrs. Benson. A fetal heart deceleration of uniform shape, beginning just as the contraction is under way and returning to the baseline at the end of the contraction, is detected. Which of the following nursing actions is most appropriate?
    ○ 1. Administer O_2.
    ○ 2. Turn the mother on her left side.
    ○ 3. Notify the physician.
    ○ 4. No action is necessary.

83. The fetal monitor begins to show late decelerations. Which of the following should the nurse do first?
    ○ 1. Decrease the Pitocin drip.
    ○ 2. Put her in Trendelenburg's position.
    ○ 3. Turn her on her left side.
    ○ 4. Inform the attending physician.

84. The nurse administers methylergonavine (Methergine) 0.2 mg parenterally to Mrs. Benson after completion of the third stage of labor. Which of the following would indicate that this drug has produced its desired effect?
   ○ **1.** A firm fundus
   ○ **2.** Increased duration and frequency of contractions
   ○ **3.** A rise in blood pressure
   ○ **4.** An increase in the respiratory rate

85. Mrs. Benson delivers a 7 lb 8 oz boy. Which of the following descriptions would best describe a postmature infant?
   ○ **1.** "Wide-eyed" with downy hair
   ○ **2.** Long finger nails and increased subcutaneous fat
   ○ **3.** Long, coarse hair and meconium-stained skin
   ○ **4.** Parchmentlike skin and thick coating of vernix

86. Thirty minutes after her delivery, the nurse makes the following assessment: fundus firm, 1 inch below the umbilicus; lochia rubra; complains of thirst; slight tremors of lower extremities. Analysis of these data is most suggestive of
   ○ **1.** impending shock.
   ○ **2.** circulatory overload.
   ○ **3.** sub-involution.
   ○ **4.** normal postpartum adjustment.

87. Two hours postdelivery, Mrs. Benson complains of severe perineal pain. Which nursing action should take highest priority?
   ○ **1.** Administer prescribed pain medication.
   ○ **2.** Administer a sitz bath immediately.
   ○ **3.** Inspect the perineum.
   ○ **4.** Instruct client in perineal muscle exercises.

88. Which of the following indicates bladder distension after Mrs. Benson's normal vaginal delivery?
   ○ **1.** Poor abdominal muscle tone
   ○ **2.** Increased lochia rubra with clots
   ○ **3.** Uterus contracted below umbilicus
   ○ **4.** Uterus soft to the right of midline

Gina Venters is a 21-year-old college student who has just learned that she contracted genital herpes from her sexual partner.

89. After completing the initial history and assessment for Miss Venters, the nurse will have data concerning areas pertinent to the disease. Which of the following would be *unnecessary* to include at this point?
   ○ **1.** Voiding patterns
   ○ **2.** Characteristics of lesions
   ○ **3.** Vaginal discharge
   ○ **4.** Prior history of varicella

90. Which of the following nursing diagnoses would most likely apply to Miss Venters as she copes with this disease?
   ○ **1.** Altered sexuality patterns
   ○ **2.** Impaired physical mobility
   ○ **3.** Diversional activity deficit
   ○ **4.** Disturbance in self-concept: personal identity

91. Miss Venters questions the reason why sexually transmitted diseases have reached epidemic proportions lately. Which of the following is the best explanation of the increased incidence?
   ○ **1.** Sexual permissiveness and promiscuity have increased.
   ○ **2.** Use of birth control pills has decreased because of better public education of their side effects.
   ○ **3.** The incidence of these diseases has increased because prostitutes transmit them.
   ○ **4.** The condom has become the primary method of birth control.

92. Miss Venters requests a shot of penicillin to cure her and promises to continue taking medication faithfully at home. How should the nurse respond to this client?
   ○ **1.** "I'll prepare the shot for you, as long as you continue the oral medication for 10 days."
   ○ **2.** "You will need to return for more penicillin if a lesion appears."
   ○ **3.** "Unfortunately, genital herpes is a lifelong disease, which at present has no cure."
   ○ **4.** "Tetracycline is the drug of choice for genital herpes."

93. Which of the following techniques would *not* aid in preventing the spread of genital herpes to others?
   ○ **1.** Refrain from sexual intercourse while lesions are present.
   ○ **2.** Restrict sexual contact to others already exposed to herpes.
   ○ **3.** Have sexual intercourse only in a darkened environment.
   ○ **4.** Use condoms during intercourse.

94. Why is it particularly difficult to assess females for gonorrhea?
○ **1.** They rarely have early distressing symptoms of the disease.
○ **2.** They are less likely to seek medical attention for diseases.
○ **3.** Cultures from the cervix cannot be utilized for diagnostic purposes.
○ **4.** They have a lower incidence of cystitis than males.

95. Syphilis may often go undetected without a thorough sexual history. Why is this so?
○ **1.** The disease is usually asymptomatic.
○ **2.** Symptoms disappear after some months, even if syphilis is not treated.
○ **3.** Symptoms appear the day after sexual contact.
○ **4.** The disease first attacks internal organs.

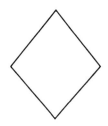

Test 1, Book III
Answers with Rationales

1. **#1.** The medulla may also be affected along with cranial nerves, but respiratory symptoms generally are not the result of increased intracranial pressure. ANALYSIS (ADULT/SAFETY AND SECURITY)

2. **#3.** The motor division of cranial nerve VII is specific; it controls the musculature of the face. ASSESSMENT (ADULT/SAFETY AND SECURITY)

3. **#1.** Treatment is symptomatic and supportive. The primary role of the nurse with these clients is careful observation and prevention of complications. PLAN (ADULT/SAFETY AND SECURITY)

4. **#1.** Ninety percent of people with this diagnosis make a complete recovery. The other options are inappropriate or inaccurate. IMPLEMENTATION (ADULT/SAFETY AND SECURITY)

5. **#2.** The client may burn or injure an extremity if sensory alteration is present. Special care to avoid injury is needed. IMPLEMENTATION (ADULT/SAFETY AND SECURITY)

6. **#4.** Conversion reaction is the loss or alteration of physical function that is not explained by any physical disorder or pathophysiologic mechanism. It is postulated that the behavior is reinforced by the gain it represents to the client, by repressing some unacceptable feeling or desire. ANALYSIS (PSYCHOSOCIAL, MENTAL HEALTH, PSYCHIATRIC PROBLEMS/ANXIOUS BEHAVIOR)

7. **#2.** Repression of feeling keeps anxiety controlled. The tension generated is converted into the presenting symptom, which is symbolic. A fixation at the anal stage of development produces defense mechanisms of sublimation and displacement, not conversion. Suppression of feelings is a conscious effort to eliminate feelings of discomfort. Conversion is an unconscious, intrapsychic conflict. Sublimation is a diversion of consciously unacceptable instinctual drives into personally and socially acceptable areas. ANALYSIS (PSYCHOSOCIAL, MENTAL HEALTH, PSYCHIATRIC PROBLEMS/ANXIOUS BEHAVIOR)

8. **#3.** In a conversion disorder, the client displays a level of concern disproportionate to the symptoms exhibited known as *la belle indifférence*. Ambivalence connotes simultaneous conflicting feelings or attitudes. Lability connotes mood swings. Narcissism, which is an abnormal interest in oneself, is not described here. ASSESSMENT (PSYCHOSOCIAL, MENTAL HEALTH, PSYCHIATRIC PROBLEMS/ANXIOUS BEHAVIOR)

9. **#4.** In addition to the primary gain of keeping anxiety out of her awareness, all the statements represent possible secondary gains. ANALYSIS (PSYCHOSOCIAL, MENTAL HEALTH, PSYCHIATRIC PROBLEMS/ANXIOUS BEHAVIOR)

10. **#3.** It is important to minimize the physical complaints and stress the positive aspects of her behavior to avoid reinforcement of the sick role. Confrontation will increase defensiveness and will meet resistance because of the client's need for denial. Supportive measures may provide secondary gain and increase dependency. The client is not psychotic; therefore, such medication is not indicated. IMPLEMENTATION (PSYCHOSOCIAL, MENTAL HEALTH, PSYCHIATRIC PROBLEMS/ANXIOUS BEHAVIOR)

11. **#4.** Sitting upright, leaning forward with mouth open, drooling, and dysphagia are classic signs of epiglottitis. ANALYSIS (CHILD/OXYGENATION)

12. **#1.** An adequate airway is the primary objective in treating epiglottitis because this child is in imminent danger of complete airway blockage. PLAN (CHILD/OXYGENATION)

13. **#3.** A change in heart rate, i.e., increasing heart rate, is an early sign of hypoxia. Options #2 and #4 are signs of lower airway involvement; #1 is characteristic of spasmodic croup. ASSESSMENT (CHILD/OXYGENATION)

14. **#1.** Determine Mark's hypersensitivity to the medication. Penicillin products are at high risk for causing allergic (and life-threatening) reactions. IMPLEMENTATION (CHILD/OXYGENATION)

15. #4. The Croupette concentrates the cool mist. This facilitates the heavy, cool water droplets reaching deeper into the respiratory tract to reduce edema and soothe irritated mucous membranes. While the Croupette will also accomplish options #1, #2, and #3 to some extent, they are not the primary goals. PLAN (CHILD/OXYGENATION)

16. #3. Loosely tucking the tent edges will allow oxygen to escape; edges should be firmly tucked around the mattress. All other options are necessary because of his age and his problem. IMPLEMENTATION (CHILD/OXYGENATION)

17. #2. A specific gravity of 1.005 indicates adequate hydration status. The other options measure parameters that do not influence hydration. ASSESSMENT (CHILD/OXYGENATION)

18. #2. Imaginary friends are normal for this age group. Because this is normal behavior, the other options are not warranted. IMPLEMENTATION (CHILD/HEALTHY CHILD)

19. #2. Tieing shoelaces, jumping rope, and walking backward are activities performed by a 5-year-old. ASSESSMENT (CHILD/HEALTHY CHILD)

20. #1. Levels of pain will vary in the foot and leg. However, as the gangrenous area develops, pain decreases because of the nerve destruction that occurs. Despite the occurrence of gangrene, infection, or inflammation, pain may be totally absent in the client with advanced neuropathy. ASSESSMENT (ADULT/NUTRITION AND METABOLISM)

21. #4. An immediate priority for the nurse is to determine the client's psychologic response to the physiologic happening: in this case, the death of a part of his body. Three ways of assessing this response are included in this option. ASSESSMENT (ADULT/NUTRITION AND METABOLISM)

22. #2. A footboard is not used for the same reasons that ambulation is not allowed. The nursing actions are directed at promoting circulation by preventing pressure areas from developing in dependent areas. PLAN (ADULT/NUTRITION AND METABOLISM)

23. #3. Fluids would be increased, not decreased, for a client on bed rest in order to prevent urinary stasis. PLAN (ADULT/NUTRITION AND METABOLISM)

24. #2. Keeping the area dry prevents moisture from promoting the growth of infection and macerating the skin. The other options would interfere with this. PLAN (ADULT/NUTRITION AND METABOLISM)

25. #2. The correct actions are stated in this option. Dakin's solution is used to debride the area, and petroleum jelly is a precautionary and preventive measure to protect the healthy tissue. ANALYSIS (ADULT/NUTRITION AND METABOLISM)

26. #3. Infection will increase the blood glucose level; thus the need for insulin increases. ANALYSIS (ADULT/NUTRITION AND METABOLISM)

27. #1. It is important to determine the person's perception of the condition before any teaching takes place. Remember, assessment occurs before planning or implementing nursing care. IMPLEMENTATION (ADULT/NUTRITION AND METABOLISM)

28. #1. Maintenance of physiologic integrity takes precedence. Determining the extent of the wounds and bleeding provides the most important information about physical status initially. In an emergency situation, a nurse must provide a calm atmosphere and yet attend to the client's safety and physiologic needs first. Option #4 is a strategy that will bc used eventually. IMPLEMENTATION (PSYCHOSOCIAL, MENTAL HEALTH, PSYCHIATRIC PROBLEMS/ELATED-DEPRESSIVE BEHAVIOR)

29. #2. This response allows the client to express the unstated feelings of hopelessness. Though anger may be present, his affect suggests hopelessness. The probability of his discussing or even recognizing anger at this time is minimal. Option #1 is a form of reassurance, which is rarely therapeutic. The nurse cannot presume to know what the client will be experiencing later. #4 would reinforce the client's determination to attempt suicide and reinforce feelings of hopelessness rather than instill a sense of hopefulness that something could be different. IMPLEMENTATION (PSYCHOSOCIAL, MENTAL HEALTH, PSYCHIATRIC PROBLEMS/ELATED-DEPRESSIVE BEHAVIOR)

30. **#1.** Though all choices provide useful information to assess suicide potential, the presence of a plan that is workable greatly increases the risk. While some attempt at connecting here-and-now events with the current situation is necessary, it is not particularly helpful in deciding suicide potential. IMPLEMENTATION (PSYCHOSOCIAL, MENTAL HEALTH, PSYCHIATRIC PROBLEMS/ELATED-DEPRESSIVE BEHAVIOR)

31. **#4.** Close observation is imperative in suicide prevention. While observation may be easier on a closed unit, an open unit is satisfactory as long as the client can be watched closely. A locked psychiatric unit does not imply that the client is being closely watched. A double room would assist the client only during the time that another client were in contact with him. However, other clients cannot bear the responsibility of supervision. IMPLEMENTATION (PSYCHOSOCIAL, MENTAL HEALTH, PSYCHIATRIC PROBLEMS/ELATED-DEPRESSIVE BEHAVIOR)

32. **#4.** Amitriptyline may take 4 weeks to become effective. It is premature to conclude the drug is not effective. The side effects of Elavil are autonomic due to the anticholinergic properties; therefore, continued depression would not be a side effect. Tolerance implies that increasing amounts of the substance (drug) must be used in order to achieve desired results. Since the desired results have yet to be achieved, tolerance is not a factor yet. ASSESSMENT (PSYCHOSOCIAL, MENTAL HEALTH, PSYCHIATRIC PROBLEMS/ELATED-DEPRESSIVE BEHAVIOR)

33. **#3.** These findings are consistent with a diagnosis of a hydatidiform mole. The uterus becomes enlarged out of proportion to the duration of pregnancy. At 3 months it is the size of a 5-month pregnancy. Excessive nausea and vomiting and an intermittent or continuous brownish-red discharge by the 12th week are common. ANALYSIS (CHILDBEARING FAMILY/ANTEPARTAL CARE)

34. **#2.** Ultrasound is the most useful tool in diagnosing a molar pregnancy; no fetal skeleton is revealed. A dilatation and curettage may be used to treat the condition. A laparoscopy is used to examine the interior of the abdomen. ASSESSMENT (CHILDBEARING FAMILY/ANTEPARTAL CARE)

35. **#4.** The current methods of removing a molar pregnancy are dilatation and curettage, induced abortion, or hysterectomy. ANALYSIS (CHILDBEARING FAMILY/ANTEPARTAL CARE)

36. **#2.** Choriocarcinoma, a neoplastic process that often follows a hydatidiform mole, has a tendency to undergo rapid, widespread metastasis. The client's human chorionic gonadotropin levels will be monitored for at least 1 year. Molar pregnancies do not place the client at higher risk for the remaining options. ANALYSIS (CHILDBEARING FAMILY/ANTEPARTAL CARE)

37. **#3.** Because of the concern about choriocarcinoma, it is generally recommended that pregnancy be avoided for 1 year following a molar pregnancy. IMPLEMENTATION (CHILDBEARING FAMILY/ANTEPARTAL CARE)

38. **#3.** Oral contraceptive use is advocated to prevent another pregnancy for at least 1 year following a hydatidiform mole. EVALUATION (CHILDBEARING FAMILY/ANTEPARTAL CARE)

39. **#3.** Gout is a disease of faulty purine metabolism and is characterized by increased amounts of uric acid, which forms stones. The other options are all associated with calcium stones but not indicated by the client's history. ANALYSIS (ADULT/ELIMINATION)

40. **#2.** Hydronephrosis is caused when the ureter is obstructed, and urine backs up and distends the kidney. ANALYSIS (ADULT/ELIMINATION)

41. **#2.** Unless the pain is controlled, there is little chance the stone will be safely passed. All the other choices would be actions to take after pain is controlled. IMPLEMENTATION (ADULT/ELIMINATION)

42. **#1.** Inorganic calcium stones occur in alkaline urine and often follow a urinary tract infection. ANALYSIS (ADULT/ELIMINATION)

43. **#2.** Vitamin C, when given in large (1 gm) daily doses, is excreted through the urine, acidifying it. ANALYSIS (ADULT/ELIMINATION)

44. **#2.** Urecholine is a cholinergic drug, which increases bladder tone and promotes urination. ANALYSIS (ADULT/ELIMINATION)

45. **#4.** All options may occur, but the specific reason is to prevent loss of bladder tone. ANALYSIS (ADULT/ELIMINATION)

46. #1. The child with nephrosis usually exhibits generalized edema, ascites, an elevated urine specific gravity, and normal blood pressure. ASSESSMENT (CHILD/ELIMINATION)

47. #1. Older toddlers and preschoolers are especially fearful of procedures that threaten their body integrity, such as rectal temperatures and injections. ANALYSIS (CHILD/ILL AND HOSPITALIZED CHILD)

48. #4. The preschooler is involved in mastering a sense of initiative versus guilt. ANALYSIS (CHILD/HEALTHY CHILD)

49. #2. Prednisone should never be withheld but tapered gradually, because sudden withdrawal may precipitate an adrenal crisis. IMPLEMENTATION (CHILD/ELIMINATION)

50. #4. Semi-Fowler's position relieves the respiratory embarrassment that often occurs with ascites. PLAN (CHILD/ELIMINATION)

51. #3. This snack is highest in potassium and protein, and low in sodium. IMPLEMENTATION (CHILD/ELIMINATION)

52. #3. This activity requires little energy expenditure while Courtney is acutely ill and also increases his sense of control and security by allowing him to project his own feelings into the story. IMPLEMENTATION (CHILD/ILL AND HOSPITALIZED CHILD)

53. #3. The client with paranoid schizophrenia has increased sensitivity. Options #1, #2, and #4 are all characteristic manifestations of paranoid schizophrenia. ASSESSMENT (PSYCHOSOCIAL, MENTAL HEALTH, PSYCHIATRIC PROBLEMS/WITHDRAWN BEHAVIORS)

54. #2. The client with paranoid schizophrenia projects his fantasy world and emotions on others. Denial, rationalization, and suppression may be utilized by a paranoid schizophrenic but are not characteristically present. ASSESSMENT (PSYCHOSOCIAL, MENTAL HEALTH, PSYCHIATRIC PROBLEMS/WITHDRAWN BEHAVIOR)

55. #4. Acting out fantasy life in group therapy would give positive reinforcement to fantasy and would not teach the client to cope in the world of reality. Options #1, #2, and #3 are all appropriate goals that are achievable and will incorporate the individual into the "real world" s/he is trying to escape. PLAN (PSYCHOSOCIAL, MENTAL HEALTH, PSYCHIATRIC PROBLEMS/WITHDRAWN BEHAVIOR)

56. #4. Mutual withdrawal is a common staff problem when clients withdraw from staff; isolation should be avoided when treating schizophrenic clients. Options #1, #2, and #3 will assist the client by allowing some control over how quickly he establishes a relationship with a staff member. IMPLEMENTATION (PSYCHOSOCIAL, MENTAL HEALTH, PSYCHIATRIC PROBLEMS/WITHDRAWN BEHAVIOR)

57. #4. This option would give positive reinforcement to the client's unhealthy behaviors. It is more helpful to work with the client's healthy and adaptive behaviors. Options #1 and #2 will assist the client in focusing on reality and avoiding retreat and withdrawal. It is necessary to initially assess the content of the hallucinations to determine if the voices are directing the individual to harm himself or others. Knowing the purpose and meaning of the hallucinations assists the nurse in planning interventions to diminish the "trigger response" that occurs prior to the voices, the subsequent "listening attitude," and finally the actual experience of the "voices." Focus on the here and now to maintain reality and avoid escapism by the client. IMPLEMENTATION (PSYCHOSOCIAL, MENTAL HEALTH, PSYCHIATRIC PROBLEMS/WITHDRAWN BEHAVIOR)

58. #1. Identifying client needs for assistance is the first step in assisting a client to be self-directing with hygiene and grooming. Group work is difficult for a schizophrenic client, and doing hygiene for him makes the client more dependent and less able to do for himself. Ignoring lack of hygiene is counterproductive to the goal. IMPLEMENTATION (PSYCHOSOCIAL, MENTAL HEALTH, PSYCHIATRIC PROBLEMS/WITHDRAWN BEHAVIOR)

59. #3. Confronting and arguing with a paranoid client tends to increase the hostility and paranoia and decrease the level of trust. The other options are beneficial for managing hostile behavior. IMPLEMENTATION (PSYCHOSOCIAL, MENTAL HEALTH, PSYCHIATRIC PROBLEMS/WITHDRAWN BEHAVIOR)

60. #4. Ambivalence is not treatable with a drug. Agitation, hallucinations, and delusions are the "target" symptoms that antipsychotic agents are specifically prescribed to diminish or alleviate. ANALYSIS (PSYCHOSOCIAL, MENTAL HEALTH, PSYCHIATRIC PROBLEMS/WITHDRAWN BEHAVIOR)

61. **#4.** Thioridazine and the other antipsychotic medications are not addictive, and there is no tolerance to their antipsychotic effect. Dry mouth, constipation, and urinary hesitancy are characteristic side effects of Mellaril due to its anticholinergic properties. ASSESSMENT (PSYCHOSOCIAL, MENTAL HEALTH, PSYCHIATRIC PROBLEMS/WITHDRAWN BEHAVIOR)

62. **#3.** The only permanent damage that may result from rheumatic fever is cardiac damage. Therefore, close monitoring of cardiac status is imperative. ASSESSMENT (CHILD/OXYGENATION)

63. **#1.** Sydenham's chorea does not impair intellectual functioning. Because of the symptoms, the chief problem is one of safety for the child. ASSESSMENT (CHILD/OXYGENATION)

64. **#1.** This goal must have priority because permanent cardiac valvular damage may result from rheumatic fever. PLAN (CHILD/OXYGENATION)

65. **#4.** Jackie is on bed rest and cannot visit other children on the unit. Because of the chorea, she is unable to play Nerf basketball or write in a diary. Therefore, listening to records is the best activity at this time. IMPLEMENTATION (CHILD/OXYGENATION)

66. **#3.** Rheumatic fever does not cause albuminuria. Nephrosis and nephritis cause large amounts of protein loss. ASSESSMENT (CHILD/OXYGENATION)

67. **#2.** Long-term antibiotic therapy with penicillin or erythromycin is necessary to prevent serious cardiac damage or recurrence of rheumatic fever. EVALUATION (CHILD/OXYGENATION)

68. **#4.** Nursing notes should be clear, specific descriptions. ASSESSMENT (ADULT/OXYGENATION)

69. **#2.** A gunshot wound is grossly contaminated and an abdominal wound would bleed profusely; any clean towels would be appropriate. ANALYSIS (ADULT/OXYGENATION)

70. **#2.** Removing or disturbing the knife in a chest wound can cause severe damage or massive hemorrhage. The knife acts as a tamponade to the affected sites. IMPLEMENTATION (ADULT/OXYGENATION)

71. **#2.** Internal injury leads to an air leak within the tissues, thereby causing subcutaneous emphysema. ANALYSIS (ADULT/OXYGENATION)

72. **#3.** A ruptured bladder causes the sensation of needing to void, but urine actually is collecting in the peritoneal cavity. ANALYSIS (ADULT/OXYGENATION)

73. **#1.** This procedure is essential to prevent administration of incompatible blood, which could result in the client's death. It is essential to check the client's blood band on his arm. Just checking the chart does not ensure the client receives the correct blood. Options #3 and #4 are important but do not require 2 nurses. IMPLEMENTATION (ADULT/OXYGENATION)

74. **#3.** A history of hepatitis disqualifies a potential blood donor for life. The other options do not disqualify a person. ASSESSMENT (ADULT/OXYGENATION)

75. **#2.** Normal saline is used, because it is an isotonic solution. ANALYSIS (ADULT/OXYGENATION)

76. **#3.** Bleeding under the skin at the IV site indicates infiltration or leaking around the site. All the other options given are signs of a transfusion reaction. ASSESSMENT (ADULT/OXYGENATION)

77. **#3.** It is imperative that the blood be stopped and the IV needle be left in place and kept patent to administer fluids and medications to counteract the reaction. Option #2 is a second action, #1 is a third action. IMPLEMENTATION (ADULT/OXYGENATION)

78. **#4.** The purpose of an oxytocin challenge test is to observe fetal heart rate response to uterine contractions. ANALYSIS (CHILDBEARING FAMILY/INTRAPARTAL CARE)

79. **#1.** Risks with the administration of oxytocin are related to uterine tetany and late decelerations. ASSESSMENT (CHILDBEARING FAMILY/INTRAPARTAL CARE)

80. **#1.** If contractions exceed 90 seconds in duration, there is a danger of ruptured uterus as well as interference with placental perfusion. A decreasing blood pressure would be a cause for concern but not related to oxytocin. EVALUATION (CHILDBEARING FAMILY/INTRAPARTAL CARE)

81. #4. Acceptance is needed in time of stress. As labor progresses the client may have difficulty maintaining control. The client will require acceptance during a time of stress and assurance that she will be accepted regardless of her behavior. The nurse's competency, administration of medication, and instruction may be ineffective in controlling the client's behavior. IMPLEMENTATION (CHILDBEARING FAMILY/INTRAPARTAL CARE)

82. #4. This is a normal occurrence called an early deceleration. It is most likely due to head compression and requires no action. IMPLEMENTATION (CHILDBEARING FAMILY/INTRAPARTAL CARE)

83. #3. Late decelerations are most likely due to uteroplacental insufficiency. Turning the client on the left side to relieve pressure on the vena cava by the gravida uterus may correct the problem. If not, Pitocin should be discontinued. The physician should be notified if the heart rate is not corrected by these nursing actions. IMPLEMENTATION (CHILDBEARING FAMILY/INTRAPARTAL CARE)

84. #1. Methergine is an oxytoxic drug given to contract the uterus after placental delivery. EVALUATION (CHILDBEARING FAMILY/POSTPARTAL CARE)

85. #3. This best describes the postmature infant. Because of prolonged gestation, these infants are more alert, have decreased vernix, dry peeling skin, and long fingernails. They exhibit varying degrees of wasting and thus decreased subcutaneous fat. Meconium staining results from intrauterine hypoxia. ASSESSMENT (CHILDBEARING FAMILY/NORMAL NEWBORN)

86. #4. These are normal observations in the immediate postpartum period. ANALYSIS (CHILDBEARING FAMILY/POSTPARTAL CARE)

87. #3. Such pain may be associated with the development of a hematoma. Assessment is necessary prior to selecting an appropriate nursing action. IMPLEMENTATION (CHILDBEARING FAMILY/POSTPARTAL CARE)

88. #4. A full bladder displaces the uterus and prevents contraction. ASSESSMENT (CHILDBEARING FAMILY/POSTPARTAL CARE)

89. #4. The other three options list common reasons for which herpes clients seek care. ASSESSMENT (CHILD/SENSATION, PERCEPTION, PROTECTION)

90. #1. Having herpes leads to an alteration or limitation in sexual relationships as well as alterations in achieving perceived or desired sex roles. Other nursing diagnoses listed are not applicable. ANALYSIS (CHILD/SENSATION, PERCEPTION, PROTECTION)

91. #1. The idea underlying these social changes is that with the advent of antibiotics and the pill, people began to lose fear of untreated disease and pregnancy, leading to increased exposure to infection. The other three options listed are not true statements. ANALYSIS (CHILD/SENSATION, PERCEPTION, PROTECTION)

92. #3. Treatment for genital herpes is most often symptomatic as there is no known cure for the disease at present. IMPLEMENTATION (CHILD/SENSATION, PERCEPTION, PROTECTION)

93. #3. Prior to sexual intercourse, partners should examine themselves and each other for evidence of disease. A darkened environment is not conducive to this. PLAN (CHILD/SENSATION, PERCEPTION, PROTECTION)

94. #1. Early symptoms of gonorrhea include a slight purulent discharge, a vague feeling of fullness in the pelvis, and discomfort in the abdomen. Many women disregard these vague symptoms (if they are present) and do not seek treatment. ANALYSIS (CHILD/SENSATION, PERCEPTION, PROTECTION)

95. #2. While the symptoms of syphilis are similar to those of a host of other diseases, they disappear without treatment, providing false reassurance to the client that nothing is really wrong. ANALYSIS (CHILD/SENSATION, PERCEPTION, PROTECTION)

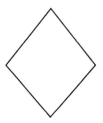

Test 1, Book IV
Questions

Ann Martin, a 47-year-old retired government employee, was admitted to the psychiatric inpatient service, accompanied by her daughter. Her admission diagnosis is a major depressive episode. She is delusional and has vegetative signs of depression.

1. Oftentimes, depression is accompanied by guilt. The multidisplinary mental health team develops a care plan that includes, ''Assist client to express guilty feelings.'' The primary nurse realizes that some clients are not aware of their guilt feelings. To implement this goal, it will be best for the nurse to have Mrs. Martin
   - ○ **1.** attend group therapy.
   - ○ **2.** explore feelings of resentment and anger.
   - ○ **3.** examine situations where she may push others away out of fear of rejection.
   - ○ **4.** participate in planning activities of daily living.

2. In which type of depression would delusions be most likely to occur?
   - ○ **1.** Transitory
   - ○ **2.** Reactive
   - ○ **3.** Psychotic
   - ○ **4.** Neurotic

3. Which of the following are specific indicators of depression?
   - ○ **1.** Crying, withdrawal
   - ○ **2.** Constipation, anorexia, hyper- or hyposomnolence
   - ○ **3.** Weakness, fatigability
   - ○ **4.** Negative view of the self and the future

4. Which of the following statements indicates most clearly that the client is suffering from a depression?
   - ○ **1.** ''I don't feel that I have any chance of a good relationship with a man. I am not very attractive or likable.''
   - ○ **2.** ''I'm a very private person and don't call my friends when I feel bad.''
   - ○ **3.** ''I don't have any appetite, I'm constipated, and I sleep too much.''
   - ○ **4.** ''I feel weak and tired all the time.''

5. Which of the following is *not* considered a sign of depression?
   - ○ **1.** Anorexia
   - ○ **2.** Impotence in men
   - ○ **3.** Morning-evening variations of mood
   - ○ **4.** Ataxia

6. Which of the following are considered vegetative signs of depression?
   - ○ **1.** Restlessness, pacing, anxiety
   - ○ **2.** Talkativeness, increased motor activity
   - ○ **3.** Haggard appearance, slowness, uncooperativeness, indecisiveness
   - ○ **4.** Argumentative, bossing staff

7. The largest number of psychiatric hospitalizations are accounted for by
   - ○ **1.** schizophrenia.
   - ○ **2.** phobic reactions.
   - ○ **3.** autism.
   - ○ **4.** depression.

8. Mrs. Martin frequently seeks out a nurse whom she resembles in height, weight, and appearance. In this nurse's presence, Mrs. Martin imitates her mannerisms and supportive ways. This defense mechanism by the client can best be described as
   - ○ **1.** idealization.
   - ○ **2.** introjection.
   - ○ **3.** identification.
   - ○ **4.** substitution.

9. During the course of her treatment, Mrs. Martin's psychiatrist orders amitriptyline HCl (Elavil) 20 mg TID PO. Which of the following side effects is *not* expected to occur?
   - ○ **1.** Excitement
   - ○ **2.** Anorexia
   - ○ **3.** Hypertension
   - ○ **4.** Nausea

10. The psychiatrist also orders isocarboxazid (Marplan) 30 mg PO daily. When recording these medication orders, the nurse should do which of the following?
    ○ **1.** Order and administer the medications.
    ○ **2.** Measure the client's blood pressure and withhold both medications if it is below 90 mm Hg systolic and 60 mm Hg diastolic.
    ○ **3.** Inquire first whether the client has had any dizziness or nausea, since both these medications could worsen these symptoms.
    ○ **4.** Call the psychiatrist and question the administration of these medications together.

11. Antidepressants may cause a number of side effects. Which of the following antidepressants may lead to hypertensive crisis and possibly a cerebrovascular accident if taken with natural foods, such as aged cheese, or alcoholic beverages, such as beer and wine?
    ○ **1.** Amitriptyline HCl (Elavil)
    ○ **2.** Imipramine HCl (Tofranil)
    ○ **3.** Lithium carbonate
    ○ **4.** Isocarboxazid (Marplan)

12. All the following assessments would be included for Mrs. Martin. Which one would be carried out first?
    ○ **1.** Degree of neglect of physical needs (e.g., fluid intake, nutrition, and elimination)
    ○ **2.** Possibility of self-harm
    ○ **3.** Willingness to attend group therapy
    ○ **4.** Response to medications

13. Which of these suicide methods has a lower rate of lethality than the others?
    ○ **1.** Ingestion of barbiturates and any sedatives
    ○ **2.** Setting herself on fire
    ○ **3.** Scratching her wrists with broken glass
    ○ **4.** Cutting the jugular vein

14. Of the following, which group has the lowest suicide risk?
    ○ **1.** Alcoholics
    ○ **2.** Depressed persons
    ○ **3.** Adolescents
    ○ **4.** Married men

Tang Phong is a 3-week-old boy brought into the emergency room by his parents. Mr. and Mrs. Phong say his vomiting has become progressively worse over the past 5 days. It is now projectile.

15. While obtaining a nursing history, which question would be *least* appropriate to ask the Phongs in order to rule out pyloric stenosis?
    ○ **1.** "Has Tang had a recent immunization?"
    ○ **2.** "Is anyone else sick at home?"
    ○ **3.** "Does Tang appear hungry after vomiting?"
    ○ **4.** "How much did Tang weigh at his last exam?"

16. Tang's condition is diagnosed as pyloric stenosis, and he is transferred to a pediatric unit. What would be the most *unexpected* finding in an infant with this condition?
    ○ **1.** A palpable, olive-shaped mass in the right upper quadrant
    ○ **2.** Visible left-to-right peristaltic waves
    ○ **3.** Stringy, frequent stools
    ○ **4.** Lethargy

17. Tang is admitted to the infant unit. Which of the following nursing actions should be implemented?
    ○ **1.** Prepare Tang and his parents for immediate surgery.
    ○ **2.** Monitor intravenous hydration.
    ○ **3.** Give diazepam (Valium) as ordered, to relax the pyloric sphincter.
    ○ **4.** Give small, frequent feedings.

18. What is the most common metabolic disturbance seen in infants who have pyloric stenosis?
    ○ **1.** Metabolic acidosis
    ○ **2.** Metabolic alkalosis
    ○ **3.** Respiratory alkalosis
    ○ **4.** Hyperkalemia

19. Tang has an IV of 5% dextrose in 0.45% saline hanging. The physician has ordered potassium chloride (KCl) to be added to the IV. What important nursing action is carried out prior to adding KCl to the IV?
    ○ **1.** Check the time of last voiding.
    ○ **2.** Look up the last serum chloride level.
    ○ **3.** Ensure that the IV is infusing through a large-bore needle.
    ○ **4.** Check skin turgor.

20. Tang is extremely restless and his repeated movements cause 2 IVs to infiltrate. Cloth extremity-restraints are applied to prevent recurrent infiltration. Which of the following measures is most important to ensure the safety of a restrained infant?
○ 1. Avoid placing padding under the restraints, since it will only increase pressure and the chance of injury.
○ 2. Fasten the restraint ties securely to the crib rails.
○ 3. Secure all 4 extremities since one loose extremity can cause the child to become entangled in the restraints.
○ 4. Check how the restraints are applied and the circulation in the extremities frequently.

21. Tang has had his pyloric stenosis surgically repaired. Which should *not* be considered when planning his post-op nursing care?
○ 1. Include parents in giving his feedings.
○ 2. Oral feedings will be started a few hours after surgery.
○ 3. Tang will be NPO for days after surgery; thus, sucking needs should be satisfied in other ways.
○ 4. Monitor Tang for signs of hypoglycemia.

22. After surgical repair of the pyloric stenosis, Tang should be placed in which position?
○ 1. High-Fowler's
○ 2. Prone
○ 3. Right side-lying
○ 4. Left side-lying

23. Which of the following post-op responses to feedings should Tang optimally exhibit?
○ 1. Immediate tolerance of oral fluids because of release of the hypertrophied muscle
○ 2. No vomiting, since the infant is NPO and is on a regimen of IVs for the first 2 to 3 days
○ 3. Tolerance for clear fluids, but frequent vomiting of formula or breast milk
○ 4. Intermittent vomiting of oral fluids that diminishes over the first 24 to 48 hours

24. Which nursing observation indicates that Tang's parents are fully prepared for his discharge?
○ 1. Tang recovers fully from surgery and his parents express happiness.
○ 2. He retains his formula after his parents feed him.
○ 3. His parents demonstrate the correct feeding technique.
○ 4. Tang gains weight appropriate for his age.

Paul Connelly, a 38-year-old bookkeeper, has suffered from chronic renal failure for 3 years. He has been maintained on outpatient hemodialysis 3 times a week while awaiting transplantation.

25. Donor-recipient compatibility must be assessed before renal transplant. Mr. Connelly asks the nurse to explain tissue typing. Which of the following statements is an *incorrect* response?
○ 1. Blood typing is the initial step in determining compatibility.
○ 2. Any natural sibling of the recipient is an ideal donor.
○ 3. Two human leukocyte antigens (HLA) are inherited from each parent.
○ 4. A mixed lymphocyte culture (MLC) requires 5 to 7 days to perform.

26. A suitable donor is located, and Mr. Connelly's transplantation is scheduled. He will receive the immunosuppressive drug azathioprine (Imuran) prior to surgery and following the transplant. What should the nurse teach him about this medication?
○ 1. Avoid crowds and contact with obviously ill people.
○ 2. The drug stimulates kidney output.
○ 3. Frequent platelet counts will be required.
○ 4. An increase in the number of circulating antibodies can be anticipated.

27. The nurse plans to observe Mr. Connelly closely following surgery for signs of rejection of the graft. Which observation is *not* associated with tissue rejection?
○ 1. Weight gain
○ 2. Irritability
○ 3. Swelling at the operative site
○ 4. Rising white blood count

28. Early post-op care for Mr. Connelly will *not* include which of the following?
○ 1. Irrigate the Foley catheter frequently.
○ 2. Maintain reverse isolation.
○ 3. Observe for symptoms of disequilibrium syndrome.
○ 4. Monitor the stool for blood.

29. Mr. Connelly's niece, Sally Burnside, aged 15, is very interested in donating her kidneys for transplant should she die unexpectedly. She asks if she can carry a donor card. Based on the Uniform Anatomical Gift Act, what can the nurse tell her?
   ○ 1. She must wait until she is 18, because she is a minor.
   ○ 2. All she needs to do is sign a card.
   ○ 3. She may carry a donor card, provided her parents have cosigned the card in the presence of witnesses.
   ○ 4. A donor card is not necessary, because her parents could give permission if the need arises.

30. Mr. Connelly returns for a follow-up visit 1 year after his transplant. He tells the nurse he feels so well he has decided to stop taking his prednisone. The nurse is concerned because he may experience
   ○ 1. infection.
   ○ 2. organ rejection.
   ○ 3. psychosis.
   ○ 4. anemia.

Rachael Carrier seeks treatment in the infertility clinic.

31. The nurse instructs Mrs. Carrier how to take her basal body temperature to identify the time of ovulation. This event can be identified by which of the following?
   ○ 1. A slight drop in temperature followed by a rise of 0.5°F to 0.7°F under the influence of progesterone
   ○ 2. An increase in temperature of 2°F under the influence of progesterone
   ○ 3. A substantial drop in temperature followed by a 0.5°F to 0.7°F rise under the influence of estrogen
   ○ 4. An increase in the temperature of 2°F under the influence of estrogen

32. At the time of ovulation, blood levels of
   ○ 1. luteinizing hormone are high.
   ○ 2. follicle-stimulating hormone-releasing factors are high.
   ○ 3. progesterone are high.
   ○ 4. estrogen are high.

33. After diagnostic testing, clomiphene (Clomid) is prescribed for Mrs. Carrier. Which of the following best describes how this drug works?
   ○ 1. Increases the estrogen-progesterone level, thereby causing ovulation
   ○ 2. Increases the amount of gonadotropin secretion, which stimulates maturation of the ovarian follicles
   ○ 3. Changes the pH of vaginal secretions to support sperm viability
   ○ 4. Stimulates the development of the endometrium to support pregnancy

Sean Collins, age 52, experiences retrosternal chest pain that radiates down his left arm when he is engaged in strenuous physical activity. A resting electrocardiagram (ECG) is normal, but a stress ECG shows ST depression.

34. As the nurse takes a history, which of the following questions is most relevant?
   ○ 1. "Can you describe the pain and the events that led up to it?"
   ○ 2. "Are you taking any medications for chest pain?"
   ○ 3. "How many packs of cigarettes do you smoke daily?"
   ○ 4. "Did the pain radiate to your jaw or neck?"

35. An ECG primarily gives information about the
   ○ 1. excitation of the myocardium.
   ○ 2. perfusion of the myocardium.
   ○ 3. contractile force of the myocardium.
   ○ 4. integrity of the myocardium.

36. Cardiac enzymes are drawn. Why were they ordered?
   ○ 1. To identify the causative organism
   ○ 2. To determine how well the blood is being oxygenated
   ○ 3. To rule out gas or indigestion
   ○ 4. To determine the presence of tissue damage

37. Based on Mr. Collins's clinical symptoms and laboratory reports, the physician makes a diagnosis of angina pectoris. Anginal pain can involve the left arm and jaw, in addition to the chest, because these areas are all supplied by the same part of the nervous system, the
   ○ 1. cranial nerve (vagus).
   ○ 2. spinal nerves.
   ○ 3. autonomic nervous system.
   ○ 4. spinal cord segment.

38. Anginal pain is caused by coronary insufficiency. The coronary arteries fill with blood when the
    ○ **1.** left ventricle contracts and the aortic valve is closed.
    ○ **2.** left ventricle contracts and the aortic valve is open.
    ○ **3.** left ventricle relaxes and the aortic valve is closed.
    ○ **4.** left ventricle relaxes and the aortic valve is open.

39. Mr. Collins is given nitroglycerin 0.4 mg to take sublingually during his angina attacks. Mr. Collins's dosage of 0.4 mg is equivalent to how many grains?
    ○ **1.** Gr 1/250
    ○ **2.** Gr 1/200
    ○ **3.** Gr 1/150
    ○ **4.** Gr 1/100

40. Nitroglycerin will produce dilation of the coronary arteries in 1 to 2 minutes after being put under the tongue. Which of these statements correctly describes the procedure for administering nitroglycerin when 1 tablet does not relieve the pain?
    ○ **1.** Administer 1 tablet q2min for 5 doses.
    ○ **2.** Administer 1 tablet q5min for 10 doses.
    ○ **3.** Administer 1 tablet q5min for 3 doses.
    ○ **4.** Administer 1 tablet q10min for 5 doses.

41. Mr. Collins should be observed for common side effects of nitroglycerin therapy. What are they?
    ○ **1.** Headache, hypotension, dizziness
    ○ **2.** Hypertension, flushing, loss of consciousness
    ○ **3.** Hypotension, shock, convulsions
    ○ **4.** Headache, hypertension, convulsions

42. What information should the nurse give to Mr. Collins about nitroglycerin?
    ○ **1.** "Take the tablets with meals."
    ○ **2.** "Take the tablets only for severe pain."
    ○ **3.** "A burning sensation under the tongue is normal."
    ○ **4.** "Call your doctor if you have a headache or flushing."

43. Which of the following would be most appropriate to teach Mr. Collins in terms of what to report immediately?
    ○ **1.** The occurrence of pain after a business meeting
    ○ **2.** A change in the pattern of pain
    ○ **3.** Pain that occurs with eating
    ○ **4.** The fact that nitroglycerin does not cause a tingling sensation under the tongue

44. Mr. Collins is also placed on a regimen of propranolol (Inderal) to control his angina. Propranolol will be contraindicated if Mr. Collins develops
    ○ **1.** myocardial infarction.
    ○ **2.** asthma.
    ○ **3.** cerebral vascular accident.
    ○ **4.** thrombophlebitis.

45. When administering a beta-blocking agent like propranolol (Inderal) for cardiac dysrhythmias, the nurse should
    ○ **1.** check the blood pressure qh.
    ○ **2.** have atropine available as an antidote.
    ○ **3.** monitor the blood pressure and peripheral pulses q4h.
    ○ **4.** make repeated counts of at least 1 full minute of both apical and radial pulses to detect any disturbances in rhythm.

46. You begin diet teaching with Mr. Collins. Which of the following is inappropriate for the teaching plan?
    ○ **1.** Eat smaller meals.
    ○ **2.** Eat snacks of cheese.
    ○ **3.** Include more fish and chicken.
    ○ **4.** Abstain from gas-forming foods.

47. Mr. Collins is discharged and referred to the outpatient clinic for a stress test and cardiac catheterization. What is the rationale for the cardiac catheterization?
    ○ **1.** To dilate the coronary blood vessels
    ○ **2.** To confirm a diagnosis of heart disease
    ○ **3.** To force oxygen under pressure to the myocardium
    ○ **4.** To bypass the diseased coronary artery

48. Mr. Collins wants to join a class on primary health care habits to prevent cardiovascular and respiratory disease, but he tells the nurse he does not plan to quit smoking. What would be the best response to Mr. Collins?
    ○ **1.** He cannot join unless he stops smoking.
    ○ **2.** He can join but cannot smoke in class.
    ○ **3.** He can join and can smoke in class.
    ○ **4.** He can join but should not attend classes on smoking.

Four-year-old Sean White was admitted to the hospital with burns received while playing with matches. His legs and lower abdomen are burned.

49. In assessing Sean's hydration status, which of the following indicates less-than-adequate fluid replacement?
   ○ 1. Decreasing hematocrit and increasing urine volume
   ○ 2. Falling hematocrit and decreasing urine volume
   ○ 3. Rising hematocrit and decreasing urine volume
   ○ 4. Stable hematocrit and increasing urine volume

50. Which symptoms indicate overhydration after the first 24 hours?
   ○ 1. Diuresis
   ○ 2. Drowsiness and lethargy
   ○ 3. Dyspnea, moist rales
   ○ 4. Warmth and redness around the intravenous site

51. Sean's burns are to be treated by the "open method." In planning his care, which of the following is *least* appropriate?
   ○ 1. Place Sean in reverse isolation.
   ○ 2. Prevent his having visitors from outside the hospital.
   ○ 3. Encourage Sean to participate in his care.
   ○ 4. Place him in a room near the nurse's station.

52. Sean's output via his Foley catheter is 10 ml/hour. What should be the first nursing action?
   ○ 1. Check the catheter to see if it is plugged.
   ○ 2. Call the physician immediately.
   ○ 3. Record the information on the chart.
   ○ 4. Increase the intravenous fluids.

53. When Sean starts oral feedings, it is particularly important that his diet have a high amount of
   ○ 1. fats and carbohydrates.
   ○ 2. minerals and vitamins.
   ○ 3. fluids and vitamins.
   ○ 4. proteins and carbohydrates.

54. What would be the best diversional activity for Sean while he is in reverse isolation?
   ○ 1. Lace leather wallets
   ○ 2. Watch television
   ○ 3. Play with puppets
   ○ 4. Use computer word games

Robert Benson, a middle-aged business executive, is admitted to the psychiatric unit. He tells the nurse that he came to the hospital because he needs a few days of relief from the constant harassment of FBI agents, who have been following him for years. The FBI, he says, wants to steal the plans he has worked out for world peace.

55. Mr. Benson's diagnosis is paranoid disorder. Which of the following is *not* characteristic of paranoia?
   ○ 1. Suspiciousness
   ○ 2. Superiority
   ○ 3. Hostility
   ○ 4. Intellectual impairment

56. Mr. Benson's behavior is most characteristic of
   ○ 1. a fixed delusional system.
   ○ 2. hallucinations.
   ○ 3. acting out.
   ○ 4. manipulation.

57. In order to help Mr. Benson, it is most important for the nurse to do which of the following?
   ○ 1. Gather more details about his problems with the FBI.
   ○ 2. Point out to him that his story is not logical.
   ○ 3. Acknowledge his feelings without agreeing with them.
   ○ 4. Explain to him that he will have to learn to live with the existing situation.

58. Mr. Benson screams at the nurse that a spy is after him. The best nursing response at this time is which of the following?
   ○ 1. "You are upset, Mr. Benson. I understand how you feel."
   ○ 2. Ignore his comment.
   ○ 3. "I am Miss Smith, a nurse on the unit."
   ○ 4. "Mr. Benson, you are in the hospital now. There are no spies here."

59. Later, Mr. Benson refuses to eat his dinner. He says he is hungry, but that his wife is trying to poison him. Taking note that Mr. Benson said he was hungry, which of the following is the best nursing action?
   ○ 1. Explain that his wife did not prepare the food.
   ○ 2. Offer to taste his food before he eats it.
   ○ 3. Call for another tray and eat with Mr. Benson.
   ○ 4. Arrange to have food in sealed containers served to Mr. Benson.

60. Mr. Benson has been placed on a regimen of chlorpromazine HCl (Thorazine). Possible side effects of the drug do *not* include
   ○ 1. agranulocytosis.
   ○ 2. photophobia.
   ○ 3. postural hypotension.
   ○ 4. dermatitis.

Betty Spaulding, aged 17, has begun to show early signs of pregnancy-induced hypertension (PIH).

61. Which of the following assessments by the nurse would most likely indicate that Betty may have PIH?
    ○ 1. A blood pressure change from 110/80 mm Hg to 120/88 mm Hg
    ○ 2. Complaints of swelling of fingers and eyelids
    ○ 3. Weight gain of 4 lb during the 8th month
    ○ 4. Presence of 1+ glucose in the urine

62. Which of the following statements best explains the pathophysiology of PIH?
    ○ 1. There is an increase in both plasma proteins and glomerular filtration.
    ○ 2. There is a decrease in aldosterone production and an increase in fluid retention.
    ○ 3. There is an increase in circulating blood volume and a decrease in cardiac output.
    ○ 4. There is a decrease in renal and uterine circulation because of vascular constriction.

63. The most likely goal of treatment for Betty, as for any mother with PIH, is to
    ○ 1. stabilize her vital signs.
    ○ 2. reduce the number and severity of headaches.
    ○ 3. increase urinary output.
    ○ 4. prevent convulsions.

64. Betty's symptoms worsen and she is admitted to the hospital. The physician orders an IV of 200 ml magnesium sulfate diluted in 10% dextrose in water. Which of the following findings would most likely lead the nurse to withhold magnesium sulfate and notify the physician?
    ○ 1. An apical pulse of 75/minute
    ○ 2. A hyperactive knee-jerk reflex
    ○ 3. A respiratory rate of less than 12/minute
    ○ 4. A urinary output of 50 ml/hour

65. Magnesium sulfate is often used in cases of severe PIH because its main action is which of the following?
    ○ 1. Central nervous system depressant
    ○ 2. Antihypertensive
    ○ 3. Diuretic
    ○ 4. Analgesic

66. Betty's labor is to be induced with 10 units of oxytocin (Pitocin). After the oxytocin is started, Betty becomes very uncomfortable during contractions and states, ''I don't think I'll be able to stand this pain.'' What would be the most appropriate initial nursing action?
    ○ 1. Call the physician.
    ○ 2. Give an analgesic.
    ○ 3. Help her try some breathing exercises.
    ○ 4. Increase the rate of the IV.

67. Betty's cervix is fully dilated. The physician makes the determination that the fetus will need to be delivered with the help of forceps. Because of the need for forceps, the nurse can expect which type of anesthesia will be used with Betty?
    ○ 1. Saddle block
    ○ 2. Paracervical block
    ○ 3. Pudendal block
    ○ 4. Local

68. Betty delivers a healthy infant of 38 weeks gestation. On Betty's first postpartum day, the nurse finds that her fundus is boggy. What is the first action the nurse should take?
    ○ 1. Lower the head of the bed.
    ○ 2. Firmly massage the fundus.
    ○ 3. Give 1 ampule of oxytocin (Pitocin) intramuscularly.
    ○ 4. Take her vital signs.

Charles Woodward, a 57-year-old salesman, has been admitted to the hospital with suspected cancer of the colon.

69. Mr. Woodward gives information for the nursing history. Which of the following is an etiologic factor strongly associated with cancer of the colon?
    ○ 1. Defecation pattern of every other day
    ○ 2. Diet high in acidic foods and low in bulk
    ○ 3. Exposure to x-rays
    ○ 4. Frequent constipation

70. Mr. Woodward is scheduled for a lower GI tract study. Which would be *inappropriate* to include in his care for this test?
    ○ 1. Breakfast of clear tea and toast, if the exam is within an hour of the test
    ○ 2. Castor oil or an enema, or both, before the test
    ○ 3. Low-cholesterol, low-fat diet 2 days prior to the test
    ○ 4. Tap water enemas till clear on the morning of the test

71. A malignant rectal tumor is diagnosed and Mr. Woodward is scheduled for surgery. Which of the following would *not* be included in Mr. Woodward's pre-op bowel preparation?
    ○ 1. Antibiotics
    ○ 2. Gastrointestinal decompression
    ○ 3. Kayexalate (sodium polystyrene sulfonate) enemas
    ○ 4. Low-residue diet

72. Mr. Woodward has an abdominoperineal resection and returns to the unit with a single-barreled sigmoid colostomy. Which of the following should the nurse expect following this surgical procedure?
    ○ 1. Continuous liquid stool until the client is discharged from the hospital
    ○ 2. Regulation of the colostomy
    ○ 3. Sanguinous drainage from the rectum mixed with feces
    ○ 4. Reconnection of the bowel after a short period of time

73. The nurse inspects the colostomy stoma as part of a post-op assessment and finds the tissue is moist with a slight bluish color. This would best be interpreted as which of the following?
    ○ 1. Early sign of necrosis
    ○ 2. Normal tissue, postsurgical trauma
    ○ 3. Infection
    4. Internal hemorrhage

74. During the first post-op day, nursing assessments of Mr. Woodward include
    ○ 1. taking rectal temperatures.
    ○ 2. noting passage of flatus.
    ○ 3. noting tolerance of oral intake.
    ○ 4. doing urine sugar and acetone test.

75. As Mr. Woodward recuperates, he begins instruction on colostomy irrigation. Which of the following should be included in the teaching?
    ○ 1. Irrigate well when diarrhea is present.
    ○ 2. Irrigate with 1,500 ml to 2,000 ml water.
    ○ 3. Lubricate the catheter tip with antibiotic ointment.
    ○ 4. Insert the catheter tip 3 to 4 inches.

76. Which of the following should be included in the teaching plan regarding common problems for the ostomate?
    ○ 1. Eat small, high-calorie meals if diarrhea occurs, until normal motility returns.
    ○ 2. Prevent hard stools with a laxative such as milk of magnesia up to 3 times per week.
    ○ 3. Colostomy odor can be reduced by taking charcoal and bismuth subcarbonate orally.
    ○ 4. Abdominal cramping can be relieved by small sips of ginger ale.

77. The effectiveness of diet teaching is evaluated as Mr. Woodward prepares for discharge. Mr. Woodward demonstrates his understanding of foods *least* likely to cause intestinal gas. Which list does he select?
    ○ 1. Canned peaches, red beets, squash
    ○ 2. Milk, lima beans, cheese
    ○ 3. Steak with onions, peas, corn
    ○ 4. Yogurt, cola, cheese

Five-year-old Tommy is scheduled for surgery to correct hypospadias.

78. In hypospadias, where is the urethral opening usually located?
    ○ 1. Anywhere along the ventral surface of the penis
    ○ 2. On the dorsal surface of the penis
    ○ 3. In the scrotal sac
    ○ 4. In the abdominal cavity

79. Which of the following signs and symptoms usually alerts the nurse to suspect hypospadias?
    ○ 1. Nausea and vomiting
    ○ 2. Urinary retention
    ○ 3. Abnormal urinary stream direction
    ○ 4. Ambiguous genitalia

80. When obtaining a health history for the child with hypospadias, it is most important to include a
    ○ 1. family history.
    ○ 2. history of childhood illnesses.
    ○ 3. history of immunizations.
    ○ 4. history of potty training techniques.

81. Pre-op nursing care should *not* include
    ○ 1. explanation to parents about the surgical procedure.
    ○ 2. explanation of the expected cosmetic results.
    ○ 3. explanation to the child about procedure.
    ○ 4. preparing the child for a nephrostomy tube.

82. Tommy's fears would most likely *not* include fear of
    ○ 1. mutilation.
    ○ 2. punishment for misdeeds.
    ○ 3. strange hospital environment.
    ○ 4. loss of sexuality.

83. Post-op care of the child with hypospadias repair does *not* include
    ○ 1. changing the surgical site dressing frequently.
    ○ 2. providing for quiet play.
    ○ 3. recording intake and output.
    ○ 4. supportive care for child and parents.

84. Postoperatively, Tommy develops a temperature of 100.4°F (38°C). Nursing actions should *not* include
    ○ 1. notifying the physician.
    ○ 2. encouraging additional oral fluid intake.
    ○ 3. providing a cool environment.
    ○ 4. starting oral penicillin.

85. Following surgical correction of hypospadias, which of the following data is *least* pertinent 3 months postoperatively?
    ○ **1.** The child is able to void in a standing position.
    ○ **2.** Genitalia appear normal or near-normal.
    ○ **3.** The organ appears to be sexually adequate.
    ○ **4.** Urinary tract infections are decreased.

Rose Potts, aged 24, has just delivered an 8 lb 4 oz boy whose Apgar scores are 8 at 1 minute and 9 at 5 minutes. She is transferred to the recovery room.

86. After several checks showed normal findings, the nurse finds the fundus is soft and 1 fingerbreadth above the umbilicus. What is the most appropriate nursing action?
    ○ **1.** Do nothing; this is normal.
    ○ **2.** Massage the fundus continuously until the physician arrives.
    ○ **3.** Place Mrs. Potts in semi-Fowler's position to compress the uterus.
    ○ **4.** Massage the fundus in a circular motion until it becomes firm.

87. The nursery brings the baby in to Mrs. Potts in order to initiate breast-feeding. How can the nurse best assist her?
    ○ **1.** Stay with her through the first feeding.
    ○ **2.** Leave her and the baby alone.
    ○ **3.** Ask her if she has any questions.
    ○ **4.** Give her a pamphlet on breast-feeding.

88. Mrs. Potts wants to know what benefits her baby derives from breast-feeding prior to the onset of milk production. What would be the nurse's best response?
    ○ **1.** "This is good practice time for the 2 of you."
    ○ **2.** "There are no particular benefits."
    ○ **3.** "The baby ingests colostrum, which contains antibodies, for the first 2 to 4 days."
    ○ **4.** "Early breast-feeding allows us to assess the infant's neurologic status."

89. What would be the best short-term goal of a teaching plan for Mrs. Potts?
    ○ **1.** Client will demonstrate confidence and relaxation during breast-feeding.
    ○ **2.** Infant will achieve a regular schedule (every 4 hours) for breast-feeding.
    ○ **3.** Client will supplement breast-feeding with formula.
    ○ **4.** Infant will nurse as long as he wishes for the first week.

90. Mrs. Potts develops postpartum cystitis. All the following nursing actions may aid in the prevention of postpartum cystitis. Which would be the *least* likely to do so?
    ○ **1.** Encourage voiding.
    ○ **2.** Ensure the first voiding postdelivery is adequate.
    ○ **3.** Give perineal care following each urination.
    ○ **4.** Provide a nutritional diet.

91. To determine whether Mrs. Potts is completely emptying her bladder, the nurse should
    ○ **1.** judge fundal height and percuss the bladder.
    ○ **2.** catheterize her after each voiding.
    ○ **3.** ask the mother whether she feels back pressure.
    ○ **4.** ask the mother to record each voiding.

Gabriel Pacetti, a 25-year-old construction worker, was injured when his foot and ankle were crushed by a heavy, jagged tool. The foot became cold and dark in color, and the pedal pulses were absent. He was scheduled for a below-the-knee amputation.

92. What instruction would the nurse give Mr. Pacetti if he were to be taught quadraceps-setting exercises preoperatively?
    ○ **1.** Alternately pinch the buttocks together and then relax them.
    ○ **2.** Lift the buttocks off the bed while lying flat.
    ○ **3.** Move the buttocks and both legs, so as to place the feet in plantar flexion.
    ○ **4.** Move the patellas proximally and press the popliteal spaces against the bed.

93. Which of the following would best be included in the plan of care for Mr. Pacetti during the first 24 hours postoperatively?
    ○ **1.** Apply a heating pad to the stump to relieve discomfort.
    ○ **2.** Have a tourniquet in view at the bedside.
    ○ **3.** Anticipate the need for large doses of narcotic analgesics.
    ○ **4.** Encourage him to look at the stump.

94. Following surgery, which is the best instruction to give Mr. Pacetti?
    ○ **1.** Keep the stump elevated on a pillow until the wound is healed.
    ○ **2.** Keep a pillow between the thighs when in a supine position.
    ○ **3.** Lie in a prone position for 30 minutes several times a day.
    ○ **4.** Apply lotion to the stump several times a day after the incision has healed.

95. Mr. Pacetti will be taught to use crutches until he can manage with a prosthesis independently. Which of the following crutch-walking instructions would be *incorrect*?

○ **1.** Extend the arms while holding weights to strengthen the triceps.

○ **2.** The crutches should be 16 inches less than the client's total height.

○ **3.** The axillary bars on the crutches should support the client's weight.

○ **4.** Both crutches and the affected leg are moved forward first, followed by the normal leg.

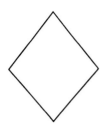

Test 1, Book IV
Answers with Rationales

1. **#2.** Anger and resentment often underlie guilt. The depressed client may not be ready to attend group therapy upon admission. When the psychiatrist orders group therapy, the client may or may not deal with her anger and resentment in that setting. Options #3 and #4 do not facilitate expression of guilty feelings. IMPLEMENTATION (PSYCHOSOCIAL, MENTAL HEALTH, PSYCHIATRIC PROBLEMS/ELATED-DEPRESSIVE BEHAVIOR)

2. **#3.** In a psychotic depression, the client loses contact with reality. This may be manifested by a fixed false belief (delusion), such as paranoid ideation that evil forces will destroy the client. Reactive depression is related to grief reactions and usually does not include distortions of thought severe enough to be considered delusions. Delusions are also not characteristic of neurotic and transitory depression. ANALYSIS (PSYCHOSOCIAL, MENTAL HEALTH, PSYCHIATRIC PROBLEMS/ELATED-DEPRESSIVE BEHAVIOR)

3. **#4.** Options #1 to #3 may apply to a number of other health care problems; #4 is specific to depression. ASSESSMENT (PSYCHOSOCIAL, MENTAL HEALTH, PSYCHIATRIC PROBLEMS/ELATED-DEPRESSIVE BEHAVIOR)

4. **#1.** The negative view of the self and the future are indicated by option #1. It is these cognitive changes that best indicate depression. #2 indicates that she at times feels bad; however, she also demonstrates awareness of her mood and her style of coping. This is not an indication of suffering from depression. Options #3 and #4 indicate a need for further assessment but do not necessarily indicate depression. ASSESSMENT (PSYCHOSOCIAL, MENTAL HEALTH, PSYCHIATRIC PROBLEMS/ELATED-DEPRESSIVE BEHAVIOR)

5. **#4.** Options #1 through #3 are commonly associated with depression. Ataxia, an inability to coordinate voluntary muscular movements, has not been reported in depression. ASSESSMENT (PSYCHOSOCIAL, MENTAL HEALTH, PSYCHIATRIC PROBLEMS/ELATED-DEPRESSIVE BEHAVIOR)

6. **#3.** The term retarded depression refers to the client who presents with general physical and cognitive slowness, head hanging, looking haggard and sitting idly. Such clients are usually indecisive and uncooperative, but not argumentative. ASSESSMENT (PSYCHOSOCIAL, MENTAL HEALTH, PSYCHIATRIC PROBLEMS/ELATED-DEPRESSIVE BEHAVIOR)

7. **#1.** Although depression is the most frequently complained of emotional illness, schizophrenia accounts for the largest number of psychiatric hospitalizations. Phobic reactions do not normally require hospitalization. Autism is not a common condition and occurs usually in childhood. While depression is a common condition, it does not often require hospitalization. ANALYSIS (PSYCHOSOCIAL, MENTAL HEALTH, PSYCHIATRIC PROBLEMS/ELATED-DEPRESSIVE BEHAVIOR)

8. **#3.** Identification means that a person takes on certain qualities associated with others. Idealization is the conscious or unconscious overestimation of another's attributes. Introjection refers to the incorporation of the traits of others, internalizing feelings toward others. Substitution refers to unconscious attempts to make up for a deficiency in one area by concentrating efforts in another area that is more attainable. ASSESSMENT (PSYCHOSOCIAL, MENTAL HEALTH, PSYCHIATRIC PROBLEMS/ELATED-DEPRESSIVE BEHAVIOR)

9. **#3.** Hypotension, not hypertension, may occur as a side effect. Options #1, #2, and #4 are side effects of Elavil and, therefore, require nurses' consideration. ASSESSMENT (PSYCHOSOCIAL, MENTAL HEALTH, PSYCHIATRIC PROBLEMS/ELATED-DEPRESSIVE BEHAVIOR)

10. **#4.** Clients who take tricyclic antidepressants such as amitriptyline HCl should not be given MAO inhibitors either simultaneously or immediately following treatment. Isocarboxid should be withheld until orders are clarified. ANALYSIS (PSYCHOSOCIAL, MENTAL HEALTH, PSYCHIATRIC PROBLEMS/ELATED-DEPRESSIVE BEHAVIOR)

11. **#4.** Marplan, as well as phenelzine (Nardil) and tranylcypromine (Parnate) are MAO inhibitors. When these drugs are combined with tyramine-containing foods, e.g., aged cheese and alcoholic beverages, the reaction cited in the question can occur. Side effects of tricyclics (Elavil and Tofranil) are associated with hyponot hypertension. Side effects of lithium are not associated with cardiovascular changes unless toxic levels are reached. Then the changes are hypotensive. IMPLEMENTATION (PSYCHOSOCIAL, MENTAL HEALTH, PSYCHIATRIC PROBLEMS/ ELATED-DEPRESSIVE BEHAVIOR)

12. **#2.** Unless the client is first assessed for self-harm or suicide potential, the staff will not observe the necessary degree of vigilance needed in the client's environment. While essential, physical needs are not the most critical concern with a depressive client. Though client may be encouraged to attend group therapy as part of the treatment plan, the client's safety takes precedence. Response to medication takes time and is not an initial concern. ASSESSMENT (PSYCHOSOCIAL, MENTAL HEALTH, PSYCHIATRIC PROBLEMS/ELATED-DEPRESSIVE BEHAVIOR)

13. **#3.** The nurse must consider the seriousness and the rapidity with which the client may die unless intervention occurs following a suicide attempt. The lethality of the method may give indications about the seriousness of the client's attempt. Following options #2 and #4, death can occur quickly and is highly likely. Following ingestion of sufficient quantities of barbiturates/sedatives, the client can also die because of central nervous system depression. Scratching one's wrists has a lower lethality than options #1, #2, and #4, and also has a lower lethality than cutting the veins of the wrist. ANALYSIS (PSYCHOSOCIAL, MENTAL HEALTH, PSYCHIATRIC PROBLEMS/ELATED-DEPRESSIVE BEHAVIOR)

14. **#4.** Specialists in suicidology have developed profiles of high-risk groups. Generally, persons cited in options #1 through #3 have a higher risk of suicide than married men. Alcoholics have a high risk associated with lack of impulse control. Women *attempt* suicide more frequently than men (3:1), but men *commit* suicide more often than women by a 3:1 ratio. Suicide rates vary according to marital status with married persons having the lowest rates, followed by the never married. Widowed or divorced persons have the highest rate. ASSESSMENT (PSYCHOSOCIAL, MENTAL HEALTH, PSYCHIATRIC PROBLEMS/ELATED-DEPRESSIVE BEHAVIOR)

15. **#1.** The immunization schedule recommended by the American Academy of Pediatrics suggests giving the first immunization at 2 months of age. ASSESSMENT (CHILD/NUTRITION AND METABOLISM)

16. **#3.** Stools usually become small and infrequent, depending on the amount of food passing through the gut. Lethargy may be present if the fluid and electrolyte imbalances are significant. ASSESSMENT (CHILD/NUTRITION AND METABOLISM)

17. **#2.** An infant with pyloric stenosis often suffers from fluid and electrolyte imbalances, primarily from vomiting. These need to be corrected prior to surgery; a child in proper acid-base and fluid balance is a much better surgical risk. PLAN (CHILD/NUTRITION AND METABOLISM)

18. **#2.** The obstruction is at the pyloric sphincter. The child becomes dehydrated from vomiting; thus, metabolic alkalosis and hypokalemia are common findings. ANALYSIS (CHILD/NUTRITION AND METABOLISM)

19. **#1.** Potassium is excreted through the kidneys. If the client is not voiding and potassium is infusing, levels rapidly become toxic. ASSESSMENT (CHILD/NUTRITION AND METABOLISM)

20. **#4.** Since restraints can severely restrict circulation and injure tissue, they must be checked frequently and regularly. IMPLEMENTATION (CHILD/NUTRITION AND METABOLISM)

21. **#3.** Feedings are usually started shortly after surgery. Parents may have become negatively conditioned to pre-op vomiting, so they need to be included in positive post-op feeding experiences. Hypoglycemia may occur as a result of pre-op depletion of hepatic glycogen. PLAN (CHILD/NUTRITION AND METABOLISM)

22. **#3.** This position facilitates emptying of the stomach by taking advantage of the normal curvature of the stomach. PLAN (CHILD/NUTRITION AND METABOLISM)

23. **#4.** The usual response following surgery for pyloric stenosis includes some vomiting up to about 48 hours post-op. ASSESSMENT (CHILD/NUTRITION AND METABOLISM)

24. **#3.** This indicates parent learning has taken place. EVALUATION (CHILD/NUTRITION AND METABOLISM)

25. **#2.** Perfect matches of all four HLAs are found in monozygotic twins and 25% of natural siblings (born of the same pair of parents). The degree of compatibility of remaining siblings varies. IMPLEMENTATION (ADULT/ELIMINATION)

26. **#1.** An immunosuppressive drug depresses the ability of the immune system to respond to infection. IMPLEMENTATION (ADULT/ELIMINATION)

27. **#4.** A rising WBC level is associated with infection. The WBCs are depressed during successful immunosuppressive therapy. ASSESSMENT (ADULT/ELIMINATION)

28. **#1.** Opening a closed urinary drainage system presents a grave risk of infection for the immunosuppressed client. PLAN (ADULT/ELIMINATION)

29. **#3.** A witnessed, cosigned donor card is appropriate for the client who is a minor. IMPLEMENTATION (ADULT/ELIMINATION)

30. **#2.** Prednisone was prescribed for its immunosuppressive effects. Withdrawal of the drug makes it more likely the body will reject the transplanted tissue. ANALYSIS (ADULT/ELIMINATION)

31. **#1.** Ovulation is believed to occur just before, at, or just after the temperature drop. Progesterone has a thermogenic effect causing a rise in temperature. ASSESSMENT (CHILDBEARING FAMILY/ANTEPARTAL CARE)

32. **#1.** Ovulation occurs 24 to 30 hours after the appearance of luteinizing hormone. ASSESSMENT (CHILDBEARING FAMILY/ANTEPARTAL CARE)

33. **#2.** Increased amounts of gonadotropins (follicle-stimulating hormone, luteinizing hormone) stimulate the maturation of the ovarian follicle, followed by ovulation, and later, development of the functioning corpus luteum. ANALYSIS (CHILDBEARING FAMILY/ANTEPARTAL CARE)

34. **#1.** To correctly evaluate chest pain, it is essential to obtain an accurate description. Also, this question can elicit the client's knowledge about heart attacks. This will provide a basis for the discharge teaching plan. IMPLEMENTATION (ADULT/OXYGENATION)

35. **#1.** An electrocardiogram reflects the electrochemical activity of the heart (i.e., the transmission of the cardiac impulse through the heart muscle). Information about heart perfusion, contraction, and integrity is inferred from this information but not measured directly. ANALYSIS (ADULT/OXYGENATION)

36. **#4.** When an organ such as the heart is damaged, it releases specific enzymes into the blood stream. ANALYSIS (ADULT/OXYGENATION)

37. **#2.** Options #1, #3, and #4 do not relate to chest pain in any way. ANALYSIS (ADULT/OXYGENATION)

38. **#3.** The coronary arteries fill, and the aortic and pulmonary valves close during ventricular diastole. ANALYSIS (ADULT/OXYGENATION)

39. **#3.** gr 1/150 = 0.4 mg. ANALYSIS (ADULT/OXYGENATION)

40. **#3.** Sublingual nitroglycerin appears in the bloodstream in about 2 minutes and peaks in 4 minutes; the effect begins to disappear in 10 minutes. IMPLEMENTATION (ADULT/OXYGENATION)

41. **#1.** Because of its dilating effect, nitroglycerin may cause headache, hypotension, and dizziness. ASSESSMENT (ADULT/OXYGENATION)

42. **#3.** Fresh nitroglycerin tablets cause a burning, tingling sensation. IMPLEMENTATION (ADULT/OXYGENATION)

43. **#2.** Pain patterns of angina vary from individual to individual but usually are the same in one individual. A change may indicate new ischemic areas. IMPLEMENTATION (ADULT/OXYGENATION)

44. **#2.** Propranolol (Inderal) is a beta-adrenergic blocking agent. As such, it blocks the bronchodilator effect of sympathetic (adrenergic) stimulation and is contraindicated for all chronic obstructive lung conditions. ANALYSIS (ADULT/OXYGENATION)

45. **#4.** All the options are important, but the underlying problem is bradycardia and heart block, detected by taking an apical pulse. IMPLEMENTATION (ADULT/OXYGENATION)

46. #2. Cheese is high in fat and sodium content, which makes it unsuitable for a cardiac client. PLAN (ADULT/OXYGENATION)

47. #2. A cardiac catheterization is done to confirm heart disease, determine the extent of heart disease, obtain pressures, measure oxygen in the blood, and inject contrast medium for angiography. ANALYSIS (ADULT/OXYGENATION)

48. #2. The client is responsible for his own health care and has a right to choose his own habits. The nurse has a right to insist on a model of health behavior in class. PLAN (ADULT/OXYGENATION)

49. #3. This is indicative of decreased total blood volume, since hematocrit is a measure of packed red blood cells per 100 ml of blood volume. ASSESSMENT (CHILD/SENSATION, PERCEPTION, PROTECTION)

50. #3. These symptoms are indicative of fluid overload resulting in congestive heart failure. ASSESSMENT (CHILD/SENSATION, PERCEPTION, PROTECTION)

51. #2. Restriction of visitors is unnecessary if they are healthy and are instructed in proper isolation technique. PLAN (CHILD/SENSATION, PERCEPTION, PROTECTION)

52. #1. Ten ml/hour is indicative of an abnormally low urinary output. However, the first measure is always to see if the catheter is patent. If it is, the next step would be to notify the physician. IMPLEMENTATION (CHILD/SENSATION, PERCEPTION, PROTECTION)

53. #4. Proteins and carbohydrates are needed for wound healing and tissue replacement. The other options do not achieve these goals primarily. PLAN (CHILD/SENSATION, PERCEPTION, PROTECTION)

54. #3. Fantasy, play therapy that allows expression of emotions, is best for preschoolers. IMPLEMENTATION (CHILD/ILL AND HOSPITALIZED CHILD)

55. #4. In areas outside their delusional system, these clients are in good contact with reality with no impairment of intellectual functioning. Suspicious behavior, superiority, and hostility are characteristics of paranoia and cause others to withdraw from such a client. ASSESSMENT (PSYCHOSOCIAL, MENTAL HEALTH, PSYCHIATRIC PROBLEMS/SUSPICIOUS BEHAVIOR)

56. #1. A fixed delusional system is characterized by a belief system that is rigid and inaccessible to reason and modification, although the basic premise on which the system is based is illogical. An hallucination is an imagined sensory perception that occurs without an external stimulus. Acting-out and manipulative behaviors occur in clients with manic-depressive disorder and personality disorders such as borderline personality disorder. ANALYSIS (PSYCHOSOCIAL, MENTAL HEALTH, PSYCHIATRIC PROBLEMS/SUSPICIOUS BEHAVIOR)

57. #3. Trying to reason with the client, correct his beliefs, or delve into the content will cause the client to work harder at improving the delusion, thereby reinforcing it and making it more entrenched. The nurse should acknowledge to Mr. Benson that it must be upsetting to feel as he does. This will promote trust by providing empathy. Thus, the nurse begins to build the relationship with the client. If the nurse focuses on the content and details of the delusion or acknowledges the delusion as reality, she gives it credibility, which reinforces it. IMPLEMENTATION (PSYCHOSOCIAL, MENTAL HEALTH, PSYCHIATRIC PROBLEMS/SUSPICIOUS BEHAVIOR)

58. #3. Presenting reality is the best response. Tell the client who you are, concisely and specifically. Communication should avoid reinforcing the client's delusion. In option #1, the nurse does not understand how the client feels and the response could be interpreted as a reinforcement of his delusional system. Ignoring his comment can cause his anxiety to rise or he may interpret the nurse's silence as agreement. Rational explanations will only make the client adhere more firmly to the delusion. IMPLEMENTATION (PSYCHOSOCIAL, MENTAL HEALTH, PSYCHIATRIC PROBLEMS/SUSPICIOUS BEHAVIOR)

59. #4. The nurse cannot talk the client out of his suspicions. Serving foods in sealed containers may diminish the client's anxiety. It is also possible that the action may not, but it allows him some control about whether to eat. Option #2 may lead the client to conclude that the nurse believes there may be some reality to his delusion *or* is refuting his belief. This is a "no-win" option. After the nurse tastes it, he can reply that the poison will be slow to kill. He may believe that you are both going to die from poisoned food. IMPLEMENTATION (PSYCHOSOCIAL, MENTAL HEALTH, PSYCHIATRIC PROBLEMS/SUSPICIOUS BEHAVIOR)

60. #2. Photosensitivity, not photophobia, is a side effect of Thorazine. Abrupt onset of sore throat, fever, malaise, and sores in the mouth may mean that agranulocytosis has occurred. A complete blood count should be done immediately to see if leukopenia is present. Postural hypotension usually occurs early in the course of treatment and disappears 1 or 2 weeks after the dose is stabilized. Pruritic maculopapular rash (dermatitis) is a common allergic response. Contact dermatitis can also occur from contact with the liquid concentrate or tablets. ASSESSMENT (PSYCHOSOCIAL, MENTAL HEALTH, PSYCHIATRIC PROBLEMS/SUSPICIOUS BEHAVIOR)

61. #2. Swelling in the upper part of the body is more significant than dependent edema of the lower extremities. The blood pressure rise in option #1 is not significant enough to indicate a problem. Protein in the urine, not glucose, would be a significant finding. ASSESSMENT (CHILDBEARING FAMILY/ANTEPARTAL CARE)

62. #4. The primary problem is a generalized vasospasm leading to uterine insufficiency. There is a decrease in plasma proteins as a result of hypoproteinemia and a decrease in glomerular filtration due to vasoconstriction. Sodium and water retention is augmented by an increase in aldosterone. Cardiac output falls as the result of hypovolemia. ANALYSIS (CHILDBEARING FAMILY/ANTEPARTAL CARE)

63. #4. There is no cure for PIH except delivery of the child. The aim of all treatment is to prevent progression of the disease to eclampsia. PLAN (CHILDBEARING FAMILY/ANTEPARTAL CARE)

64. #3. A decreased respiratory rate indicates central nervous system depression from the magnesium sulfate. The pulse rate and urinary output listed are within normal limits. The drug produces hypoactive reflexes. ASSESSMENT (CHILDBEARING FAMILY/ANTEPARTAL CARE)

65. #1. Magnesium sulfate is used to depress the central nervous system. It also reduces blood pressure and produces diuresis, but this is not its main action. ANALYSIS (CHILDBEARING FAMILY/ANTEPARTAL CARE)

66. #3. When the client seems to be losing control, the first action should be to help the client cope with the contractions through breathing and relaxation. Analgesia should not be used in early labor. IMPLEMENTATION (CHILDBEARING FAMILY/INTRAPARTAL CARE)

67. #1. A saddle block is an intradural anesthetic that affects the sensory and motor pathways. The client is therefore unable to push during the second stage of labor. This is desirable if forceps are indicated. That ability is not lost with the other types of anesthesia listed. ANALYSIS (CHILDBEARING FAMILY/INTRAPARTAL CARE)

68. #2. Firmly massaging the fundus is always the first action to take with a boggy uterus. If that is ineffective, oxytocin may need to be ordered. These measures will contract the uterus, preventing hemorrhage. IMPLEMENTATION (CHILDBEARING FAMILY/POSTPARTAL CARE)

69. #4. One theory regarding the etiology of colon cancer postulates that fecal contents are carcinogenic and that prolonged contact with the bowel wall (as in constipation) promotes cancer. Overnutrition and a diet high in fat are also linked with cancer of the colon. X-ray exposure is associated with leukemia. ASSESSMENT (ADULT/ELIMINATION)

70. #3. Preparation for a lower GI tract study includes clear liquids the day or evening prior to the test and a low-residue diet for 1 to 3 days before the test. IMPLEMENTATION (ADULT/ELIMINATION)

71. #3. Kayexalate enemas are given to reduce serum potassium levels. Cleansing enemas would be given to reduce bacteria and fecal matter in the bowel; antibiotics are given to reduce gastrointestinal flora. PLAN (ADULT/ELIMINATION)

72. #2. A single-barreled colostomy is always permanent. When the sigmoid colon has been preserved, regulation of bowel evacuation is possible, because stool is more formed here. Some such ostomates will be able to go without a colostomy bag. Others may find varying need for one, depending on their diet and success with irrigation. ANALYSIS (ADULT/ELIMINATION)

73. #1. The bluish color is a sign of decreased vascularity of the tissue. The stoma should appear pink and moist. ANALYSIS (ADULT/ELIMINATION)

74. #2. The passage of flatus signals the return of gastrointestinal motility. (Flatus may also appear as air in the colostomy bag.) Rectal temperatures are contraindicated; the rectum was removed and the anal area was sutured or packed with a dressing following an abdomino-perineal resection. Oral intake is not usually begun for several days, and sugar and acetone tests are needed only if the client is a diabetic or is receiving hyperalimentation. PLAN (ADULT/ELIMINATION)

75. #4. The irrigation catheter may be inserted up to 4 inches. Use 1,000 ml of water or less to irrigate; more may produce abdominal cramping. Do not irrigate if diarrhea is present to prevent further electrolyte imbalance. The catheter tip should be lubricated, but antibiotic preparations are not necessary. IMPLEMENTATION (ADULT/ELIMINATION)

76. #3. Ostomates sometimes find odor is reduced by taking charcoal or bismuth subcarbonate, with the physician's approval. Clear liquids such as tea and water are advised during diarrhea, and the physician should be notifed in order to monitor electrolyte imbalances. Stool softeners such as docusate sodium (Colace) can help prevent hard stools, but laxatives are not advised. Carbonated beverages can exacerbate cramping. IMPLEMENTATION (ADULT/ELIMINATION)

77. #1. These are the only foods listed that are not known gas producers. Legumes, onions, peas, cabbage, carbonated beverages, nuts, and chewing gum often cause gas. Milk can cause gas in clients with a lactose intolerance. Foods that caused gas prior to the surgery will continue to cause a problem. EVALUATION (ADULT/ELIMINATION)

78. #1. Hypospadias is located anywhere along the ventral surface of the penile shaft. In mild cases, the opening is just off center of the glans; in the most severe cases, it is on the perineum. ASSESSMENT (CHILD/ELIMINATION)

79. #3. Nausea and vomiting are unrelated to hypospadias. Urinary retention is due to obstruction of flow and is not the case with hypospadias. Ambiguous genitalia may be seen in conjunction with hypospadias in severe cases, but it is not the norm. The abnormal stream direction is often the first indication. ASSESSMENT (CHILD/ELIMINATION)

80. #1. Family history is important because certain genitourinary anomalies are familial. Childhood illness, immunizations, and potty training do not have significance for embryonic development (and detection) of these anomalies. ASSESSMENT (CHILD/ELIMINATION)

81. #4. Diversion of urinary flow is usually accomplished with an urethral-bladder catheter. A nephrostomy tube is uncommon because the kidneys are not usually involved. Explanation to child/parents is important along with explanation of expected outcome so there are no surprises. PLAN (CHILD/ELIMINATION)

82. #4. The 4-year-old has not developmentally defined completely his sexuality while fear of mutilation is common to this age group. Also, fear of punishment for misdeeds is common in the preschool child. ANALYSIS (CHILD/ELIMINATION)

83. #1. Dressings are usually not changed for several days to allow the plastic surgery repair to heal. Providing quiet play is essential for the young hospitalized child, as well as giving support to the child/family. PLAN (CHILD/ELIMINATION)

84. #4. Medications are ordered by the physician and then given by the physician or nurse. Increased fluids will help hydration and decrease the elevated temperature. Notifying the physician is appropriate. Providing a cool environment decreases fluid loss by perspiration and allows for decreased metabolic rate. IMPLEMENTATION (CHILD/ELIMINATION)

85. #4. Urinary tract infections are not a primary concern. The other data indicate the male child can function within the physical and psychosocial habits of the male sex. EVALUATION (CHILD/ELIMINATION)

86. #4. The uterus is best returned to firmness by intermittent massage. IMPLEMENTATION (CHILDBEARING FAMILY/POSTPARTAL CARE)

87. #1. An experienced nurse should be available to mothers who are beginning breast-feeding, to provide explanation and reinforcement. Written material may be helpful but is no substitute for one-on-one teaching. IMPLEMENTATION (CHILDBEARING FAMILY/POSTPARTAL CARE)

88. **#3.** Colostrum is secreted for 2 to 3 days after birth and is rich in antibodies. Early breast-feeding not only allows for practice but stimulates the production of breast milk. Neurologic status is best assessed through observation of the Moro reflex. IMPLEMENTATION (CHILDBEARING FAMILY/POSTPARTAL CARE)

89. **#1.** The let-down reflex can be influenced profoundly by the mother's emotions. An immediate short-term goal would be that the client is able to confidently initiate the process of breast-feeding. Breast-feeding is generally done on demand. Supplements are discouraged until breast-feeding is successfully established. Time the infant breast-feeds is controlled initially to prevent nipple breakdown. PLAN (CHILDBEARING FAMILY/POSTPARTAL CARE)

90. **#4.** The postpartum client is vulnerable to the development of cystitis. The diet would be least likely to prevent this condition. Keeping the bladder empty will prevent urinary stasis, a common cause of cystitis. Perineal care will reduce microorganisms that may ascend into the urinary tract. IMPLEMENTATION (CHILDBEARING FAMILY/POSTPARTAL CARE)

91. **#1.** When the bladder is not emptied, it may push the uterus upward and to the side of the abdomen. On percussion, a full bladder emits a dull sound. IMPLEMENTATION (CHILDBEARING FAMILY/POSTPARTAL CARE)

92. **#4.** This motion is the only one listed that uses the quadriceps muscles to perform. Thus it increases their strength. IMPLEMENTATION (ADULT/ACTIVITY AND REST)

93. **#2.** Hemorrhage has very serious consequences. The first post-op day is too early for the client to accept his loss (option #4), and temperature sense in the stump is too impaired to risk a hot pad. The pain after amputation is almost always quite mild. IMPLEMENTATION (ADULT/ACTIVITY AND REST)

94. **#3.** This position prevents hip contracture. Lotion is contraindicated for the stump; it keeps the skin soft with increased risk of skin breakdown. Elevating the stump after the first 24 hours results in flexion contractures and a pillow between the thighs promotes abduction fixation. Both of these result in difficulty walking with the prosthesis. IMPLEMENTATION (ADULT/ACTIVITY AND REST)

95. **#3.** Pressure on the axillae causes pressure on the brachial plexus. This can lead to paralysis of the arms. IMPLEMENTATION (ADULT/ACTIVITY AND REST)

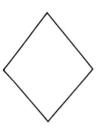

Test 2

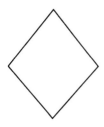

Test 2, Book I Questions

Twenty-six-month-old Crystal visits the well-child clinic for a checkup.

1. When assessing Crystal's development, the nurse should expect her to exhibit which one of the following abilities?
   - ○ 1. Dressing herself unassisted
   - ○ 2. Pointing to parts of her body when asked
   - ○ 3. Drawing a person with 3 to 6 parts
   - ○ 4. Speaking in 4- to 5-word sentences

2. During the otoscopic examination, Crystal cries loudly and tries to pull away. What is the best approach?
   - ○ 1. Explain to Crystal why you must look into her ears.
   - ○ 2. Postpone the ear exam until Crystal's next visit when she will be older.
   - ○ 3. Say to her, "I thought you were a big girl, Crystal."
   - ○ 4. Get someone to restrain Crystal and proceed with the exam.

3. Crystal's mother mentions that she and her husband have been trying to toilet train Crystal because she seems interested. Which of the following would *not* facilitate this process?
   - ○ 1. Give Crystal a toy to play with while she sits on the potty.
   - ○ 2. Dress her in clothing with Velcro fasteners.
   - ○ 3. Provide her with her own potty chair.
   - ○ 4. Respond matter-of-factly when Crystal has an "accident."

4. Crystal's mother tells you, "Crystal just doesn't seem to eat enough; I don't know where she gets all her energy." After assessing the child's condition and finding no evidence of nutritional deficiency, the nurse's best response is which of the following?
   - ○ 1. "You may want to increase her milk intake to be sure she gets enough calories."
   - ○ 2. "Why don't you double her daily vitamin and mineral dose for your peace of mind?"
   - ○ 3. "Try giving her small portions of a variety of foods and allow her to decide which of those foods she will eat."
   - ○ 4. "It's best at this age to insist that she take at least 2 bites of the foods you offer her to be sure she is getting enough to eat."

Andrew Goll, a 56-year-old rancher, is admitted for an episode of acute pancreatitis. This is Mr. Goll's eighth admission for this disorder over the past 3 years.

5. Pancreatitis can best be described as an
   - ○ 1. infectious disease of the pancreas primarily seen in the black population.
   - ○ 2. inherited disease affecting the pancreas and is primarily seen in the black population.
   - ○ 3. inflammation of the pancreas resulting in obstruction and edema.
   - ○ 4. outpouching of the pancreas.

6. The nurse knows that the pancreas is responsible for secreting
   - ○ 1. sucrose, peptidase, lipase, and amylase.
   - ○ 2. amylase, lactase, trypsin, and chymotrypsin.
   - ○ 3. amylase, lipase, pepsin, and peptidase.
   - ○ 4. amylase, lipase, trypsin, and chymotrypsin.

7. Which of the following would be an unlikely finding with pancreatitis?
   - ○ 1. Hypoglycemia
   - ○ 2. Extreme epigastric pain
   - ○ 3. Elevated serum and urine amylase
   - ○ 4. Abdominal distension

8. Mr. Goll's laboratory values show hypocalcemia as a result of the inadequate metabolism of
   - ○ 1. fat.
   - ○ 2. protein.
   - ○ 3. starch.
   - ○ 4. glucose.

9. In planning for adequate nutrition for Mr. Goll, which of the following would be considered *inappropriate*?
   - ○ 1. Administer cholinergic drugs.
   - ○ 2. Supplement nutrition with IV fluids.
   - ○ 3. Give clear liquids after inflammation subsides.
   - ○ 4. Include a bland diet in the teaching plan.

10. Mr. Goll is complaining of severe pain. The physician has ordered meperidine (Demerol) and morphine. The nurse chooses meperidine. The best reason for selecting meperidine is that
    ○ 1. meperidine depresses respirations less than morphine.
    ○ 2. meperidine exerts its effects on striated muscles.
    ○ 3. morphine has a tendency to produce spasms of the sphincter of Oddi.
    ○ 4. morphine has less effect on smooth muscle.

Tim Lampert, a 52-year-old alcoholic, has been drinking excessively for 20 years. He drinks 2 pints of whiskey daily. For the last 2 days, he has cut his drinking back to 1 pint per day. While he plans to stop drinking, he decided to keep drinking 1 pint a day to avoid withdrawal symptoms.

11. Mr. Lampert comes to the emergency room of his community hospital with an elevated blood pressure, tremors, and ''nervousness.'' He tells the nurse his drinking history and how he cut back, but did not stop, drinking. The nurse needs to be most alert for which of the following?
    ○ 1. Increased withdrawal symptoms
    ○ 2. Possible stroke
    ○ 3. Cardiac arrest
    ○ 4. Increased anxiety reactions

12. While in the hospital, Mr. Lampert is believed to be in the early stages of Korsakoff's syndrome. Which of the following symptoms is most common with this disease?
    ○ 1. Chronic gastritis
    ○ 2. Excessive perspiration
    ○ 3. Confabulation
    ○ 4. Fatty liver

13. Mr. Lampert tells the nurse that the effects of alcohol on his body frighten him. He wants to quit but is afraid he cannot do it. Which of the following nursing actions would be most helpful at this point in the treatment program?
    ○ 1. Discuss coping mechanisms he might use under stress other than alcohol.
    ○ 2. Discuss ways to decrease the number of his social contacts.
    ○ 3. Find ways he can decrease the amount of emotional support he needs from others.
    ○ 4. Recommend psychoanalysis as part of discharge planning.

14. Mr. Lampert starts his disulfiram (Antabuse) regimen while in the hospital. The nurse, when teaching him what may occur if he ingests alcohol, will tell him to be aware of
    ○ 1. increased blood pressure, pulse, and respirations.
    ○ 2. headache, pallor, vomiting.
    ○ 3. nausea and vomiting, flushed face, decreased blood pressure.
    ○ 4. ataxia, muscle contractions, dilated pupils.

15. Mr. Lampert and his family have agreed to start family therapy. The nurse should tell them to expect that the focus of the therapy would primarily be on
    ○ 1. Mr. Lampert's drinking problem.
    ○ 2. Mrs. Lampert and the ways in which her behavior may cause her husband to drink.
    ○ 3. increasing communication between the family members.
    ○ 4. teaching the family members to be more like each other.

Annie Daugherty is a 28-year-old multigravida admitted to the labor room in active labor. The nurse admitting Mrs. Daugherty determines that her cervix is 90% effaced and the fetus is in left occiput posterior position, with a fetal heart rate of 136. The cervix is 4 cm dilated, and the fetus is at −1 station.

16. Which type of breathing and relaxation techniques would be appropriate for Mrs. Daugherty to use at this time?
    ○ 1. Panting
    ○ 2. Candle blowing
    ○ 3. Accelerated
    ○ 4. Slow abdominal

17. Fetal heart rate is being evaluated by the use of a fetoscope. When is the most appropriate time to listen to fetal heart sounds?
    ○ 1. During uterine contractions
    ○ 2. 60 seconds after uterine contractions
    ○ 3. During and immediately following uterine contractions
    ○ 4. Immediately following uterine contractions

18. Mrs. Daugherty complains of severe back pain. Which nursing action would be best?
    ○ 1. Apply a warm pad to the sacral area.
    ○ 2. Encourage her to bear down.
    ○ 3. Keep her flat with a pillow under her head.
    ○ 4. Turn her to Sims's position and apply sacral pressure.

19. Mrs. Daugherty's membranes rupture spontaneously. In addition to assessing the color of the fluid, what is the most important nursing action at that time?
   ○ 1. Call the physician.
   ○ 2. Take the fetal heart rate.
   ○ 3. Time the contractions.
   ○ 4. Move her to the delivery room.

20. Which of the following most likely indicates that the third stage of labor is coming to an end?
   ○ 1. The episiotomy is being performed.
   ○ 2. Dilatation and effacement are complete.
   ○ 3. The birth of the baby is completed.
   ○ 4. There is a gush of blood from the vagina and a lengthening of the cord.

Jennifer Theil, a 60-year-old homemaker, was admitted to the orthopedic unit and is scheduled for a left, total hip replacement in 3 days. She states that she has had severe pain in the hip for several years and takes large doses of aspirin. She says she has no other health problems.

21. Which of the following would normally *not* be included as part of her pre-op lab work?
   ○ 1. Blood type and crossmatch
   ○ 2. Prothrombin time
   ○ 3. Sedimentation rate
   ○ 4. Bence Jones protein

22. Which of the following would be *inappropriate* to include in Mrs. Theil's plan of care preoperatively?
   ○ 1. Teach her to use the trapeze.
   ○ 2. Measure her for antiembolic hose.
   ○ 3. Restrict her to bed rest.
   ○ 4. Teach her the bedpan exercise.

23. Mrs. Theil is at risk of an infection developing in the operative site. Which of the following measures will *not* prevent this complication?
   ○ 1. Scrub the leg BID before surgery with a bacteriostatic soap.
   ○ 2. Caution the client not to shave any part of the body.
   ○ 3. Use reverse isolation for 3 days preoperatively.
   ○ 4. Restrict in-and-out traffic in the surgical suite during the operation.

24. Which of the following nursing measures would be *inappropriate* for Mrs. Theil postoperatively?
   ○ 1. Schedule active range of motion to both ankles.
   ○ 2. Remind her to keep her toes pointed outward.
   ○ 3. Assist her to pivot on the unaffected foot.
   ○ 4. Remind her not to cross her legs.

25. Your post-op assessment of circulation would include the blanching sign. What is the best definition of blanching?
   ○ 1. It is a test of adequate venous circulation.
   ○ 2. The pink color returns in 2 seconds after pressure on the nail bed is released.
   ○ 3. It is the absence of color from the nail bed when pressure is applied.
   ○ 4. It is a test for adequate arterial blood flow.

26. Mrs. Theil has a wound drain connected to suction. During the first 8 hours, there were 100 ml of bright bloody drainage. She is alert and her vital signs are stable. Which of the following nursing actions would be most appropriate?
   ○ 1. Notify the physician.
   ○ 2. Apply a pressure dressing to the wound.
   ○ 3. Continue to observe and record the amount of drainage.
   ○ 4. Anticipate a stat order for a transfusion by ordering up a unit of blood.

27. Which of the following is a common sequela of a total hip replacement within the first post-op week?
   ○ 1. Urinary retention
   ○ 2. Contractures
   ○ 3. Weight loss
   ○ 4. Incontinence, especially with coughing

28. A serious complication of a total hip replacement is displacement of the prosthesis. What is the primary sign of displacement?
   ○ 1. Pain on movement and weight bearing
   ○ 2. Hemorrhage
   ○ 3. The affected leg will be 1 to 2 inches longer
   ○ 4. Edema in the area of the incision

29. Mrs. Theil has an abductor splint in place. What is the best guide to the placement of the splint?
   ○ 1. Fasten the splint firmly in place.
   ○ 2. Position the splint so that it does not interfere with the use of the bedpan.
   ○ 3. Position the strap so that it is not directly over the peroneal nerve.
   ○ 4. Position the proximal strap just above the knee.

30. The nurse evaluates the client's readiness for discharge. Mrs. Theil identifies which of the following as being *incorrect* behavior?
  ○ 1. Use a rocking chair or reclining chair when sitting for an extended period of time.
  ○ 2. Continue to sleep with a pillow between the knees.
  ○ 3. Take antibiotics prophylactically when dental work is being done.
  ○ 4. Hyperextend the affected leg while flexing the other one when retrieving objects from the floor.

Gerald Schmidt, a 36-year-old veteran of the Vietnam War, comes to the Veterans Administration Hospital saying he "cannot go on like this" and requests admission. He states he has not slept in days and that his wife has left him. He has been unable to work for 2 weeks. The admitting physician diagnoses post-traumatic stress disorder.

31. During Mr. Schmidt's admission interview, 3 of the following symptoms are noted. Which one would the nurse *not* likely assess?
  ○ 1. Recurrent nightmares reliving various Vietnam experiences
  ○ 2. Feelings of numbness toward previously enjoyed experiences
  ○ 3. Active hallucinations of insects crawling on his legs
  ○ 4. Difficulty concentrating on current activities

32. Mr. Schmidt is admitted to the crisis unit. He is assigned to a primary nurse, who establishes a relationship with him. In helping Mr. Schmidt to establish a therapeutic relationship, the nurse should
  ○ 1. provide support to help him believe that the nurse is understanding and cares about him.
  ○ 2. explore the coping behaviors that he used in the past that were not successful and decide on new coping techniques.
  ○ 3. teach him relaxation techniques to help reduce his anxiety.
  ○ 4. arrange a meeting between Mr. Schmidt and his wife to establish a support system.

33. The nurse needs to use a variety of creative techniques in assisting Mr. Schmidt to cope with his stress. Which of the following nursing actions would be *least* helpful?
  ○ 1. Encourage him to describe his experiences in Vietnam.
  ○ 2. Encourage him to express the relationship between his experiences in Vietnam and his present life.
  ○ 3. Encourage expression of the anger and rage he feels toward society for sending him to Vietnam.
  ○ 4. Communicate confidence that the nurse will assist him in finding solutions to his problems.

34. Mr. Schmidt and the nurse develop a plan to be implemented after he is discharged. Which one of the following would be most helpful for Mr. Schmidt to use to reduce stress after discharge?
  ○ 1. Move back with his wife
  ○ 2. Attend a support group of Vietnam veterans
  ○ 3. Take diazepam (Valium) as needed
  ○ 4. Begin a job-training program

Four-year-old Steffan is admitted for a tonsillectomy.

35. When preparing Steffan for surgery, it is most important for the nurse to check his chart for which of the following laboratory values?
  ○ 1. Hematocrit and hemoglobin
  ○ 2. Urinalysis
  ○ 3. Bleeding and clotting times
  ○ 4. White blood cell count

36. When preparing a child for surgery, it is especially important to check for loose teeth in which age group?
  ○ 1. Older infant
  ○ 2. Toddler-preschool
  ○ 3. School-age
  ○ 4. Adolescent

37. Which of the following best describes the nursing rationale for providing Steffan with role playing as part of his pre-op preparation?
  ○ 1. To ensure compliant behavior
  ○ 2. To minimize Steffan's need to express his feelings verbally
  ○ 3. As a means of permitting physical expression of feelings that Steffan cannot express verbally
  ○ 4. As a teaching strategy and to decrease anxiety

38. When Steffan is ready to be taken to the operating room, the nurse should *not* implement which of the following nursing actions?
    ○ **1.** Tell Steffan's parents to wait in his hospital room so he will not become distraught on his way to the operating room.
    ○ **2.** Allow Steffan to take his stuffed tiger with him.
    ○ **3.** Allow Steffan to wear his underwear to surgery.
    ○ **4.** Have a familiar nurse stay with Steffan in the operating room until he is asleep.

39. Twelve hours following Steffan's surgery, the nurse should be most concerned about observing which one of the following signs or symptoms?
    ○ **1.** Fever of 100°F (37.8°C)
    ○ **2.** Respirations 24/minute and shallow
    ○ **3.** Frequent swallowing
    ○ **4.** Complaint of a sore throat

40. The nurse should implement which of the following nursing measures to promote Steffan's comfort postoperatively?
    ○ **1.** Apply an ice collar.
    ○ **2.** Administer 5 gr aspirin orally.
    ○ **3.** Have Steffan gargle with normal saline.
    ○ **4.** Encourage Steffan to drink some hot chocolate.

41. The nurse is aware that certain factors may lead children to deny the existence of actual pain. Which of the following is *not* one of these factors?
    ○ **1.** Fear of an injection
    ○ **2.** Better tolerance for pain than adults
    ○ **3.** Lack of understanding of what ''pain'' means
    ○ **4.** Attempts to meet expectations of others

42. Which of the following data is most helpful to the nurse in evaluating a young child's pain status?
    ○ **1.** A verbal statement of pain
    ○ **2.** Physiologic changes
    ○ **3.** Behavioral changes
    ○ **4.** Parental comments

Gordon Isaac has cancer of the bladder. He has been admitted for a cystectomy and urinary diversion.

43. Most clients are curious about the appearance and placement of the stoma of their urinary diversion. What area of the abdomen is usually used?
    ○ **1.** Right side, 1 to 2 inches below the waist
    ○ **2.** Superior, anterior region of the iliac crest
    ○ **3.** Left side, just above the waist
    ○ **4.** Area near the umbilicus

44. During this critical period immediately postoperatively, the nurse would be especially observant of the client's general condition. What is the most critical sign/symptom Mr. Isaac could exhibit?
    ○ **1.** Absence of urinary output over a period of 1 to 2 hours
    ○ **2.** Pain along the incision site
    ○ **3.** Increased pulse rate to 100/minute
    ○ **4.** Serous drainage from the incision line

45. Mr. Isaac has an ileostomy bag fastened around the stoma. Select the most common problem that the nurse is trying to prevent with the use of this bag.
    ○ **1.** Infection of the stoma
    ○ **2.** Skin excoriation
    ○ **3.** Stricture of the ileal stoma
    ○ **4.** Ammonia odor from the stoma

46. What is the most important reason for attaching the ileostomy bag to gravity drainage at night?
    ○ **1.** To prevent infection of the stoma resulting from urinary stasis in the bag
    ○ **2.** To prevent leakage of urine around the bag on the skin that can be caused by overdistension of the bag
    ○ **3.** To facilitate the normal urinary method of excretion
    ○ **4.** To prevent reflux of urine into the renal pelvis

47. Mr. Isaac needs adequate teaching before his discharge. In doing discharge teaching, which complication needs to be emphasized?
    ○ **1.** Recurrent bladder infection
    ○ **2.** Possible intestinal obstruction
    ○ **3.** Ileal stoma dilation
    ○ **4.** Inflammation and infection of the kidney

Maria Cordobas, a 26-year-old woman in computer sales, was raped on her way home from work one evening. The rape occurred in the parking lot where she was employed. A passerby found her lying on the ground. She told him, in a very calm voice, that she had been raped. He brought her to an emergency room. Although she was in physical pain, her condition was not serious.

48. Which of the following actions is the most important for the emergency room nurse to take?
    ○ **1.** Call the police.
    ○ **2.** Call a psychiatrist.
    ○ **3.** Provide emotional support.
    ○ **4.** Offer protection from pregnancy.

49. The nurse in the emergency room can provide the best emotional support to Miss Cordobas by
    ○ **1.** asking her questions to help her talk about the rape.
    ○ **2.** telling her it is very important that she discuss the rape now while it is still fresh in her mind.
    ○ **3.** telling her that at some point she may feel angry, afraid, or sad, and that these feelings are normal.
    ○ **4.** explaining that since her initial reaction is different from other victims, she probably will not have problems coping.

50. A coworker tells the nurse, "Miss Cordobas is so calm, I bet she wasn't even raped." The source of the coworker's response is probably reflected in which of the following statements?
    ○ **1.** She knows the client personally and knows she may be lying.
    ○ **2.** She may know the rapist and is trying to protect him.
    ○ **3.** The client's rape reminds her that she is also vulnerable to rape.
    ○ **4.** She correctly knows that rape victims are hysterical after a rape, not calm.

51. After the physical exam is finished, Miss Cordobas quietly and calmly asks the nurse if she can see the psychiatric clinical specialist. The clinical specialist provides crisis intervention. This type of therapy is most appropriate for which of the following reasons?
    ○ **1.** It will help the client gain insightful understanding about her feelings.
    ○ **2.** It will help her to understand childhood conflicts brought into awareness by this trauma.
    ○ **3.** It provides the long-term therapy needed for an event this serious.
    ○ **4.** It may prevent serious psychiatric symptoms.

52. The clinical specialist assesses Miss Cordobas. Which of the following will *not* necessarily be important for Miss Cordobas at this stage?
    ○ **1.** An identified support system
    ○ **2.** A positive response to the significant others who come to pick her up at the hospital
    ○ **3.** An ability to maintain some level of control over her care
    ○ **4.** An awareness of how she might prevent a rape in the future

53. When the clinical specialist tries to talk with Miss Cordobas, the client angrily tells her, "You certainly took long enough. No one cares enough here to provide decent support." The clinical specialist knows that the staff had dealt with Miss Cordobas gently and supportively. Which of the following statements most accurately describes the source of Miss Cordobas's anger?
    ○ **1.** She is angry at her rapist for what he did to her.
    ○ **2.** She is angry at the staff for hurting her during the examination.
    ○ **3.** She may have been raped as a child, and this rape brings up memories.
    ○ **4.** She is angry because it happened to her and not someone else.

54. Which of the following is the best response the clinical specialist could make to Miss Cordobas's angry remark?
    ○ **1.** "I think you're angry at something else and not myself or the staff."
    ○ **2.** "You sound angry."
    ○ **3.** "I'd rather talk with you about the rape."
    ○ **4.** "It is not productive being angry with me and the staff."

55. According to the community mental health model, Miss Cordobas's rape would be considered a crisis if which of the following conditions occurred?
    ○ **1.** Her supports were excessive and overpowered the stress of the event.
    ○ **2.** Her defense mechanisms were not adequate for the situation.
    ○ **3.** The stress caused by the rape was great, and she could not contain it unless she stayed with a friend.
    ○ **4.** The stress generated was much greater than her support systems could handle.

56. Crisis-intervention therapy is considered to be
    - ○ 1. secondary prevention.
    - ○ 2. tertiary prevention.
    - ○ 3. insight-oriented therapy.
    - ○ 4. long-term therapy.

57. Primary prevention for the community problem of rape would best be achieved by which of the following?
    - ○ 1. Emergency care after the rape
    - ○ 2. A class by policewomen on how to avoid rape
    - ○ 3. Hospitalization for the rape victim
    - ○ 4. A long jail sentence for the rapist
    - ○ 4. The client verbalizes that she will never return from a pass in such a state again.

Flora Robinson has missed 2 menstrual periods and has experienced some nausea in the mornings. She comes in to the health clinic to confirm her suspicion that she might be pregnant.

58. Mrs. Robinson's urine specimen was positive for human chorionic gonadotropin. Which of the following physical signs might be observed on the initial examination?
    - ○ 1. Palpation of the outline of the fetus
    - ○ 2. Softening of the lower uterine segment
    - ○ 3. Fetal heart sounds
    - ○ 4. Effacement of the cervix

59. While the nurse is taking a history, Mrs. Robinson tells the nurse that she has 4 children at home, that this baby will be her fifth child, and that, in addition, she has had 2 miscarriages, both at 8 weeks gestation. Based upon this information, what would the nurse record?
    - ○ 1. Gravida 4, para 2
    - ○ 2. Gravida 7, para 5
    - ○ 3. Gravida 5, para 2
    - ○ 4. Gravida 7, para 4

60. Mrs. Robinson asks what she can do to eliminate her nausea. Which of the following should the nurse suggest?
    - ○ 1. "Avoid foods that are high in fiber."
    - ○ 2. "Drink a glass of water before getting out of bed."
    - ○ 3. "Eat some crackers before getting up."
    - ○ 4. "Eliminate breakfast and eat a large lunch."

61. During the eighth month of pregnancy, Mrs. Robinson returns for a prenatal visit. As part of her assessment, the nurse performs Leopold's maneuver. What is the best explanation the nurse can give Mrs. Robinson about this procedure?
    - ○ 1. Helps push the fetus into the pelvis
    - ○ 2. Helps to turn the baby around
    - ○ 3. Helps to determine fetal abnormalities
    - ○ 4. Helps to determine the baby's position

62. Mrs. Robinson tells the nurse that she has been having painless uterine contractions occurring at irregular intervals, which are relieved by walking. Based on this information, what would the nurse best conclude?
    - ○ 1. This is a pathologic sign.
    - ○ 2. This is a sign of true labor.
    - ○ 3. These are Braxton Hicks' contractions.
    - ○ 4. This is a sign of impending fetal distress.

63. During this visit, the nurse listens to the fetal heart tones and determines that the rate is 96 beats/minute and the heart sound is strong. How should the nurse best interpret these data?
    - ○ 1. Consider this normal.
    - ○ 2. Take the mother's blood pressure.
    - ○ 3. Take the mother's pulse.
    - ○ 4. Notify the physician immediately.

64. Mrs. Robinson is scheduled for a nonstress test when she is 36 weeks pregnant. Which of the following is true regarding a nonstress test?
    - ○ 1. An IV of Pitocin is started to stimulate mild contractions.
    - ○ 2. The test determines the gestational age of the fetus.
    - ○ 3. Late decelerations in relation to contractions are monitored.
    - ○ 4. The test relates fetal heart rates to fetal movement to assess the adequacy of the fetal-placental reserve.

Three-month-old Heather has cystic fibrosis. As a neonate, she had surgery for meconium ileus.

65. Heather's parents were told that meconium ileus was related to cystic fibrosis, but they state that they do not understand why. Which of the following nursing explanations is most accurate?
    ○ **1.** The bile ducts become obstructed with tenacious mucus.
    ○ **2.** The intestinal cilia are blunted and prevent meconium from passing through the intestinal tract.
    ○ **3.** The small intestine is constricted, resulting in meconium impaction.
    ○ **4.** The pancreas is unable to secrete the enzymes necessary for digestion.

66. Heather's parents also ask what test was used to diagnose Heather's condition. Which one of the following tests is used to diagnose cystic fibrosis?
    ○ **1.** Stool exam for trypsin, amylase, and lipase
    ○ **2.** Sweat chloride test
    ○ **3.** Chest x-ray
    ○ **4.** Stool exam for fat content

67. Heather is hospitalized with pneumonia in the right lower lobe. Which of the following nursing orders concerning Heather's chest physical therapy is indicated?
    ○ **1.** To right lower lobe qh
    ○ **2.** To right lung q2h
    ○ **3.** To all lobes q2h to q4h
    ○ **4.** To all lobes once each shift

68. Ampicillin 100 mg IV q6h has been prescribed for Heather. The ampicillin vial contains 250 mg per 1.2 ml when reconstituted. How much should be administered?
    ○ **1.** 0.25 ml
    ○ **2.** 0.48 ml
    ○ **3.** 0.75 ml
    ○ **4.** 2.5 ml

69. A developmental assessment indicates that Heather is developing at an age-appropriate level. Which of the following actions will best promote her continued development?
    ○ **1.** Provide bright-colored objects within reach.
    ○ **2.** Provide space for her to practice crawling.
    ○ **3.** Offer her small objects to improve her pincer grasp.
    ○ **4.** Teach her to play pat-a-cake.

70. Heather is receiving pancreatic enzymes to aid digestion. Her parents should be instructed to administer the enzymes in which of the following ways?
    ○ **1.** Add it to her formula.
    ○ **2.** Put it in a small amount of pureed apple sauce.
    ○ **3.** Mix it with an ounce of orange juice.
    ○ **4.** Mix it with water in a syringe.

71. Which one of the following is the best indicator of a successful outcome of Heather's treatment plan?
    ○ **1.** Growth rate within normal limits
    ○ **2.** Achievement of developmental milestones
    ○ **3.** Ability to digest a variety of foods
    ○ **4.** Decrease in incidence of respiratory infections

72. Heather's mother asks what the risk is of having another child with cystic fibrosis, since she and her husband are ''thinking about having another baby someday.'' What is the best nursing response?
    ○ **1.** ''It's probably best if you don't have any more children.''
    ○ **2.** ''Your next child may be a carrier but won't have the disease.''
    ○ **3.** ''You can have an amniocentesis in early pregnancy to detect whether the baby has cystic fibrosis and, if so, you may choose to have a therapeutic abortion.''
    ○ **4.** ''I'd like to refer you to the genetic counselor on our staff, who can discuss with you the probability of your second child's having cystic fibrosis.''

Joseph Fenter, a 55-year-old black man, was admitted to the hospital with a diagnosis of hypertension. While taking his history, the nurse learns that he is employed as a sales manager for a large video business. His hypertension was discovered on a routine visit to the medical department at work.

73. On admission, Mr. Fenter would most likely be expected to make which of these statements?
    ○ **1.** ''I don't know why I am here. There is nothing wrong with me.''
    ○ **2.** ''I have been having numerous episodes of nausea and vomiting.''
    ○ **3.** ''I have been experiencing dizzy spells.''
    ○ **4.** ''I am here because I have hypertension.''

74. Which of these findings would constitute a significant index of hypertension?
    ○ **1.** A pulse pressure of 10 mm Hg
    ○ **2.** A regular pulse of 90 beats/minute
    ○ **3.** A sustained diastolic pressure greater than 90 mm Hg
    ○ **4.** A systolic pressure fluctuating between 140 and 150 mm Hg

75. Mr. Fenter is to receive a diet low in fat, sodium, and cholesterol. His knowledge of foods lowest in these elements would be good if he selected which of these menus?
    ○ **1.** Beans, ham, rye bread, a carrot
    ○ **2.** Cold baked chicken, tomatoes, apple sauce
    ○ **3.** Cold cuts, salad with blue cheese dressing, custard pie
    ○ **4.** Cheese sandwich, cream of mushroom soup, chocolate pie

76. When teaching Mr. Fenter about his diet, the nurse should include which of these instructions?
    ○ **1.** Season meats with lemon juice.
    ○ **2.** Drink decaffeinated coffee.
    ○ **3.** Eat a lot of canned foods.
    ○ **4.** Restrict green vegetable intake.

77. Mr. Fenter is taking the medication isosorbide dinitrate (Isordil) for symptoms of angina. Discharge teaching about Isordil should include information that this drug is
    ○ **1.** a non-nitrite preparation that will not cause dilation of peripheral vessels.
    ○ **2.** a nitrite preparation that will constrict both small and large vessels.
    ○ **3.** a vasodilator that will cause an increase in vascular resistance.
    ○ **4.** a nitrite preparation that will dilate both large and small vessels.

78. Mr. Fenter has a prescription for metoprolol (Lopressor) to control his hypertension. This drug reduces blood pressure by which of the following mechanisms?
    ○ **1.** Decreases cardiac output and suppresses renin activity
    ○ **2.** Increases cardiac output and suppresses aldosterone activity
    ○ **3.** Depletes norepinephrine from the heart and peripheral organs
    ○ **4.** Suppresses norepinephrine secretion from the medulla of the brain

79. Which one of the following types of adrenergic-blocking agents is particularly useful in producing vasodilation?
    ○ **1.** Alpha-blocking agents
    ○ **2.** Beta-blocking agents
    ○ **3.** Adrenergic neuron-blocking agents
    ○ **4.** Gamma-blocking agents

Gladys Stein is admitted to the postpartal unit following delivery of her second child.

80. Which of the following mothers on the postpartum unit is at greatest risk for potential infection?
    ○ **1.** A client who delivered vaginally with marginal placenta previa
    ○ **2.** Woman who had rupture of membranes 36 hours before delivery
    ○ **3.** A mother delivered by cesarian section because of cephalopelvic disproportion
    ○ **4.** A multigravida delivered of twins by low forceps

81. While caring for Mrs. Stein on the second postpartal day following a normal spontaneous delivery, the nurse notes each of the following is on the chart. Which requires immediate notification of the physician?
    ○ **1.** White blood cell count of 11,000
    ○ **2.** Oral temperature of 101°F (38.3°C)
    ○ **3.** Slight diaphoresis
    ○ **4.** Urinating large quantitites

82. Cervical culture indicates a strep infection; a diagnosis of endometritis is confirmed. Isolation precautions are initiated and the infant is separated from the mother. Mrs. Stein is upset about this and promises to wash her hands carefully if she can be allowed to be with the infant. What action would best meet her needs at this time?
    ○ **1.** Remind her that the isolation is required by the health department.
    ○ **2.** Suggest she discuss options with the physician and pediatrician.
    ○ **3.** Encourage her to verbalize her feelings about the separation.
    ○ **4.** Offer her opportunities for diversional activities at the bedside.

83. Ampicillin 1 gm is to be administered in 50 ml of 5% dextrose in water every 6 hours. The drop factor of the infusion set is 10 drops per ml. The medication is to infuse over 30 minutes. What is the rate of infusion?
    ○ **1.** 6 drops per minute
    ○ **2.** 60 drops per minute
    ○ **3.** 16 drops per minute
    ○ **4.** 1.6 drops per minute

The school nurse is asked to teach the school staff about inspecting the children for head lice. This infestation has recently become prevalent in the community.

84. Head lice and dandruff look very similar. How can the school nurse best determine that a child has lice instead of dandruff?
    - ○ 1. Preadolescents rarely have dandruff.
    - ○ 2. Areas of alopecia on the nape of the neck indicate lice.
    - ○ 3. Children scratch more with lice than with dandruff.
    - ○ 4. Nits will not fall off the hair shaft when it is moved.

85. In addition to explaining how to look for the ova (nits) on the hair shafts, the nurse should instruct the staff to assess for which one of the following?
    - ○ 1. Honey-colored vesicles
    - ○ 2. Enlarged cervical lymph nodes
    - ○ 3. Alopecia
    - ○ 4. Ringlike lesions

86. Several cases of head lice are discovered in the school. The nurse telephones the children's parents to inform them. Each of the infested children is treated with Kwell shampoo. What is the most important information to give their parents?
    - ○ 1. Follow shampoo directions explicitly.
    - ○ 2. Cut the children's hair short.
    - ○ 3. Prevent the children from scratching their heads.
    - ○ 4. Launder or disinfect the children's clothing and bedding.

87. One of the mothers states she prides herself on keeping a spotlessly clean house and cannot imagine how her daughter got the lice. Knowing how lice are transmitted, the nurse identifies which of the following as the most likely source?
    - ○ 1. Letting her cat sleep on her bed
    - ○ 2. Walking to school with someone who has lice
    - ○ 3. Sharing her friend's pretty new hat
    - ○ 4. Playing with the neighbor's dog

88. One child's parents asks when her child can return to school. What should be the nurse's response?
    - ○ 1. "After she has been shampooed 3 times with Kwell."
    - ○ 2. "When all the nits are gone, following 1 shampoo with Kwell."
    - ○ 3. "After you cut her hair short all over."
    - ○ 4. "In 2 weeks."

Fernando Cruz, 21 years old, sustained a compound, comminuted fracture in the distal portion of the left femur while learning to ride his new motorcycle. He was placed in skeletal traction with a Thomas splint and a Pearson attachment with a 20 lb weight. A Steinman pin was inserted into the femur, distal to the fracture.

89. Which of the following is a definition of a compound, comminuted fracture?
    - ○ 1. The fracture is associated with injury to surrounding tissue and structures.
    - ○ 2. Bone fragments are forcibly driven into one another.
    - ○ 3. The bone is splintered into fragments that extend through the skin.
    - ○ 4. The line of the fracture forms a spiral that encircles the bone.

90. Mr. Cruz is admitted to the orthopedic unit. The nursing care plan should include which of the following?
    - ○ 1. Ensure the sole of the affected foot is supported against the foot of the bed.
    - ○ 2. Instruct the client to move about in bed as little as possible.
    - ○ 3. Position the Thomas splint around the upper thigh without putting pressure on the groin.
    - ○ 4. Place and remove the bedpan from the affected side.

91. Which of the following statements made by Mrs. Cruz indicates a need for further teaching or discussion?
    - ○ 1. "A diet high in roughage and fiber will prevent constipation."
    - ○ 2. "Maintaining a positive nitrogen balance is important."
    - ○ 3. "Mr. Cruz needs an increased calcium intake."
    - ○ 4. "The 2,000-calorie diet should provide nutrients that promote healing."

92. To maintain traction there must be countertraction. How is countertraction best applied to Mr. Cruz's leg?
    - ○ 1. By raising the head of the bed to a 45° angle
    - ○ 2. By elevating the foot of the bed on 6 inch shock blocks
    - ○ 3. By using 20 lb of weight supported by the Steinman pin
    - ○ 4. By keeping the Thomas splint in an inclined position

93. Because a Steinman pin has been inserted, Mr. Cruz is at risk of acquiring
    ○ 1. flexion contracture of the knee.
    ○ 2. impaired skin sensations.
    ○ 3. addiction to pain medication.
    ○ 4. osteomyelitis.

94. Mr. Cruz complains that the ropes hurt his thigh. Which of the following would be the most appropriate nursing action?
    ○ 1. Replace the spreader bar with a wider one.
    ○ 2. Place padding between the thigh and the rope.
    ○ 3. Employ distraction techniques.
    ○ 4. Medicate with a mild analgesic.

95. What is the purpose of the Pearson attachment on Mr. Cruz's traction?
    ○ 1. To support the lower part of the leg
    ○ 2. To support the upper part of the leg
    ○ 3. To provide traction to the fracture
    ○ 4. To prevent flexion contracture of the ankle

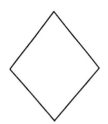

Test 2, Book I
Answers with Rationales

1. **#2.** Most toddlers are able to point to their body parts by 15 to 18 months of age. All other options are too advanced for a toddler. ASSESSMENT (CHILD/HEALTHY CHILD)

2. **#4.** Toddlers will resist invasive procedures, so it is best to proceed confidently. Obtain assistance to restrain the child and be matter-of-fact, so the child does not feel that what is happening is a punishment or the result of being "bad." The child is too young to benefit from options #1 and #3. Deferring the exam is not appropriate. IMPLEMENTATION (CHILD/HEALTHY CHILD)

3. **#1.** Playing with a toy will divert Crystal's attention from the task of learning independent toileting skills. IMPLEMENTATION (CHILD/HEALTHY CHILD)

4. **#3.** The toddler often has physiologic anorexia and is more likely to accept small portions of a variety of foods. This approach also allows the toddler to exert autonomy by making choices. IMPLEMENTATION (CHILD/HEALTHY CHILD)

5. **#3.** Pancreatitis is an inflammation of the pancreas, which results in obstruction and edema. ANALYSIS (ADULT/NUTRITION AND METABOLISM)

6. **#4.** The enzymes secreted by the pancreas are trypsin, chymotrypsin, nucleases, carboxypeptidase, pancreatic lipase, and pancreatic amylase. ANALYSIS (ADULT/NUTRITION AND METABOLISM)

7. **#1.** Chronic pancreatitis causes degeneration of the islet cells, thereby decreasing production and secretion of insulin, which elevates the blood glucose level. ASSESSMENT (ADULT/NUTRITION AND METABOLISM)

8. **#1.** Fats are incompletely metabolized and calcium ions are bound to fats; thus calcium ions are not absorbed in normal amounts. ANALYSIS (ADULT/NUTRITION AND METABOLISM)

9. **#1.** Clients with pancreatitis are given anticholinergic drugs to decrease secretions and relax spasms. PLAN (ADULT/NUTRITION AND METABOLISM)

10. **#3.** Meperidine is preferred for the treatment of the pain of pancreatitis, because it produces less spasm of the sphincter of Oddi. ANALYSIS (ADULT/NUTRITION AND METABOLISM)

11. **#1.** Withdrawal can occur if the client cuts back the amount of alcohol consumed as well as if drinking is stopped altogether. Emergency room nurses must always evaluate cardiovascular status; however, Mr. Lampert's history and presenting clinical picture are more consistent with withdrawal. Increased anxiety is only 1 symptom of alcohol withdrawal. ASSESSMENT (PSYCHOSOCIAL, MENTAL HEALTH, PSYCHIATRIC PROBLEMS/SUBSTANCE USE DISORDERS)

12. **#3.** Since Korsakoff's syndrome causes gaps in the client's memory, confabulation is used to fill in these gaps with relevant, but untrue, pieces of information. Alcoholics often suffer from chronic gastritis and fatty liver; however, Korsakoff's syndrome is an organic brain syndrome associated with vitamin B_1 deficiency. Excessive perspiration is often experienced in alcohol detoxification, but is usually noted about 72 hours after cessation of drinking. ASSESSMENT (PSYCHOSOCIAL, MENTAL HEALTH, PSYCHIATRIC PROBLEMS/SUBSTANCE USE DISORDERS)

13. **#1.** Working with the client to find new ways of handling difficult situations without alcohol is a long-term goal of treatment. Short-term goals would include learning to handle specific situations. Mr. Lampert needs the support from his friends and family and increased emotional support to assist him through this difficult time. Psychoanalysis has not been found to be very effective in treating alcoholism. IMPLEMENTATION (PSYCHOSOCIAL, MENTAL HEALTH, PSYCHIATRIC PROBLEMS/SUBSTANCE USE DISORDERS)

14. **#3.** While Antabuse does cause tachycardia, it also causes a drop, not an increase, in blood pressure and respiratory depression. A pulsating headache (from dilation of peripheral blood vessels) and vomiting do occur; however, a generalized flushing becomes apparent rather than pallor. While ataxia and blurred vision do occur, dry skin does not as the person experiences profuse sweating. IMPLEMENTATION (PSYCHOSOCIAL, MENTAL HEALTH, PSYCHIATRIC PROBLEMS/)

15. **#3.** Family therapy looks upon the presenting problem as a family problem. Family therapy does not focus on any 1 individual; instead, it aims at getting a better understanding of the relationship between the alcoholic and members of his/her family. Its goal is to help the family members communicate more effectively in order to find healthy ways to meet their needs. The family therapy sessions would not be centered on getting Mr. Lampert to stop drinking, but on having the members express themselves clearly on important matters, including the drinking issue, and on helping the members to listen carefully to what each member is saying. PLAN (PSYCHOSOCIAL, MENTAL HEALTH, PSYCHIATRIC PROBLEMS/SUBSTANCE USE DISORDERS)

16. **#4.** A slow breathing pattern is desirable in early labor to ensure adequate oxygenation to the fetus. Candle blowing and accelerated breathing are useful in active labor. Panting is carried out when the client has the desire to push when it is not indicated. IMPLEMENTATION (CHILDBEARING FAMILY/INTRAPARTAL CARE)

17. **#3.** Decelerations can be detected early only if fetal heart tones are evaluated during and soon after contractions, as they occur at this time. ANALYSIS (CHILDBEARING FAMILY/INTRAPARTAL CARE)

18. **#4.** The fetus is in a posterior presentation, resulting in fetal pressure on the mother's back. This can be relieved by side-lying, tailor-sitting, or having the client crouch on her hands and knees. Sacral pressure can also be an effective comfort measure. IMPLEMENTATION (CHILDBEARING FAMILY/INTRAPARTAL CARE)

19. **#2.** The fetal heart rate should be checked every 5 minutes for 15 minutes after rupture of the membranes, because of the possibility of cord prolapse, an emergency that can be detected by a changed fetal heart rate pattern. IMPLEMENTATION (CHILDBEARING FAMILY/INTRAPARTAL CARE)

20. **#4.** These signs are indicative of delivery of the placenta, which signals the end of the third stage. Other signs of placental separation include a firmly contracting uterus, a change in its shape from discoid to globular, and a lengthening of the umbilical cord. ANALYSIS (CHILDBEARING FAMILY/INTRAPARTAL CARE)

21. **#4.** The Bence Jones protein is a test for multiple myeloma. A type and crossmatch would be done because of anticipated blood loss, which is substantial in bone or joint surgery. The prothrombin time is required because she has been taking large doses of aspirin. A sedimentation rate can rule out the possibility of infection. ASSESSMENT (ADULT/ACTIVITY AND REST)

22. **#3.** Clients should not be exposed to the risks of immobility when it is not necessary. PLAN (ADULT/ACTIVITY AND REST)

23. **#3.** Reverse isolation is not used, but the other interventions listed are done in an effort to prevent infection. PLAN (ADULT/ACTIVITY AND REST)

24. **#2.** The client should keep her toes pointed toward the ceiling to prevent adduction or external rotation. PLAN (ADULT/ACTIVITY AND REST)

25. **#2.** This option provides the best definition of blanching. ANALYSIS (ADULT/ACTIVITY AND REST)

26. **#3.** Wound drainage of 100 ml post-hip replacement over an 8-hour period is not unusual. ASSESSMENT (ADULT/ACTIVITY AND REST)

27. **#1.** Urinary retention is a common problem after a total hip replacement, because of the recumbent position. In the elderly male client, prostatic enlargement can also be a contributing factor. ANALYSIS (ADULT/ACTIVITY AND REST)

28. **#1.** Pain on movement and weight bearing indicates pressure on the nerves and/or muscles caused by the dislocation. ASSESSMENT (ADULT/ACTIVITY AND REST)

29. **#3.** Pressure on the peroneal nerve places the client at risk for foot drop to occur. IMPLEMENTATION (ADULT/ACTIVITY AND REST)

30. **#1.** Rocking chairs and recliners are difficult to get out of and cause the hip to be flexed beyond the safe limits. EVALUATION (ADULT/ACTIVITY AND REST)

31. #3. This client is experiencing severe anxiety and stress. Recurrent nightmares, feelings of numbness, and difficulty in concentration are all symptoms commonly found in post-traumatic stress disorder. Hallucinations that involve insects are generally a part of toxic reactions such as alcohol withdrawal. ASSESSMENT (PSYCHOSOCIAL, MENTAL HEALTH, PSYCHIATRIC PROBLEMS/ANXIOUS BEHAVIOR)

32. #1. The client experiencing post-traumatic stress disorder has a sense of isolation, believes he is alone and that no one understands the pain he is experiencing. In establishing a relationship, the nurse must demonstrate that s/he is on the client's side and will be a helping person. It is important to identify past coping behaviors and to teach the client relaxation techniques; however, this will prove easier after a therapeutic relationship has been established. Until the client and his wife gain insight into the cause of their difficulties, their relationship will probably not be a source of support for the client. IMPLEMENTATION (PSYCHOSOCIAL, MENTAL HEALTH, PSYCHIATRIC PROBLEMS/ANXIOUS BEHAVIOR)

33. #3. While encouraged ventilation of feelings might include crying or an angry outburst, the continued expression of anger and rage can lead the client to lose self-control or to experience increased tension and anxiety, rather than help to reduce it. Encourage the client to describe his thoughts rather than his feelings. He should think through how his Vietnam experiences affect his current relationships in society. Assist him by discussing ways to control anger and gain a perspective on his experiences. As the nurse communicates confidence that s/he will help him find solutions, the client gains a sense of the ''normalcy'' of his reactions and that his problems are not insurmountable. IMPLEMENTATION (PSYCHOSOCIAL, MENTAL HEALTH, PSYCHIATRIC PROBLEMS/ANXIOUS BEHAVIOR)

34. #2. The client will need continued support after he leaves the hospital. Self-help groups are an effective way to decrease feelings of loneliness, integrate past experiences into present life, and explore new coping methods and solutions to problems. Unless both the client and his wife have had an opportunity to explore the reason for their separation, moving back with his wife might cause increased stress for the client. Diazepam might be useful as adjunctive therapy for reduction of anxiety, but it is not the best long-term solution for the client. Since the client's job is probably not what has caused the increase in his anxiety, a job-training program might not be necessary after the client's emotional state is stabliized. EVALUATION (PSYCHOSOCIAL, MENTAL HEALTH, PSYCHIATRIC PROBLEMS/ANXIOUS BEHAVIOR)

35. #3. Hemorrhage is the most common complication following tonsillectomy. Bleeding and clotting times are necessary to determine whether the child is at risk for hemorrhage and to serve as a baseline value postoperatively. ASSESSMENT (CHILD/SENSATION, PERCEPTION, PROTECTION)

36. #3. During the school-age period, most children lose their primary teeth and develop their permanent teeth. By adolescence, all deciduous teeth should be gone. Options #1 and #2 are periods when deciduous teeth are erupting. ANALYSIS (CHILD/SENSATION, PERCEPTION, PROTECTION)

37. #4. The use of play to prepare a child for surgery is an effective teaching strategy and helps to decrease anxiety. While there is some truth to option #3, option #4 describes a wider application of play. PLAN (CHILD/ILL AND HOSPITALIZED CHILD)

38. #1. Allow Steffan's parents to accompany him to the operating room door because of the heightened fears of this age group. IMPLEMENTATION (CHILD/ILL AND HOSPITALIZED CHILD)

39. #3. Frequent swallowing is often an early sign of bleeding from the operative site post-tonsillectomy. ASSESSMENT (CHILD/SENSATION, PERCEPTION, PROTECTION)

40. #1. An ice collar decreases the risk of hemorrhage and provides soothing relief from throat discomfort as well. The other measures increase the risk of bleeding. IMPLEMENTATION (CHILD/ILL AND HOSPITALIZED CHILD)

41. **#2.** This statement is a myth. ANALYSIS (CHILD/ILL AND HOSPITALIZED CHILD)

42. **#3.** Behavioral manifestations are most frequently noted in children experiencing pain. This is especially true of young children who may not have the vocabulary to communicate pain, and in children who fear injections for pain relief. EVALUATION (CHILD/ILL AND HOSPITALIZED CHILD)

43. **#1.** This is the best position both anatomically (near the terminal ileum) and for the client. It will be visible for self-care but will not interfere with clothing. ANALYSIS (ADULT/ELIMINATION)

44. **#1.** Urine output of at least 30 ml per hour is vital to show adequate renal perfusion. Because there is no bladder, urine output becomes evident immediately. ASSESSMENT (ADULT/ELIMINATION)

45. **#2.** Skin excoriation is caused when urine remains in contact with the skin, and the appliance prevents this contact. ANALYSIS (ADULT/ELIMINATION)

46. **#4.** Although leakage could occur, the most important reason is to prevent reflux, which predisposes the client to pyelonephritis. ANALYSIS (ADULT/ELIMINATION)

47. **#4.** This is the most common long-term problem other than skin excoriation. PLAN (ADULT/ELIMINATION)

48. **#3.** Of the options provided, #3 is most crucial. In high stress situations, it is important for the nurse to provide emotional support as a key part of the care. Notifying the police is important, but of a lower priority. The client may or may not need a psychiatrist. Crisis intervention includes emotional support and is part of the emergency room nurse's or clinical specialist's role. Pregnancy concerns can be dealt with later. IMPLEMENTATION (PSYCHOSOCIAL, MENTAL HEALTH, PSYCHIATRIC PROBLEMS/SOCIALLY MALADAPTIVE BEHAVIOR)

49. **#3.** It is important to give the client an opportunity to talk if she wishes. If she does not want to talk, then a statement or 2 preparing her for some of the feelings she may experience later may help her. Offering a telephone number she may call for help if she wishes is another way to provide support. Multiple questions are inappropriate and tire a client. It is not important that the client discuss the rape at this time unless she wishes to do so. Not all rape victims want to discuss the rape. How a client copes does not depend on what her initial reaction is like. IMPLEMENTATION (PSYCHOSOCIAL, MENTAL HEALTH, PSYCHIATRIC PROBLEMS/SOCIALLY MALADAPTIVE BEHAVIOR)

50. **#3.** Staff will sometimes minimize or deny the seriousness of a traumatic event to decrease their own anxiety that it may also happen to them. Sometimes staff will look for ways in which the client did something to "cause" the rape. This too helps them feel they have control over such a traumatic event. However, it is much better for a nurse to accept that people are vulnerable and to be aware of the emotional pain that awareness can cause. This self-awareness can increase the nurses' effectiveness in providing emotional support. Options #1 and #2 are not likely; people rarely lie about being raped. Responses to rape vary and include both high anxiety behavior and a calm external demeanor. ANALYSIS (PSYCHOSOCIAL, MENTAL HEALTH, PSYCHIATRIC PROBLEMS/SOCIALLY MALADAPTIVE BEHAVIOR)

51. **#4.** The purpose of crisis-intervention therapy is to return clients to a level of functioning equal to or better than that prior to the crisis. Crisis intervention can be effective whether or not the client develops insightful understanding about her feelings. It deals with the immediate event and does not aim at understanding earlier conflicts. Should a better understanding occur, it is incidental rather than directly intended. Crisis intervention is brief; the focus is on the present; treatment is short term and time limited. PLAN (PSYCHOSOCIAL, MENTAL HEALTH, PSYCHIATRIC PROBLEMS/SOCIALLY MALADAPTIVE BEHAVIOR)

52. #4. The early phase of a crisis is a time when here-and-now issues are dealt with by the client. The client becomes very focused on the present. Options #1, #2, and #3 are all important and necessary components of the assessment. Successful weathering of a crisis is most dependent upon the client's ability to cope with the situation. The support of significant others helps a client cope better. ASSESSMENT (PSYCHOSOCIAL, MENTAL HEALTH, PSYCHIATRIC PROBLEMS/SOCIALLY MALADAPTIVE BEHAVIOR)

53. #1. Clients may find the crisis situation too difficult to examine and misdirect their anger at staff, family, or friends. There is no data to suggest that the staff hurt her. The present situation is generating the client's anger at this time. There is no data to suggest that she is angry because the rape did not happen to someone else. An early response may be, ''Why me?'' but does not usually include ''Why not someone else?''. ANALYSIS (PSYCHOSOCIAL, MENTAL HEALTH, PSYCHIATRIC PROBLEMS/SOCIALLY MALADAPTIVE BEHAVIOR)

54. #2. This option allows the client to focus on her feelings without judging her or pushing her to discuss issues she is not comfortable talking about. It will not be therapeutic to push the client to identify a particular person and may make her feel defensive and ashamed. Such an approach could stifle her anger or even enrage her. Option #3 avoids dealing with the client's anger and is not therapeutic. #4 tries to talk the client out of her anger rather than permitting and encouraging her to express angry feelings. IMPLEMENTATION (PSYCHOSOCIAL, MENTAL HEALTH, PSYCHIATRIC PROBLEMS/SOCIALLY MALADAPTIVE BEHAVIOR)

55. #4. Rape is not a crisis situation for every victim, as defined by the community mental health model. Sometimes the victim may have adequate coping mechanisms and social supports to handle the trauma. Option #1 describes conditions that lessen the potential for crisis. Defense mechanism is a term from Freudian theory. Coping mechanisms and social supports are terms used in crisis theory. If the client stayed with a friend and was able to contain the stress, a crisis would not occur. ANALYSIS (PSYCHOSOCIAL, MENTAL HEALTH, PSYCHIATRIC PROBLEMS/SOCIALLY MALADAPTIVE BEHAVIOR)

56. #1. Secondary prevention refers to early treatment to prevent long-term illness. Crisis-intervention therapy helps the client during the acute phase of the problem. Tertiary prevention refers to treatment of chronic, long-term problems. Crisis intervention does not aim for insight although insights may occur. Crisis intervention is a kind of brief psychotherapy. ANALYSIS (PSYCHOSOCIAL, MENTAL HEALTH, PSYCHIATRIC PROBLEMS/SOCIALLY MALADAPTIVE BEHAVIOR)

57. #2. Preventing a rape would be primary prevention. Emergency care after the rape is an example of secondary prevention. Hospitalization is considered to be tertiary prevention. Option #4 is a legal action and not a type of prevention. ANALYSIS (PSYCHOSOCIAL, MENTAL HEALTH, PSYCHIATRIC PROBLEMS/SOCIALLY MALADAPTIVE BEHAVIOR)

58. #2. About the sixth week of pregnancy, the lower uterine segment becomes much softer than the cervix (Hegar's sign). Palpation of the fetal outline is possible at approximately 26 weeks. Fetal heart tones are obtained at 10 to 12 weeks with ultrasound, and at 17 to 24 weeks with a fetal stethoscope. ASSESSMENT (CHILDBEARING FAMILY/ANTEPARTAL CARE)

59. #4. The term gravida refers to the number of a woman's pregnancies regardless of their duration. The term para refers to the number of past pregnancies that have produced an infant of viable age, whether the infant is alive or dead at birth. ANALYSIS (CHILDBEARING FAMILY/ANTEPARTAL CARE)

60. #3. Eating dry carbohydrates such as crackers before getting out of bed in the morning may decrease nausea. IMPLEMENTATION (CHILDBEARING FAMILY/ANTEPARTAL CARE)

61. #4. In the second half of pregnancy, palpation of the uterus using Leopold's maneuver determines the position of the fetus. IMPLEMENTATION (CHILDBEARING FAMILY/ANTEPARTAL CARE)

62. #3. Contractions that occur at irregular intervals and are relieved by walking are Braxton Hicks' contractions. ANALYSIS (CHILDBEARING FAMILY/ANTEPARTAL CARE)

63. #3. This rate is too slow to be a fetal heart rate. The nurse is most likely hearing a uterine souffle as blood rushes through the placenta. This rate is the same as the mother's pulse. If the mother's pulse rate is not 96, further assessment would be required. ANALYSIS (CHILD-BEARING FAMILY/ANTEPARTAL CARE)

64. #4. The oxytocin challenge test uses medication to assess fetal response to maternal contractions. Ultrasound is used to determine gestational age. ANALYSIS (CHILDBEARING FAMILY/ANTEPARTAL CARE)

65. #4. Pancreatic ducts are clogged with mucus and, thus, enzymes needed for digestion are not secreted into the small intestine. IMPLEMENTATION (CHILD/NUTRITION AND METABOLISM)

66. #2. An elevated sweat chloride level is the definitive diagnostic test for cystic fibrosis. ASSESSMENT (CHILD/NUTRITION AND METABOLISM)

67. #3. Chest physical therapy should be done q4h prophylactically for the child with cystic fibrosis and more frequently when the child has a respiratory infection. Percuss and drain all lobes of both lungs. PLAN (CHILD/NUTRITION AND METABOLISM)

68. #2. $\dfrac{250 \text{ mg}}{1.2 \text{ ml}} = \dfrac{100 \text{ mg}}{x \text{ ml}} \qquad \dfrac{100(1.2)}{250} = .48 \text{ ml}$

IMPLEMENTATION (CHILD/NUTRITION AND METABOLISM)

69. #1. A 3-month-old is able to focus the eyes on objects, likes bright colors, and is ready to begin practicing reaching for objects. PLAN (CHILD/NUTRITION AND METABOLISM)

70. #2. Apple sauce helps disguise the taste of the enzymes; also, the cellulose in the apple sauce retards the otherwise instant action of the enzymes. IMPLEMENTATION (CHILD/NUTRITION AND METABOLISM)

71. #4. Pulmonary involvement is the leading cause of illness and death in children with cystic fibrosis. The major goal is to decrease the incidence of pulmonary infections in order to promote adequate oxygenation and increase life expectancy. EVALUATION (CHILD/NUTRITION AND METABOLISM)

72. #4. Refer families with children who have inherited disorders such as cystic fibrosis for genetic counseling. There is currently no screening test for the prenatal detection of cystic fibrosis. IMPLEMENTATION (CHILD/NUTRITION AND METABOLISM)

73. #1. Denial of illness and fear of losing control are predominant when clients discover they have a chronic disease. ASSESSMENT (ADULT/OXYGENATION)

74. #3. The normal blood pressure ranges from 115 to 120 mm Hg systolic over 75 to 80 mm Hg diastolic. A sustained diastolic pressure of greater than 90 mm Hg is defined as hypertension by the American Heart Association. ASSESSMENT (ADULT/OXYGENATION)

75. #2. Foods low in fat, sodium, and cholesterol include baked chicken (fowl), raw vegetables, and raw fruits. EVALUATION (ADULT/OXYGENATION)

76. #1. Lemon juice and vinegar are acceptable to season foods when no added salt is allowed in the diet. IMPLEMENTATION (ADULT/OXYGENATION)

77. #4. Isordil, a nitrite preparation, dilates small and large blood vessels. IMPLEMENTATION (ADULT/OXYGENATION)

78. #1. Lopressor is a beta-adrenergic blocking agent that reduces blood pressure by its action on the beta receptors in the heart. ANALYSIS (ADULT/OXYGENATION)

79. #1. Alpha-blocking agents are nonspecific and produce significant vasodilation. ANALYSIS (ADULT/OXYGENATION)

80. #2. Both mother and neonate are at risk, because of prolonged labor after membrane rupture. Because of the high risk of amnionitis following early rupture of membranes, labor is induced within 72 hours if it does not occur spontaneously. ASSESSMENT (CHILDBEARING FAMILY/POSTPARTAL CARE)

81. #2. All other assessments are normal in the postpartal period. A temperature elevated above 100.4°F (38°C) indicates sepsis. Leucocytosis normally occurs after delivery and may be related to the stress of labor and delivery. A process of diuresis begins 2 to 4 days after delivery. The client eliminates excess fluid via the skin and urinary tract in an attempt to return to normal water metabolism. ASSESSMENT (CHILDBEARING FAMILY/POSTPARTAL CARE)

82. #3. While isolation is required, the client needs an opportunity to talk about her feelings at this time. IMPLEMENTATION (CHILDBEARING FAMILY/POSTPARTAL CARE)

83. #3. $$\frac{\text{Amount to be infused} \times \text{gtt factor}}{\text{total time in minutes}}$$
$$=\frac{50 \text{ ml} \times 10 \text{ gtt/ml}}{30 \text{ minutes}} = 16$$

IMPLEMENTATION (ADULT/SURGERY)

84. #4. Lice nits attach firmly to the hair shaft; dandruff flakes off easily. Lice do not cause areas of alopecia (ringworm does). Itching can occur with lice or dandruff. ASSESSMENT (CHILD/SENSATION, PERCEPTION, PROTECTION)

85. #2. Enlarged lymph nodes often accompany head lice. Honey-colored vesicles are characteristic of impetigo. Alopecia and ringlike lesions are characteristic of ringworm (tinea). ASSESSMENT (CHILD/SENSATION, PERCEPTION, PROTECTION)

86. #1. Kwell shampoo can cause neurotoxicity if used more often than prescribed. The shampoo directions explicitly state not to shampoo more frequently than once a week. IMPLEMENTATION (CHILD/SENSATION, PERCEPTION, PROTECTION)

87. #3. Lice are most often spread by sharing personal articles (e.g., comb, hat). ANALYSIS (CHILD/SENSATION, PERCEPTION, PROTECTION)

88. #2. A single shampoo with Kwell kills the ova in nearly all cases. If observable nits are no longer present, the nurse and parent can safely assume the child's condition is no longer communicable. IMPLEMENTATION (CHILD/SENSATION, PERCEPTION, PROTECTION)

89. #3. Option #1 describes a closed fracture; #2, an impacted fracture; #4, a spiral fracture. ANALYSIS (ADULT/ACTIVITY AND REST)

90. #3. The splint tends to dig into the groin, causing irritation. The foot plate is attached to the Pearson splint. Immobility is not likely to be a problem, because balanced traction allows a great deal of freedom to move. Bedpan use is easier from the unaffected side. PLAN (ADULT/ACTIVITY AND REST)

91. #3. Calcium is lost from the bone following a fracture. Serum calcium levels are increased, and the potential for renal calculi is increased. Thus, a normal or decreased calcium intake is indicated along with sufficient fluids. EVALUATION (ADULT/ACTIVITY AND REST)

92. #2. Raising the foot of the bed enables the client's body weight to oppose the traction. The body weight is the countertraction. PLAN (ADULT/ACTIVITY AND REST)

93. #4. The pin enters the bone, providing an opening for bacteria. The pin does not inhibit knee joint movement or cause nerve damage. ANALYSIS (ADULT/ACTIVITY AND REST)

94. #1. A narrow spreader bar allows the ropes to rub against the outer aspect of the thigh. Placing padding would still result in pressure on the skin. Options #3 and #4 are inappropriate because if the ropes are correctly positioned, the client will not be uncomfortable. IMPLEMENTATION (ADULT/ACTIVITY AND REST)

95. #1. The skeletal traction and Thomas splint provide traction and support of the upper leg. ANALYSIS (ADULT/ACTIVITY AND REST)

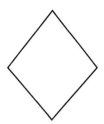

Test 2, Book II Questions

Marsha Hanover is admitted to rule out cholecystitis. She is 40 years old, 5 ft 2 in, 215 lb. She is a homemaker with 2 teenage children.

1. Which of the following statements is *incorrect* about obesity and its treatment?
   - 1. Exercise is the most practical method of weight control.
   - 2. Obesity tends to run in families because of eating habits.
   - 3. Food can become an individual's major source of gratification.
   - 4. Obese children tend to become obese adults.

2. Mrs. Hanover is scheduled for an upper gastrointestinal series. Which of the following will be used to prepare her?
   - 1. Clear liquids for breakfast the day of the exam
   - 2. A cleansing enema the morning of the exam
   - 3. Food and fluids withheld 10 to 12 hours prior to the exam
   - 4. Radiopaque tablets given the evening before the exam

3. The physician schedules Mrs. Hanover for a gastric analysis with a nasogastric tube. Which of the following nursing actions would be essential when preparing a client for gastric analysis?
   - 1. Force fluids for 24 hours preceding the test.
   - 2. Administer enemas on the preceding evening.
   - 3. Withhold food the morning of the analysis.
   - 4. Record the pulse rate when beginning the test.

4. Which of the following findings from gastric analysis would best support the diagnosis of a peptic ulcer?
   - 1. Absence of gastric secretion
   - 2. Increased hydrochloric acid
   - 3. Lack of intrinsic factor
   - 4. Decreased gastric motility

5. A tubeless gastric analysis test is used to specifically determine which of the following?
   - 1. Absence of hydrochloric acid
   - 2. The amount of hydrochloric acid secreted
   - 3. The pH of gastric secretion
   - 4. Amount of diagnex blue that can be excreted

6. Mrs. Hanover's test results indicate a duodenal ulcer. She is discharged with a prescription for a 1,500-calorie diet with no coffee or hot spices and cimetidine (Tagamet) 300 mg TID. What is the therapeutic effect of this drug?
   - 1. Neutralizes gastric acid
   - 2. Inhibits gastric secretions
   - 3. Slows digestion
   - 4. Reduces gastric motility

7. In spite of conservative treatment, Mrs. Hanover's ulcer perforates and an emergency vagotomy and pyloroplasty are performed. What is the expected outcome following the vagotomy?
   - 1. An increase in the blood supply to the stomach
   - 2. A decrease in gastric secretions and motility
   - 3. A decrease in the epigastric pain postoperatively
   - 4. An increase in gastric emptying and motility

8. Mrs. Hanover returns to her room with an IV and a nasogastric tube attached to suction. That evening she is ambulated to the bathroom and returned to bed. Suddenly she begins to gag and has dry heaves. What is the nurse's initial action?
   - 1. Splint her abdomen and turn her head to the side.
   - 2. Check her abdomen to see if an evisceration has occurred.
   - 3. Check the nasogastric tube and suction equipment for kinks or malfunction.
   - 4. Irrigate the nasogastric tube with 50 ml of normal saline.

Mary Washington, a 34-year-old unemployed secretary, has been admitted to the psychiatric unit with a diagnosis of hypochondriasis. She was brought in by her sister who states Miss Washington has a history of severe headaches for which she has sought help in many hospitals and clinics.

9. What is the best definition of hypochondriasis?
   ○ 1. A morbid concern with one's physical health
   ○ 2. A morbid concern with one's mental health
   ○ 3. An organic loss of physical functioning
   ○ 4. A category of psychosis characterized by sensory or motor disturbances

10. Which ego-defense mechanism is most frequently demonstrated in this disorder?
   ○ 1. Substitution resulting in adaptation
   ○ 2. Suppression resulting in physical symptoms
   ○ 3. Rationalization resulting in justification of behavior
   ○ 4. Displacement producing symptoms in an effort to manage anxieties

11. The best action to use in caring for Miss Washington would be which of the following?
   ○ 1. Allow her to talk about her headaches, since ventilation is therapeutic.
   ○ 2. Minimize the care given for physical symptoms, so that her attention to them will be decreased.
   ○ 3. Avoid discussion of physical symptoms since additional information may encourage her to develop further symptoms.
   ○ 4. Allow her to discuss her feelings and concerns without focusing on physical symptoms.

Su-Jen Chang delivered her first child, a boy, 24 hours ago. She had a normal vaginal delivery with a midline episiotomy and is breast-feeding her baby.

12. Which one of the following assessments on the first postpartal day would most likely indicate normal adjustment?
   ○ 1. Fundus 2 finger breadths above the umbilicus
   ○ 2. Breasts tender and engorged
   ○ 3. Moderate, steady flow of lochia serosa
   ○ 4. Lack of bowel movement since delivery

13. Instructions to Mrs. Chang regarding care of the perineal area should include which of the following?
   ○ 1. Separate the labia while cleansing.
   ○ 2. Cleanse the perineum with soap and water after elimination.
   ○ 3. Pour sterile water over the perineum after elimination.
   ○ 4. Perform perineal care only if an episiotomy was performed.

14. Which one of the following behaviors best indicates Mrs. Chang has understood the nurse's instructions to prevent cracked nipples while breast-feeding?
   ○ 1. She uses an alcohol swab to cleanse nipples prior to feeding.
   ○ 2. She air dries her nipples 15 minutes after feeding.
   ○ 3. She cleanses her nipples daily with soap and water.
   ○ 4. She allows the baby to nurse 15 minutes on each breast on her first postpartum day.

15. Which of the following behaviors would indicate Mrs. Chang is in the taking-hold phase of the postpartum period?
   ○ 1. Talking about the details of her labor and delivery experience
   ○ 2. Asking questions about normal growth and development
   ○ 3. Requesting the nurse to return the baby to the nursery immediately after feeding
   ○ 4. Asking to do a return demonstration of cord and circumcision care for her baby

16. Mrs. Chang asks the nurse when it is safe to resume sexual intercourse after she goes home. Which of the following is *not* appropriate information to give her?
   ○ 1. Resumption is safe by the 3rd to 4th week, if lochia has stopped.
   ○ 2. Resumption is safe by the 3rd to 4th week, if the episiotomy has healed.
   ○ 3. Refrain from intercourse until after the 6-week checkup.
   ○ 4. Avoid intercourse in the event of a hematoma or infection.

17. Mrs. Chang is 2 days postpartum. In addition to an elevated temperature and chills, which assessment finding would most likely suggest Mrs. Chang has acquired postpartal endometritis?
    ○ 1. Complaint of increased thirst
    ○ 2. Lochia change from rubra to serosa
    ○ 3. Uterus very tender when palpated abdominally
    ○ 4. Diastasis recti detected on abdominal palpation

Erma Olin, an 86-year-old widow, was brought to the emergency room by ambulance after suffering a fall at home. She was accompanied by a neighbor who told the admitting nurse that Mrs. Olin was active in church, and several senior citizen groups. She is self-sufficient and financially secure. She has a history of heart problems and is taking medication.

18. When approaching Mrs. Olin, what should be the nurse's first action?
    ○ 1. Explain the emergency room procedures.
    ○ 2. Tell her that a physician will be in to examine her shortly.
    ○ 3. Introduce him/herself.
    ○ 4. Apply electrode patches to monitor her cardiac activity.

19. When applying electrode patches to monitor Mrs. Olin's cardiac activity, which of the following assessments will the nurse *not* be able to make?
    ○ 1. Level of consciousness and orientation
    ○ 2. Skin color and temperature
    ○ 3. Muscle tension and motor activity
    ○ 4. Cardiac output

20. A complete 12-lead ECG on Mrs. Olin shows that she has a rate of 48 beats per minute. She is given a diagnosis of sinus bradycardia. The most common cause of this condition is
    ○ 1. stress, excitement.
    ○ 2. severe pain.
    ○ 3. digitalis toxicity.
    ○ 4. hyperthyroidism.

21. When planning care for Mrs. Olin, what would the primary goal be at this stage of her illness?
    ○ 1. Client will be free from further damage to her myocardium.
    ○ 2. Client will maintain optimum cardiac output.
    ○ 3. Client will experience a decrease in environmental and emotional stimuli.
    ○ 4. Client will maintain close communication with her significant others.

22. The laboratory report indicated that the cause of Mrs. Olin's condition was digitalis toxicity and an acceleration of cardiac atherosclerosis. She is scheduled for an insertion of a permanent pacemaker. The nurse assigned to prepare Mrs. Olin should remember that
    ○ 1. a planned, systematic approach to teaching a client to live with a pacemaker is a vital part of nursing care.
    ○ 2. Mrs. Olin will easily adjust to a pacemaker, because she has had a heart problem for 20 years.
    ○ 3. Mrs. Olin probably already has some information about pacemakers, from discussion in the media.
    ○ 4. it is the physician's responsibility to teach Mrs. Olin about her pacemaker.

23. Which of the following precautions would *not* need to be considered for Mrs. Olin's safety during the first 48 hours post-op?
    ○ 1. Use nonelectric beds.
    ○ 2. Use battery-run radios.
    ○ 3. Properly ground the electric equipment.
    ○ 4. Disconnect the television set.

24. Discharge planning for Mrs. Olin would *not* include
    ○ 1. activity and exercise.
    ○ 2. awareness of environmental hazards that might interfere with the function of the pacemaker.
    ○ 3. how to take a radial pulse daily.
    ○ 4. how to care for a permanently implanted pacemaker.

Two siblings, Bobby, aged 5, and Tina, aged 2, are admitted to the hospital with a diagnosis of chronic lead poisoning.

25. Which of the following assessments are especially important to conduct on Bobby and Tina?
    ○ 1. Pulse and respiratory rates
    ○ 2. Urinary output
    ○ 3. Dietary habits
    ○ 4. Neurologic status

26. To best promote Bobby's and Tina's adaptation to being in the hospital, which nursing action should be implemented?
    ○ 1. Insist that one of their parents stay with them.
    ○ 2. Give each of them a new stuffed animal.
    ○ 3. Take them to the playroom to get acquainted with the other children.
    ○ 4. Place them together in the same hospital room.

27. Both children are receiving injections of EDTA and dimercaprol (BAL). Which of the following observations indicate a toxic response to these drugs?
    ○ **1.** Seizures
    ○ **2.** Long-bone pain
    ○ **3.** Oliguria
    ○ **4.** Anemia

28. The nurse should prepare to administer Tina's injection in which of the following sites?
    ○ **1.** The gluteus medius muscle
    ○ **2.** The deltoid muscle
    ○ **3.** The vastus lateralis muscle
    ○ **4.** The subcutaneous tissue of the abdomen

29. As the nurse prepares to administer Bobby's injections, he begins to cry and kick. What is the best nursing response to Bobby?
    ○ **1.** ''Bobby, Tina is going to get an injection, too.''
    ○ **2.** ''Bobby, you can cry as much as you want, but you must hold still.''
    ○ **3.** ''Be a big boy now, Bobby, and this will be over in a minute.''
    ○ **4.** ''Bobby, this will just feel like a little stick in your leg.''

30. When assessing the possible source of the lead poisoning, the nurse *not* need to determine
    ○ **1.** the type of home the family lives in.
    ○ **2.** the children's eating habits.
    ○ **3.** the family's income level.
    ○ **4.** how closely the children are supervised.

31. Which of the following menus is most appropriate to serve Bobby and Tina?
    ○ **1.** Hamburger and bun, peas, milk, orange slices
    ○ **2.** Spaghetti, lettuce, grape juice, gelatin with bananas
    ○ **3.** Peanut butter sandwich, raw carrots, apple juice, vanilla pudding
    ○ **4.** Liver, broccoli, bread and butter, milk, cookie

32. Bobby and Tina are discharged to return to the clinic in 2 weeks. When they come to clinic, which of the following laboratory tests is *not* likely to be ordered?
    ○ **1.** Blood lead level
    ○ **2.** Hematocrit and hemoglobin
    ○ **3.** Urinalysis
    ○ **4.** Clotting and bleeding times

33. Which of the following outcomes is the best long-term indicator of successful treatment of Bobby and Tina?
    ○ **1.** Physical growth within normal limits
    ○ **2.** Adequate dietary intake of essential nutrients
    ○ **3.** Age-appropriate achievement of developmental milestones
    ○ **4.** Normal sleep patterns

Esteban Caliente, aged 71, is brought to the psychiatric unit by his son. The police found him wandering along the highway a mile from home. This is the fourth time Mr. Caliente has wandered away. His son states his father is becoming increasingly confused and unkempt, and he is no longer able to care for his father at home.

34. Which factor is most relevant concerning the behavior Mr. Caliente is likely to exhibit in the hospital?
    ○ **1.** The amount of alcohol he has ingested in the last 50 years
    ○ **2.** The amount of brain damage he shows
    ○ **3.** The degree of orientation he shows at the time of admission
    ○ **4.** His specific personality traits

35. In checking Mr. Caliente's orientation, the nurse will most likely find that he knows
    ○ **1.** what day it is.
    ○ **2.** where he is.
    ○ **3.** who he is.
    ○ **4.** how old he is.

36. In planning for Mr. Caliente's care, what will be most helpful?
    ○ **1.** Schedule him for as many activities as possible, so that he will not have time to miss his family.
    ○ **2.** Ensure that he meets everyone on the ward right away, so he will feel more at home.
    ○ **3.** Vary his schedule every day to prevent boredom.
    ○ **4.** Adhere to the same schedule every day to provide structure and security.

37. The information Mr. Caliente gives you about his past varies from day to day. Filling in the gaps caused by memory loss is known as which of the following?
    ○ **1.** Amnesia
    ○ **2.** Confabulation
    ○ **3.** Flashbacks
    ○ **4.** Free association

38. Mr. Caliente's son and daughter-in-law come to visit. He does not recognize them. Which response by the nurse would be most appropriate for these relatives?
    ○ 1. "He is disoriented because of his new surroundings. He will know who you are tomorrow."
    ○ 2. "There is no need for you to visit very often, since he probably won't recognize you most of the time."
    ○ 3. "I know this is difficult for you. I hope you will continue to visit as often as possible."
    ○ 4. "Perhaps you could send other family members to visit. He might recognize them."

39. One evening as the nurse is helping him prepare for bed, Mr. Caliente says, "Why didn't I get my supper?" The nurse knows he received his meal and that this client is exhibiting
    ○ 1. circumstantiality.
    ○ 2. manipulation.
    ○ 3. memory loss for recent events.
    ○ 4. retardation of thought.

40. One day the nurse finds Mr. Caliente standing in the doorway of his room. He has soiled his clothing. Which is the best response for the nurse to make?
    ○ 1. "Why didn't you let me know you had to go to the bathroom, Mr. Caliente?"
    ○ 2. "How can we keep this from happening, Mr. Caliente?"
    ○ 3. "Go in and change your clothes, Mr. Caliente."
    ○ 4. "Let me help you change, Mr. Caliente. I know this upsets you."

41. Mr. Caliente says to the nurse, "I have to meet a client in an hour." Which response shows the best understanding of his condition on the part of the nurse?
    ○ 1. "Your client just called and said he was sick today, Mr. Caliente."
    ○ 2. "I understand you were a stockbroker, Mr. Caliente. Tell me about that."
    ○ 3. "You can't meet a client, Mr. Caliente. You're in the hospital now."
    ○ 4. "You don't have to go, Mr. Caliente. Someone else is going to see him."

Jack Reynolds is a 45-year-old, unemployed engineer. He was admitted to the hospital 2 days ago with acute gastrointestinal bleeding. Two years ago, cirrhosis was diagnosed; he has been a heavy drinker for many years. Although Mr. Reynolds stopped drinking several months ago, he has had 2 recent admissions for bleeding esophageal varices.

42. An emergency endoscopy was performed on Mr. Reynolds. Following this procedure, what would be the nurse's primary concern?
    ○ 1. Urinary output
    ○ 2. Respiratory pattern
    ○ 3. Level of consciousness
    ○ 4. Gag reflex

43. The endoscopy revealed bleeding esophageal varices. A Sengstaken-Blakemore tube was inserted to control the bleeding. What is most important to remember in caring for a client with this tube?
    ○ 1. Both esophageal and gastric outlets are attached to suction.
    ○ 2. Pressure on the gastric balloon can be maintained for no more than 4 hours at a time.
    ○ 3. Iced saline lavages can be discontinued after the tube is inserted.
    ○ 4. Traction can be discontinued when the bloody drainage is less than 50 ml/hour.

44. Which of the following laboratory tests is most helpful in determining the excretory function of the liver?
    ○ 1. Albumin/globulin ratio
    ○ 2. Alkaline phosphatase
    ○ 3. Prothrombin time
    ○ 4. Bromsulphthalein test (BSP)

45. The nurse assesses Mr. Reynolds's ascites. Which of the following does *not* contribute to the ascites?
    ○ 1. Decreased plasma proteins
    ○ 2. Increased portal pressure
    ○ 3. Inability of liver to detoxify aldosterone
    ○ 4. Inability of kidneys to handle the solute load

46. What is the diuretic of choice for Mr. Reynolds?
    ○ 1. Furosemide (Lasix)
    ○ 2. Hydrochlorothiazide (HydroDIURIL)
    ○ 3. Ethacrynic acid (Edecrin)
    ○ 4. Spironolactone (Aldactone)

47. Mr. Reynolds is being considered as a candidate for a portacaval shunt. What is the primary purpose of this operation?
    ○ 1. Eliminate the incidence of further bleeding episodes
    ○ 2. Restore hepatic function
    ○ 3. Reduce portal hypertension and congestion
    ○ 4. Decrease further hepatic degeneration

48. Mr. Reynolds is at high risk for infection. Protecting him is a major nursing goal. To achieve this goal, the nurse should
    ○ 1. discourage ambulating in the corridor.
    ○ 2. initiate cooling measures for any temperature above 100°F (37.6°C).
    ○ 3. discourage visitors from coming to see him at this time.
    ○ 4. change his IV tubing and dressing q24–48h.

49. The nurse caring for Mr. Reynolds assesses that he is slightly confused and has flapping tremors of his hands. She reports this to his physician. The physician will most likely order which of the following?
    ○ 1. Increased sodium via IV route
    ○ 2. Diazepam (Valium) to decrease tremors
    ○ 3. Neomycin by mouth
    ○ 4. A CT scan to rule out any neurologic complications

50. Mr. Reynolds's daughter comes to the nurse saying, "I know Daddy is going to die. If only I'd done more to help him." The nurse might best respond by saying which of the following?
    ○ 1. "Why do you think your father is going to die?"
    ○ 2. "You must not feel guilty for your actions."
    ○ 3. "Have you shared your feelings with your father?"
    ○ 4. "I can understand your feelings. Would you like to talk?"

51. It is often difficult for the nurse to help the alcoholic client explore behavioral alternatives. An effective initial step for the nurse is to
    ○ 1. enlist the family's support.
    ○ 2. assess the client's motivation.
    ○ 3. explore his or her own feelings and attitudes about alcohol.
    ○ 4. acquire knowledge about community treatment programs.

Four-month-old Emalee is brought to the clinic for a checkup and immunizations.

52. When assessing Emalee's development, the nurse should be most concerned about which one of the following observations?
    ○ 1. Visually follows objects 180°.
    ○ 2. Does not attempt to transfer a toy from one hand to the other.
    ○ 3. Is unable to roll from back to front.
    ○ 4. Does not turn her head to locate sounds.

53. Emalee is scheduled to receive her second diphtheria/pertussis/tetanus and polio immunizations today. She has a slight cough, a runny nose, and a temperature of 100.4°F (38°C). Which of the following nursing actions is most appropriate?
    ○ 1. Advise parents of possible side effects of immunizations.
    ○ 2. Give the immunizations and recommend use of a mild analgesic as soon as they get home.
    ○ 3. Postpone the immunizations.
    ○ 4. Advise the parents to notify their physician.

54. Emalee's parents state that she does not like cereal, because she always spits it out when they try to feed it to her. What is the most appropriate nursing response to the parents?
    ○ 1. "Discontinue cereal and try fruit instead."
    ○ 2. "You may need to position her differently during meals."
    ○ 3. "She will outgrow this in a month or so."
    ○ 4. "When she is hungry enough she will eat."

55. Emalee's parents have been planning a second honeymoon in Bermuda. They want to leave the baby with an adult relative. At what age will Emalee tolerate this absence with the least amount of emotional trauma?
    ○ 1. 5 months
    ○ 2. 7 months
    ○ 3. 9 months
    ○ 4. 11 months

56. In anticipation of Emalee's next stage of development, which of the following toys and games encourage her developmental progress?
    ○ 1. Let her throw and retrieve objects.
    ○ 2. Play peek-a-boo.
    ○ 3. Play a music box.
    ○ 4. Let her bang on pots and pans.

57. In providing the parents with anticipatory guidance for Emalee, it is important that they know the common causes of mortality and morbidity in her age group. Next to birth defects, which of the following problems results in the highest death rate in infants?
    ○ 1. Drowning
    ○ 2. Accidents
    ○ 3. Child abuse and neglect
    ○ 4. Communicable disease

Arnold Hindricks is a 30-year-old college graduate, who has been employed as a manager of a print shop for the past 5 years. In the past 9 months, he has gradually become less effective in his performance, demonstrating an inability to communicate clearly and a deterioration in appearance. His wife accompanies him to the unit where he states, "They keep telling me I'm the one who did it." He is admitted with a diagnosis of schizophrenia, paranoid type.

58. When planning for activities and therapy for Mr. Hindricks, the nurse should know that which statement is characteristic of the schizophrenic client?
    ○ **1.** He is very receptive to the attention of others.
    ○ **2.** He will respond very rapidly to hospitalization and psychotropic medications.
    ○ **3.** He is very sensitive to what others are feeling.
    ○ **4.** He will require electroconvulsive therapy to disrupt the pattern of psychosis.

59. Mr. Hindricks is experiencing sensory perceptions without external stimuli. Which of the following does this best describe?
    ○ **1.** A delusion
    ○ **2.** An illusion
    ○ **3.** An hallucination
    ○ **4.** A loose association

60. Which of the following would be the best response by the nurse to Mr. Hindricks's statement?
    ○ **1.** "I don't hear the voices. What else do they say to you?"
    ○ **2.** "I don't hear the voices. They seem to frighten you."
    ○ **3.** "I don't hear the voices. It is time for you to go to occupational therapy now."
    ○ **4.** "I don't hear the voices. They are only in your head."

61. As a result of withdrawing from reality, Mr. Hindricks exhibits preoccupation with ideas and fantasies that have meaning only to him. This is an example of
    ○ **1.** adaptation.
    ○ **2.** ambivalence.
    ○ **3.** apathy.
    ○ **4.** autism.

62. One day while watching TV, Mr. Hindricks suddenly runs over and states to the announcer, "I told you before, I am not a homosexual." This behavior best describes
    ○ **1.** an idea of influence.
    ○ **2.** an idea of reference.
    ○ **3.** introjection.
    ○ **4.** labeling.

63. Mr. Hindricks is to start taking fluphenazine (Prolixin) 5 mg BID, PO. Which side effect is he most likely to experience from this drug?
    ○ **1.** Hypotension
    ○ **2.** Hypothermia
    ○ **3.** Impotence
    ○ **4.** Nausea and vomiting

64. After taking fluphenazine for 1 week, Mr. Hindricks is restless. The nurse notices that he is moving his hands and mouth and pacing in the hallway. What is the term used to describe these side effects of fluphenazine?
    ○ **1.** Akinesia
    ○ **2.** Akathesia
    ○ **3.** Catatonia
    ○ **4.** Dyskinesia

65. Which of the following drugs and dose would be most appropriate to alleviate Mr. Hindricks's symptoms?
    ○ **1.** Benztropine mesylate (Cogentin) 1 mg BID, PO
    ○ **2.** Trihexyphenidyl (Artane) 15 mg BID, PO
    ○ **3.** Chlordiazepoxide (Librium) 25 mg BID, PO
    ○ **4.** Diazepam (Valium) 5 mg TID, PO

66. Mr. Hindricks will remain on a fluphenazine regimen after discharge. What is the primary advantage of this drug for outpatient use?
    ○ **1.** It is safer than other phenothiazines.
    ○ **2.** It has fewer side effects than other phenothiazines.
    ○ **3.** It is less addicting than other phenothiazines.
    ○ **4.** It is available in a long-acting form.

67. Mr. Hindricks participates in milieu therapy on the unit. Milieu therapy manipulates the hospital environment in order to provide
    ○ **1.** positive living and learning experiences.
    ○ **2.** a safe atmosphere.
    ○ **3.** an opportunity for improvement of socialization skills.
    ○ **4.** the opportunity to learn new skills through adjunctive therapies.

68. Mr. and Mrs. Hindricks plan to go to family therapy. What is the main objective of this therapy?
- ○ **1.** Client will verbalize the cause of the illness.
- ○ **2.** Client will reestablish effective communication patterns.
- ○ **3.** Client will avoid rehospitalization.
- ○ **4.** Client's children will remain free of the symptoms of schizophrenia.

Daniel Jackowitz has just been born. He weighs 8 lb and appears to be normal. He is being breast-fed.

69. Silver nitrate or penicillin drops are used in a baby's eyes at birth to prevent
- ○ **1.** retrolental fibroplasia.
- ○ **2.** ophthalmia neonatorum.
- ○ **3.** treponema pallidium.
- ○ **4.** chemical conjunctivitis.

70. Baby Daniel's Apgar score was 9 because of acrocyanosis. This condition in newborns is a result of
- ○ **1.** retained amniotic fluid in the lungs.
- ○ **2.** failure to breathe within the expected amount of time.
- ○ **3.** sluggish peripheral circulation.
- ○ **4.** increased hormonal levels in the mother.

71. What should the nurse expect Baby Daniel's stool to look like at 1 week?
- ○ **1.** Black and tarry
- ○ **2.** Green and seedy
- ○ **3.** Light yellow and mushy
- ○ **4.** Bright yellow and formed

72. When testing a breast-fed neonate for phenylketonuria, a false-negative result is most often the result of which condition?
- ○ **1.** Decreased vitamin K level
- ○ **2.** Inadequate fluid intake
- ○ **3.** Increased serum bilirubin
- ○ **4.** Insufficient protein absorption

73. The admitting nurse would most likely need to include assessment of which of the following to determine Baby Daniel's gestational age?
- ○ **1.** Body temperature
- ○ **2.** Amount of vernix and lanugo
- ○ **3.** Heart rate
- ○ **4.** Laboratory values

74. Baby Daniel has a core temperature of 100.4°F (38°C). The temperature of the Isolette reads 98°F (36.6°C). The neonate's fever is most probably a result of
- ○ **1.** an infection.
- ○ **2.** the temperature of the Isolette.
- ○ **3.** a maternal infection.
- ○ **4.** a neonatal abnormality.

75. Baby Daniel is now 2 days old and weighs 7 lb 9 oz. He is voiding 8 times a day and breast-feeds every 3 to 4 hours around the clock. Which nursing action would probably be appropriate at this time?
- ○ **1.** Consult with the physician about adding supplementary formula to his diet.
- ○ **2.** Weigh him before and after breast-feeding.
- ○ **3.** Continue to support his mother's breast-feeding efforts.
- ○ **4.** Observe him for signs of impending dehydration.

76. Circumcision without a local anesthetic was performed on Baby Daniel. Care of this newly circumcised infant within the first 4 hours would *not* include which of the following?
- ○ **1.** Inspect the site every hour for excessive bleeding.
- ○ **2.** Withhold feeding immediately after the procedure.
- ○ **3.** Monitor and record first voiding.
- ○ **4.** Apply fresh, sterile petroleum-jelly dressing with each diaper change.

77. Which of the following assessments is the most important after phototherapy is initiated?
- ○ **1.** Appearance of the sclera
- ○ **2.** Estimated urinary output
- ○ **3.** Number and type of stools
- ○ **4.** Daily weight

Bert Arnold, aged 36, is a sales representative for a large computer corporation. Three years ago, an ulcer was diagnosed, and he was advised to find more time for rest and relaxation. He did not comply and, in the last month, has had more epigastric pain.

78. Which of the following would be the most realistic short-term goal to help Mr. Arnold begin to deal with his stress?
- ○ **1.** Express emotions directly
- ○ **2.** Decrease workload
- ○ **3.** Use relaxation techniques daily
- ○ **4.** Decrease social commitments

79. When Mr. Arnold's ulcer was diagnosed 3 years ago, his physician prescribed cimetidine (Tagamet). However, Mr. Arnold reports that he has not taken it. Which of the following approaches would be *least* effective in helping Mr. Arnold comply?
- ○ **1.** Help him set up a medical-reminder schedule.
- ○ **2.** Educate him about ulcer complications.
- ○ **3.** Suggest he enlist the help of his wife and coworkers.
- ○ **4.** Explain that taking the medication will help decrease his pain.

80. Perforation is a major complication of a duo-
    denal ulcer. When this has occurred, what is
    the initial nursing priority?
    ○ 1. Insert a nasogastric tube.
    ○ 2. Start an IV and infuse fluids.
    ○ 3. Administer a high dose of an antibiotic.
    ○ 4. Teach turning, coughing, and deep
         breathing.

81. Mr. Arnold is taught that he should not take
    any medications before checking with his phy-
    sician, since there are many drugs that can ag-
    gravate his ulcer. An example of one of these
    drugs is
    ○ 1. indomethacin (Indocin).
    ○ 2. magnesium and aluminum hydroxide (Maa-
         lox).
    ○ 3. atropine.
    ○ 4. acetaminophen (Tylenol).

*Nine-month-old Bradley has been admitted to the pe-
diatric unit with vomiting, colicky abdominal pain, and
abdominal distension. A tentative diagnosis of intussusception is made.*

82. When assessing Bradley, which type of stool
    indicates a worsening of Bradley's condition?
    ○ 1. Fatty, bulky, foul-smelling
    ○ 2. Dark red, jellylike
    ○ 3. Ribbonlike, dark green
    ○ 4. Clay colored

83. Bradley is *not* likely to exhibit which of the
    following behaviors?
    ○ 1. Loud crying when his parents leave him
    ○ 2. Fear of strangers
    ○ 3. Searching for hidden objects
    ○ 4. Saying at least 3 words besides ''mama''
         and ''dada''

84. Bradley is scheduled for surgery. His parents
    are anxious and ask what will be done in sur-
    gery. Which explanation should be given?
    ○ 1. The sigmoid colon will be resected with a
         pull-through anastomosis.
    ○ 2. The obstruction will be corrected by manual
         reduction.
    ○ 3. The affected portion of the intestine will be
         resected with an end-to-end anastomosis.
    ○ 4. The ileum will be resected and a permanent
         ileostomy created.

85. Bradley's parents ask what is wrong with his
    intestines. Which statement best describes
    Bradley's condition?
    ○ 1. A telescoping of one part of the bowel into
         a more distal part
    ○ 2. Malrotation of the small intestine
    ○ 3. Atresia of the intestinal tract
    ○ 4. Absence of parasympathetic ganglion cells

86. Preoperatively, the priority nursing goal for
    Bradley is to
    ○ 1. maintain Bradley's attachment to his par-
         ents.
    ○ 2. meet Bradley's needs for sucking and com-
         fort while he is NPO.
    ○ 3. maintain adequate hydration.
    ○ 4. promote adequate rest and sleep.

87. Following surgery, Bradley returns to the unit.
    He is fussy and seems to be in discomfort. The
    nurse palpates his abdomen and notes some dis-
    tension. Which action should be implemented
    first?
    ○ 1. Call the surgeon to report this observation.
    ○ 2. Insert a rectal tube.
    ○ 3. Sit Bradley upright and pat him on the
         back.
    ○ 4. Check the nasogastric tube for patency.

88. What is potentially the greatest threat to Brad-
    ley's continued development while he is hospi-
    talized?
    ○ 1. Developing mistrust of the nursing staff
    ○ 2. Separation from his parents
    ○ 3. Restricted mobility
    ○ 4. Disruption in his sleeping and eating rou-
         tines

89. Bradley is recovering well, and his IV and na-
    sogastric tube have been discontinued. He is
    taking half-strength formula feedings. Assum-
    ing Bradley's development is average for his
    age, which toy would be most appropriate for
    him at this time?
    ○ 1. An activity box for his crib
    ○ 2. A fuzzy stuffed animal
    ○ 3. A small toy truck
    ○ 4. A music box

90. Bradley is ready for discharge. The nurse discusses his nutritional habits with his mother. Bradley has been taking a commercial iron-fortified formula and juices from a bottle, also cereal, strained fruits, and vegetables, which his parents feed him. Which anticipatory instruction is *not* appropriate to give Bradley's mother at this time?
    ○ **1.** Switch Bradley to whole milk and give him supplemental vitamins and minerals.
    ○ **2.** Begin introducing chopped meats, egg yolk, and breads such as zwieback, one at a time, to Bradley's diet.
    ○ **3.** Introduce a cup for drinking juices and water.
    ○ **4.** Give Bradley foods he can feed himself with his fingers or a spoon.

Robert Heil, aged 55, is admitted to the hospital with complaints of nausea and vomiting and dull, wavelike abdominal pains. He appears malnourished and has a markedly enlarged abdomen. The physician suspects cirrhosis and has ordered a liver biopsy to make a definitive diagnosis.

91. The nurse charts the following observations of the admitting physical assessment. Which of the following would *not* be a symptom of cirrhosis?
    ○ **1.** Jaundiced sclera
    ○ **2.** Irregular pulse
    ○ **3.** Edema of the ankles
    ○ **4.** Patches of ecchymosis in the extremities

92. Why does Mr. Heil have a tendency to bleed as manifested by abnormal bruising?
    ○ **1.** Inadequate vitamin K absorption
    ○ **2.** Inadequate vitamin A absorption
    ○ **3.** Depressed production of platelets
    ○ **4.** Depressed production of red blood cells

93. What is the most appropriate nursing action for a client undergoing a liver biopsy?
    ○ **1.** Explain to the client that he may resume his bathroom privileges after the procedure.
    ○ **2.** Position the client in a semi-Fowler's position for the procedure.
    ○ **3.** Turn the client on his left side following the procedure.
    ○ **4.** Assess the client for complaints of abdominal pain postprocedure for at least 24 hours.

94. Which of the following diets would the nurse encourage Mr. Heil to select, in order to best meet his nutritional needs?
    ○ **1.** High-protein foods
    ○ **2.** Low-protein foods
    ○ **3.** Low-calorie foods
    ○ **4.** High-sodium foods

95. What nursing action would best promote adequate respiratory function?
    ○ **1.** Instruct client to cough and deep breathe qh.
    ○ **2.** Ambulate client frequently.
    ○ **3.** Maintain client in a high-Fowler's position in bed.
    ○ **4.** Provide postural drainage and percussion q2h.

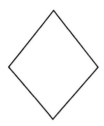

Test 2, Book II
Answers with Rationales

1. **#1.** As a method of weight loss, exercise alone is not practical, because of the large amount of exercise needed to lose 1 lb. ANALYSIS (ADULT/NUTRITION AND METABOLISM)

2. **#3.** An upper gastrointestinal series and barium swallow must be done on an empty stomach. Food and fluids are withheld for several hours. Cleansing enemas are given prior to large bowel exams. Radiopaque tablets are for gallbladder x-rays. PLAN (ADULT/NUTRITION AND METABOLISM)

3. **#3.** A fasting specimen of hydrochloric acid is used to obtain baseline data. Eating stimulates acid production. PLAN (ADULT/NUTRITION AND METABOLISM)

4. **#2.** Peptic ulcers are directly related to high levels of hydrochloric acid. Option #1 is too vague. Lack of intrinsic factor results in anemia. Decreased motility is not related to ulcers. ANALYSIS (ADULT/NUTRITION AND METABOLISM)

5. **#3.** The tubeless gastric analysis determines the pH by measuring the excretion of diagnex blue via the urinary system. ANALYSIS (ADULT/NUTRITION AND METABOLISM)

6. **#2.** Cimetidine (Tagamet) is a histamine antagonist that blocks histamine-stimulated gastric secretions. Antacids (e.g., Maalox) neutralize acids in the stomach. Smooth muscle relaxants decrease motility. ANALYSIS (ADULT/NUTRITION AND METABOLISM)

7. **#2.** A vagotomy is done to eliminate the acid-secreting stimulus of the gastric cells. It has no effect on post-op pain or stomach perfusion. ANALYSIS (ADULT/NUTRITION AND METABOLISM)

8. **#3.** Nausea and gagging may be due to kinks or a nonpatent tube, which can cause an increased volume of retained gastric secretions and pressure on the anastomosis. The risk of evisceration usually occurs later, once the sutures are removed. Option #4 may be a second action if there is an order. IMPLEMENTATION (ADULT/NUTRITION AND METABOLISM)

9. **#1.** There is no attending organic pathologic condition or actual loss of function. Clients with hypochondriasis will deny any relationship between their symptoms and their mental health. Hypochondriasis is not a psychotic disorder. ASSESSMENT (PSYCHOSOCIAL, MENTAL HEALTH, PSYCHIATRIC PROBLEMS/ANXIOUS BEHAVIOR)

10. **#4.** Anxieties are displaced onto the body in an effort to cope. While hypochondriasis is a replacement of behavior, it does not produce adaptation. It is not a voluntary exclusion of anxiety from the conscious level as in suppression. Hypochondriacs do not attempt to justify their behavior, nor do they have a conscious understanding about their behavior. ANALYSIS (PSYCHOSOCIAL, MENTAL HEALTH, PSYCHIATRIC PROBLEMS/ANXIOUS BEHAVIOR)

11. **#4.** Symptoms occur as an attempt to cope with stressful situations, and the ability to gain insight may decrease the need for secondary gain. Allowing her to talk about her physical symptoms provides secondary gain and reinforces continuing concern. Physical symptoms must be assessed and treated, not minimized or avoided. IMPLEMENTATION (PSYCHOSOCIAL, MENTAL HEALTH, PSYCHIATRIC PROBLEMS/ANXIOUS BEHAVIOR)

12. **#4.** A spontaneous bowel movement may be delayed until several days after delivery. Within 24 hours following delivery the fundus should have begun involution and be located below the umbilicus. The breasts should be soft at this time as breast milk does not come in until 2 to 3 days after delivery. Lochia rubra is typical at this time. ASSESSMENT (CHILDBEARING FAMILY/POSTPARTAL CARE)

13. **#2.** The labia should not be separated as this would result in a greater possibility of introducing microorganisms. Perineal care is carried out even if an episiotomy was not performed in order to decrease microorganisms. IMPLEMENTATION (CHILDBEARING FAMILY/POSTPARTAL CARE)

14. #2. To prevent nipple cracking, air drying after each nursing period is suggested. Soap and alcohol cause drying of the nipples, increasing the chance of breakdown. Breast-feeding is begun gradually starting with 3 minutes on each breast. EVALUATION (CHILDBEARING FAMILY/ POSTPARTAL CARE)

15. #4. The mother begins to be the initiator in the taking-hold phase. Her early mothering tasks are especially important to her. This is considered the optimal time for teaching. ASSESSMENT (CHILDBEARING FAMILY/POSTPARTAL CARE)

16. #3. It is safe to resume sexual intercourse by the third or fourth week if bleeding has stopped and the episiotomy has healed. Most couples resume intercourse before the 6-week checkup. IMPLEMENTATION (CHILDBEARING FAMILY/POSTPARTAL CARE)

17. #3. This is another sign of endometritis. Lochia would have a red-brown color and may be either foul smelling or odorless. An increase in thirst is most likely due to dehydration. Diastasis recti is separation of the abdominal muscle due to weakened muscles. ASSESSMENT (CHILDBEARING FAMILY/POSTPARTAL CARE)

18. #3. This is a basic principle when approaching a client for the first time. It establishes rapport and communicates respect for the individual. IMPLEMENTATION (ADULT/OXYGENATION)

19. #4. When applying electrodes, an assessment using touch can be done concurrently to determine skin and muscle conditions. Level of consciousness and orientation are assessed when evaluating her response to the explanation of electrode application. Cardiac output is determined by actual monitoring, either noninvasively by blood pressure or invasively by arterial line or central line (e.g., Swan-Ganz). ASSESSMENT (ADULT/OXYGENATION)

20. #3. Stress, severe pain, and hyperthyroidism are causes of tachycardia. Sinus bradycardia in clients over age 65 is usually due to medications, especially digoxin. Remember that digitalis toxicity can also result in a heart rate greater than 100 beats per minute. ANALYSIS (ADULT/OXYGENATION)

21. #2. Bradycardia results in a decrease in cardiac output; therefore all nursing activity would be directed at maintaining the best possible cardiac output. Options #1 and #3 are related to this primary goal. PLAN (ADULT/OXYGENATION)

22. #1. A planned, systematic approach to client teaching is essential when a major alteration in activities of daily living and life-style will be the outcome of an illness. Options #2 and #3 are assumptions that cannot be made. Patient education is a shared responsibility. PLAN (ADULT/OXYGENATION)

23. #4. The electrical conduits of a television set are all well grounded in hospitals and will not interfere with pacemaker activity. The other precautions must be taken to avoid electrical interference with the pacemaker. PLAN (ADULT/OXYGENATION)

24. #4. Permanently implanted pacemakers require no physical or technical care. Teaching must focus on any adjustments to be made in activities of daily living. PLAN (ADULT/OXYGENATION)

25. #4. The major and potentially most serious effects of chronic lead poisoning are neurologic. Therefore, frequent assessment of neurologic status is imperative. ASSESSMENT (CHILD/SENSATION, PERCEPTION, PROTECTION)

26. #4. Allowing Bobby and Tina to room together will promote security for each of them, because they are familiar with each other. IMPLEMENTATION (CHILD/SENSATION, PERCEPTION, PROTECTION)

27. #3. EDTA is potentially toxic to the kidneys and can cause damage that can result in oliguria. ASSESSMENT (CHILD/SENSATION, PERCEPTION, PROTECTION)

28. #3. In the toddler, EDTA and BAL should be administered intramuscularly in the anteriolatteral thigh (vastus lateralis muscle). IMPLEMENTATION (CHILD/SENSATION, PERCEPTION, PROTECTION)

29. #2. This tells Bobby what is expected of him but also gives him an outlet for his fears. The other options either increase fear or belittle him. IMPLEMENTATION (CHILD/SENSATION, PERCEPTION, PROTECTION)

30. #3. The family's income level has no bearing on the risk of lead poisoning. If the family lives in an old house, there may be lead paint chips. Any history of pica is important to ascertain. Also, if the children are not properly supervised in a potentially unsafe environment, the risk of lead poisoning is increased. ASSESSMENT (CHILD/SENSATION, PERCEPTION, PROTECTION)

31. **#1.** This menu is highest in vitamin D, calcium, and phosphorus, which are needed to aid in the excretion of lead from the bones. IMPLEMENTATION (CHILD/SENSATION, PERCEPTION, PROTECTION)

32. **#4.** Lead does not interfere with platelet production or bleeding and clotting mechanisms. ANALYSIS (CHILD/SENSATION, PERCEPTION, PROTECTION)

33. **#3.** Achievement of age-appropriate developmental milestones indicates there has been no permanent neurologic damage. EVALUATION (CHILD/SENSATION, PERCEPTION, PROTECTION)

34. **#4.** An exaggeration of personality traits determines the behaviors exhibited in chronic organic brain syndrome. There is no correlation between the amount of brain damage and amount of alcohol ingested to the severity of psychologic symptoms. The degree of orientation the client shows at the time of admission may change for the better or worse. ASSESSMENT (PSYCHOSOCIAL, MENTAL HEALTH, PSYCHIATRIC PROBLEMS/CONFUSED BEHAVIOR)

35. **#3.** Deterioration in knowledge of time occurs first, then confusion of place, and finally, confusion of person. ASSESSMENT (PSYCHOSOCIAL, MENTAL HEALTH, PSYCHIATRIC PROBLEMS/CONFUSED BEHAVIOR)

36. **#4.** It is beneficial to reinforce reality by providing structure and order in as many areas of the client's life as possible. In coordinating the client's schedule, it is important to avoid excessive stimulation and variations, which might only serve to confuse the client further. Making numerous introductions may be futile because of the client's loss of memory for recent events. IMPLEMENTATION (PSYCHOSOCIAL, MENTAL HEALTH, PSYCHIATRIC PROBLEMS/CONFUSED BEHAVIOR)

37. **#2.** Confabulation is a process whereby experiences are imagined to fill in memory blanks. It is a form of protection against anxiety. Amnesia is loss or lack of memory. Flashbacks are a sudden sense of "reliving" past experiences, especially those which were painful or traumatic. Free association is a process whereby the client is encouraged to describe thoughts or feelings as they occur. IMPLEMENTATION (PSYCHOSOCIAL, MENTAL HEALTH, PSYCHIATRIC PROBLEMS/CONFUSED BEHAVIOR)

38. **#3.** Continued contact is important for both father and son. The client with organic brain syndrome will be aware of a caring person even though he may not always display recognition. While it is true that Mr. Caliente is probably disoriented by his new surroundings, chances are that he will still not know his son or any other family members tomorrow because of the nature of organic brain syndrome. IMPLEMENTATION (PSYCHOSOCIAL, MENTAL HEALTH, PSYCHIATRIC PROBLEMS/CONFUSED BEHAVIOR)

39. **#3.** Poor memory of recent events is common in this condition. Circumstantiality is a symptom whereby the client introduces into the conversation details which have little if anything to do with the conversation. It is possible that manipulation is part of the client's normal coping skills, but it is more likely that the client is confused rather than manipulative. Retardation of thought refers to a slowing down of thought processes. ANALYSIS (PSYCHOSOCIAL, MENTAL HEALTH, PSYCHIATRIC PROBLEMS/CONFUSED BEHAVIOR)

40. **#4.** Incontinence may occur frequently in a client with this syndrome. The nurse needs to demonstrate understanding as well as institute nursing measures that will decrease its incidence. Options #1, #2, and #3 convey a lack of understanding of organic brain syndrome, plus an unnecessary annoyance with the client that is nontherapeutic. He will probably be unable to work with the nurse to discover how to prevent his incontinence or change his clothes and clean up. IMPLEMENTATION (PSYCHOSOCIAL, MENTAL HEALTH, PSYCHIATRIC PROBLEMS/CONFUSED BEHAVIOR)

41. **#2.** Encouraging clients to reminisce is valuable in maintaining their sense of value. It also helps decrease feelings of isolation and promotes a sense of continuity. Options #1, #3, and #4 reflect his disorientation; the nurse should not "play along" with the client but, rather, reorient him to the present. IMPLEMENTATION (PSYCHOSOCIAL, MENTAL HEALTH, PSYCHIATRIC PROBLEMS/CONFUSED BEHAVIOR)

42. **#4.** Local anesthesia is used for this procedure; testing for the gag reflex is necessary to prevent aspiration. PLAN (ADULT/NUTRITION AND METABOLISM)

43. #1. Both esophageal and gastric outlets are attached to suction to drain blood from the gastrointestinal system. As long as there are bloody returns in the aspirate, iced lavage is continued. Traction is maintained for a period of time to ensure control of bleeding. It should not be maintained longer than 72 hours, or esophageal necrosis may result. PLAN (ADULT/NUTRITION AND METABOLISM)

44. #4. Of the options listed, only the bromsulfophthalein test measures liver excretory function. ASSESSMENT (ADULT/NUTRITION AND METABOLISM)

45. #4. Increased hydrostatic pressure from portal hypertension and the diminished synthesis of albumin by the liver result in ascites. The inability of the liver to break down aldosterone also contributes to the process. Thus, increased aldosterone levels result in sodium reabsorption. ANALYSIS (ADULT/NUTRITION AND METABOLISM)

46. #4. Spironolactone would be the first choice, as its action is to block aldosterone, which the liver cannot detoxify. ANALYSIS (ADULT/NUTRITION AND METABOLISM)

47. #3. The operation diverts the blood from the portal circulation, thus decreasing some of the portal hypertension. It cannot prevent bleeding, nor does it facilitate liver regeneration. ANALYSIS (ADULT/NUTRITION AND METABOLISM)

48. #4. Any opening in the skin is a portal of entry for bacteria. Cooling measures will do nothing to decrease or prevent infection and generally will not be initiated until the temperature has gone above 101°F (38.3°C) or 102°F (38.8°C). IMPLEMENTATION (ADULT/NUTRITION AND METABOLISM)

49. #3. In Mr. Reynolds, encephalopathy is likely to develop because of his recent bleeding. Neomycin is given to decrease the ammonia production in the intestines, as increased ammonia levels are believed to bring on symptoms of hepatic encephalopathy. ANALYSIS (ADULT/NUTRITION AND METABOLISM)

50. #4. She needs an opportunity to express feelings and receive some support. Eventually she will need to discuss things with her father. IMPLEMENTATION (ADULT/NUTRITION AND METABOLISM)

51. #3. Frequently, nurses have been directly or indirectly affected by problems associated with alcohol and are not able to assist the client in a helping manner until they discern their own attitudes. IMPLEMENTATION (ADULT/NUTRITION AND METABOLISM)

52. #4. Turning the head to locate sounds should be present before 4 months of age. All other options are age appropriate. ASSESSMENT (CHILD/HEALTHY CHILD)

53. #3. Immunizations should be postponed if the child has a febrile illness. This is a nursing decision. The child's symptoms do not warrant referral to a physician at this time. IMPLEMENTATION (CHILD/HEALTHY CHILD)

54. #3. The extrusion reflex is present until approximately 4 months of age. Although the infant may be hungry, she cannot bring solids to the back of her mouth yet. The child will outgrow this with practice. Altering eating patterns or foods because of this may establish poor feeding habits. IMPLEMENTATION (CHILD/HEALTHY CHILD)

55. #1. After 7 months of age, stranger anxiety sets in and makes separation from parents very difficult. ANALYSIS (CHILD/HEALTHY CHILD)

56. #2. This game teaches a sense of object permanence, which gradually develops from 4 to 8 months. The other activities listed are more appropriate for older ages. PLAN (CHILD/HEALTHY CHILD)

57. #2. Accidents are the second leading cause of death in Emalee's age group. ANALYSIS (CHILD/HEALTHY CHILD)

58. #3. Even the most withdrawn client is very sensitive to what others are feeling, even though they themselves communicate very little verbally and may be unaware of their feelings. Clients diagnosed with paranoid schizophrenia generally demonstrate social isolation related to impaired ability to trust and are unreceptive to receiving attention from others. Response to treatment is generally slow due to the client's protectiveness and impaired ability to trust. Electroconvulsive therapy is most successfully used with depressed clients and is usually not effective in disrupting psychosis. ASSESSMENT (PSYCHOSOCIAL, MENTAL HEALTH, PSYCHIATRIC PROBLEMS/WITHDRAWN BEHAVIOR)

59. **#3.** Auditory hallucinations are the most common. Hallucinations temporarily decrease anxiety by delaying interaction with someone real. Delusion is a fixed, false belief that may be persecutory, grandiose, or somatic in nature, and cannot be corrected with reasoning. Illusion is a misinterpretation of a real sensory experience. Loose association is a communication pattern characterized by lack of clarity of connection between one thought and the next. ANALYSIS (PSYCHOSOCIAL, MENTAL HEALTH, PSYCHIATRIC PROBLEMS/WITHDRAWN BEHAVIOR)

60. **#2.** This statement points out reality, but acknowledges the feelings of the client. While the other options reinforce the reality that the nurse does not perceive the voices, #1 focuses attention on and gives importance to the voices, #3 avoids discussing the client's feelings, and #4 will escalate the client's anxiety level making him more committed to the hallucinations. IMPLEMENTATION (PSYCHOSOCIAL, MENTAL HEALTH, PSYCHIATRIC PROBLEMS/WITHDRAWN BEHAVIOR)

61. **#4.** The private reality of the schizophrenic is derived from internal ideas and desires not shared by others. Adaptation is the capability of the body/mind to cope with any type of increased demand made upon it. Ambivalence is having simultaneous conflicting feelings or attitudes toward a person or object. Apathy is a lack of interest and concern. ANALYSIS (PSYCHOSOCIAL, MENTAL HEALTH, PSYCHIATRIC PROBLEMS/WITHDRAWN BEHAVIOR)

62. **#2.** An idea of reference is a belief that certain events or statements relate directly to the individual when they do not. Idea of influence is when the individual feels as though s/he has influence over other individuals. Introjection is a type of identification in which the client incorporates qualities or values of another person or group into his/her own ego structure. Labeling is to describe or designate with a label. ANALYSIS (PSYCHOSOCIAL, MENTAL HEALTH, PSYCHIATRIC PROBLEMS/WITHDRAWN BEHAVIOR)

63. **#1.** Changes in blood pressure are common with this drug. Instruct clients to rise slowly from a sitting or lying position. The other options are all noted side effects of phenothiazines; however, the most common side effect is orthostatic hypotension due to the interference with dopamine reception or synthesis at the neural synapse. ASSESSMENT (PSYCHOSOCIAL, MENTAL HEALTH, PSYCHIATRIC PROBLEMS/WITHDRAWN BEHAVIOR)

64. **#2.** Akathesia is evidenced by motor restlessness. Akinesia is a lethargic, subjective sense of fatigue and muscle weakness that is a side effect of antipsychotic medication. Catatonia is a state of psychologically induced immobility at times interrupted by episodes of agitation. Dyskinesia is associated with the long-term use of high-dose phenothiazine drugs, and is characterized by involuntary, jerking, and uncoordinated movements. ANALYSIS (PSYCHOSOCIAL, MENTAL HEALTH, PSYCHIATRIC PROBLEMS/WITHDRAWN BEHAVIOR)

65. **#1.** Cogentin is effective in relieving the symptoms of parkinsonism caused by antipsychotic medications. This is an appropriate dosage and can be given parenterally if indicated. Artane is another good antiparkinson drug; however, the dose is 5 mg BID, not 15 mg. The use of a benzodiazepine (e.g., Librium, Valium) is not appropriate because these drugs do not have a direct effect on the extrapyramidal system. ANALYSIS (PSYCHOSOCIAL, MENTAL HEALTH, PSYCHIATRIC PROBLEMS/WITHDRAWN BEHAVIOR)

66. **#4.** Fluphenazine is used parenterally every 7 to 21 days for outpatients. The other statements are false. Fluphenazine has a mild anticholinergic sedating effect and extrapyramidal effect. Tolerance and addiction to antipsychotics are not substantiated in the literature, although mild withdrawal symptoms (e.g., headaches, irritability, nausea) can present with rapid discontinuation. ANALYSIS (PSYCHOSOCIAL, MENTAL HEALTH, PSYCHIATRIC PROBLEMS/WITHDRAWN BEHAVIOR)

67. **#1.** Milieu therapy provides the opportunity to improve the physical and emotional condition of the client by providing positive living experiences. The other options are an integral part of milieu therapy but not the overall goal. PLAN (PSYCHOSOCIAL, MENTAL HEALTH, PSYCHIATRIC PROBLEMS/WITHDRAWN BEHAVIOR)

68. **#2.** Family therapy is helpful to improve communication and acceptance of differences among members. The cause of schizophrenia is unknown. Family therapy in conjunction with drug therapy could prevent rehospitalization. Schizophrenia is not known to be inherited; however, Mr. Hindricks's children could well benefit from family therapy. PLAN (PSYCHOSOCIAL, MENTAL HEALTH, PSYCHIATRIC PROBLEMS/WITHDRAWN BEHAVIOR)

69. #2. Ophthalmia neonatorum is an eye disease of infants that causes blindness. It is passed from mother to infant through a birth canal infected with gonorrhea. Silver nitrate or penicillin drops prevent this. ANALYSIS (CHILD-BEARING FAMILY/NORMAL NEWBORN)

70. #3. Acrocyanosis is blue hands and feet and is due to poor peripheral circulation. ANALYSIS (CHILDBEARING FAMILY/NORMAL NEWBORN)

71. #3. When breast-fed, an infant's stool is light yellow and mushy. Stools go through a transitional process from black meconium in the first 24 hours to a greenish yellow (transitional) color to a breast- or bottle-fed stool on the 5th day of life. ASSESSMENT (CHILDBEARING FAMILY/NORMAL NEWBORN)

72. #4. Phenylalanine is an amino acid found in milk. Often the mother's breast milk is not sufficiently established at the time of testing to give an accurate result. Therefore, it may be necessary to retest the infant at a later date. ANALYSIS (CHILDBEARING FAMILY/NORMAL NEWBORN)

73. #2. The amount of vernix and lanugo decreases with increasing gestational age. Term infants usually have vernix only in the skin creases, and lanugo tends to be found only over the shoulders. The determination of gestational age by physical examination most often utilizes the tool described by Dubowitz. ASSESSMENT (CHILDBEARING FAMILY/NORMAL NEWBORN)

74. #2. An Isolette should be maintained at a temperature of 92° to 94°F (33.3° to 34.4°C). An infection in the neonate, not the mother, may be accompanied by an elevated temperature. ASSESSMENT (CHILDBEARING FAMILY/NORMAL NEWBORN)

75. #3. Newborns lose up to 10% of their birth weight in the first few days after birth. As this is expected weight loss, support the mother in her efforts to breast-feed. The normal neonate will void 6 to 10 times/day. This is indicative of adequate hydration. IMPLEMENTATION (CHILDBEARING FAMILY/NORMAL NEWBORN)

76. #2. Feeding the baby who has just been circumcised is comforting and essential, as it is recommended that feedings be withheld for several hours prior to the procedure. The penis is checked hourly for bleeding and pressure is applied should it occur. Voiding is monitored to determine complications with the procedure. Vaseline gauze promotes healing. IMPLEMENTATION (CHILDBEARING FAMILY/NORMAL NEWBORN)

77. #3. Phototherapy may result in dehydration. Watery stools are common. Fluid loss is replaced by increasing fluid volume offered to the neonate by 25%. ASSESSMENT (CHILDBEARING FAMILY/NORMAL NEWBORN)

78. #3. All the other options are appropriate for Mr. Arnold, but use of the relaxation techniques can be started immediately and can be very beneficial. PLAN (ADULT/NUTRITION AND METABOLISM)

79. #2. Information about the complications of ulcer may not be helpful. He has not experienced the complications, so he can use denial and choose not to comply. IMPLEMENTATION (ADULT/NUTRITION AND METABOLISM)

80. #2. Hypovolemic shock can occur very quickly following a perforation, so fluid replacement must be done first and quickly. Options #1, #3, and #4 are all appropriate once the client is safe and stable. IMPLEMENTATION (ADULT/NUTRITION AND METABOLISM)

81. #1. Indocin is very irritating to the stomach and duodenum and can cause or aggravate ulcers. ANALYSIS (ADULT/NUTRITION AND METABOLISM)

82. #2. Dark red, "currant jelly" stools indicate the onset of bowel necrosis from gangrene. ASSESSMENT (CHILD/ELIMINATION)

83. #4. The average 9-month-old infant may be able to say "mama" or "dada" but has not learned to articulate other words yet. ASSESSMENT (CHILD/HEALTHY CHILD)

84. #3. Only the affected portion of the intestine is resected, and an end-to-end anastomosis of the remaining healthy intestinal segments is done. IMPLEMENTATION (CHILD/ELIMINATION)

85. #1. Intussusception is the telescoping or invagination of one part of the intestine into a more distal portion. IMPLEMENTATION (CHILD/ELIMINATION)

86. **#3.** Although all these goals are important, Bradley is especially at risk for dehydration and electrolyte imbalance because of vomiting associated with intussusception. PLAN (CHILD/ELIMINATION)

87. **#4.** The nasogastric tube may be obstructed, causing the abdominal distension. Inserting a rectal tube is contraindicated because Bradley has had lower intestinal tract surgery. IMPLEMENTATION (CHILD/ELIMINATION)

88. **#2.** Separation anxiety begins at about 8 months of age and can cause extreme distress for the infant in this age group. ANALYSIS (CHILD/ELIMINATION)

89. **#1.** An activity box will promote continued development of fine motor skills and hand-eye coordination, and allow Bradley some activity within the confines of his hospital crib. IMPLEMENTATION (CHILD/ELIMINATION)

90. **#1.** Infants should not be switched to whole milk (or 2% low-fat milk) until 1 year of age. IMPLEMENTATION (CHILD/ELIMINATION)

91. **#2.** An irregular pulse is characteristic of a disturbance of electrical stimulation or conduction in the heart. This is more commonly found in clients with heart disease. ASSESSMENT (ADULT/NUTRITION AND METABOLISM)

92. **#1.** Clients with liver disease have an increased tendency to bleed. This is caused either by a failure to absorb vitamin K or because the liver is unable to utilize vitamin K to form prothrombin. If the client's bile duct is obstructed, absorption of vitamin K is reduced. Even if vitamin K is absorbed, damaged liver cells cannot synthesize adequate amounts. ANALYSIS (ADULT/NUTRITION AND METABOLISM)

93. **#4.** A complication of this procedure is accidental penetration of a blood vessel causing hemorrhage, or penetration of a biliary vessel causing chemical peritonitis from leakage of bile into the abdominal cavity. These complications would be manifested as abdominal pain and unstable vital signs. Pressure to the biopsy site can be applied by positioning the client on his right side after the procedure. The client remains on strict bed rest for 24 hours after the procedure. PLAN (ADULT/NUTRITION AND METABOLISM)

94. **#1.** Cellular function in the liver depends upon tissue-building materials supplied by amino acids derived from proteins. Clients with liver disease with no evidence of encephalopathy need high-protein, high-calorie, low-sodium diets. PLAN (ADULT/NUTRITION AND METABOLISM)

95. **#3.** Clients with ascites experience dyspnea, resulting from pressure exerted against the diaphragm. A high-Fowler's position reduces this pressure. The client needs rest to reduce metabolic demands on the liver and should keep activities to a minimum by resting quietly in bed most of the day. IMPLEMENTATION (ADULT/NUTRITION AND METABOLISM)

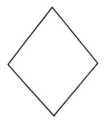

Test 2, Book III Questions

Monica Corley enters the labor and delivery unit at 40 weeks gestation. Her cervix is 2 cm dilated and 80% effaced. Her contractions are 3 to 5 minutes apart and are associated with mild discomfort.

1. Based upon the information presented, which of these assessments of Mrs. Corley's phase of labor is most accurate?
   - ○ 1. First stage, latent phase
   - ○ 2. First stage, active phase
   - ○ 3. First stage, deceleration phase
   - ○ 4. Second stage of labor

2. Mrs. Corly is restless and complaining of severe pain. Her cervix is 5 cm dilated and 90% effaced. The vertex is at 0 station. She requests pain medication, and the physician has ordered meperidine (Demerol) 75 mg. Which of the following nursing actions is most appropriate?
   - ○ 1. Give her the Demerol, as it is an optimal time to do so.
   - ○ 2. Try to have her wait until her cervix is at least 6 cm dilated and the vertex is at 1+ station.
   - ○ 3. Tell her the Demerol will cause her baby to be "sleepy" when it is born.
   - ○ 4. Give her one-half dose of the medication.

3. The medication contains 100 mg Demerol/ml. How many ml will the nurse administer?
   - ○ 1. 1.0
   - ○ 2. 0.5
   - ○ 3. 0.75
   - ○ 4. 1.5

4. Which of the following principles accurately explains the effects on the fetus of analgesics and anesthetics administered to the mother during the intrapartum period?
   - ○ 1. Medication effects are generally negligible if they are administered 2 or more hours before delivery.
   - ○ 2. Medication effects are related to the duration of labor.
   - ○ 3. Medication effects are time, dose, and route related.
   - ○ 4. Medication effects are related to maternal age and weight.

5. What is the primary rationale for administering an antacid during labor?
   - ○ 1. To settle the laboring mother's stomach
   - ○ 2. To increase digestion during labor
   - ○ 3. To prevent pneumonia in case of aspiration during use of general anesthesia
   - ○ 4. To lower the pH of the blood in cases of possible hyperventilation

6. Mrs. Corley states she heard someone say her baby is "ROP" and asks what that means. What would be the best response?
   - ○ 1. "Your baby is fine. Those initials simply refer to the baby's position in the birth canal."
   - ○ 2. "ROP stands for right occiput posterior. This means your baby is head down, with the back of its head pointing toward your right flank."
   - ○ 3. "ROP means your baby is bottom down and turned the opposite direction from the way most babies are turned. This does not mean you will not be able to deliver vaginally."
   - ○ 4. "ROP stands for right orbital presentation. This means your baby's head is extended and will need to flex before delivery can be completed."

7. In planning care for Mrs. Corley, the nurse will need to take into account the typical consequences of fetal malpresentation. Which of the following consequences is most pertinent to the care of Mrs. Corley?
   - ○ 1. Malpresentation frequently slows the dilatation of the cervix.
   - ○ 2. Malpresentation does not increase the risk of fetal trauma when the head is the presenting part.
   - ○ 3. Because labor is more efficient in multiparas, malpresentation does not have a significant impact on the effectiveness of the contractions.
   - ○ 4. Regardless of presentation, the cardinal movements of labor remain the same.

Mary Smith is brought to the emergency room by a friend. Mrs. Smith is tense, shaking, and pale. When the nurse touches her to guide her to a chair, the nurse notes that Mrs. Smith's skin is cool and clammy. The friend reports that Mrs. Smith is a graduate student at the university and that she has been preparing for her oral examinations for her doctoral degree. When the nurse asks Mrs. Smith how she is feeling, Mrs. Smith says, "How do you think I feel?" She bursts into tears, then says, "I'm sorry. I'm just so scared. I feel like something awful is about to happen to me."

8. What level of anxiety is the client experiencing?
   - ○ 1. Mild
   - ○ 2. Moderate
   - ○ 3. Severe
   - ○ 4. Panic

9. What is the most appropriate immediate goal for the nurse to set for the client?
   - ○ 1. Client will develop a trusting relationship with the nurse.
   - ○ 2. Client will gain insight into her problems.
   - ○ 3. Client will demonstrate alternate methods of coping.
   - ○ 4. Client will reduce anxiety at least 1 level.

10. Which of the following is appropriate to try with Mrs. Smith in her current state?
    - ○ 1. Recognize and reflect the feelings client is experiencing and indicate that the nurse will be there to help her.
    - ○ 2. Leave her alone until she feels more like being around other persons.
    - ○ 3. Reassure her that nothing bad is going to happen to her.
    - ○ 4. Encourage her to act out anxiety by moving around or to express her feelings verbally.

11. When the physician on duty sees Mrs. Smith, she orders 5 mg of diazepam (Valium) IM and asks the nurse to stay with the client until she becomes less anxious. When the nurse prepares to administer the medication, Mrs. Smith becomes more agitated and says, "You're not going to make a junkie out of me!" Which of the following is the best response?
    - ○ 1. "The doctor wouldn't have ordered something that was going to hurt you. You need this to calm down."
    - ○ 2. "It will help you calm down, but I won't give it to you until you are ready."
    - ○ 3. "No one is trying to turn you into a junkie. You are so upset that you are confused."
    - ○ 4. "You can't become a junkie from just one shot. Please let me give you this shot to help you."

12. When Mrs. Smith's friend urges her to take the medication, she consents to do so. Which of the following would be the best way to begin interviewing Mrs. Smith?
    - ○ 1. "How do you usually cope with anxiety?"
    - ○ 2. "You must be really upset about your doctoral work."
    - ○ 3. "Tell me about what happened about the time that you started feeling anxious."
    - ○ 4. "What can I do to help you?"

13. About 30 minutes after the diazepam was administered, Mrs. Smith asks to lie down because she feels dizzy and faint. Which of the following is the most likely cause of these symptoms?
    - ○ 1. Her level of anxiety
    - ○ 2. An allergic response to the drug
    - ○ 3. Common side effects of the drug
    - ○ 4. Her state of exhaustion

Jorge Benton is a newborn with a bilateral cleft lip and a cleft palate.

14. Jorge's parents are young but seem very concerned and willing to learn about his care. Which of the following would be *inappropriate* to include in the teaching plan for the parents?
    - ○ 1. Remove the nipple frequently when feeding Jorge.
    - ○ 2. Encourage mother to breast-feed.
    - ○ 3. Jorge's security needs can be met other than by sucking.
    - ○ 4. Jorge's mental functioning should be normal.

15. When Jorge is 2½ months old, he is hospitalized for repair of his cleft lip. Preoperatively, which of the following nursing actions is most important for Jorge?
    - ○ 1. Burp him frequently during feedings.
    - ○ 2. Offer him small, frequent feedings so as not to tire him.
    - ○ 3. Hold him in a low or flat position to facilitate swallowing.
    - ○ 4. Offer thickened bottle feedings to increase his intake.

16. When Jorge is 13 months old, he is admitted for repair of his cleft palate. What is the best reason for the palate to be repaired at this age?
    - ○ 1. To give Jorge a chance to develop basic speech patterns
    - ○ 2. To prevent damaging tooth buds
    - ○ 3. To allow better cooperation from Jorge post-op
    - ○ 4. So Jorge can be weaned from breast-feeding

17. Jorge's long-range nursing care plans should include follow-up and referral for several potential problems. Which of the following problems will Jorge's mother be most likely to observe?
    ○ **1.** Headaches and malocclusion
    ○ **2.** Dental caries and emotional problems
    ○ **3.** Contractures of the mandible
    ○ **4.** Speech problems and otitis media

Ann Duke, aged 60, was admitted to the hospital after complaining of right-sided weakness, slurring of speech, dysphagia, and some visual disturbances. She has a history of hypertension. The admitting diagnosis is a cerebrovascular accident.

18. What is the most probable cause of the admitting symptoms?
    ○ **1.** Transient ischemic attack
    ○ **2.** Cerebral aneurysm
    ○ **3.** Cerebral hemorrhage
    ○ **4.** Meningitis

19. The client has a positive Babinski's reflex. This is indicated by
    ○ **1.** dorsiflexion of the great toe when the sole is scratched.
    ○ **2.** tremor of the foot following brisk, forceful dorsiflexion.
    ○ **3.** extension of the leg when the patellar tendon is struck.
    ○ **4.** plantar flexion of the great toe when the sole is scratched.

20. Mrs. Duke was incontinent during the first few days of her hospitalization. What would be the most satisfactory means of handling this problem?
    ○ **1.** Restrict oral fluid intake.
    ○ **2.** Insert an indwelling catheter.
    ○ **3.** Offer the bedpan q4h.
    ○ **4.** Apply disposable diapers.

21. While you are bathing Mrs. Duke, she begins to mutter something unintelligible about the "plant," while pointing excitedly at a glass of water on the bedside stand. She indicates in pantomime that she wants a drink of water. This behavioral observation is most characteristic of which of the following types of aphasia?
    ○ **1.** Visual
    ○ **2.** Hysterical
    ○ **3.** Receptive
    ○ **4.** Expressive

22. This type of aphasia occurs when the injury is in the speech center. Where in the brain is the speech center located?
    ○ **1.** Medulla oblongata
    ○ **2.** Around the central fissure (Broca's area)
    ○ **3.** Occipital lobe
    ○ **4.** Parietal lobe

23. What would be the most therapeutic nursing approach when Mrs. Duke's aphasia is severe?
    ○ **1.** Anticipate her wishes, so she will not need to talk.
    ○ **2.** Communicate by means of questions that can be answered by shaking her head.
    ○ **3.** Keep up a steady flow of talk to minimize her silence.
    ○ **4.** Encourage her to speak at every possible opportunity.

24. When Mrs. Duke is attempting to speak, she becomes frustrated. Her family asks you how to deal with this problem. What is your best advice?
    ○ **1.** They should continue to encourage her.
    ○ **2.** It may be their frustration rather than Mrs. Duke's.
    ○ **3.** It will help if they anticipate her needs more.
    ○ **4.** Be patient with her and do not expect too much progress at this time.

25. Mrs. Duke still has some dysphagia, but she is beginning to eat solid foods. What is the most important aspect when assisting her to eat?
    ○ **1.** Use a bulb syringe when giving fluids.
    ○ **2.** Praise her consistently if she can feed herself.
    ○ **3.** Keep her positioned in a semi-Fowler's position.
    ○ **4.** Allow her to attempt to feed herself.

26. Mr. Duke asks whether the right arm and leg will always be paralyzed. The nurse's answer is primarily based on knowledge that
    ○ **1.** much of the initial paralysis is due to edema of brain tissue.
    ○ **2.** strokes are characterized by functional, rather than organic, changes.
    ○ **3.** new neurons will be regenerated to replace the damaged ones.
    ○ **4.** her future neurologic status cannot be predicted this early.

27. When is the best time to begin a rehabilitation plan for Mrs. Duke?
   ○ **1.** When the physician orders it
   ○ **2.** 24 hours after the critical phase of the illness
   ○ **3.** Upon admission to the hospital
   ○ **4.** When the entire health team can meet and decide on a comprehensive program

28. Which one of the following would be considered most vital to success or failure of a rehabilitation program?
   ○ **1.** Physicians
   ○ **2.** Nursing staff
   ○ **3.** Significant others or family members
   ○ **4.** Physical therapist

29. Mrs. Duke has been taking anticoagulant medication. She will be discharged on a regimen of warfarin (Coumadin) 10 mg daily. What instructions should her family receive?
   ○ **1.** Ensure weekly partial thromboplastin times (PTT) are done.
   ○ **2.** Eat foods that are high in vitamin K.
   ○ **3.** Do daily checks of Mrs. Duke's skin.
   ○ **4.** Expect to see pink urine for several days.

Sally, age 2 years, has eczema.

30. In which age group is eczema most frequently seen?
   ○ **1.** Infancy
   ○ **2.** Childhood
   ○ **3.** Adolescence
   ○ **4.** It is seen equally in all age groups.

31. The primary objective of nursing care of the infant/child with eczema is
   ○ **1.** treatment of pruritus.
   ○ **2.** identification of the allergen.
   ○ **3.** giving treated baths.
   ○ **4.** education for diet regimen.

32. Sally's parents say she is irritable and does not sleep well. What is the most likely cause of Sally's irritability and lack of sleep?
   ○ **1.** Pruritus
   ○ **2.** Pain
   ○ **3.** Teething
   ○ **4.** Hunger

33. When planning to give Sally a bath, which of the following baths should the nurse recommend?
   ○ **1.** Warm water and soap
   ○ **2.** Cool water and soap
   ○ **3.** Tepid water only
   ○ **4.** Warm water with lipid soap

34. Which activity would be most appropriate for Sally?
   ○ **1.** Playing with clay
   ○ **2.** Naming pictures in a book/magazine
   ○ **3.** Building a column with plastic building blocks
   ○ **4.** Drawing pictures of familiar objects with crayons

35. When instructing Sally's parents about skin care at home, which of the following instructions is *not* appropriate?
   ○ **1.** Provide a cool, dry environment.
   ○ **2.** Use wool clothing in the winter to allow for air circulation.
   ○ **3.** Rinse clothes twice during washing.
   ○ **4.** Prevent scratching.

36. Which of the following responses indicates that Sally's parents do *not* fully understand how to prevent their daughter's scratching?
   ○ **1.** ''Sally wears elbow restraints when we can't directly supervise her.''
   ○ **2.** ''Sometimes Sally wears cotton gloves so she won't irritate her rash.''
   ○ **3.** ''We've been dressing her in 1-piece outfits.''
   ○ **4.** ''Sally wears close-fitting clothes.''

37. To help Sally's parents promote her nutrition, which of the following observations indicates a need for teaching?
   ○ **1.** Sally is fed after her rest period.
   ○ **2.** She takes vitamin and mineral supplements.
   ○ **3.** Her parents occasionally allow her to have a favorite restricted food to encourage her eating.
   ○ **4.** Sally's parents allow her to feed herself.

38. Sally is placed on a hypoallergenic diet. Which of the following foods is *least* likely to be allowed?
   ○ **1.** Turkey
   ○ **2.** Soy milk
   ○ **3.** Pancakes
   ○ **4.** Peaches

Renata Jones is a 44-year-old woman whose divorce was final 2 months ago. She is having trouble sleeping, is unable to eat, and reports having very little energy. She has been having trouble taking care of her house.

39. The symptoms that Mrs. Jones describes are most likely a manifestation of
   ○ **1.** depression.
   ○ **2.** anxiety.
   ○ **3.** psychosis.
   ○ **4.** paranoia.

40. Which of the following is the most appropriate goal for Mrs. Jones?
   ○ **1.** Client will be free of signs of suspicious behavior after 1 month.
   ○ **2.** Client will resume activities of daily living within 1 month.
   ○ **3.** Client will be able to distinguish between what is real and what is not real within 2 weeks.
   ○ **4.** Client will demonstrate more calm and rational behavior within 2 weeks.

41. Which of the following best explains Mrs. Jones's symptoms?
   ○ **1.** She has lost a sense of reality orientation.
   ○ **2.** Her symptoms result from stimulation of the sympathetic nervous system related to high stress levels.
   ○ **3.** She lacks a feeling of trust in people.
   ○ **4.** She is angry at the loss of her husband and is taking out the anger on herself.

42. During an interview with the nurse, Mrs. Jones begins to cry. The appropriate nursing response is
   ○ **1.** "Don't cry, Mrs. Jones. You'll feel better in a day or so."
   ○ **2.** to leave her alone and check on her in 15 minutes.
   ○ **3.** "This is really a difficult time for you, isn't it Mrs. Jones."
   ○ **4.** to force her to talk and reveal her feelings.

43. Mrs. Jones appears to be feeling much better the next day, when the nurse talks with her. Mrs. Jones asks to be discharged stating, "I can handle it on my own now. You've helped me so much." The nurse knows that the appropriate response to such a request is to
   ○ **1.** deny discharge, suspecting that she may have made the decision to attempt suicide.
   ○ **2.** discharge her.
   ○ **3.** permit her a 2-day pass to see how she gets along.
   ○ **4.** permit her a 2-hour pass.

44. The next week, Mrs. Jones is irritable. She is criticizing the staff and their treatment of her. The nurse is most likely to evaluate this behavior as
   ○ **1.** regression.
   ○ **2.** dangerous to the staff.
   ○ **3.** improvement.
   ○ **4.** suicidal.

45. Which of the following would the nurse consider when evaluating Mrs. Jones's progress?
   ○ **1.** Her ability to deal with stress
   ○ **2.** Her reality orientation
   ○ **3.** Her preoccupation with suspicious thoughts
   ○ **4.** Her handling of activities of daily living

Gladys Witt, aged 70, is undergoing hemodialysis for acute renal failure following a hysterectomy. An arteriovenous (AV) shunt has been placed in her right forearm.

46. Which of the following is the *least* likely cause of prerenal azotemia, such as Miss Witt is most likely experiencing?
   ○ **1.** Hypovolemia
   ○ **2.** Severe crush injuries
   ○ **3.** Shock
   ○ **4.** Poisons

47. What is the most important indication for hemodialysis?
   ○ **1.** To prepare the client for renal transplant
   ○ **2.** To control a high and rising serum potassium level
   ○ **3.** To increase the life span of a client with chronic renal failure
   ○ **4.** To avoid excessive diet and fluid restrictions

48. Which of the following is *not* an aim of hemodialysis?
   ○ **1.** To restore fluid and electrolyte balance
   ○ **2.** To correct acid-base imbalance
   ○ **3.** To replace the endocrine functions of the kidneys
   ○ **4.** To remove the nitrogenous by-products of protein metabolism

49. Miss Witt says she's concerned about needing to be on the kidney machine. Which is the most appropriate response?
   ○ **1.** "Don't worry. I'm sure your Medicare will cover the cost."
   ○ **2.** "We can teach you to do your own treatments at home."
   ○ **3.** "Do you have family who can learn to do your dialysis?"
   ○ **4.** "It's unlikely you'll need long-term dialysis, and we'll keep you informed about how your kidneys are recovering."

50. The nurse plans to observe Miss Witt carefully for symptoms of disequilibrium syndrome during dialysis and immediately following. Which is *not* a symptom of this complication?
   ○ **1.** Agitation
   ○ **2.** Lethargy
   ○ **3.** Muscle twitching
   ○ **4.** Convulsions

51. During hemodialysis, the nurse is most concerned about observing for
    ○ 1. anuria.
    ○ 2. infection.
    ○ 3. uremic intoxication.
    ○ 4. hypovolemic shock.

52. Why is regional heparinization used during the dialysis procedure?
    ○ 1. To retard clotting in the cannula
    ○ 2. To prevent clotting in the dialyzer
    ○ 3. To minimize intravascular thrombosis
    ○ 4. To decrease embolization of clots from the cannula

53. Which action is *inappropriate* when caring for the arteriovenous shunt?
    ○ 1. Palpate to assess blood flow.
    ○ 2. Apply a tight dressing to prevent cannula dislodgement.
    ○ 3. Avoid blood pressure readings in the affected limb.
    ○ 4. Apply antibiotic ointment to the shunt site.

Baby Girl Ortiz, 39-weeks gestation, has been admitted to the observation nursery. She weighs 7 lb 1 oz and had Apgar scores of 9 at 1 minute and 10 at 5 minutes.

54. The nurse admitting the infant to the nursery notes a temperature of 96.8°F (36°C) on admission. Which nursing action is most appropriate at this time?
    ○ 1. Chart the temperature reading.
    ○ 2. Call the pediatrician to check the infant.
    ○ 3. Place the infant in a warmed incubator.
    ○ 4. Administer oxygen by mask.

55. If the temperature remains at 96.8°F (36°C) after 5 hours, which condition would the infant be most prone to develop?
    ○ 1. Respiratory acidosis
    ○ 2. Bilirubinemia
    ○ 3. Polycythemia
    ○ 4. Hyperglycemia

56. The nurse does a complete assessment. All of the following are noted. Which requires immediate attention?
    ○ 1. Cephalohematoma
    ○ 2. Milia
    ○ 3. Moro's reflex
    ○ 4. Expiratory grunting

57. What is the major reason why an injection of vitamin K is given to newborns in the nursery?
    ○ 1. It helps conjugate bilirubin in the infant.
    ○ 2. It prevent Rh sensitization in the infant.
    ○ 3. It reduces the possibility of hemorrhage in the infant.
    ○ 4. It increases the infant's resistance to infection.

58. While performing a newborn assessment, the nurse observes the following: respiratory rate 44 and irregular, and apical heart rate 148, bluish hands and feet. How should the nurse interpret these data?
    ○ 1. Possible cardiovascular problem. Call the physician.
    ○ 2. Respiratory distress. Administer oxygen.
    ○ 3. Normal newborn. Continue to observe.
    ○ 4. Cold stress. Place infant in heated Isolette.

59. Which of the following observations is considered normal?
    ○ 1. Heart rate of 90/minute
    ○ 2. Jaundice in the first 24 hours
    ○ 3. Nasal flaring
    ○ 4. Uncoordinated eye movements

60. Mrs. Ortiz is worried because her 2-day-old infant has lost 5 oz since birth. How should the nurse respond?
    ○ 1. "Try giving her formula more frequently."
    ○ 2. "The nurse probably made a mistake while weighing your baby."
    ○ 3. "The nurses will feed your baby for you for a few days."
    ○ 4. "It is normal for an infant to lose up to 10% of her weight in the first few days."

61. The nurse observes signs of jaundice in Baby Ortiz on the third day of her life. What is the most likely explanation?
    ○ 1. Liver failure
    ○ 2. Physiologic jaundice
    ○ 3. Erythroblastosis fetalis
    ○ 4. Sepsis

Mike Lane, an acutely ill 10-year-old, is hospitalized with an upper respiratory infection and right otitis media. He is pale and lethargic and has a low-grade fever. Mike's condition is diagnosed as lymphoblastic leukemia.

62. Mike's initial pallor and lethargy are most likely the result of

○ **1.** an accumulation of toxic wastes in body tissues caused by poor kidney functioning.

○ **2.** body tissues being deprived of oxygen because of a decrease in the number of red blood cells.

○ **3.** excessive needs for energy because of Mike's respiratory and ear infections.

○ **4.** a slower than normal blood flow to body tissues caused by a decreased heart rate.

63. The nurse notes that Mike has petechiae; bleeding from his gums, lips, and nose; and bruises on various parts of his body. Which one of the laboratory findings should the nurse expect to find?

○ **1.** Low serum calcium level

○ **2.** Faulty thrombin production

○ **3.** Decreased platelet count

○ **4.** Elevated partial thromboplastin time

64. Which of the following nursing measures is *contraindicated* for Mike?

○ **1.** Alternate medications between oral and intramuscular route.

○ **2.** Handle his extremities with care while turning him.

○ **3.** Use stool softeners prn.

○ **4.** Provide frequent oral hygiene.

65. Which statement best indicates that Mike understands the use of chemotherapy for treatment?

○ **1.** "I must be getting worse, because the drugs make me so sick."

○ **2.** "I won't be able to return to school until my disease-fighting cells increase."

○ **3.** "I can tolerate the nausea, because I know the drugs will kill all the cancer cells."

○ **4.** "I don't want a wig, because boys don't lose their hair."

66. Mike returns to the hospital 2 years later in a terminal stage. His parents decide to remain with him continuously. What is the most reasonable nursing plan?

○ **1.** Be available to the Lanes for emotional support while providing most of Mike's care.

○ **2.** Leave the Lanes alone with Mike to help them work through their grief.

○ **3.** Provide all meals and sleeping accommodations for the Lanes.

○ **4.** Teach the Lanes to give Mike most of his care.

Jane Smith, a 35-year-old single parent, has been hospitalized as the result of a court order for psychiatric evaluation and treatment, following continuing physical violence toward her 3-year-old daughter. History indicates that she has been fired 3 times from waitress positions for "refusing to do things that are beneath me, like clearing off the table for those fat slobs. I told them that they are pigs and they could clear their own messy table." Miss Smith's mother states that the client has no friends, probably because "she tricks people so much and hurts their feelings." While being evaluated in the emergency room, the client screams that her back is hurting her and refuses to be admitted to the psychiatric unit. She is first admitted to the orthopedic unit to assess her back problem.

67. While making rounds on nights, the nurse observes that Miss Smith has diaphoresis and mild tremors. At 8:00 A.M. the following day, the client complains of nervousness and is noted to be grossly disoriented and hyperactive. What substance has most likely been abused by Miss Smith?

○ **1.** Valium

○ **2.** Alcohol

○ **3.** Barbiturates

○ **4.** Marijuana

68. Miss Smith tells one of the primary nurses that another nurse, Miss Levy, "is a royal ass. I like you, because you're a good nurse. You're the only one who really understands me. Miss Levy isn't a good nurse." Which of the following does the client's remark best indicate?

○ **1.** Ability to detect staff weaknesses

○ **2.** Thought disorder

○ **3.** Rigid defense mechanism

○ **4.** Manipulative behavior

69. Which of the following characteristics is most likely to suggest a personality disorder?

○ **1.** Complies readily and passively with hospital rules and regulations

○ **2.** Minimal insight and poor impulse control

○ **3.** Demonstrates ego disintegration and impaired thought processes

○ **4.** Delusional and acting-out behavior

70. When dealing with clients with personality disorders, staff most often experience which of the following emotional states?

○ **1.** Anger, helplessness

○ **2.** Apathy, boredom

○ **3.** Confusion, mild irritability

○ **4.** Curious absence of feelings

71. In addition to psychiatric evaluation, one of the goals of Miss Smith's hospitalization is that she will recognize and abide by the limits set on her behavior in her interactions with other clients and with staff. Which of the following approaches is the most therapeutic way for staff to deal with her behavior?
    ○ **1.** Provide her with attention when she is not manipulating others.
    ○ **2.** Do not intervene in Miss Smith's interactions with other clients.
    ○ **3.** Make decisions as soon as possible after she makes a request.
    ○ **4.** Give detailed explanations about what she is expected to do.

Rena Klein is a 73-year-old, retired telephone operator who had a hemorrhoidectomy this morning. She has just returned from the recovery room, has an IV infusing, and is alert and oriented.

72. What step should the nurse take after checking her vital signs?
    ○ **1.** Auscultate her chest.
    ○ **2.** Check for excess bleeding.
    ○ **3.** Check her abdomen for distension.
    ○ **4.** Percuss her bladder.

73. Six hours after her surgery, Mrs. Klein has not voided. What is the most appropriate nursing action to take at this time?
    ○ **1.** Ask her if she needs to urinate.
    ○ **2.** Catheterize her.
    ○ **3.** Help her to the bathroom.
    ○ **4.** Run warm water over her fingers.

74. Mrs. Klein progresses well on her second post-op day. What care is appropriate?
    ○ **1.** Encourage Mrs. Klein to lie on her back when in bed.
    ○ **2.** Encourage Mrs. Klein to sit up for as long as possible.
    ○ **3.** Have Mrs. Klein sit on a rubber ring when in a chair.
    ○ **4.** Take Mrs. Klein's temperature orally.

75. Mrs. Klein tells the nurse that she is worried about having her first bowel movement. What is the best response?
    ○ **1.** "All hemorrhoid patients are concerned about that."
    ○ **2.** "What concerns you about it?"
    ○ **3.** "Are you afraid that it will be painful?"
    ○ **4.** "Don't worry. Your doctor has ordered medication to make it as painless as possible."

76. Which of the following instructions would be best to give Mrs. Klein in order to help avoid post-op infection?
    ○ **1.** "Do perineal care with antiseptic solution after every stool and take as many sitz baths as you need to clean the incision."
    ○ **2.** "Do perineal care every morning and every evening and take sitz baths as necessary to clean the incision."
    ○ **3.** "Do perineal care with antiseptic solution every evening and take 3 sitz baths every day."
    ○ **4.** "Do perineal care with plain soap and water after every stool and take a sitz bath 4 times a day."

77. Which of the following is important to tell Mrs. Klein in preparation for discharge?
    ○ **1.** "Limit your fluid intake."
    ○ **2.** "Notify your doctor if you have increased pain when having a bowel movement."
    ○ **3.** "Notify your doctor when you have your first bowel movement."
    ○ **4.** "Stay with a low-residue, soft diet for 3 weeks."

Jimmy Baker, aged 1½, is brought to the emergency room by his mother. He has a skull fracture and multiple body bruises. Child abuse is suspected.

78. Assessing the situation, the nurse should find what information most useful?
    ○ **1.** The interaction between Jimmy and his mother
    ○ **2.** When the accident occurred
    ○ **3.** Presence of other children in the family
    ○ **4.** Age of Jimmy's mother

79. Which of the following actions should be taken by hospital personnel when child abuse is suspected?
    ○ **1.** Confront Jimmy's mother.
    ○ **2.** Notify the police.
    ○ **3.** Notify the child protective services.
    ○ **4.** Do nothing until the diagnosis is certain.

80. Before an effective working relationship with Jimmy's mother can be established, which of the following is most important for the nurse to do?
    ○ **1.** Identify personal feelings regarding child abuse.
    ○ **2.** Learn to deal with negative feelings about abusive care givers.
    ○ **3.** Review the family history thoroughly.
    ○ **4.** Identify referral sources for abusive care givers.

81. A nursing goal for Mrs. Baker is that she will develop more adaptive parenting skills. Which of the following indicates that she has, at least partially, met this goal?
○ **1.** She attends Parents Anonymous group meetings.
○ **2.** She brings Jimmy presents in the hospital.
○ **3.** She calls the hospital several times a day to check on Jimmy's progress.
○ **4.** After discharge, she brings Jimmy to the clinic for his immunizations.

Jack Silsbe is a 64-year-old client with a 30-year history of cigarette smoking. A chest x-ray, bronchoscopy, and biopsy confirm oat-cell carcinoma.

82. Mr. Silsbe's cancer is inoperable. External radiation is prescribed as a palliative measure. What side effect is Mr. Silsbe most likely to experience?
○ **1.** Alopecia
○ **2.** Bone-marrow suppression
○ **3.** Stomatitis
○ **4.** Dyspnea

83. Nursing management of Mr. Silsbe's irradiated skin will *not* include
○ **1.** applying A and D Ointment to relieve dry skin.
○ **2.** cleansing the skin with tepid water and a soft cloth.
○ **3.** avoiding direct exposure to the sun.
○ **4.** redrawing the skin markings if they are accidentally removed.

84. Mr. Silsbe tells you that he fears he is radioactive and a danger to his family and friends. How should the nurse dispel his fears?
○ **1.** Inform him that radiation machines are risk free.
○ **2.** Explain that once the machine is off, radiation is no longer emitted.
○ **3.** Avoid telling him that his fears are in fact true.
○ **4.** Instruct him to spend short periods of time with his family and friends.

85. Fatigue is part of a radiation syndrome not related to the site of therapy. How might the nurse best ensure that Mr. Silsbe receives adequate rest?
○ **1.** Schedule all Mr. Silsbe's hospital activities early in the morning, so that he has the remainder of the day to rest.
○ **2.** Encourage Mr. Silsbe's family to carry out all his activities for him, so that he will not overexert himself.
○ **3.** Keep Mr. Silsbe on bed rest with bathroom privileges only.
○ **4.** Balance Mr. Silsbe's daily activities with frequent rest periods.

Jim Taylor, a 6-month-old infant, is admitted to the hospital with diarrhea of 2 days duration. The physician suspects the infant has eaten something contaminated by salmonella.

86. Which of the following foods or fluids are most likely to be contaminated by salmonella?
○ **1.** Water, fruits
○ **2.** Eggs and poultry
○ **3.** Milk, vegetables
○ **4.** Beef, pork

87. At Jim's age, what is the most critical clinical manifestation of the degree of dehydration?
○ **1.** Sunken fontanel
○ **2.** Weight loss
○ **3.** Decreased urine output
○ **4.** Dry skin

88. Jim has a potassium deficit. Which of the following is *not* a symptom of this?
○ **1.** Muscle weakness
○ **2.** Hunger
○ **3.** Anorexia
○ **4.** Cardiac dysrhythmias

89. Which of the following is *not* an appropriate nursing order for Jim?
○ **1.** Monitor intake and output.
○ **2.** Restrain the limb with the IV infusion.
○ **3.** Maintain bed rest; do not pick up.
○ **4.** Observe activity and alertness.

Cathy Lubbick, a 32-year-old woman, reports to her gynecologist for her yearly Pap test. She states she has been in good health but complains of a watery vaginal discharge. She is concerned because there is a family history of cancer.

90. Assessing Mrs. Lubbick, you keep in mind the early signs of cancer. Which of the following are early signs of cancer of the cervix?
   ○ 1. A dark, foul-smelling discharge
   ○ 2. Pressure on the bladder or bowel or both
   ○ 3. Pain and weight loss
   ○ 4. Watery vaginal discharge

91. While assessing Mrs. Lubbick, the nurse considers the possibility of endometrial cancer. Which of the following statements is *incorrect* concerning endometrial cancer?
   ○ 1. Diagnosis is most frequently established by a dilatation and curettage (D&C).
   ○ 2. Prolonged use of exogenous estrogen increases the occurrence.
   ○ 3. The first and most important symptom is abnormal bleeding.
   ○ 4. This malignancy tends to spread rapidly to other organs.

92. The Pap smear reveals that Mrs. Lubbick has cancer of the cervix. The mode of treatment is an abdominal hysterectomy. She voices concern about undergoing menopause. In counseling her, which of the following statements would be most appropriate?
   ○ 1. A surgical menopause will occur, and treatment with estrogen therapy will be necessary.
   ○ 2. The ovaries will continue to function and produce estrogen, thus preventing menopause.
   ○ 3. Ovarian hormone secretion ceases, but the hypothalamus will continue to secrete FSH, preventing menopause.
   ○ 4. The ovaries will cease functioning; thus, it will be necessary to administer estrogen.

93. Estrogen therapy is often prescribed to suppress the symptoms experienced by the menopausal client. Which of the following symptoms would *not* be characteristic of menopause?
   ○ 1. Anxiety, nervousness
   ○ 2. Vasomotor instability
   ○ 3. Osteoporosis resulting in backache
   ○ 4. Dysmenorrhea and mittelschmerz

94. Following the hysterectomy, which of the following symptoms would most likely indicate that Mrs. Lubbick is experiencing a serious complication of a hysterectomy?
   ○ 1. Gas pains and difficulty defecating
   ○ 2. Moderate amount of serosanguinous drainage on the perineal pad
   ○ 3. Low back pain, decreased urinary output
   ○ 4. Incisional pain requiring narcotic administration for relief

95. In providing post-op discharge instructions for Mrs. Lubbick, the nurse should *not* include which of the following?
   ○ 1. Return to the clinic in 10 days for the removal of the vaginal packing.
   ○ 2. Carry out abdominal strengthening exercises.
   ○ 3. Expect to experience periodic crying spells.
   ○ 4. Avoid activities that increase pelvic congestion.

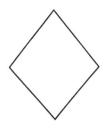

Test 2, Book III
Answers with Rationales

1. **#1.** Latent phase, stage 1 generally spans from 0 to 3 or 4 cm dilation and is accompanied by minimal discomfort in most women. ANALYSIS (CHILDBEARING FAMILY/INTRAPARTAL CARE)

2. **#1.** Demerol should be given late enough in the labor so as not to slow the labor, yet not so late as to cause the newborn to be "sleepy" when delivered. The situation given describes the optimum time to administer the pain medication. IMPLEMENTATION (CHILDBEARING FAMILY/INTRAPARTAL CARE)

3. **#3.** $\dfrac{100 \text{ mg}}{1 \text{ ml}} \times \dfrac{75 \text{ mg}}{X \text{ ml}} = 100 \text{ X} = 0.75$

   OR

   $75/100 \text{ ml} \times 1 \text{ ml} = 75/100 = 0.75 \text{ ml}$
   IMPLEMENTATION (CHILDBEARING FAMILY/ INTRAPARTAL CARE)

4. **#3.** The effects of selected medications on the fetus are generally heightened by increasing the dosage, giving the drug intravenously, and administering the agent close to delivery. ANALYSIS (CHILDBEARING FAMILY/INTRAPARTAL CARE)

5. **#3.** Gastrointestinal absorption is decreased during labor. Food ingested several hours earlier may remain in the client's stomach undigested. Antacids may neutralize the highly acidic gastric juice and thereby prevent a fatal chemical pneumonitis if aspiration occurs. ANALYSIS (CHILDBEARING FAMILY/INTRAPARTAL CARE)

6. **#2.** Occiput refers to vertex presentation; the words right and posterior refer to those portions of the maternal pelvis. Option #1 is correct but does not answer the client very specifically; #3 and #4 are incorrect. IMPLEMENTATION (CHILDBEARING FAMILY/INTRAPARTAL CARE)

7. **#1.** A major consequence of malpresentation is the lengthening of labor through decreased efficiency of contractions, longer time for the presenting part to descend, and weaker forces working on the cervix, all of which slow dilatation. Nursing actions should be designed to provide physical comfort and emotional support when labor is prolonged. IMPLEMENTATION (CHILDBEARING FAMILY/INTRAPARTAL CARE)

8. **#4.** All the client's symptoms are typical of panic. Mild anxiety does not produce the discomfort that this client is experiencing; it motivates growth and creativity. Moderate anxiety, which narrows the perceptual field, can be redirected with help and clients can feel challenged to cope. The severely anxious person has a greatly reduced perceptual field and develops a denial of existing feelings with selective inattention. While problem solving is difficult, it is not impossible. ANALYSIS (PSYCHOSOCIAL, MENTAL HEALTH, PSYCHIATRIC PROBLEMS/ANXIOUS BEHAVIOR)

9. **#4.** The highest priority is to reduce the client's panic. Priorities differ in the emergency room as opposed to a long-term setting. The focus is not immediately on relationship, although trust in relationships with helpers will occur. An immediate goal of gaining insight is impossible since she is now in a panic level of anxiety where cognitive functioning is blocked. This client is not capable of making behavioral changes while she is in a panic state. PLAN (PSYCHOSOCIAL, MENTAL HEALTH, PSYCHIATRIC PROBLEMS/ANXIOUS BEHAVIOR)

10. **#1.** Persons in a panic state need to feel that someone understands their terror and that they will not be left alone. Reassurance negates the experience and discounts the terror of the present. Clients in panic must not be left alone because panic is experienced as dread and terror. Acting out and/or verbal expression of true feelings of anger and helplessness would be blocked. IMPLEMENTATION (PSYCHOSOCIAL, MENTAL HEALTH, PSYCHIATRIC PROBLEMS/ANXIOUS BEHAVIOR)

11. **#2.** Clients may not want medication but come to recognize their need for it and, therefore, ready themselves. Respond to the anxiety, not to the content of the client's remark. The first remark is authoritarian and defensive. It makes an assumption that client cannot refuse ordered medication. #2 and #3 are patronizing and discount the client's fear of addiction. IMPLEMENTATION (PSYCHOSOCIAL, MENTAL HEALTH, PSYCHIATRIC PROBLEMS/ANXIOUS BEHAVIOR)

12. #3. Orient assessment toward finding out the factors that precipitated the client's present stage of anxiety. Be specific. Clients in a panic state need great assistance in staying focused. Option #1 is very generalized and assumes a high level of awareness on the part of the client. #2 assumes a connection between client's present situation and her anxiety with little input from client. If the client knew how to be helped, she would not be in the emergency room. People seek assistance from health providers because they do not know how to help themselves. ASSESSMENT (PSYCHOSOCIAL, MENTAL HEALTH, PSYCHIATRIC PROBLEMS/ANXIOUS BEHAVIOR)

13. #3. Drowsiness, vertigo, and dizziness are the most common side effects of diazepam. Her level of anxiety (panic) does not manifest itself in faintness and dizziness. Allergic responses to diazepam are skin rash, urticaria, fever, angioneurotic edema, and bronchial spasms. There is no indication from data presented that she has been sleepless or experiencing exhaustion. ANALYSIS (PSYCHOSOCIAL, MENTAL HEALTH, PSYCHIATRIC PROBLEMS/ANXIOUS BEHAVIOR)

14. #1. Removing the nipple frequently while feeding breaks the suction causing the child to swallow more air. This also frustrates the child, and crying further aggravates the problem. Breast-feeding is permitted if the mother wants to, but is more difficult. IMPLEMENTATION (CHILD/NUTRITION AND METABOLISM)

15. #1. This child will swallow a lot of air because of the abnormal openings. The other answers are contraindicated. PLAN (CHILD/NUTRITION AND METABOLISM)

16. #1. Most surgeons prefer to repair the palate before the child develops faulty speech patterns. By 12 to 18 months of age, palatal growth has progressed enough to allow surgery. Although some surgeons prefer to wait until 4 or 5 years of age to allow complete palatal development, by that age the child's speech will have been permanently affected by the deformity. ANALYSIS (CHILD/NUTRITION AND METABOLISM)

17. #4. Speech and hearing problems are common after this repair because of the necessary change in the palate arch and concomitant change in eustachian tubes. Contractures of the mandible are unrelated to this repair. ANALYSIS (CHILD/NUTRITION AND METABOLISM)

18. #3. With her history of hypertension, cerebral hemorrhage is the probable cause of the cardiovascular accident. ANALYSIS (ADULT/SAFETY AND SECURITY)

19. #1. The normal response to scratching the sole is to plantar flex the foot. ASSESSMENT (ADULT/SAFETY AND SECURITY)

20. #3. Offering the bedpan q4h is the first step in initiating bladder training, which is part of rehabilitation. Catheters can cause bladder infections and should be avoided when possible. Wearing a diaper may cause embarrassment and skin breakdown. PLAN (ADULT/SAFETY AND SECURITY)

21. #4. In expressive aphasia, the client is able to recognize objects but is unable to use the correct words. ANALYSIS (ADULT/SAFETY AND SECURITY)

22. #2. The occipital lobe holds the visual center; the medulla deals with essential functions (e.g., temperature); the parietal lobe deals mainly with sensory function. ANALYSIS (ADULT/SAFETY AND SECURITY)

23. #4. Encourage her to speak at any possible opportunity. Although time consuming, it is more therapeutic for the client. Options #1 to #3 actually discourage the rehabilitation of verbal communication. IMPLEMENTATION (ADULT/SAFETY AND SECURITY)

24. #1. Have the family continue to encourage Mrs. Duke's efforts. If the aphasia is expressive, she may be able to choose another word to communicate her needs. IMPLEMENTATION (ADULT/SAFETY AND SECURITY)

25. #3. Keeping Mrs. Duke positioned in semi-Fowler's position is important to prevent aspiration, a frequent complication post-CVA. While the other options may be appropriate, client safety comes first. PLAN (ADULT/SAFETY AND SECURITY)

26. #1. Initial damage to any tissue creates edema and impairs functioning. As the cerebral edema decreases, muscle function begins to return and can improve for a period of up to 6 months. ANALYSIS (ADULT/SAFETY AND SECURITY)

27. #3. Rehabilitation is a goal that is worked on as soon as the planning of care begins (i.e., upon admission to the hospital). PLAN (ADULT/SAFETY AND SECURITY)

28. **#3.** With the help of significant others or family, rehabilitation efforts are continued over the long term, resulting in a more optimal recovery. ANALYSIS (ADULT/SAFETY AND SECURITY)

29. **#3.** Daily skin checks are done to note any potential bleeding. Pink urine may be from hematuria and must be reported immediately. Foods high in vitamin K will enhance the clotting mechanism and counteract the effects of the drug. Prothrombin levels, not partial thromboplastin times, are measured in clients receiving warfarin (Coumadin). IMPLEMENTATION (ADULT/SAFETY AND SECURITY)

30. **#1.** Eczema is most often seen in infancy. The most frequent cause is cow's milk and egg albumin allergy. The infant is at highest risk for developing an allergic response because the immune system is still not fully mature. ASSESSMENT (CHILD/SENSATION, PERCEPTION, PROTECTION)

31. **#2.** Before treatment can be effective, the allergen that is causing the problem must be identified. PLAN (CHILD/SENSATION, PERCEPTION, PROTECTION)

32. **#1.** Pruritus is the most difficult symptom of eczema to control. It causes infants/children to be irritable and interferes with sleep. Eczema is not usually painful unless infection occurs. While teething is common at age 2 years, it does not cause long periods of irritability and sleeplessness. Hunger is unrelated but may be manifested by a diet that is restrictive to the point that the child does not like any of the foods allowed. ANALYSIS (CHILD/SENSATION, PERCEPTION, PROTECTION)

33. **#3.** Soaps are drying agents and not used. Lipid lotions/agents are not good cleansing agents. Warm water increases itching; cool water promotes chilling and loss of body heat. Tepid baths soothe irritated skin and decrease itching. PLAN (CHILD/SENSATION, PERCEPTION, PROTECTION)

34. **#2.** This is an age-appropriate activity that would provide a distraction for Sally without giving her anything to scratch with. Working with clay requires more coordination than the average 2-year-old has; additionally, the clay may prove irritating to Sally's skin condition. Although building columns with blocks is age appropriate for Sally, she may use the blocks to scratch or irritate her eczema. Until her eczema clears, Sally should play with safe objects with rounded edges. Although the average 2-year-old is able to hold a crayon and make circular and linear lines, they do not typically associate these markings with specific objects. IMPLEMENTATION (CHILD/SENSATION, PERCEPTION, PROTECTION)

35. **#2.** Wool is not used because it can irritate the skin. Synthetic materials are substituted for wool in coats, hats, gloves, etc. IMPLEMENTATION (CHILD/SENSATION, PERCEPTION, PROTECTION)

36. **#4.** Close-fitting clothes cause irritation, perspiration, and increased itching. These should be avoided. Loose-fitting, 1-piece clothing prevents access for itching. EVALUATION (CHILD/SENSATION, PERCEPTION, PROTECTION)

37. **#3.** Allowing restricted foods, even occasionally, can cause the exacerbation of eczema. Options #1, #2, and #4 encourage intake in a toddler. EVALUATION (CHILD/SENSATION, PERCEPTION, PROTECTION)

38. **#3.** Pancakes are not included because they are usually made from wheat flour. Soy milk is used if there is an allergy to cow's milk. Turkey/chicken are permitted, as are bland fruits (e.g., apples, pears, peaches, bananas). PLAN (CHILD/SENSATION, PERCEPTION, PROTECTION)

39. **#1.** Reactive depression is characterized by a loss, sleeping disorder, eating disorder, decreased energy. She may be experiencing anxiety about being alone, but the symptoms indicate depression. Psychosis would include more severe symptoms such as a thought disorder. Paranoia would include symptoms of a rigid belief system and delusions of persecution. ANALYSIS (PSYCHOSOCIAL, MENTAL HEALTH, PSYCHIATRIC PROBLEMS/ELATED-DEPRESSIVE BEHAVIOR)

40. #2. One indication of increased well-being in the client is resumption of activities of daily living. There is no evidence in the situation to suggest that the client is suspicious or has a thought disorder. When Mrs. Jones starts taking better care of herself, it will indicate that the immobility imposed by the depression is lifting. Options #1 and #3 reflect a person with a psychosis; and #4 reflects a goal for a person with anxiety. PLAN (PSYCHOSOCIAL, MENTAL HEALTH, PSYCHIATRIC PROBLEMS/ELATED-DEPRESSIVE BEHAVIOR)

41. #4. Reactive depression is characterized by an identifiable loss of some type. In Mrs. Jones's case, it is the loss of a relationship with her husband. The anger at the loss of her husband is not directly expressed externally or verbally. It is turned inward; she takes the anger out on herself and becomes depressed. Option #1 reflects a person with a psychosis, #2 reflects an anxiety disorder, and #3 reflects a person with paranoia. ANALYSIS (PSYCHOSOCIAL, MENTAL HEALTH, PSYCHIATRIC PROBLEMS/ELATED-DEPRESSIVE BEHAVIOR)

42. #3. This response is client centered and reflects the nurse's empathy. Option #1 gives false reassurance and ignores the client's feelings and situation. #2 may help the nurse feel better by getting her/him out of the situation, but may not meet the client's need. The nurse can offer to help the client discharge feelings, but should not force the client to talk. IMPLEMENTATION (PSYCHOSOCIAL, MENTAL HEALTH, PSYCHIATRIC PROBLEMS/ELATED-DEPRESSIVE BEHAVIOR)

43. #1. Clients who are depressed and suddenly get better may have made the decision to commit suicide or may now be feeling better and have the energy to make a suicide attempt. Discharging her or giving her a pass as soon as she feels better is premature. ANALYSIS (PSYCHOSOCIAL, MENTAL HEALTH, PSYCHIATRIC PROBLEMS/ELATED-DEPRESSIVE BEHAVIOR)

44. #3. When Mrs. Jones becomes irritable, it is a sign that the anger is moving from being inwardly directed to being directed out. This is a sign that the depression is lifting. An indication of regression would be acting childish. Mrs. Jones is not threatening the staff, nor is she acting suicidal. EVALUATION (PSYCHOSOCIAL, MENTAL HEALTH, PSYCHIATRIC PROBLEMS/ELATED-DEPRESSIVE BEHAVIOR)

45. #4. Improved mental well-being of a client is evidenced by an increased ability to carry out activities of daily living. When the depression is less incapacitating, the client has more energy to act. Option #1 reflects improvement from an anxiety disorder, #2 reflects improvement from psychosis, and #3 reflects improvement from paranoia. EVALUATION (PSYCHOSOCIAL, MENTAL HEALTH, PSYCHIATRIC PROBLEMS/ELATED-DEPRESSIVE BEHAVIOR)

46. #4. Prerenal azotemia refers to causes outside the kidneys; poisons cause renal azotemia. ANALYSIS (ADULT/ELIMINATION)

47. #2. Hyperkalemia is an immediate and life-threatening problem associated with renal failure. PLAN (ADULT/ELIMINATION)

48. #3. The hemodialysis machine works on the simple physical principles of filtration, osmosis, and diffusion. It cannot duplicate the complex endocrine functions of the kidneys (e.g., the production of erythropoietin). PLAN (ADULT/ELIMINATION)

49. #4. Post-op renal shutdown is usually reversible. IMPLEMENTATION (ADULT/ELIMINATION)

50. #2. Lethargy is a symptom of a high BUN. Disequilibrium syndrome is caused by a rapid decline of electrolytes or wastes. ASSESSMENT (ADULT/ELIMINATION)

51. #4. The shift of too much blood to the dialyzer produces symptoms of hypovolemic shock. Accidental disconnection of the tubing also results in rapid exsanguination and hypovolemic shock. PLAN (ADULT/ELIMINATION)

52. #2. Regional heparinization prevents clotting in the hemodialyzer without subjecting the client to the risks of systemic anticoagulation. PLAN (ADULT/ELIMINATION)

53. #2. Blood flow must be maintained in the cannula to prevent clotting. A tight dressing constricts flow. IMPLEMENTATION (ADULT/ELIMINATION)

54. #3. The infant's temperature normally drops immediately after birth if the infant is not dried and well wrapped. The large body surface area and the difference in external temperature from the mother's internal temperature predispose the infant to chilling. The infant must be warmed immediately. The easiest way to do this is placement in a warmed incubator. IMPLEMENTATION (CHILDBEARING FAMILY/NORMAL NEWBORN)

55. **#1.** Cold increases an infant's metabolic rate because of inability to shiver. This increases both oxygen and calorie consumption, necessitating the administration of more oxygen and calories. If they are unavailable, the infant develops metabolic acidosis, which is manifested by lowered blood pH. ANALYSIS (CHILDBEARING FAMILY/NORMAL NEWBORN)

56. **#4.** Grunting is an abnormal breathing pattern, usually indicative of respiratory distress. Cephalohematoma, a collection of blood between the bone and periosteum, is the result of pressure sustained at birth, usually requiring no treatment. Milia, due to blocked sebaceous glands, is a normal newborn characteristic, as is the Moro or startle reflex. ASSESSMENT (CHILDBEARING FAMILY/NORMAL NEWBORN)

57. **#3.** Synthesis of vitamin K by *E. coli* bacteria occurs in the intestinal tract. Newborns have a sterile intestinal tract and lack the vitamin, which is essential in the formation of prothrombin and for normal blood clotting. ANALYSIS (CHILDBEARING FAMILY/NORMAL NEWBORN)

58. **#3.** Acrocyanosis is usually present in a normal neonate because of immature peripheral circulation. Average pulse rate is 100 to 160, respirations 30 to 60 and irregular. ANALYSIS (CHILDBEARING FAMILY/NORMAL NEWBORN)

59. **#4.** Uncoordinated eye movements are a normal finding in full-term neonates, because they have poor control of eye muscles. The normal heart rate is 100 to 160. Jaundice in the first 24 hours is considered pathologic. Nasal flaring is a sign of respiratory distress. ASSESSMENT (CHILDBEARING FAMILY/NORMAL NEWBORN)

60. **#4.** During the first few days after birth, the infant may lose 5% to 10% of her birth weight, because of loss of excess fluid and minimal intake of nutrients. IMPLEMENTATION (CHILDBEARING FAMILY/NORMAL NEWBORN)

61. **#2.** Approximately 50% of full-term newborns develop jaundice around the third day of life in the absence of disease or a specific cause. This is called physiologic jaundice due to the rapid breakdown of fetal cells resulting in an increase in bilirubin. This subsides approximately 5 to 7 days after birth. ANALYSIS (CHILDBEARING FAMILY/NORMAL NEWBORN)

62. **#2.** The immense metabolic needs of the proliferating leukemic cells cause bone-marrow depression and reduce red blood cell production. ANALYSIS (CHILD/CELLULAR ABERRATION)

63. **#3.** Platelets are involved in clotting and coagulation and are decreased in number because of leukocytosis. ASSESSMENT (CHILD/CELLULAR ABERRATION)

64. **#1.** Intramuscular injections can precipitate bleeding and are to be avoided. PLAN (CHILD/CELLULAR ABERRATION)

65. **#2.** This indicates that he is aware that myelosuppression occurs and is temporary. EVALUATION (CHILD/CELLULAR ABERRATION)

66. **#1.** This is the most realistic because it is supportive to the family without overburdening them. Options #2, #3, and #4 place too much responsibility on the family and do not allow them a respite. PLAN (CHILD/CELLULAR ABERRATION)

67. **#2.** Alcohol withdrawal involves 4 stages. Signs and symptoms occurring in Stage I (8 hours plus after cessation of drinking) include mild tremors and nervousness. In Stage II, symptoms include hyperactivity and disorientation. Miss Smith was admitted on the previous day and sufficient time had elapsed without alcohol ingestion, resulting in several signs of alcohol withdrawal. Signs of Valium withdrawal are tremors, abdominal and muscle cramps, and convulsions. Barbiturate withdrawal would manifest with nausea, vomiting, diarrhea, sleep disturbance, diaphoresis, irritability, hostility, and agitation. Marijuana does not produce withdrawal symptoms. ANALYSIS (PSYCHOSOCIAL, MENTAL HEALTH, PSYCHIATRIC PROBLEMS/ SUBSTANCE USE DISORDERS)

68. **#4.** Clients with personality disorders "use" or manipulate other persons for their own motives. They have a tendency to ascribe their own motivations and behaviors to others. In psychiatric settings, these clients consistently try to split the staff by complaining about one staff member to another and by flattering some staff members. Miss Smith is describing her reaction to Miss Levy, not identifying her weaknesses. Manipulative behavior is well thought out and deliberate, not irrational as with a thought disorder or unconscious as with a defense mechanism. ANALYSIS (PSYCHOSOCIAL, MENTAL HEALTH, PSYCHIATRIC PROBLEMS/SOCIALLY MALADAPTIVE BEHAVIOR)

69. #2. Clients with personality disorders have no impairment of thought, no ego disintegration, and no delusional behavior the way psychotic clients do. The client with a personality disorder has minimal insight and poor impulse control, which results in acting-out behavior. Compliance and passivity are seen in clients with low self-esteem who wish to please others to be liked. ASSESSMENT (PSYCHOSOCIAL, MENTAL HEALTH, PSYCHIATRIC PROBLEMS/SOCIALLY MALADAPTIVE BEHAVIOR)

70. #1. Clients with personality disorders consistently arouse uncomfortable feelings of anger, frustration, helplessness, and defensiveness in staff. The deliberate, manipulative behaviors are blatant enough that there is no confusion about what is happening. An absence of feelings is sometimes seen in response to schizophrenic clients, and boredom can be experienced with withdrawn, depressed clients. ASSESSMENT (PSYCHOSOCIAL, MENTAL HEALTH, PSYCHIATRIC PROBLEMS/SOCIALLY MALADAPTIVE BEHAVIOR)

71. #1. Because staff feel so angry and helpless with clients with personality disorders, these clients are rarely sought out. Reinforcing positive behavior is an effort to reward the client with attention. Options #2 through #4 tend to foster the client's chronic manipulative behavior. IMPLEMENTATION (PSYCHOSOCIAL, MENTAL HEALTH, PSYCHIATRIC PROBLEMS/SOCIALLY MALADAPTIVE BEHAVIOR)

72. #2. Checking for excess bleeding is the next priority. IMPLEMENTATION (ADULT/ELIMINATION)

73. #1. Post-op clients should void within 8 to 12 hours after surgery. At this time, it is appropriate to assess her status by asking her if she needs to urinate. IMPLEMENTATION (ADULT/ELIMINATION)

74. #4. Mrs. Klein's temperature should be taken orally, not rectally. Avoid the supine position, sitting for prolonged periods, and sitting on rubber rings, all of which increase venous stagnation in the rectal area. IMPLEMENTATION (ADULT/ELIMINATION)

75. #2. This option gives Mrs. Klein the opportunity to voice her concerns. The other options assume the cause of the client's worry. IMPLEMENTATION (ADULT/ELIMINATION)

76. #1. In order to avoid post-op infection, Mrs. Klein should do perineal care with an antiseptic solution after each stool, and she may have sitz baths as needed to clean the incision. IMPLEMENTATION (ADULT/ELIMINATION)

77. #2. Increased pain with bowel movements is a symptom of anal stricture and Mrs. Klein should notify her physician. She should drink 2,500 to 3,000 ml of fluid daily and eat a low-residue, soft diet for the first post-op week. Mrs. Klein will have had her first bowel movement before she is discharged. IMPLEMENTATION (ADULT/ELIMINATION)

78. #1. Observe the interaction between Jimmy and his mother. Abusers frequently do not offer appropriate comfort or support to the distressed child. The abused child frequently appears wary of the care givers or does not seek them out for comfort and affection. Options #2, #3, and #4 may prove useful, but #1 will provide the most important information to assess child abuse. ASSESSMENT (PSYCHOSOCIAL, MENTAL HEALTH, PSYCHIATRIC PROBLEMS/SOCIALLY MALADAPTIVE BEHAVIOR)

79. #3. All suspected cases of child abuse must be reported to the child welfare, protective services agency. Personnel cannot be prosecuted for defamation of character if their suspicions prove to be incorrect. Option #1 is not helpful at this time and would create further problems. The law requires the use of protective services rather than the police directly. If nothing is done, the child's life will continue to be endangered. IMPLEMENTATION (PSYCHOSOCIAL, MENTAL HEALTH, PSYCHIATRIC PROBLEMS/SOCIALLY MALADAPTIVE BEHAVIOR)

80. #2. While identification of one's feelings is a necessary first step, the ability to deal with any negative feelings is imperative in establishing a working relationship. Family history does have value, but it has a lower priority and is more likely to be obtained after a relationship is established. Option #4 has a lower priority and does not necessarily facilitate an effective working relationship. IMPLEMENTATION (PSYCHOSOCIAL, MENTAL HEALTH, PSYCHIATRIC PROBLEMS/SOCIALLY MALADAPTIVE BEHAVIOR)

81. **#1.** Attendance at a parent-support group indicates that Mrs. Baker is willing to invest her time, and that there is at least a minimal level of motivation to change. Bringing gifts to Jimmy and calling the hospital do not necessarily indicate a commitment to furthering parenting skills. Although having Jimmy immunized indicates attention to his physical care, attendance at the parents' group (which deals with feelings and needs of parents and children) demonstrates interest, motivation, and commitment. EVALUATION (PSYCHOSOCIAL, MENTAL HEALTH, PSYCHIATRIC PROBLEMS/SOCIALLY MALADAPTIVE BEHAVIOR)

82. **#4.** The majority of side effects of external radiation are dependent on the specific site being radiated. Because the client's site is the lung, radiation will result in irritation of the lung mucosa, resulting in dyspnea. ASSESSMENT (ADULT/CELLULAR ABERRATION)

83. **#4.** Skin markings must not be removed in any way. If they are inadvertently washed off, markings are redrawn only by the radiation technician. PLAN (ADULT/CELLULAR ABERRATION)

84. **#2.** It is important to understand the difference between external and internal radiation, so that the nurse can be accurate when correcting the client's misconceptions. He is not radioactive and does not need to limit contact with others. Option #1 is incorrect. IMPLEMENTATION (ADULT/CELLULAR ABERRATION)

85. **#4.** Encourage the client to participate in his own care as much as possible, but provide periods of uninterrupted rest in a quiet environment. PLAN (ADULT/CELLULAR ABERRATION)

86. **#2.** The most common sources of salmonella infection are poultry and eggs. Other sources may be dogs, cats, hamsters, pet turtles. ANALYSIS (CHILD/NUTRITION AND METABOLISM)

87. **#2.** The posterior fontanel is closed by 2 months and the anterior closes at 12 to 18 months, but is usually covered with hair. While the anterior fontanel can be an indicator of dehydration at 6 months, the weight of the infant is a more reliable sign of fluid loss and dehydration. ASSESSMENT (CHILD/NUTRITION AND METABOLISM)

88. **#2.** The infant with a potassium deficit has decreased peristalsis and abdominal distension; irritability and poor eating due to anorexia are common problems. ASSESSMENT (CHILD/NUTRITION AND METABOLISM)

89. **#3.** It is important to hold and touch an infant with an IV infusion; not picking up a child with an IV who is on bed rest is usually inappropriate. PLAN (CHILD/NUTRITION AND METABOLISM)

90. **#4.** The first symptoms to occur with cancer of the cervix are metrorrhagia and a watery vaginal discharge. ASSESSMENT (ADULT/CELLULAR ABERRATION)

91. **#4.** Cancer of the endometrium tends to be slow spreading. Once it has spread to the cervix, invaded the myometrium, or spread outside the uterus, the prognosis is poor. ANALYSIS (ADULT/CELLULAR ABERRATION)

92. **#2.** Menstruation will cease following a hysterectomy, but as long as the ovaries are left in place, they will continue to function, and surgical menopause will not occur. IMPLEMENTATION (ADULT/CELLULAR ABERRATION)

93. **#4.** Menstrual irregularities occur with menopause, but these do not include dysmenorrhea and mittelschmerz. ANALYSIS (ADULT/CELLULAR ABERRATION)

94. **#3.** A serious complication of a hysterectomy is the accidental ligation of the ureter during surgery. These symptoms would be found if such had occurred. ASSESSMENT (ADULT/CELLULAR ABERRATION)

95. **#1.** Vaginal packing is not used following an abdominal hysterectomy. IMPLEMENTATION (ADULT/CELLULAR ABERRATION)

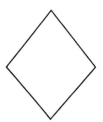

Test 2, Book IV
Questions

Mary Phillips, 28 years old, is admitted to your unit with the following complaints: urgency, frequency, dysuria, suprapubic pain, and hematuria. Her admitting diagnosis is cystitis.

1. What is the most likely cause of Miss Phillips's urgency?
   - ○ **1.** Contracted bladder
   - ○ **2.** Inflamed bladder
   - ○ **3.** Enlarged bladder
   - ○ **4.** Increased vascularity in the bladder

2. Fluids should be encouraged for this client, especially those that can aid in altering the urinary pH. Her nurse should advise her to take liberal quantities of which of the following?
   - ○ **1.** Apple juice
   - ○ **2.** Tea and coffee
   - ○ **3.** Cranberry juice
   - ○ **4.** Orange juice

3. Miss Phillips will be given a drug that acts only on bacteria in the urine and is not absorbed systemically. This drug is
   - ○ **1.** sulfisoxazole (Gantrisin).
   - ○ **2.** pencillin.
   - ○ **3.** ampicillin.
   - ○ **4.** tetracycline.

4. What organism is this drug most effective against?
   - ○ **1.** *E. coli*
   - ○ **2.** *Pseudomonas*
   - ○ **3.** *Salmonella*
   - ○ **4.** *Klebsiella*

Eight-year-old Randall, a third grader, visits his pediatrician for an annual health checkup and a camp physical examination. The nurse begins a history and exam.

5. When obtaining a nursing history from Randall and his mother, the nurse questions Randall about his school activities and achievement. This is important because, according to Erikson's stages of development, Randall should be developing a sense of
   - ○ **1.** initiative.
   - ○ **2.** industry.
   - ○ **3.** generativity.
   - ○ **4.** identity.

6. Randall's weight is at the 95th percentile and his height is at the 75th percentile. Based on this information, which of the following conclusions is most warranted?
   - ○ **1.** Randall is overweight and should be referred to the dietitian for nutrition counseling.
   - ○ **2.** Randall's weight is disproportionate to his height, and he should be counseled to reduce his caloric intake.
   - ○ **3.** Randall's weight and height indicate he is growing normally.
   - ○ **4.** Additional information should be collected before drawing conclusions.

7. The nurse screens Randall's vision using the Snellen alphabet chart. The results show Randall has 20/30 vision in his left eye and 20/40 vision in his right eye. Corneal light reflex and cover tests are normal. Which follow-up action is most indicated?
   - ○ **1.** Rescreen Randall in 1 month.
   - ○ **2.** Test Randall for color blindness.
   - ○ **3.** Discuss with the physician a referral to an ophthalmologist or optometrist.
   - ○ **4.** Counsel Randall's mother that the findings are normal.

8. Randall's camp administrator requires that his immunizations be up-to-date. Prior to today, Randall had received the full recommended series of childhood immunizations. Which of the following would be appropriate to administer to Randall?
   - ○ **1.** No immunization
   - ○ **2.** A tetanus booster
   - ○ **3.** Diphtheria (adult type) and tetanus booster
   - ○ **4.** Measles and mumps vaccines

9. The nurse takes this opportunity to discuss general safety with Randall's mother. Which of the following approaches to encourage safety is *not* appropriate?
   ○ 1. Live safely to show the child how it is done.
   ○ 2. Anticipate that fatigue and strong emotions may increase the danger of accidents.
   ○ 3. Comply with local laws and support law enforcement in action and attitude.
   ○ 4. Restrict the child from experience with fire, tools, electrical appliances.

Jerry Hall is a handsome, bright young man who has just been admitted to the psychiatric unit after 1 week in the alcohol withdrawal unit. He has a history of several marriages in the last 5 years, 2 children he does not support, and a criminal record. On the unit, he has been observed to be charming and helpful; he says he is doing fine and hopes to be discharged soon. His diagnosis is borderline personality disorder.

10. Which of the following is most characteristic of the client with borderline personality disorder?
    ○ 1. Poor impulse control because of inadequate internal control
    ○ 2. Realistic appraisal of others
    ○ 3. Ritualistic behavior
    ○ 4. Unfounded, morbid fear of a seemingly harmless object

11. Which of the following statements most often applies to clients with borderline personality disorder?
    ○ 1. Will be helped greatly by psychotropic drugs
    ○ 2. Will be given electroconvulsive therapy
    ○ 3. Will not be given psychotropic drugs
    ○ 4. Will be given antidepressants

12. In the initial stages of the therapeutic relationship, the nurse should be aware that Mr. Hall may most likely
    ○ 1. ruminate.
    ○ 2. hallucinate.
    ○ 3. manipulate.
    ○ 4. lose contact with reality.

13. Which of the following nursing actions would be inappropriate?
    ○ 1. Set limits on behavior.
    ○ 2. Maintain a firm, consistent, and positive attitude.
    ○ 3. Expect Mr. Hall to act in a realistic, mature way, knowing that he will not always fulfill this expectation.
    ○ 4. Encourage Mr. Hall to assist staff with some of the more withdrawn clients.

14. Which of the following would be the most effective approach to attain the goal of, "Client will strengthen ability to relate to others in socially acceptable ways"?
    ○ 1. Allow the client to set his own standards of behavior on the unit.
    ○ 2. Accept the client's evaluation of social problem areas.
    ○ 3. Include the client in mixed-diagnosis group for group therapy, so that he learns to get along with different kinds of people.
    ○ 4. Set rules for the client's behavior on the unit and treat infractions of rules with loss of privileges.

15. Mr. Hall attends the daily discussion group, focuses group work on other clients' problems, and states, "My problems are over; I just want to help others." The nurse should be aware that the client is probably demonstrating which of the following behaviors?
    ○ 1. Learning social skills
    ○ 2. Impulse control
    ○ 3. Learning problem-solving skillls
    ○ 4. Avoiding working on his own problems

16. Mr. Hall stays late in the exercise yard and states that he forgot his appointment to talk with his primary nurse. Which response would be the most effective at this time?
    ○ 1. "If you don't talk with me, I'll call your doctor."
    ○ 2. Accept his excuse and ask to have the client assigned to another staff member.
    ○ 3. Ignore the forgotten appointment and act as if it never happened.
    ○ 4. Go to the exercise yard and state, "You and I are scheduled to talk for awhile now."

17. Mr. Hall tells his primary nurse on the 3-to-11 shift that the only help he is getting is from her. He complains that the day staff are too task oriented, and that the night staff ignore his requests and stay in the nurses' station drinking coffee and chatting. Which of the following would be the most appropriate response?
    ○ 1. Confront the night shift with these complaints.
    ○ 2. Report the night shift behaviors to the 11-to-7 supervisor.
    ○ 3. Collect data on staff behavior from other clients at the evening, client-government group.
    ○ 4. Bring this information to daily staff conference to discuss the situation and decide on an approach to the client.

18. Which of the following is *not* an effective action to cope with the client who attempts to split the staff?
    ○ 1. Review requests made by client with other staff before permission is granted.
    ○ 2. Be flexible and let client make own rules.
    ○ 3. Hold daily staff conference to discuss, set approach, and inform all staff of approaches and limits with client.
    ○ 4. Utilize written care plans for consistent approach.

Betty Pohl, 35 years old, is admitted to your unit for diagnostic tests. She is 5 ft 2 in tall and weighs 120 lb. She appears acutely ill and complains of pain and stiffness of the joints in her hands, feet, and knees. She says she is becoming dependent on her family for her activities of daily living. The tentative diagnosis is rheumatoid arthritis.

19. Which of the following is most characteristic of rheumatoid arthritis?
    ○ 1. It most often occurs in women between the ages of 40 and 80.
    ○ 2. Nonsystemic involvement is most common in rheumatoid arthritis.
    ○ 3. Joints are affected bilaterally and symmetrically.
    ○ 4. It first occurs in a joint following a traumatic injury.

20. Which one of the following lab values would most confirm Mrs. Pohl's diagnosis?
    ○ 1. Elevated sedimentation rate
    ○ 2. Decreased WBC count in the synovial fluid
    ○ 3. Normal hematocrit and hemoglobin
    ○ 4. Absence of rheumatoid factor in the serum

21. The nurse is about to take Mrs. Pohl's history. Which of the following assessment findings would *not* be typical?
    ○ 1. A recent weight loss and anorexia
    ○ 2. Stiffness that becomes more pronounced later in the day
    ○ 3. Tender, hot, and red joints
    ○ 4. Low-grade fever

22. Which of the following would be *inappropriate* to include in a plan of care for Mrs. Pohl?
    ○ 1. Schedule her activities to allow for at least 8 to 10 hours of sleep every night, plus naps during the day.
    ○ 2. Educate the client and family to avoid quackery.
    ○ 3. Put the head of the bed in high position when assisting her out of bed.
    ○ 4. Assist her to select a high-calorie, high-protein, and high-calcium diet.

23. Preventing deformities is a major goal for Mrs. Pohl. Which of the following nursing actions would be *inappropriate* to achieve this goal?
    ○ 1. Place pillows under the major joints.
    ○ 2. Encourage her to lie prone several times a day.
    ○ 3. Place a pillow between the legs when positioned on the side.
    ○ 4. Provide her with a small pillow for her head.

24. Another goal is to assist Mrs. Pohl to be as pain free as possible. Which of the following is an *incorrect* method of relieving pain?
    ○ 1. Apply hot, moist packs to the affected joints.
    ○ 2. Apply cold packs to the affected joints.
    ○ 3. Give analgesics on a regular schedule every 3 to 4 hours.
    ○ 4. Massage the joints when they ache.

25. Exercise is an important treatment modality for clients with arthritis. Which of the following responses by Mrs. Pohl indicates the need for further teaching regarding physical exercise guidelines?
    ○ 1. "Exercise only to the point of pain, never beyond."
    ○ 2. "Refrain from exercising affected joints until pain and swelling subside."
    ○ 3. "Isometric exercises can be done independently and without supervision."
    ○ 4. "An ongoing regimen of exercise at all times for all joints is essential."

26. Phenylbutazone (Butazolidin) was prescribed for its anti-inflammatory actions. What instructions should be given to Mrs. Pohl regarding this drug?
    ○ 1. Take the drug 2 hours before and 2 hours after eating.
    ○ 2. Take alternately with aspirin.
    ○ 3. Examine the stools and urine for blood.
    ○ 4. You may need to take the drug indefinitely.

27. Mrs. Pohl tells you that the physician may prescribe a gold preparation if the present medications are not effective. What is a major *disadvantage* of gold preparations?
    ○ 1. They must be administered several months before benefits can be determined.
    ○ 2. They must be given intravenously.
    ○ 3. The urine will turn green.
    ○ 4. Serious adverse effects commonly occur during the first week.

Julie Carter, aged 36, has just had her first pregnancy confirmed. She has been married 5 years and appears excited and nervous after hearing she is pregnant.

28. In performing an initial assessment of Mrs. Carter during the first trimester, what is most appropriate for the nurse to assess?
    ○ **1.** Fetal heart rate
    ○ **2.** Fetal movement
    ○ **3.** Plans for childbirth preparation
    ○ **4.** Past medical history

29. When a nursing history is taken, Mrs. Carter asks the nurse, "How soon can I find out if I'm carrying a normal baby?" Which response by the nurse would be most appropriate?
    ○ **1.** "A 24-hour estriol can be done now."
    ○ **2.** "An amniocentesis can be done at 14 weeks."
    ○ **3.** "An oxytocin challenge test can be done at 16 weeks."
    ○ **4.** "A nonstress test can be done immediately."

30. Mrs. Carter's history reveals she smokes a pack of cigarettes per day. Which of the following problems should the nurse discuss with her that might occur as a result of smoking?
    ○ **1.** Small-for-gestational-age infant
    ○ **2.** Large-for-gestational-age infant
    ○ **3.** Fetal limb anomalies
    ○ **4.** Reduced maternal weight gain in pregnancy

31. Mrs. Carter's blood work at this visit demonstrated the following results: blood type A, Rh negative, rubella titer 1:64, hemoglobin 14 gm, hematocrit 37%, serology for syphilis: nonreactive. How should the nurse interpret these data?
    ○ **1.** Rubella vaccine should be given.
    ○ **2.** Iron supplements are needed.
    ○ **3.** Mr. Carter should be checked for the Rh factor.
    ○ **4.** Baby Carter could acquire congenital syphilis.

32. The nurse should provide Mrs. Carter with 3 of the following pieces of advice about rest and exercise. Which one is *not* appropriate?
    ○ **1.** Avoid standing or sitting for long periods of time.
    ○ **2.** Prevent fatigue, as pregnant women tire more readily.
    ○ **3.** Continue usual exercise regimen.
    ○ **4.** Begin a new active exercise program, such as jogging.

33. Mrs. Carter has active genital herpes simplex type 2. What kind of a delivery will she have if she still has active lesions at the time of delivery?
    ○ **1.** Low-segment cesarean section
    ○ **2.** Vaginal delivery with low forceps
    ○ **3.** Induction at 36 weeks gestation
    ○ **4.** Method selected by client

34. Mrs. Carter is scheduled to have an amniocentesis. Which of the following test results would most likely indicate that she has a mature fetus in good condition?
    ○ **1.** Falling estriol levels
    ○ **2.** Lecithin/sphingomyelin (L/S) ratio of 1:5 to 1
    ○ **3.** Creatinine of 2 mg/100 ml amniotic fluid
    ○ **4.** An increase in alphafetoprotein

35. Mrs. Carter is now 7 months pregnant. She complains of severe leg cramps, especially at night. When the nurse is instructing her on ways of alleviating this problem, which of the following is the most appropriate action to advise?
    ○ **1.** Walk briskly around the room.
    ○ **2.** Get up and drink a cup of tea.
    ○ **3.** Straighten her leg and dorsiflex her ankle.
    ○ **4.** Rub her leg until the pain subsides.

36. Mrs. Carter is now in her eighth month of pregnancy. She is in conference with the nurse at her antepartal visit. Which of the following would indicate that Mrs. Carter understands how to obtain relief from the discomfort of the varicosities in her legs?
    ○ **1.** She is presently sitting with her legs crossed at the knees.
    ○ **2.** She is presently wearing knee-high hose with stretch bands.
    ○ **3.** She states she frequently elevates her legs above her hips when lying down or sitting.
    ○ **4.** She is still employed as a secretary and remains sedentary most of her work day.

37. At Mrs. Carter's next antepartal visit, the nurse notes that she has gained 3 lb since her last visit 2 weeks ago and is complaining that her wedding ring is tight. Her urine shows 1 + proteinuria, and her blood pressure is markedly increased from baseline. The probable cause of these findings is which of the following factors?

○ **1.** Normal fluid retention of pregnancy
○ **2.** Normal cardiovascular alterations of pregnancy
○ **3.** Pathologic changes accompanying polyhydramnios
○ **4.** Pathologic changes of mild preeclampsia

Twenty-month-old Ryan Shore has a diagnosis of iron-deficiency anemia.

38. Which of the following is most likely to be the cause of iron-deficiency anemia in a toddler?

○ **1.** Excessive milk intake, which decreases the intake of solid foods
○ **2.** Insufficient iron stores at birth
○ **3.** Refusal to eat iron-rich foods, because of their unappealing taste
○ **4.** A normal physiologic occurrence during the toddler years

39. Which of the following signs and symptoms should the nurse expect her assessment of Ryan to reveal?

○ **1.** Overweight, normal exercise tolerance, flushed face
○ **2.** Pallor, fatigue, irritability
○ **3.** Pallor, average muscle tone, accelerated growth rate
○ **4.** Exercise tolerance, good muscle tone, average growth rate

40. Mrs. Shore has been taught how to administer Ryan's oral iron preparation at home. Which statement by Mrs. Shore indicates the need for clarification by the nurse?

○ **1.** ''I'll give Ryan his medicine between meals with fruit or juice.''
○ **2.** ''I'll use a straw, syringe, or dropper placed to the back of Ryan's mouth when I give him his medicine.''
○ **3.** ''I'll help Ryan brush his teeth after he takes the medicine to decrease the likelihood of staining his teeth.''
○ **4.** ''I'll expect the color of Ryan's stool to change to a dark yellow.''

41. As a result of Ryan's increased mobility and developmental curiosity, which medication should Mrs. Shore keep in her medicine cabinet?

○ **1.** Tylenol
○ **2.** Milk of magnesia
○ **3.** Syrup of ipecac
○ **4.** Baby aspirin

Andrea Stuben is admitted to the psychiatric unit with a diagnosis of reactive depression. She is 26 years old. She was severely injured in an automobile accident 2 months ago. Her husband and 3-year-old daughter were killed in the same accident. Because of her injuries, she was unable to attend their funeral. She is in 2 full-leg casts, is thin, and apathetic.

42. Which is the best explanation for Mrs. Stuben's behavior?

○ **1.** She is in poor physical condition from the accident.
○ **2.** The inability to attend the funeral has probably affected the process of grieving.
○ **3.** The realization she will not see her daughter grow up was overwhelming.
○ **4.** She is experiencing unbearable loneliness.

43. Mrs. Stuben has had a 10-lb weight loss since the accident. Which would be the most helpful for her?

○ **1.** Have her eat with a client who is recovering from depression.
○ **2.** Serve a tray in her room, so others will not observe her poor appetite.
○ **3.** Allow her to eat in the cafeteria, so she can select food that appeals to her.
○ **4.** Have the dietitian prepare special trays to ensure the inclusion of all food groups.

44. Mrs. Stuben has difficulty falling asleep. It is most appropriate to

○ **1.** allow her to exercise the upper part of her body 20 minutes every night at 9:00 P.M.
○ **2.** provide a cool sponge bath and a cup of tea at bedtime.
○ **3.** allow her to watch TV every night until midnight.
○ **4.** provide a warm sponge bath and a warm glass of milk at bedtime.

45. Since there are variations in energy level in depressed clients, at what time of day would it be best to schedule Mrs. Stuben's activities?

○ **1.** Morning
○ **2.** Noon
○ **3.** Afternoon
○ **4.** Evening

46. Which of the following behaviors will demonstrate to the nurse that Mrs. Stuben is progressing in the resolution of her grief?

○ **1.** She reduces the amount of time spent crying.

○ **2.** She begins to talk about both the positive and negative aspects of relationships with the deceased.

○ **3.** She begins to demonstrate increased self-control by becoming more detached.

○ **4.** She begins to notice hospital staff members and seeks them out to discuss her concerns.

Harlan King, aged 68, sustained a left-sided cerebro-vascular accident 4 weeks ago. He has been transferred to a rehabilitation unit. He is able to communicate by minimal verbal expression and gesturing that he intends to walk again and use his right arm. His wife expresses the same goals.

47. In making assessments and initiating a program for Mr. King, what must all rehabilitation team members consider?

○ **1.** Initial assessments will need to be modified throughout the first week or 2, because the transfer to a new environment and the client's fatigue during this period will affect the accuracy of assessments.

○ **2.** Try to accomplish as much as possible with this client in the first 2 weeks; after that, motivation will generally decrease and gains made thereafter will be minimal.

○ **3.** Mrs. King will need to find something to do outside the rehabilitation setting. Mr. King needs to concentrate on his rehabilitation program at this point, and too much stimulation from family members will confuse him.

○ **4.** While making diagnostic assessments, give the client as many cues as possible, so that he will perform optimally.

48. Safety precautions are an important part of Mr. King's care. His right arm and leg have decreased sensation, along with the paresis, and could easily be injured. Based on these data, the plan of care would be to

○ **1.** protect these extremities with an arm sling and bivalved leg cast.

○ **2.** instruct Mr. King to observe his affected arm and leg frequently for positioning and to become aware of any movements that might injure them.

○ **3.** concentrate on the positives; do not talk about the paralyzed extremities and depress the client.

○ **4.** place any equipment, food tray, etc., on Mr. King's right side, so he can help himself safely and gain self-esteem through increasing independence.

49. Mr. King is having difficulty attaining sufficient nutritional intake. He has some trouble swallowing and has choked while eating. How can eating be facilitated?

○ **1.** Teach him to eat slowly and place food in the paralyzed side of his mouth.

○ **2.** Instruct Mrs. King to feed her husband after ensuring all food is cut into bite-sized pieces.

○ **3.** Assist him to a sitting position, place food in the unparalyzed side of his mouth, and have him concentrate on swallowing.

○ **4.** Restrict his intake to liquids until his chewing and swallowing capacities are fully restored.

50. It is important to minimize deformities in clients who have sustained brain damage. How is this best accomplished?

○ **1.** Set up a program with the client and let him be responsible for doing range-of-motion exercises on his own.

○ **2.** Schedule daily visits to physical therapy while the client is in the rehabilitation setting.

○ **3.** Remind Mr. King that he has flaccid paralysis of his right side and needs to prevent subluxation of his right shoulder by exercise.

○ **4.** Establish a schedule to exercise his right side with his unaffected side.

51. Which behavior best typifies the client with right-sided hemiplegia?
    ○ 1. Unaware of limitations; plunges into activities unaware of safety factors
    ○ 2. Anxious, approaches tasks in a halting, fearful way; may respond best to simple gestures
    ○ 3. Content with verbal directives, feels gestures and pantomime are demeaning
    ○ 4. Especially prone to spatial-perceptual problems

52. Mr. King spends a lot of time sitting in a chair. Where do decubitus ulcers most often develop when clients spend most of their time sitting?
    ○ 1. Over the sacrum
    ○ 2. Over the coccyx
    ○ 3. Over the ischial tuberosities
    ○ 4. Heels

Twelve-year-old Zachary has newly diagnosed insulin-dependent diabetes. He is on the pediatric unit.

53. Which of the following would *not* be an expected finding in Zachary's nursing history?
    ○ 1. Rapid weight gain
    ○ 2. Drinking large amounts of fluids
    ○ 3. Lethargic and tired
    ○ 4. Sudden return of bed-wetting

54. Zachary is admitted in ketoacidosis. The physician orders insulin "IV push." Which type of insulin should the nurse anticipate the physician will order?
    ○ 1. Lente
    ○ 2. Regular
    ○ 3. NPH
    ○ 4. PZI

55. Zachary has an order for an 1,800-calorie, diabetic exchange diet. The nurse explains to Zachary and his parents that this means Zachary
    ○ 1. can eat what he wants as long as he avoids concentrated sweets.
    ○ 2. can substitute items on one food list with other items from the same food list.
    ○ 3. can substitute any food item for any other as long as his total daily calorie intake remains the same.
    ○ 4. must carefully weigh or measure all portions of his food intake.

56. When teaching Zachary and his parents about insulin shock, the nurse emphasizes which of the following signs as indicating impending insulin shock?
    ○ 1. Acetone breath
    ○ 2. Slowed respirations
    ○ 3. Tremors
    ○ 4. Increased thirst

57. It is also important to teach Zachary and his parents about situations that will increase Zachary's insulin requirements. Which of the following will *not*?
    ○ 1. Increased exercise
    ○ 2. Increased food intake
    ○ 3. Infectious disease
    ○ 4. Changes associated with puberty

58. While being taught to administer his own insulin, Zachary becomes frustrated, throws down the syringe, and says, "I wish I could just forget this stuff!" What is the best explanation for this behavior?
    ○ 1. Zachary lacks confidence in himself.
    ○ 2. Zachary is not emotionally mature enough to assume full responsibility for his own insulin administration.
    ○ 3. Zachary is having difficulty coping with the knowledge and implications of having a chronic illness.
    ○ 4. Zachary is angry with the nurse.

59. How should the nurse respond to Zachary's behavior?
    ○ 1. Discuss this reaction with Zachary's parents and physician.
    ○ 2. Ask a 13-year-old boy on the unit who also has insulin-dependent diabetes to talk with Zachary.
    ○ 3. Refer Zachary to the staff psychologist.
    ○ 4. Tell Zachary, "You'll get used to this eventually and it won't seem difficult."

Theodore Eliasson, a 32-year-old advertising executive, has had surgery for the removal of a peptic ulcer. He states he has been under increasing stress in his employment and is very concerned about being able to continue in his position.

60. Which of the following statements most accurately describes Mr. Eliasson's condition?
○ 1. The stress of his environment has contributed to a physical condition of known organic origin.
○ 2. Although there is stress in his environment, it is not a direct contributing cause of his physical problem.
○ 3. His basic personality is the most influential factor in the cause of his physical problem.
○ 4. Hereditary factors are the most important cause of his physical problem.

61. The principal ego-defense mechanism utilized by Mr. Eliasson is which of the following?
○ 1. Rationalization
○ 2. Reaction formation
○ 3. Regression
○ 4. Repression

62. A condition such as Mr. Eliasson's differs from malingering in which of the following ways?
○ 1. The malingerer cooperates more readily in the treatment plan.
○ 2. The malingerer unconsciously develops symptoms to avoid an undesirable situation.
○ 3. The malingerer consciously develops symptoms to avoid an undesirable situation.
○ 4. The malingerer does not adapt as easily to illness.

63. The nurse will need to take into consideration Mr. Eliasson's diagnosis when developing a treatment plan. For this reason, the nurse will assess 3 of the following behavioral characteristics. Which characteristic will *not* be evident?
○ 1. Dependency issues
○ 2. Difficulty with decision making
○ 3. Excessive controlling behavior
○ 4. Poor reality orientation

64. In the assessment, the nurse finds that Mr. Eliasson has difficulty with decision making. One of the main goals of nursing care will be to have
○ 1. Mrs. Eliasson assume more responsibility for her husband's meals.
○ 2. Mr. Eliasson follow the physician's orders more closely.
○ 3. Mr. Eliasson work with the nurse to plan his care.
○ 4. Mr. Eliasson suggest to his wife what to make for his meals.

65. Mr. Eliasson tells the nurse he will be unable to walk down the hall today, because he has a headache. When the nurse states it's necessary for him to do so for his recovery, he yells, "You're the only nurse who makes me do that. You are cruel and heartless, and I refuse to be pushed around by you anymore." The nurse is surprised by his outburst, as he had not done it before. Which of the following responses would best meet Mr. Eliasson's nursing needs at this point?
○ 1. "All right, if no one else does, then I won't either."
○ 2. "I don't care what everyone else does, when I take care of you, you'll walk in the hall."
○ 3. "You seem very angry, and I'm not sure what about."
○ 4. "Don't yell at me. Talk to me in a civilized tone or don't talk at all."

66. After a few days, the nurse notices that Mr. Eliasson begins to have frequent violent outbursts at the staff when he does not want to do something. The nurse sees these outbursts as Mr. Eliasson's way of gaining control over his environment. The best nursing approach would be to
○ 1. explain to him that yelling is not permitted and that staff members will leave the room when he yells.
○ 2. allow him to yell, as he needs to feel some control while in the hospital.
○ 3. take away his television until he has not yelled for an entire day.
○ 4. allow him to yell at the staff, because they really have no right to yell back at him.

67. The most important contribution to the improvement of Mr. Eliasson's health is likely to be
○ 1. taking time for more leisure activities so that stress will be reduced.
○ 2. appropriately sharing concerns and feelings, so that emotional tensions are rechanneled.
○ 3. getting back to work, so there is less time to focus on physical symptoms.
○ 4. realizing that emotions affect physical conditions.

Bonnie Turner, aged 28, is suffering from metrorrhagia.

68. Mrs. Turner should be encouraged to seek medical assistance primarily because
○ **1.** excessive bleeding during menses may lead to anemia.
○ **2.** bleeding between periods may be the only early sign of cancer.
○ **3.** this is often symptomatic of a serious psychosomatic problem.
○ **4.** this is the main cause of failure to begin menses by 18 years of age.

69. In counseling Mrs. Turner, the nurse tells her that a yearly Pap smear is essential for which of the following reasons?
○ **1.** When uterine abnormalities are identified early, surgical treatment can be avoided.
○ **2.** Cervical cancer is usually curable in the preinvasive stage.
○ **3.** The Pap test is very reliable in diagnosing endometrial cancer.
○ **4.** The death rate for uterine cancer has steadily increased in recent years.

70. Mrs. Turner has had a Pap smear. The results reveal a stage 0, carcinoma in situ. It is decided that a conization will be the only treatment necessary. What is the major advantage of this procedure?
○ **1.** The procedure can be carried out on an outpatient basis.
○ **2.** Surgery carries less risk than the use of radiation.
○ **3.** The client retains the capacity to reproduce.
○ **4.** Leaving the ovaries intact while removing the uterus will prevent surgical menopause.

Colleen Green is in her third postpartum day. She has 2 children at home, aged 7 and 2. She is breast-feeding for the first time.

71. Mrs. Green was unsuccessful in breast-feeding her first baby. Which of the following actions would be most beneficial in assisting her to achieve her goal?
○ **1.** Explore the reasons why she failed the first time.
○ **2.** Tell her that it is easier with this baby as she is used to handling infants.
○ **3.** Stay with her and assist her with feeding the infant.
○ **4.** Ask her to put the call light on if she needs help.

72. Mrs. Green's infant is having difficulty grasping the nipple because of engorgement. The best initial nursing action is to tell the client to
○ **1.** use a nipple shield.
○ **2.** discontinue breast-feeding.
○ **3.** express some milk manually before each feeding.
○ **4.** breast-feed more frequently.

73. Fundal height is measured daily to monitor the involution of the uterus. When would an *inaccurate* reading be obtained?
○ **1.** Just after Mrs. Green has nursed her baby
○ **2.** If Mrs. Green has a full bladder
○ **3.** If Mrs. Green takes methylergonovine (Methergine)
○ **4.** If the baby is large (over 10 lb)

74. Mrs. Green is having severe afterpains. What is the most appropriate explanation to give her?
○ **1.** "It is very individual. One cannot predict what the nature of the pains might be."
○ **2.** "Afterpains increase with each pregnancy. Breast-feeding also increases the intensity of the pains."
○ **3.** "They are not usual. I will call your doctor."
○ **4.** "Afterpains are due to clots within the uterus. The uterus contracts trying to expel them."

75. Mrs. Green does not like to drink milk and wonders whether she can continue to nurse her baby. What is the best explanation the nurse can give?
○ **1.** "Breast-feeding will have to be discontinued; milk is essential in the diet to produce milk."
○ **2.** "When you don't like milk, it is very important to eat dark green vegetables as a source of calcium."
○ **3.** "Fruit juices can be used instead of drinking milk."
○ **4.** "There is no real advantage to drinking milk when lactating."

76. Mrs. Green has learned about the let-down reflex. Which one of the following statements most enables the nurse to conclude that Mrs. Green understands the nature of the reflex?
    ○ 1. "I have excess milk now, but the quantity will adjust itself depending on the baby's needs."
    ○ 2. "If I use a bottle often, I will stop secreting adequate milk for the baby."
    ○ 3. "When milk drips from my other breast, I know that my baby is getting milk."
    ○ 4. "The more the baby sucks and stimulates my breast, the more I will produce."

77. Mrs. Green is concerned that her 2-year-old daughter will want to try to breast-feed. She asks the nurse what she might do. The nurse should suggest which of the following?
    ○ 1. Explain that breast milk is only for little babies and that the 2-year-old can have the bottle.
    ○ 2. Allow her to try, as she is testing her mother. Soon she will stop being interested in it.
    ○ 3. Feed the baby in a room where the 2-year-old will not be able to watch.
    ○ 4. Give the 2-year-old a doll and ask her to feed it "just like mom."

Alex Frankl is a 23-month-old boy with tetralogy of Fallot. At this time, he is admitted to the hospital for further evaluation and possible surgery.

78. During the initial nursing assessment of Alex, the nurse would most likely expect to find which of the following signs and symptoms of tetralogy of Fallot?
    ○ 1. Bradycardia, dependent edema, slow weight gain
    ○ 2. Pale, scrawny appearance; machinery murmur; feeding difficulties
    ○ 3. Higher blood pressure in the arms than the legs, weak pedal pulses, epistaxis
    ○ 4. Clubbing of the fingers and toes, tachycardia, cyanosis

79. A child with tetralogy of Fallot is prone to several complications. The nurse should be alert for
    ○ 1. brain abscess.
    ○ 2. air emboli.
    ○ 3. cerebral emboli.
    ○ 4. all the above conditions.

80. Alex suddenly begins to choke and cough, and he turns cyanotic. What should the nurse do first?
    ○ 1. Help Alex assume a squatting position.
    ○ 2. Put a Venturi mask over Alex's nose and mouth.
    ○ 3. Place Alex upside down and pat his back vigorously.
    ○ 4. Determine if Alex is trying to use his condition to gain attention.

81. The physician orders 65 mcg of digoxin for Alex at 8:00 A.M. and 8:00 P.M. What would be the best method for giving Alex his medicine?
    ○ 1. Mix the digoxin with milk.
    ○ 2. Allow Alex to drink the digoxin himself from a plastic medicine cup.
    ○ 3. Use the dropper from the bottle.
    ○ 4. Offer Alex a reward if he takes his medicine without difficulty.

82. Alex has an order for a low-sodium diet. Which one of the following foods would be most *inappropriate* for his diet?
    ○ 1. Eggs
    ○ 2. Fruited yogurt
    ○ 3. Cottage cheese
    ○ 4. Cheddar cheese

Jane Johnson, 22 years old, is admitted to the hospital for a diagnostic workup. For the past 2 months, she has been irritable and argumentative with her boyfriend. At other times, she has been almost euphoric. She has been depressed about recent body changes. She has gained 15 lb; her face is puffy and flushed. She has also noted numerous bruises over her body; and while her abdomen has begun to protrude, her legs have become thin. Miss Johnson is admitted with the tentative diagnosis of Cushing's syndrome.

83. Assessments that would commonly lead the nurse to suspect a client has Cushing's syndrome include
    ○ 1. low blood sugar and tachycardia.
    ○ 2. thickening of the skin and bruising.
    ○ 3. weight loss and sodium retention.
    ○ 4. delayed wound healing and osteoporosis.

84. What test results are most indicative of Cushing's syndrome?
    ○ 1. Increased serum sodium and urinary 17-ketosteroids
    ○ 2. Decreased serum potassium and BUN
    ○ 3. Increased serum epinephrine and norepinephrine
    ○ 4. Decreased urinary 17-ketosteroids and 17-hydroxysteroids

85. Which of the following would *not* be the possible etiology of Cushing's syndrome in this client?
    ○ 1. Adrenal tumor
    ○ 2. Ectopic source of ACTH
    ○ 3. Pituitary tumor
    ○ 4. Adrenal atrophy

86. When Miss Johnson has been admitted to the hospital, the immediate nursing priority is
    ○ 1. decrease stress in the environment.
    ○ 2. encourage liberal amounts of fluids.
    ○ 3. explain tests and procedures.
    ○ 4. provide diversional activities.

87. Which of the following fluid and electroyte problems is most likely to occur with Miss Johnson?
    ○ 1. Hyperkalemia
    ○ 2. Increased output of dilute urine
    ○ 3. Sodium and H_2O retention
    ○ 4. Decreased serum calcium

88. The physician has ordered a plasma cortisol test. A positive test in a client with Cushing's syndrome would indicate elevated cortisol levels at what time of day?
    ○ 1. Morning
    ○ 2. Afternoon
    ○ 3. Evening
    ○ 4. Morning and evening

89. Miss Johnson is constantly hungry and is quite concerned that she cannot stop eating. This is probably occurring for which of the following reasons?
    ○ 1. She is stressed and is compensating by eating.
    ○ 2. She is hypoglycemic and the body compensates with hunger.
    ○ 3. She has increased cortisol levels that accelerate gluconeogenesis.
    ○ 4. She has had an increase in energy output and requires more calories.

90. Miss Johnson's diet needs to be modified. Which of the following would be a good choice for lunch?
    ○ 1. Chicken, brown rice, sliced oranges
    ○ 2. Tomato soup, tuna fish sandwich, vanilla pudding
    ○ 3. Macaroni and cheese, tomato salad, baked apple
    ○ 4. Broiled steak, green beans, ice cream

91. The diagnosis of Cushing's disease has been confirmed. A bilateral adrenalectomy is scheduled. Client teaching will include which of the following?
    ○ 1. Lifelong replacement of corticosteroids will be required.
    ○ 2. She will need to have weekly ACTH injections.
    ○ 3. Cortisol will be required in stress situations.
    ○ 4. No replacement therapy will be necessary.

92. Preoperatively, the client says to the nurse, ''I want to have this operation so I will look like my old self again.'' What would be an appropriate response?
    ○ 1. ''It will take several months before the changes are reversed.''
    ○ 2. ''I can see this is bothering you. Can you tell me what concerns you the most?''
    ○ 3. ''Adjusting to body changes is never easy to do.''
    ○ 4. ''Have you discussed this with your boyfriend?''

93. The most important post-op adrenalectomy assessment is
    ○ 1. type of nasogastric drainage.
    ○ 2. presence of drainage on abdominal dressing.
    ○ 3. heart rate.
    ○ 4. blood pressure.

94. On her third post-op day, Miss Johnson shows signs and symptoms of a mild addisonian crisis. Why is this considered a medical emergency?
    ○ 1. The increased cortisol levels can result in a hyperosmolar coma.
    ○ 2. Loss of sodium and increased potassium levels can cause life-threatening fluid and electrolyte imbalances.
    ○ 3. Increased aldosterone levels can trigger cardiac failure.
    ○ 4. The posterior pituitary gland cannot produce enough antidiuretic hormone (ADH).

95. Miss Johnson continues to convalesce without any further complications. What is the most important point to be included in her discharge teaching?
    ○ 1. Meticulous skin care
    ○ 2. Relaxation techniques
    ○ 3. Diet teaching
    ○ 4. Medication administration

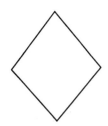

Test 2, Book IV
Answers with Rationales

1. **#2.** An inflamed mucosa is the most likely cause of the spasms that lead to symptoms of urgency. ANALYSIS (ADULT/ELIMINATION)

2. **#3.** Cranberry juice is the only choice given that will acidify urine. IMPLEMENTATION (ADULT/ELIMINATION)

3. **#1.** Sulfa drugs are excreted by the kidneys and not absorbed and are, therefore, more active in the urine than other antibiotics. ANALYSIS (ADULT/ELIMINATION)

4. **#1.** *E. coli* is the most common cause of urinary tract infections and is very sensitive to sulfa drugs. ANALYSIS (ADULT/ELIMINATION)

5. **#2.** The school-age child is developing a sense of industry (doing, accomplishing, achieving) to gain control through mastery and to build a positive self-concept. All the other options are too advanced for him. ANALYSIS (CHILD/HEALTHY CHILD)

6. **#4.** There is not enough information to make a judgment about Randall's growth. Information concerning his previous growth pattern, his dietary habits and exercise patterns, and hereditary influences (growth of family members) is needed before conclusions can be drawn. ANALYSIS (CHILD/HEALTHY CHILD)

7. **#3.** Results of visual-acuity testing are abnormal for Randall's age, and he should be referred for a more comprehensive evaluation at once. Option #4 is wrong; options #1 and #2 are inappropriate. PLAN (CHILD/HEALTHY CHILD)

8. **#1.** Since Randall has had the full recommended series, he will not need any additional immunizations until he is 14 to 16 years old. PLAN (CHILD/HEALTHY CHILD)

9. **#4.** Restricting a school-age child from experiences with fire, tools, and electrical appliances allows no opportunity to learn safety rules with these important objects. The child will remain unsafe. IMPLEMENTATION (CHILD/HEALTHY CHILD)

10. **#1.** Such clients make unrealistic appraisals of others and usually do not demonstrate ritualistic or fearful behaviors. Most characteristic of a borderline personality is the poor impulse control because of inadequate internal control. Ritualistic behavior is seen in compulsive personalities. Morbid fear of a seemingly harmless object is true of a phobic. ASSESSMENT (PSYCHOSOCIAL, MENTAL HEALTH, PSYCHIATRIC PROBLEMS/SOCIALLY MALADAPTIVE BEHAVIOR)

11. **#3.** Psychotropic drugs, electroconvulsive therapy, and antidepressants have not been found helpful in borderline personality disorder. Psychotropic drugs are used to treat psychotic disorders. Electroconvulsive therapy and antidepressants are used for clients with depression. ANALYSIS (PSYCHOSOCIAL, MENTAL HEALTH, PSYCHIATRIC PROBLEMS/SOCIALLY MALADAPTIVE BEHAVIOR)

12. **#3.** Manipulation is characteristic behavior of clients like Mr. Hall. These clients seldom ruminate, lose contact with reality, or have ritualistic behavior. Rumination occurs mostly in depressed clients. Hallucinations occur in psychotic individuals and clients using street drugs (e.g., cocaine, PCP). Although depersonalization and splitting occur and are serious distortions of reality, actual psychosis is the exception rather than the rule. ASSESSMENT (PSYCHOSOCIAL, MENTAL HEALTH, PSYCHIATRIC PROBLEMS/SOCIALLY MALADAPTIVE BEHAVIOR)

13. **#4.** Since clients with borderline personality disorder have a tendency to manipulate and use others, they should not be asked to assist staff with other clients. Mr. Hall requires firm limits on his behavior since he has little inner control. A firm, consistent, and positive attitude will help strengthen the client's ego, which will help him deal with the emotional discomfort of psychotherapy. Clients with borderline disorders regress quickly in the hospital. By expecting the client to act in a realistic, mature way, less regression should occur. IMPLEMENTATION (PSYCHOSOCIAL, MENTAL HEALTH, PSYCHIATRIC PROBLEMS/SOCIALLY MALADAPTIVE BEHAVIOR)

14. **#4.** Consistent limit setting is necessary in order to teach the client with borderline personality disorder to relate to others in socially acceptable ways. The client has little internal control and needs to learn control of impulsivity and acting-out behavior. Borderline clients often use flippancy and a light affect to minimize their desperation and pain. They often distort social problem areas and blame others for their problems. This client will antagonize others with critical and hostile complaints and verbal abuse. IMPLEMENTATION (PSYCHOSOCIAL, MENTAL HEALTH, PSYCHIATRIC PROBLEMS/SOCIALLY MALADAPTIVE BEHAVIOR)

15. **#4.** Clients with borderline personality disorder manipulate to avoid facing and working on their own problems. Genuine social skill development occurs very slowly. Impulse control is demonstrated when client shows restraint, not when focusing on other clients' problems. There is no evidence that the client is learning problem-solving skills. EVALUATION (PSYCHOSOCIAL, MENTAL HEALTH, PSYCHIATRIC PROBLEMS/SOCIALLY MALADAPTIVE BEHAVIOR)

16. **#4.** This approach is demonstrating consistent limit-setting in a matter-of-fact way. A firm and consistent approach is necessary so it is important not to ignore the incident. The nurse is responsible and accountable for meeting with the client. The nurse has been manipulated and is experiencing a common negative countertransference reaction to the borderline client, that of aversion. This behavior by the nurse results in abandonment feelings in the client. IMPLEMENTATION (PSYCHOSOCIAL, MENTAL HEALTH, PSYCHIATRIC PROBLEMS/SOCIALLY MALADAPTIVE BEHAVIOR)

17. **#4.** Daily staff conferences must be held to discuss client behaviors and plan consistent approach for all 3 shifts; clients with borderline personality disorder have an amazing ability to split staffs. The possibility exists that the night shift may behave as described. If so, clinical and managerial aspects of the matter must be explored by nursing management. Better methods than that described in option #3 can be taken if staff behavior appears to be a problem. IMPLEMENTATION (PSYCHOSOCIAL, MENTAL HEALTH, PSYCHIATRIC PROBLEMS/SOCIALLY MALADAPTIVE BEHAVIOR)

18. **#2.** The client with borderline personality disorder needs limits and does not have the ability to adaptively set his own limits and rules. Reviewing requests, holding daily staff conferences, and utilizing written care plans are very effective in decreasing manipulation and consequently staff anger, as well as preventing splitting of staff. IMPLEMENTATION (PSYCHOSOCIAL, MENTAL HEALTH, PSYCHIATRIC PROBLEMS/SOCIALLY MALADAPTIVE BEHAVIOR)

19. **#3.** The other options are characteristic of osteoarthritis. ASSESSMENT (ADULT/ACTIVITY AND REST)

20. **#1.** The sedimentation rate is elevated and is the most consistent lab finding in rheumatoid arthritis. The white blood cell count is usually slightly elevated; the client is usually anemic; and protein antibodies are present in 80% of clients. ASSESSMENT (ADULT/ACTIVITY AND REST)

21. **#2.** Stiffness is more pronounced in the early morning; it diminishes with use of the joint. ASSESSMENT (ADULT/ACTIVITY AND REST)

22. **#4.** The client's weight is within normal limits. Increasing calories and weight would place extra stress on joints. Added calcium would cause serum calcium to be high with increased risk of frozen joints. PLAN (ADULT/ACTIVITY AND REST)

23. **#1.** Pillows under major joints contribute to the complication of flexion contractures. Options #2 and #4 prevent contractures. Option #3 maintains skin integrity. IMPLEMENTATION (ADULT/ACTIVITY AND REST)

24. **#4.** Massage tends to further traumatize swollen, inflamed joints. Heat or cold can both be used effectively. IMPLEMENTATION (ADULT/ACTIVITY AND REST)

25. **#4.** Inflamed joints should not be exercised. An appropriate exercise regimen must be flexible and adjustable. EVALUATION (ADULT/ACTIVITY AND REST)

26. **#3.** Phenylbutazone causes bleeding; thus, stools and urine should be examined. Since acetylsalicylic acid (aspirin) also has an ulcerogenic effect, it should be avoided when taking phenylbutazone. IMPLEMENTATION (ADULT/ACTIVITY AND REST)

27. **#1.** Several months of therapy are required before effectiveness can be determined. The drug is given deep intramuscularly. Adverse effects most commonly occur late, often after treatment has been discontinued. ANALYSIS (ADULT/ACTIVITY AND REST)

28. **#4.** The client, by virtue of age, is a high-risk client. A medical history would be important to further assess for conditions affecting the course of pregnancy. As she is in the first trimester, fetal heart tones and movement of fetus would not be expected. Plans for childbirth would be appropriate, but not as critical as the initial medical history. ASSESSMENT (CHILDBEARING FAMILY/ANTEPARTAL CARE)

29. **#2.** Although a vast majority of birth defects will not be detected by amniocentesis as early as 14 weeks of gestation when adequate amniotic fluid can be obtained, this procedure can be used to assess specific disorders common in clients of advanced maternal age. The oxytocin challenge test, nonstress test, and urine estriols are carried out to determine fetal and placental functioning rather than chromosomal disorders. IMPLEMENTATION (CHILDBEARING FAMILY/ANTEPARTAL CARE)

30. **#1.** Women who smoke give birth to small-for-gestational-age infants at a rate almost twice that of women who do not smoke. Smoking causes constriction in the vasculature of the mother as well as of the placenta. Fewer nutrients are thus delivered to the fetus. Smoking does not reduce maternal weight gain. ANALYSIS (CHILDBEARING FAMILY/ANTEPARTAL CARE)

31. **#3.** Maternal isoimmunization in the Rh-negative expectant mother may occur if the baby inherits the father's Rh factor; therefore, it should be determined if Mr. Carter is Rh positive. All other data would require no action. ANALYSIS (CHILDBEARING FAMILY/ANTEPARTAL CARE)

32. **#4.** Strenuous new exercise should not be started during pregnancy. Current research indicates most fetuses can tolerate strenuous maternal exercise if the mother was previously conditioned to that level of activity. Jogging is also a controversial issue among physicians. IMPLEMENTATION (CHILDBEARING FAMILY/ANTEPARTAL CARE)

33. **#1.** The baby will contract the herpes through the birth canal if delivered vaginally. This virus has a devastating effect on newborns and many will die if infected. IMPLEMENTATION (CHILDBEARING FAMILY/ANTEPARTAL CARE)

34. **#3.** A creatinine of 2 mg/100 ml of amniotic fluid is indicative of a mature fetus. However, this test should not be used as a sole indicator. It should be used in conjunction with other test results. The L/S ratio is considered most important. A ratio of 2:1 indicates maturity. Falling estriol levels obtained by urine or blood samples indicate fetal compromise. An increase in alphafetoprotein is indicative of neural defects in the fetus. ASSESSMENT (CHILDBEARING FAMILY/ANTEPARTAL CARE)

35. **#3.** This is the only remedy known to eliminate the cramp quickly. The other methods listed do not work. IMPLEMENTATION (CHILDBEARING FAMILY/ANTEPARTAL CARE)

36. **#3.** Swelling and discomfort from varicosities caused by impeding venous return can be decreased by lying down or sitting with the legs elevated. Relief measures are aimed at promoting venous return. Thus, increased periods of sitting (causing popliteal pressure) or constricting garments should be avoided. EVALUATION (CHILDBEARING FAMILY/ANTEPARTAL CARE)

37. **#4.** Preeclampsia is the development of hypertension with proteinuria, edema, or both after the 20th week of gestation. Normal fluid retention is reflected in lower extremity edema in late pregnancy. Blood pressure should remain within normal limits. Data do not support a diagnosis of polyhydramnios. ANALYSIS (CHILDBEARING FAMILY/ANTEPARTAL CARE)

38. **#1.** Excessive milk intake limits ingestion of iron-rich foods. ASSESSMENT (CHILD/OXYGENATION)

39. **#2.** Iron-deficiency anemia can cause symptoms including pallor, fatigue, irritability, decreased exercise tolerance, decreased growth rate, and poor muscle tone. ASSESSMENT (CHILD/OXYGENATION)

40. **#4.** Stools, after administration of an oral iron preparation, will become a tarry-green color. EVALUATION (CHILD/OXYGENATION)

41. **#3.** Accidents, including ingestion of toxic substances, are the leading cause of death, once the child begins walking. IMPLEMENTATION (CHILD/SENSATION, PERCEPTION, PROTECTION)

42. **#2.** Clients are often prevented from beginning resolution of their grief when they are unable to attend funerals of loved ones. Options #1, #3, and #4 are all possible explanations for why she is thin and apathetic, but she is having a delayed grief response because her physical condition prevented her from going through the normal funeral ritual. ANALYSIS (PSYCHOSOCIAL, MENTAL HEALTH, PSYCHIATRIC PROBLEMS/ELATED-DEPRESSIVE BEHAVIOR)

43. **#3.** Independence is encouraged by allowing her to select foods that appeal to her. Option #1 imposes another person upon her and places a burden on the other client. #2 causes isolation. #4 is a good second choice if she will not select her own foods. IMPLEMENTATION (PSYCHOSOCIAL, MENTAL HEALTH, PSYCHIATRIC PROBLEMS/ELATED-DEPRESSIVE BEHAVIOR)

44. **#4.** These are appropriate nursing measures to promote sleep. Options #1, #2, and #3 are all stimulating actions that would increase arousal. IMPLEMENTATION (PSYCHOSOCIAL, MENTAL HEALTH, PSYCHIATRIC PROBLEMS/ELATED-DEPRESSIVE BEHAVIOR)

45. **#1.** In reactive depression, the client usually feels best in the morning and worse as the day progresses. PLAN (PSYCHOSOCIAL, MENTAL HEALTH, PSYCHIATRIC PROBLEMS/ELATED-DEPRESSIVE BEHAVIOR)

46. **#2.** Resolution of grief is demonstrated by the ability to reminisce about both the positive and negative aspects of a relationship in a realistic manner. Crying is a normal response but will occur less often and for shorter periods. Detachment is a sign of abnormal grieving. Being able to talk about her concerns shows an ability to deal with the reality of the loss but does not show resolution; it shows the beginning of the working phase in dealing with the grief. EVALUATION (PSYCHOSOCIAL, MENTAL HEALTH, PSYCHIATRIC PROBLEMS/ELATED-DEPRESSIVE BEHAVIOR)

47. **#1.** A change in environment affects concentration, but confusion is usually minimal unless the client is fatigued. The unfamiliar is overwhelming to a person with brain damage. The client's level of fatigue must be considered to obtain accurate assessment data. ASSESSMENT (ADULT/SAFETY AND SECURITY)

48. **#2.** Involve the client in his care with mutual goal setting and by promoting self-responsibility. These actions can enhance client compliance. Use arm sling and leg cast only during transport; these restrict range of motion if used continuously. Food trays and equipment should be positioned on the client's unaffected side. PLAN (ADULT/SAFETY AND SECURITY)

49. **#3.** This is the optimal way to facilitate eating. Feeding clients increases dependency. Chewing and swallowing may never be completely restored. IMPLEMENTATION (ADULT/SAFETY AND SECURITY)

50. **#4.** A cerebrovascular accident is an upper motor neuron lesion; therefore, spastic paralysis is present. Clients should participate in exercises but cannot be expected to initiate and remember their own exercise program. PLAN (ADULT/SAFETY AND SECURITY)

51. **#2.** These behaviors are characteristic of left-brain lesions. ASSESSMENT (ADULT/SAFETY AND SECURITY)

52. **#3.** Most pressure is on the ischial tuberosities when sitting. Any redness that does not resolve 20 minutes after the pressure is relieved is at risk for tissue breakdown. ASSESSMENT (ADULT/SAFETY AND SECURITY)

53. **#1.** Weight loss is typical of diabetes in children. Since glucose is unable to enter the cells, the body quickly is in a state of starvation. ASSESSMENT (CHILD/NUTRITION AND METABOLISM)

54. **#2.** Regular insulin is the only type given intravenously, because it can act quickly to reduce the blood glucose level. ANALYSIS (CHILD/NUTRITION AND METABOLISM)

55. **#2.** Zachary can exchange food items within each list (e.g., one vegetable for another vegetable from the same list), but he cannot exchange a vegetable for another food (e.g., meat or fruit). PLAN (CHILD/NUTRITION AND METABOLISM)

56. **#3.** Tremors or a shaky feeling indicate hypoglycemia and impending insulin shock. ASSESSMENT (CHILD/NUTRITION AND METABOLISM)

57. **#1.** Increased exercise will decrease Zachary's insulin requirements. IMPLEMENTATION (CHILD/NUTRITION AND METABOLISM)

58. **#3.** Zachary is expressing his frustration over his lack of control of the situation and the realization of the long-term nature of his illness. ANALYSIS (CHILD/NUTRITION AND METABOLISM)

59. **#2.** Peers are very important at this age, and talking with another boy with the same illness may help Zachary see things from a more positive perspective. IMPLEMENTATION (CHILD/NUTRITION AND METABOLISM)

60. **#1.** The diagnosis of psychosomatic disorder is used when there is evidence of a relationship between the environment and its meaning to the client, and the initiation or exacerbation of a physical condition. The client is not always aware of the relationship. Personality and hereditary factors may have contributed to his physical problem, but the condition has been exacerbated by a stressful working environment. ANALYSIS (PSYCHOSOCIAL, MENTAL HEALTH, PSYCHIATRIC PROBLEMS/ANXIOUS BEHAVIOR)

61. **#4.** The repression of emotional tension is unconsciously channeled through visceral organs. Rationalization is the falsification of experience by the construction of logically or socially approved explanations of behavior. Reaction formation is the development of conscious attitudes and behavior patterns that are opposite to what one really feels or would like to do. Regression is a retreat to earlier patterns of behavior. ANALYSIS (PSYCHOSOCIAL, MENTAL HEALTH, PSYCHIATRIC PROBLEMS/ANXIOUS BEHAVIOR)

62. **#3.** The malingerer consciously produces symptoms so that some recognizable goal can be achieved. The malingerer does not cooperate with the treatment plan, fears getting well, and is more comfortable with the sick role. The malingerer is aware of his behavior and the environment and its effect. ANALYSIS (PSYCHOSOCIAL, MENTAL HEALTH, PSYCHIATRIC PROBLEMS/ANXIOUS BEHAVIOR)

63. **#4.** Poor reality testing is a problem for clients with a psychotic disorder; it is not a symptom of a psychosomatic disorder. Dependency issues, indecision, and excessive controlling behavior are all characteristic of clients with peptic ulcers. ASSESSMENT (PSYCHOSOCIAL, MENTAL HEALTH, PSYCHIATRIC PROBLEMS/ANXIOUS BEHAVIOR)

64. **#3.** Working cooperatively with another person, such as the nurse, is an effective way for a client to receive help in decision making. Taking an excessively assertive stand with clients is an ineffective way to teach them how to make decisions. Giving more responsibility to the client's wife will not help. A client is less likely to follow orders when he has not actively participated in their development. PLAN (PSYCHOSOCIAL, MENTAL HEALTH, PSYCHIATRIC PROBLEMS/ANXIOUS BEHAVIOR)

65. **#3.** This response by the nurse encourages the client to express his feelings and redirects him from blaming her to discussing what is bothering him. This response does not blame or judge. To back down because of an angry outburst will encourage further use of that behavior in difficult situations. Option #2 introduces a power struggle between the client and the nurse. #4 is a parent-to-child communication and leaves the client feeling more frustrated. IMPLEMENTATION (PSYCHOSOCIAL, MENTAL HEALTH, PSYCHIATRIC PROBLEMS/ANXIOUS BEHAVIOR)

66. **#1.** This response by the nurse sets limits on the client's outbursts, protects the staff in their need not to be yelled at, and does not cause the client to feel judged or demeaned. Yelling is not a constructive method of communicating in any environment and does not enhance one's feeling of control. Removal of the television is a punitive measure and is not related to his yelling. Clients do not have the right to abuse staff members; the client needs to be taught how to successfully relate to others to have his needs met. IMPLEMENTATION (PSYCHOSOCIAL, MENTAL HEALTH, PSYCHIATRIC PROBLEMS/ANXIOUS BEHAVIOR)

67. **#2.** Participation in group or individual therapy and reevaluation of family relationships would help him understand his condition so that management of the environment can become more effective. Leisure activities may help to reduce the client's stress, but psychosomatic illnesses will recur if the client does not learn how to express his feelings and concerns constructively. Continued repression of emotional tension in a stressful environment will enhance the probability of a recurrence of his illness. Option #4 is a good first step, but the client needs to learn how to express his emotions. EVALUATION (PSYCHOSOCIAL, MENTAL HEALTH, PSYCHIATRIC PROBLEMS/ANXIOUS BEHAVIOR)

68. #2. Metrorrhagia is bleeding between periods. It may be the first sign of cervical cancer. ANALYSIS (CHILDBEARING FAMILY/POSTPARTAL CARE)

69. #2. When cervical cancer is diagnosed in the preinvasive stage, it carries a 95% to 100% cure rate. IMPLEMENTATION (CHILDBEARING FAMILY/POSTPARTAL CARE)

70. #3. Conization may be the only type of therapy needed if an area of normal tissue surrounds the malignancy. Other treatments are hysterectomy and radiation, both of which result in infertility. Option #1 is an advantage, but not the primary one. ANALYSIS (CHILDBEARING FAMILY/POSTPARTAL CARE)

71. #3. The fact that the first experience was unsatisfactory calls for supportive nursing action. IMPLEMENTATION (CHILDBEARING FAMILY/POSTPARTAL CARE)

72. #3. Manual expression of breast milk prior to feeding will decrease engorgement and allow the baby to latch on to the nipple with greater ease. If this measure is unsuccessful, a nipple shield may be recommended. IMPLEMENTATION (CHILDBEARING FAMILY/POSTPARTAL CARE)

73. #2. The uterus is displaced by a full bladder. Both nursing the infant and the administration of Methergine will cause the uterus to contract; a large baby may result in decreased tone in the uterus. However, these factors will not result in an inaccurate assessment. ASSESSMENT (CHILDBEARING FAMILY/POSTPARTAL CARE)

74. #2. Afterpains are uterine contractions that cause involution. The oxytocin released during breast-feeding intensifies the contractions. Afterbirth pains are more common in the multipara and breast-feeding mother. IMPLEMENTATION (CHILDBEARING FAMILY/POSTPARTAL CARE)

75. #2. Dark green vegetables are higher in calcium than most foods other than milk and milk products. IMPLEMENTATION (CHILDBEARING FAMILY/POSTPARTAL CARE)

76. #3. The let-down reflex causes milk to be pushed through the lacteal ducts. Oxytocin is released from the posterior pituitary for action on the myoepithelial cells of the mammary glands. As these cells contract, milk moves from the duct system to the lactiferous sinuses for ultimate delivery to the infant. The other options listed do not relate to the let-down reflex. EVALUATION (CHILDBEARING FAMILY/POSTPARTAL CARE)

77. #2. The 2-year-old requires the security and confidence that her mother loves her in spite of the newcomer. Options #1 and #4 are not developmentally appropriate for a 2-year-old. IMPLEMENTATION (CHILD/HEALTHY CHILD)

78. #4. As one of the cyanotic heart defects, tetralogy of Fallot is characterized by cyanosis. Clubbing is due to chronic hypoxia, and tachycardia is an attempt by the heart to compensate for lack of oxygen. ASSESSMENT (CHILD/OXYGENATION)

79. #4. When a right-to-left shunt is present, the macrophage-filtering system of the lungs is bypassed. This gives bacteria and air access to the systemic circulation. Clients with congenital heart disease have areas of turbulent blood flow. These clients are more susceptible to the formation and deposition of clots or vegetative matter at these sites. ANALYSIS (CHILD/OXYGENATION)

80. #1. Squatting alters the cardiovascular dynamics and improves pulmonary blood flow, thereby alleviating the symptoms of a choking spell. It is the position of choice often assumed spontaneously by these children. IMPLEMENTATION (CHILD/OXYGENATION)

81. #3. Because the dose of digoxin must be measured so exactly, this is the recommended method of administration. IMPLEMENTATION (CHILD/OXYGENATION)

82. #4. Because the child with heart disease is vulnerable to cardiac stress or failure, a restricted-sodium diet may be prescribed. Foods allowed in the cheese group on a low-sodium diet include unsalted cottage, pot, and low-sodium dietetic cheese. Cheddar cheese contains a high amount of sodium and is contraindicated. IMPLEMENTATION (CHILD/OXYGENATION)

83. #4. Cushing's syndrome is characterized by excessive amounts of cortisone. This delays wound healing (anti-inflammatory) and interferes with calcium metabolism leading to osteoporosis. ASSESSMENT (ADULT/NUTRITION AND METABOLISM)

84. #1. Increased cortisone leads to sodium retention and higher excretion of ketosteroids. ASSESSMENT (ADULT/NUTRITION AND METABOLISM)

85. #4. Adrenal atrophy results in hypocorticism (Addison's disease). ANALYSIS (ADULT/NUTRITION AND METABOLISM)

86. **#1.** Because of increased cortisol levels, clients with Cushing's disease have a low tolerance for stress; in addition, the accuracy of diagnostic tests performed is dependent upon minimizing stress. PLAN (ADULT/NUTRITION AND METABOLISM)

87. **#3.** Increased amounts of glucocorticoids will cause increased sodium and water retention. ANALYSIS (ADULT/NUTRITION AND METABOLISM)

88. **#4.** Normally, cortisol levels are highest during the waking hours and decrease during the evening hours. A client with Cushing's disease will have elevated levels regardless of wake/sleep pattern or time. ASSESSMENT (ADULT/NUTRITION AND METABOLISM)

89. **#3.** Cushing's disease results in increased gluconeogenesis; hyperglycemia occurs resulting in a diabetic state, and polyphagia is not uncommon. ANALYSIS (ADULT/NUTRITION AND METABOLISM)

90. **#1.** Diet should be high in protein, low in calories and sodium, and high in potassium. Complex carbohydrates should be included. IMPLEMENTATION (ADULT/NUTRITION AND METABOLISM)

91. **#1.** Cortisone, the glucocorticoid of choice, will be taken on a daily basis for the rest of her life. When there is an increase in stress, the dosage may need to be temporarily increased. With total removal of a gland, replacement therapy is indicated. With partial removal, follow-up without replacement is possible. IMPLEMENTATION (ADULT/NUTRITION AND METABOLISM)

92. **#2.** Having the client verbalize the meaning of the body changes is essential before care can be planned. IMPLEMENTATION (ADULT/NUTRITION AND METABOLISM)

93. **#4.** Following the stress of surgery, addisonian crisis is a possibility if there has not been adequate steroid replacement. Change in blood pressure, a first indication of this problem, must be reported immediately. ASSESSMENT (ADULT/NUTRITION AND METABOLISM)

94. **#2.** Decreased steroid production following an adrenalectomy can result in loss of sodium and water in copious amounts. In the absence of aldosterone, sodium is lost. Hypovolemic shock can occur quickly if the crisis is untreated. Also, potassium levels rise to dangerous levels causing life-threatening dysrhythmias. ANALYSIS (ADULT/NUTRITION AND METABOLISM)

95. **#4.** Miss Johnson needs to know all the precautions about steroid therapy. Stress the importance of taking medications daily and informing a physician about the medication when ill or having surgery so that the dosage can be temporarily increased. IMPLEMENTATION (ADULT/NUTRITION AND METABOLISM)

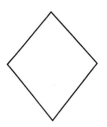

Appendices

Editor's Note

There are two components of the NCLEX-RN Test Plan: Nursing Process and Client Needs. Nursing process is composed of 5 steps: assessment, analysis, plan, implementation, and evaluation. Four client needs have been identified: environmental safety, physiologic integrity, psychosocial integrity, and health promotion. The practice of nursing requires knowledge in all these areas.

The following Appendices list the categories of nursing process and client needs assigned to all the questions in this book. Assignment of categories was made by item writers and nurse editors after consultation with the NCLEX-RN. Precise delineation of the categories is an evolving process and, as such, assignment of categories is also evolving.

The Appendices are provided for you should you wish to use them. Remember that your test will be scored on your ability to answer a given question correctly and not on your ability to correctly assign a category to a given question.

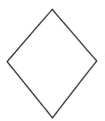

Nursing Process Categories

Section 2: Nursing Care of the Client with Psychosocial, Psychiatric/Mental Health Problems

Assessment

11,	18,	19,	22,	28,	31,	33,	34,	38,
45,	53,	54,	55,	70,	78,	81,	89,	96,
99,	104,	110,	118,	119,	121,	147,	149,	152,
153,	154,	159,	165,	166,	172,	173,	180,	189,
208,	210,	222,	230					

Analysis

2,	5,	10,	15,	16,	26,	37,	42,	43,
44,	58,	62,	71,	77,	82,	86,	95,	98,
111,	113,	116,	122,	123,	124,	127,	130,	133,
143,	144,	148,	156,	158,	168,	177,	178,	181,
184,	187,	190,	191,	197,	198,	200,	221,	227,
229,	235,	236,	247,	248,	249,	254		

Plan

8,	14,	30,	39,	46,	47,	48,	69,	87,
92,	100,	105,	134,	163,	171,	174,	182,	194,
203,	216,	217,	223,	244,	251			

Implementation

1,	3,	4,	6,	7,	9,	13,	17,	20,
21,	23,	24,	25,	27,	29,	32,	35,	40,
49,	50,	57,	59,	60,	61,	63,	64,	65,
66,	67,	68,	72,	73,	74,	75,	76,	79,
80,	83,	84,	85,	88,	90,	93,	94,	97,
101,	102,	103,	106,	107,	108,	109,	112,	113,
115,	117,	120,	125,	126,	128,	129,	131,	135,
136,	137,	138,	139,	140,	141,	142,	145,	146,
150,	155,	157,	160,	161,	162,	167,	169,	170,
175,	176,	179,	183,	185,	186,	192,	193,	195,
196,	199,	201,	202,	204,	205,	206,	209,	211
212,	213,	214,	215,	218,	219,	220,	224,	225,
226,	228,	231,	232,	234,	237,	238,	239,	240,
241,	242,	243,	245,	246,	250,	252,	253	

Evaluation

36,	41,	51,	52,	91,	151,	164,	188,	207,
233								

Section 3: Nursing Care of the Adult

Assessment

5	7,	10,	14,	31,	39,	44,	50,	51,
56,	57,	59,	67,	71,	75,	76,	82,	84,
85,	86,	87,	90,	94,	97,	101,	105,	108,
114,	116,	117,	123,	137,	144,	146,	147,	149,
151,	157,	162,	168,	169,	182,	187,	190,	191,
192,	196,	200,	202,	206,	211,	213,	214,	224,
227,	229,	232,	236,	239,	240,	245,	247,	251,
255,	271,	272,	277,	288,	292,	293,	294,	295,
299,	311,	320,	321,	335,	336,	340,	342,	349,
352,	362,	363,	367,	372,	373,	376,	381,	382,
385,	387,	392,	401,	402,	412,	414,	417,	429,

439,	444,	449,	450,	452,	455,	467,	477,	478,
490,	491,	500,	503					

Analysis

3,	6,	8,	9,	12,	13,	15,	16,	17,
18,	19,	20,	21,	22,	25,	26,	28,	32,
33,	34,	35,	36,	37,	38,	43,	46,	47,
48,	49,	52,	54,	55,	58,	61,	63,	69,
72,	74,	77,	78,	80,	81,	83,	89,	91,
93,	95,	96,	98,	100,	102,	103,	106,	107,
111,	112,	119,	122,	126,	127,	128,	129,	130,
131,	132,	133,	134,	135,	136,	138,	140,	141,
142,	152,	156,	158,	160,	165,	170,	171,	175,
179,	180,	183,	188,	193,	194,	195,	198,	204,
207,	208,	209,	210,	212,	238,	244,	248,	249,
252,	256,	257,	258,	259,	260,	261,	268,	275,
276,	282,	289,	290,	291,	296,	302,	304,	305,
306,	307,	310,	312,	319,	322,	326,	329,	331,
332,	333,	334,	337,	338,	341,	344,	346,	347,
354,	355,	356,	357,	358,	359,	360,	365,	371,
374,	379,	380,	383,	388,	389,	391,	393,	394,
395,	397,	400,	403,	405,	407,	411,	413,	415,
419,	420,	422,	430,	433,	434,	438,	443,	448,
454,	456,	457,	458,	461,	462,	470,	473,	479,
481,	482,	483,	488,	489,	495,	501,	502,	504,
506								

Plan

4,	42,	62,	68,	88,	104,	109,	118,	145,
159,	163,	164,	166,	177,	184,	185,	197,	215,
225,	226,	254,	264,	274,	281,	283,	303,	316,
317,	318,	323,	324,	339,	343,	351,	353,	364,
368,	369,	370,	384,	386,	398,	399,	404,	406,
409,	410,	416,	418,	423,	424,	426,	431,	432,
437,	440,	459,	460,	471,	480,	484,	487,	505,
508								

Implementation

1,	2,	23,	24,	27,	29,	40,	41,	45,
53,	60,	64,	65,	66,	70,	73,	79,	92,
99,	110,	113,	120,	121,	124,	125,	139,	143,
150,	153,	154,	155,	167,	172,	173,	174,	176,
178,	181,	186,	189,	199,	201,	203,	205,	216,
218,	219,	220,	221,	222,	223,	228,	230,	231,
235,	237,	241,	242,	243,	246,	250,	253,	262,
263,	265,	266,	267,	269,	273,	278,	279,	280,
284,	285,	286,	287,	297,	298,	300,	308,	309,
313,	315,	325,	327,	328,	330,	345,	348,	350,
361,	377,	378,	396,	408,	421,	425,	427,	428,
435,	436,	441,	442,	445,	446,	447,	451,	453,
463,	464,	465,	466,	468,	476,	485,	486,	492,
493,	494,	496,	497,	498,	499,	507,	509,	510,
511								

Evaluation

11,	30,	115,	148,	161,	233,	234,	270,	314,
366,	375,	390,	469,	474				

Section 4: Nursing Care of the Childbearing Family

Assessment

1,	7,	10,	13,	16,	17,	20,	23,	38,
39,	46,	47,	59,	64,	68,	71,	74,	77,
82,	84,	92,	95,	106,	109,	110,	111,	122,

	132,	134,	136,	142,	149,	150,	152,	155,	156,
	157,	158,	159,	160,	165,	166,	172,	173	

Analysis	2,	3,	8,	11,	27,	33,	37,	40,	41,
	49,	50,	55,	57,	62,	66,	70,	72,	76,
	79,	89,	90,	91,	94,	100,	107,	114,	117,
	119,	124,	128,	133,	138,	139,	141,	145,	151,
	167,	169,	176,	177,	178,	179			

Plan	21,	54,	60,	61,	67,	147

Implementation	4,	5,	6,	9,	12,	15,	18,	22,	24,
	25,	26,	29,	30,	32,	34,	35,	36,	42,
	43,	44,	45,	48,	51,	52,	53,	56,	58,
	63,	65,	69,	75,	78,	80,	83,	85,	87,
	88,	93,	96,	97,	98,	99,	101,	102,	103,
	104,	105,	108,	112,	113,	115,	116,	118,	120,
	121,	123,	125,	126,	127,	129,	130,	135,	137,
	140,	143,	144,	146,	148,	153,	154,	161,	163,
	164,	168,	170,	171,	174,	180			

Evaluation	14,	19,	28,	31,	73,	81,	86,	131

Section 5: Nursing Care of the Child

Assessment	2,	14,	17,	34,	36,	40,	49,	50,	61,
	67,	75,	80,	81,	84,	90,	93,	99,	100,
	103,	109,	110,	111,	116,	134,	140,	142,	152,
	165,	166,	170,	172,	182,	183,	185,	190,	191,
	196,	205,	213						

Analysis	3,	5,	19,	23,	24,	29,	31,	33,	35,
	42,	54,	46,	65,	68,	73,	76,	86,	88,
	92,	96,	105,	107,	117,	118,	119,	124,	125,
	126,	133,	135,	139,	143,	148,	149,	173,	174,
	179,	192,	193,	195,	201,	206,	207,	209,	212

Plan	6,	16,	21,	22,	25,	26,	30,	37,	43,
	47,	55,	58,	63,	69,	70,	77,	78,	79,
	82,	83,	85,	97,	104,	121,	130,	136,	153,
	154,	162,	169,	171,	177,	184,	200,	208,	215,
	216,	217							

Implementation	1,	4,	7,	8,	9,	10,	11,	12,	13,
	15,	18,	20,	27,	28,	32,	38,	39,	41,
	44,	45,	46,	51,	52,	53,	57,	59,	60,
	62,	64,	66,	72,	87,	89,	91,	94,	95,
	98,	101,	102,	106,	112,	113,	114,	115,	120,
	122,	123,	127,	128,	129,	132,	137,	138,	144,
	146,	147,	150,	151,	155,	156,	157,	158,	159,
	160,	161,	163,	164,	167,	168,	175,	176,	178,
	180,	186,	188,	189,	194,	197,	198,	199,	202,
	203,	204,	211,	214,	218				

Evaluation	48,	71,	74,	108,	131,	141,	181,	187

Section 6: Sample Tests
Test 1, Book I

Assessment	1,	2,	6,	12,	24,	29,	30,	45,	48,
	49,	50,	57,	61,	62,	77,	90		
Analysis	5,	8,	9,	13,	15,	16,	23,	31,	34,
	35,	36,	37,	39,	43,	47,	52,	53,	66,
	67,	68,	69,	71,	75,	76,	86,	87,	89,
	91,	94,	95						
Plan	4,	17,	19,	51,	59,	74,	81,	93	
Implementation	3,	7,	14,	18,	21,	22,	25,	26,	27,
	28,	32,	33,	38,	40,	41,	42,	44,	46,
	54,	56,	58,	60,	63,	64,	65,	72,	73,
	78,	79,	80,	84,	85,	88,	92		
Evaluation	10,	11,	55,	70,	82				

Test 1, Book II

Assessment	5,	7,	11,	18,	20,	22,	31,	36,	38,
	39,	40,	53,	58,	60,	63,	69,	89	
Analysis	2,	4,	6,	8,	10,	13,	14,	15,	16,
	17,	21,	26,	28,	29,	32,	43,	44,	54,
	59,	62,	65,	74,	75,	76,	83,	87,	91,
	94,	95							
Plan	9,	30,	34,	41,	42,	46,	47,	55,	56,
	64,	68,	70,	71,	84,	90			
Implementation	1,	3,	12,	19,	23,	24,	25,	27,	33,
	37,	45,	48,	49,	50,	51,	57,	61,	67,
	72,	73,	77,	78,	79,	81,	82,	85,	88,
	92,	93							
Evaluation	35,	52,	66,	80,	86				

Test 1, Book III

Assessment	2,	8,	13,	17,	19,	20,	21,	32,	34,
	46,	53,	54,	61,	62,	63,	66,	68,	74,
	76,	79,	85,	88,	89				
Analysis	1,	6,	7,	9,	11,	25,	26,	33,	35,
	36,	39,	40,	42,	43,	44,	45,	47,	48,
	60,	69,	71,	72,	75,	78,	86,	90,	91,
	94,	95							
Plan	3,	12,	15,	22,	23,	24,	50,	55,	64,
	93								
Implementation	4,	5,	10,	14,	16,	18,	27,	28,	29,
	30,	31,	37,	41,	49,	51,	56,	57,	58,
	59,	65,	70,	73,	77,	81,	82,	83,	87,
	92								

| **Evaluation** | 38, | 67, | 80, | 84 | | | | | |

Test 1, Book IV

Assessment	3,	4,	5,	6,	8,	9,	12,	14,	15,
	16,	19,	23,	27,	31,	32,	41,	· 49,	50,
	61,	64,	69,	78,	79,	80			

Analysis	2,	7,	10,	13,	18,	30,	33,	35,	36,
	37,	38,	39,	44,	47,	56,	62,	65,	67,
	72,	73,	82						

| **Plan** | 17, | 21, | 28, | 46, | 48, | 51, | 53, | 63, | 71, |
| | 74, | 81, | 83, | 89 | | | | | |

Implementation	1,	11,	20,	25,	26,	29,	34,	40,	42,
	43,	45,	52,	54,	57,	58,	59,	66,	68,
	70,	75,	76,	84,	86,	87,	88,	90,	91,
	92,	93,	94,	95					

| **Evaluation** | 24, | 77, | 85 | | | | | | |

Test 2, Book I

Assessment	1,	7,	11,	12,	21,	26,	28,	31,	35,
	39,	44,	52,	58,	66,	73,	74,	80,	81,
	84,	85							

Analysis	5,	8,	10,	17,	20,	25,	27,	36,	41,
	43,	45,	46,	50,	53,	55,	56,	57,	59,
	62,	63,	64,	78,	79,	87,	89,	93,	95

| **Plan** | 9, | 15, | 22, | 23, | 24, | 37, | 47, | 51, | 67, |
| | 69, | 90, | 92 | | | | | | |

Implementation	2,	3,	4,	13,	14,	16,	18,	19,	29,
	32,	33,	38,	40,	48,	49,	54,	60,	61,
	65,	68,	70,	72,	76,	77,	82,	83,	86,
	88,	94							

| **Evaluation** | 30, | 34, | 42, | 71, | 75, | 91 | | | |

Test 2, Book II

Assessment	9,	12,	15,	17,	19,	25,	27,	30,	34,
	35,	44,	52,	58,	63,	71,	73,	74,	77,
	82,	83,	91						

Analysis	1,	4,	5,	6,	7,	10,	20,	32,	39,
	45,	46,	47,	49,	55,	57,	59,	61,	62,
	64,	65,	66,	69,	70,	72,	81,	88,	92

| **Plan** | 2, | 3, | 21, | 22, | 23, | 24, | 42, | 43, | 56, |
| | 67, | 68, | 78, | 86, | 93, | 94 | | | |

Implementation	8,	11,	13,	16,	18,	26,	28,	29,	31,
	36,	37,	38,	40,	41,	48,	50,	51,	53,
	54,	60,	75,	76,	79,	80,	84,	85,	87,
	89,	90,	95						

Evaluation   14,   33

Test 2, Book III

| **Assessment** | 12, | 19, | 30, | 50, | 56, | 59, | 63, | 69, | 70, |
| | 78, | 82, | 87, | 88, | 90, | 94 | | | |

Analysis	1,	4,	5,	8,	13,	16,	17,	18,	21,
	22,	26,	28,	32,	39,	41,	43,	46,	55,
	57,	58,	61,	62,	67,	68,	86,	91,	93

| **Plan** | 9, | 15, | 20, | 25, | 27, | 31, | 33, | 38, | 40, |
| | 47, | 48, | 51, | 52, | 64, | 66, | 83, | 85, | 89 |

Implementation	2,	3,	6,	7,	10,	11,	14,	23,	24
	29,	34,	35,	42,	49,	53,	54,	60,	71,
	72,	73,	74,	75,	76,	77,	79,	80,	84,
	92,	95							

| **Evaluation** | 36, | 37, | 44, | 45, | 65, | 81 | | | |

Test 2, Book IV

Assessment	10,	12,	19,	20,	21,	28,	34,	38,	39,
	47,	51,	52,	53,	56,	63,	73,	78,	83,
	88,	93							

Analysis	1,	3,	4,	5,	6,	11,	27,	30,	31,
	37,	42,	54,	58,	60,	61,	62,	68,	70,
	79,	85,	87,	89,	94				

| **Plan** | 7, | 8, | 22, | 45, | 48, | 50, | 55, | 64, | 86 |

Implementation	2,	9,	13,	14,	16,	17,	18,	23,	24,
	26,	29,	32,	33,	35,	41,	43,	44,	49,
	57,	59,	65,	66,	69,	71,	72,	74,	75,
	77,	80,	81,	82,	90,	91,	92,	95	

| **Evaluation** | 15, | 25, | 36, | 40, | 46, | 67, | 76 | | |

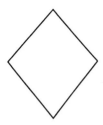

Client Needs Categories

Section 2: Nursing Care of the Client with Psychosocial, Psychiatric/Mental Health Problems

Environmental Safety

1,	2,	4,	8,	29,	30,	46,	47,	57,
73,	79,	80,	83,	86,	87,	88,	93,	97,
100,	105,	112,	117,	120,	130,	131,	133,	136,
160,	162,	170,	172,	173,	174,	177,	178,	182,
185,	188,	193,	194,	203,	212,	215,	217,	223,
225,	241							

Physiologic Integrity

15,	17,	28,	40,	56,	64,	74,	77,	85,
89,	94,	101,	102,	119,	122,	123,	124,	132,
137,	147,	148,	149,	157,	158,	159,	165,	168,
169,	184,	187,	200,	201,	208,	210,	211,	226,
228,	231,	234,	238,	240,	243,	247,	250,	254

Psychosocial Integrity

3,	5,	6,	7,	9,	10,	14,	20,	21,
24,	26,	27,	31,	32,	33,	34,	35,	36,
37,	38,	39,	41,	42,	43,	44,	45,	48,
49,	50,	51,	52,	54,	55,	58,	59,	60,
61,	62,	63,	66,	67,	70,	71,	78,	81,
82,	84,	92,	95,	98,	99,	104,	106,	108,
110,	111,	113,	115,	116,	118,	121,	126,	127,
129,	135,	139,	141,	142,	143,	144,	145,	152,
153,	154,	156,	161,	166,	167,	176,	180,	181,
183,	189,	190,	195,	196,	197,	198,	199,	212,
204,	205,	206,	209,	213,	214,	218,	219,	220,
221,	222,	224,	227,	236,	237,	239,	242,	245,
248,	249,	251,	252,	253				

Health Promotion

11,	12,	13,	16,	18,	19,	22,	25,	53,
65,	68,	69,	75,	76,	91,	103,	107,	109,
114,	125,	128,	138,	140,	150,	155,	163,	164,
171,	175,	179,	191,	192,	207,	216,	232,	233,
235,	244,	246						

Section 3: Nursing Care of the Adult

Environmental Safety

53,	64,	73,	88,	92,	93,	113,	126,	143,
145,	151,	154,	156,	163,	166,	167,	172,	173,
174,	177,	185,	189,	193,	197,	201,	203,	205,
206,	225,	226,	236,	237,	239,	250,	254,	265,
272,	273,	277,	278,	280,	281,	284,	285,	286,
297,	298,	300,	308,	323,	330,	342,	343,	348,
369,	370,	386,	398,	404,	408,	416,	421,	425,
431,	436,	437,	444,	445,	446,	459,	460,	468,
471,	480,	484,	485,	497,	504,	505,	506,	508

Physiologic Integrity

1,	2,	3,	4,	5,	6,	7,	8,	9,
10,	11,	12,	13,	14,	15,	16,	17,	18,
19,	20,	21,	22,	23,	24,	25,	26,	29,

30,	31,	32,	33,	34,	35,	36,	37,	38,
39,	40,	44,	46,	47,	48,	50,	52,	54,
55,	56,	57,	58,	59,	60,	61,	62,	63,
67,	68,	69,	70,	71,	72,	74,	75,	76,
77,	78,	79,	80,	81,	82,	83,	84,	85,
86,	87,	89,	90,	91,	94,	95,	96,	97,
98,	100,	101,	102,	103,	104,	105,	106,	107,
108,	109,	110,	111,	112,	114,	115,	116,	117,
119,	121,	122,	123,	127,	128,	129,	130,	131,
132,	133,	134,	135,	136,	137,	138,	140,	141,
142,	144,	146,	147,	149,	150,	152,	153,	155,
157,	158,	159,	160,	161,	162,	164,	165,	168,
169,	170,	171,	175,	176,	179,	180,	181,	182,
183,	184,	187,	188,	190,	191,	192,	194,	195,
196,	198,	200,	202,	204,	207,	208,	210,	211,
213,	214,	215,	217,	218,	220,	221,	224,	227,
229,	231,	232,	238,	240,	242,	243,	244,	245,
246,	247,	248,	249,	251,	252,	255,	256,	257,
258,	259,	260,	261,	262,	263,	264,	266,	267,
268,	271,	274,	275,	276,	279,	282,	287,	288,
289,	290,	291,	292,	293,	294,	295,	296,	299,
301,	304,	305,	306,	307,	309,	310,	311,	312,
313,	316,	317,	318,	319,	320,	321,	322,	324,
325,	326,	327,	328,	329,	330,	331,	332,	333,
334,	335,	336,	337,	338,	340,	341,	344,	345,
346,	347,	349,	351,	352,	353,	354,	355,	356,
357,	358,	359,	362,	363,	364,	365,	366,	367,
368,	371,	372,	373,	374,	375,	376,	378,	379,
381,	382,	383,	384,	385,	387,	388,	389,	390,
391,	392,	393,	394,	395,	396,	397,	399,	400,
401,	402,	403,	406,	411,	412,	413,	414,	415,
417,	419,	420,	422,	426,	427,	429,	430,	432,
433,	435,	438,	441,	442,	443,	447,	448,	449,
450,	452,	453,	454,	455,	456,	457,	458,	461,
462,	463,	467,	470,	479,	481,	482,	483,	487,
488,	489,	490,	491,	493,	498,	500,	502,	509

Psychosocial Integrity

28,	51,	216,	219,	230,	241,	303,	315,	465,
466,	486,	492,	494,	496,	501,	503		

Health Promotion

27,	41,	42,	43,	45,	65,	66,	99,	118,
120,	124,	125,	139,	148,	178,	186,	199,	209,
212,	222,	223,	228,	233,	234,	235,	253,	269,
270,	283,	302,	314,	350,	360,	361,	377,	380,
405,	409,	410,	418,	423,	424,	428,	434,	439,
440,	451,	464,	469,	472,	473,	474,	475,	476,
477,	478,	495,	499,	507,	510,	511		

Section 4: Nursing Care of the Childbearing Family

Environmental Safety

16,	17,	24,	25,	31,	36,	43,	44,	48,
53,	54,	58,	60,	61,	67,	75,	87,	88,
89,	102,	103,	105,	106,	108,	112,	118,	125,
126,	144,	147,	168,	171				

Physiologic Integrity

1,	2,	3,	6,	7,	8,	9,	10,	11,
13,	20,	23,	28,	32,	33,	34,	37,	38,
39,	40,	41,	42,	46,	47,	49,	50,	51,
52,	55,	56,	57,	59,	62,	64,	65,	66,

70,	71,	72,	74,	77,	82,	83,	84,	85,
86,	90,	91,	92,	93,	94,	95,	96,	97,
98,	99,	100,	104,	107,	109,	110,	111,	114,
116,	117,	119,	122,	123,	124,	127,	128,	129,
132,	133,	134,	135,	136,	138,	140,	141,	142,
145,	149,	151,	152,	155,	156,	157,	158,	159,
160,	162,	165,	166,	167,	169,	172,	173,	175,
176,	177,	178,	179					

Psychosocial Integrity

15,	22,	26,	27,	45,	68,	69,	76,	78,
79,	81,	113,	120,	121,	123,	139,	174,	180

Health Promotion

4,	5,	12,	14,	18,	19,	21,	29,	30,
35,	63,	73,	80,	101,	115,	130,	131,	137,
143,	146,	148,	150,	153,	154,	161,	163,	164,
170								

Section 5: Nursing Care of the Child

Environmental Safety

25,	27,	28,	30,	32,	55,	58,	60,	78
80,	97,	101,	136,	137,	146,	157,	158,	159
162,	175,	186,	199					

Physiologic Integrity

2,	11,	14,	16,	29,	31,	34,	35,	36,
37,	40,	42,	43,	45,	46,	48,	50,	54,
61,	62,	63,	64,	65,	66,	67,	68,	69,
70,	73,	75,	76,	77,	79,	81,	82,	85,
86,	87,	88,	89,	90,	92,	94,	99,	100,
103,	105,	106,	107,	110,	111,	116,	117,	118,
121,	122,	123,	124,	125,	126,	127,	128,	134,
145,	152,	153,	154,	155,	156,	160,	161,	163,
164,	166,	170,	172,	173,	176,	177,	178,	179,
180,	181,	182,	183,	184,	185,	187,	188,	189,
191,	195,	196,	200,	202,	203,	204,	206,	207,
208,	209,	210,	211,	212,	213,	215,	216	

Psychosocial Integrity

13,	18,	23,	24,	33,	56,	57,	72,	74,
95,	96,	104,	113,	114,	115,	129,	132,	133,
139,	140,	143,	144,	148,	149,	150,	151,	174,
192,	193,	198						

Health Promotion

1,	3,	4,	5,	6,	7,	8,	9,	10,
12,	15,	17,	19,	20,	21,	22,	26,	38,
39,	41,	44,	47,	49,	51,	52,	53,	59,
60,	71,	83,	84,	91,	93,	98,	102,	108,
109,	112,	119,	120,	130,	131,	135,	138,	141,
142,	147,	165,	167,	168,	169,	171,	190,	194,
197,	201,	205,	214,	217,	218			

Section 6: Sample Tests
Test 1, Book I

Environmental Integrity

1,	3,	4,	7,	17,	19,	33,	51,	59,
62,	78,	88						

Physiologic Integrity

2,	12,	13,	14,	15,	16,	18,	20,	21,
22,	23,	24,	26,	29,	30,	31,	32,	34,
35,	45,	46,	47,	48,	49,	50,	52,	53,

57, 60, 61, 65, 66, 67, 68, 69, 71,
72, 73, 74, 84, 85, 90, 91, 92, 93,
94, 95

Psychosocial Integrity 5, 6, 8, 9, 10, 11, 36, 37, 38,
39, 40, 41, 42, 43, 44, 56, 75, 76,
77, 79, 80, 81, 82, 83, 86, 89

Health Promotion 25, 27, 28, 54, 55, 58, 63, 64, 70

Test 1, Book II

Environmental Safety 1, 23, 30, 41, 46, 55, 61, 67, 71,
84

Physiologic Integrity 2, 3, 4, 5, 6, 7, 10, 11, 12,
13, 14, 15, 16, 17, 18, 19, 20, 21,
22, 25, 28, 29, 31, 32, 34, 36, 37,
38, 39, 40, 42, 54, 60, 62, 63, 64,
65, 66, 68, 69, 70, 74, 75, 76, 82,
83, 85, 86, 87, 88, 89, 90, 91, 93,
94, 95

Psychosocial Integrity 9, 26, 27, 44, 45, 47, 48, 49, 50,
51, 52, 57, 72, 73, 77, 78, 79, 80

Health Promotion 8, 24, 33, 35, 43, 53, 56, 58, 81,
92

Test 1, Book III

Environmental Safety 3, 14, 16, 22, 23, 28, 30, 31, 50,
55, 64, 73, 77

Physiologic Integrity 1, 2, 11, 12, 13, 15, 17, 20, 21,
24, 25, 26, 32, 33, 34, 35, 36, 37,
39, 40, 41, 42, 43, 44, 45, 46, 49,
51, 60, 61, 62, 63, 65, 66, 68, 69,
70, 71, 72, 74, 75, 76, 78, 79, 80,
82, 83, 84, 85, 86, 87, 88, 89, 90,
91, 92, 93, 94, 95

Psychosocial Integrity 4, 6, 7, 8, 9, 10, 18, 29, 47,
53, 54, 56, 57, 58, 59, 81

Health Promotion 5, 19, 38, 48, 52, 67

Test 1, Book IV

Environmental Safety 20, 51, 54, 63, 75, 87, 89

Physiologic Integrity 9, 10, 11, 14, 16, 17, 18, 19, 21,
22, 23, 25, 27, 28, 30, 32, 33, 34,
35, 36, 37, 38, 39, 40, 41, 44, 45,
47, 49, 50, 52, 53, 60, 61, 62, 63,
64, 65, 67, 68, 69, 70, 71, 72, 73,
74, 78, 79, 80, 81, 83, 84, 85, 86,
88, 90, 91, 92, 93, 94

| **Psychosocial Integrity** | 1, | 2, | 3, | 4, | 5, | 6, | 7, | 8, | 12, |
| | 13, | 14, | 55, | 56, | 57, | 58, | 59, | 66, | 82 |

| **Health Promotion** | 24, | 26, | 29, | 31, | 42, | 43, | 46, | 48, | 76, |
| | 77, | 95 | | | | | | | |

Test 2, Book I

| **Environmental Safety** | 22, | 23, | 36, | 37, | 76, | 86, | 90, | 94 | |

Physiologic Integrity	5,	6,	7,	8,	9,	10,	11,	12,	13,
	16,	17,	18,	19,	20,	21,	24,	25,	26,
	27,	28,	29,	35,	39,	40,	41,	42,	43,
	44,	45,	46,	58,	59,	60,	61,	62,	63,
	64,	65,	66,	67,	68,	70,	74,	77,	78,
	79,	80,	81,	83,	84,	85,	87,	89,	92,
	93,	95							

| **Psychosocial Integrity** | 2, | 13, | 15, | 31, | 32, | 33, | 38, | 48, | 49, |
| | 50, | 51, | 52, | 53, | 54, | 55, | 56, | 73, | 82 |

| **Health Promotion** | 1, | 3, | 4, | 30, | 34, | 47, | 57, | 69, | 71, |
| | 72, | 75, | 88, | 91 | | | | | |

Test 2, Book II

| **Environmental Safety** | 13, | 21, | 22, | 23, | 43, | 48, | 57, | 67, | 84, |
| | 86, | 93 | | | | | | | |

Physiologic Integrity	1,	2,	3,	4,	5,	6,	7,	8,	12,
	17,	19,	20,	25,	27,	28,	32,	44,	47,
	49,	53,	63,	64,	65,	66,	69,	70,	71,
	72,	73,	74,	75,	76,	77,	80,	81,	82,
	85,	87,	91,	92,	94,	95			

Psychosocial Integrity	9,	10,	11,	15,	18,	26,	29,	34,	35,
	36,	37,	39,	40,	41,	51,	58,	59,	60,
	61,	62,	78,	79					

| **Health Promotion** | 14, | 16, | 24, | 30, | 31, | 33, | 38, | 50, | 52, |
| | 54, | 55, | 56, | 68, | 83, | 88, | 89, | 90 | |

Test 2, Book III

| **Environmental Safety** | 9, | 14, | 23, | 25, | 40, | 65, | 89 | | |

Physiologic Integrity	1,	2,	3,	4,	5,	6,	7,	13,	15,
	16,	18,	19,	20,	21,	22,	26,	27,	29,
	30,	31,	32,	33,	38,	46,	47,	48,	50,
	51,	52,	53,	54,	55,	56,	57,	58,	59,
	60,	61,	62,	63,	64,	67,	72,	73,	74,
	75,	82,	83,	85,	86,	87,	88,	90,	91,
	92,	93,	94						

| **Psychosocial Integrity** | 8, | 10, | 11, | 12, | 39, | 41, | 42, | 43, | 44, |
| | 45, | 49, | 68, | 69, | 70, | 71, | 78, | 80, | 84 |

| **Health Promotion** | 17, | 24, | 28, | 34, | 35, | 36, | 37, | 66, | 76, |
| | 77, | 81, | 95 | | | | | | |

Test 2, Book IV

Environmental Safety	9,	22,	23,	45,	47,	48,	50,	55,	56,
	64,	71,	76,	91,	92				
Physiologic Integrity	1,	2,	3,	4,	6,	7,	8,	19,	20,
	21,	24,	26,	27,	28,	29,	30,	31,	33,
	34,	35,	36,	37,	38,	39,	41,	43,	44,
	49,	51,	52,	53,	54,	60,	68,	70,	72,
	73,	74,	75,	78,	79,	80,	81,	82,	83,
	84,	85,	86,	87,	88,	89,	90,	93,	94
Psychosocial Integrity	10,	11,	12,	13,	14,	15,	16,	17,	18,
	42,	46,	58,	59,	61,	62,	63,	65,	66
Health Promotion	5,	25,	32,	40,	57,	67,	69,	77,	95

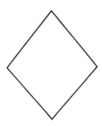

Nursing Process and Client Needs Categories

AS = Assessment
AN = Analysis
PL = Plan
IM = Implementation
EV = Evaluation

E = Environmental Safety
PS = Physiologic Integrity
PC = Psychosocial Integrity
H = Health Promotion

Section 2: Nursing Care of the Client With Psychosocial, Mental Health/Psychiatric Problems

1. IM	E	42. AN	PC	83. IM	E	124. AN	PS	165. AS	PC
2. AN	E	43. AN	PC	84. IM	PC	125. IM	H	166. AS	PC
3. IM	PC	44. AN	PC	85. IM	PS	126. IM	PC	167. IM	PC
4. IM	E	45. AS	PC	86. AN	E	127. AN	PC	168. AN	PS
5. AN	PC	46. PL	E	87. PL	E	128. IM	H	169. IM	PS
6. IM	PC	47. PL	E	88. IM	E	129. IM	PC	170. IM	E
7. IM	PC	48. PL	PC	89. AS	PS	130. AN	E	171. PL	H
8. PL	E	49. IM	PC	90. IM	PS	131. IM	E	172. AS	E
9. IM	PL	50. IM	PC	91. EV	H	132. IM	PS	173. AS	E
10. AN	PL	51. EV	PC	92. PL	PC	133. AN	E	174. PL	E
11. AS	H	52. EV	PC	93. IM	E	134. PL	E	175. IM	H
12. AN	H	53. AS	H	94. IM	PS	135. IM	PC	176. IM	PC
13. IM	H	54. AS	PC	95. AN	PC	136. IM	E	177. AN	E
14. PL	PC	55. AS	PC	96. AS	PC	137. IM	PS	178. AN	E
15. AN	PS	56. IM	PS	97. IM	E	138. IM	H	179. IM	H
16. AN	H	57. IM	E	98. AN	PC	139. IM	PC	180. AS	PC
17. IM	PS	58. AN	PC	99. AS	E	140. IM	PC	181. AN	PC
18. AS	H	59. IM	PC	100. PL	E	141. IM	PC	182. PL	E
19. AS	H	60. IM	PC	101. IM	PS	142. IM	PC	183. IM	PC
20. IM	PC	61. IM	PC	102. IM	PS	143. AN	PC	184. AN	PS
21. IM	PC	62. AN	PC	103. IM	H	144. AN	PC	185. IM	E
22. AS	H	63. IM	PC	104. AS	PC	145. IM	PC	186. IM	E
23. IM	H	64. IM	PS	105. PL	E	146. IM	PC	187. AN	PS
24. IM	PC	65. IM	H	106. IM	PC	147. AS	PS	188. EV	E
25. IM	H	66. IM	PC	107. IM	H	148. AN	PS	189. AS	PC
26. AN	PC	67. IM	PC	108. IM	PC	149. AS	PS	190. AN	PC
27. IM	PC	68. IM	H	109. IM	H	150. IM	H	191. AN	H
28. AS	PS	69. PL	H	110. AS	PC	151. EV	H	192. IM	H
29. IM	E	70. AS	PC	111. AN	E	152. AS	PC	193. IM	E
30. PL	E	71. AN	PC	112. IM	E	153. AS	PC	194. PL	E
31. AS	PC	72. IM	PC	113. AN	PC	154. AS	PC	195. IM	PC
32. IM	PC	73. IM	E	114. IM	H	155. IM	H	196. IM	PC
33. AS	PC	74. IM	PS	115. IM	PC	156. AN	PC	197. AN	PC
34. AS	PC	75. IM	H	116. AN	PC	157. IM	PS	198. AN	PC
35. IM	PC	76. IM	H	117. IM	E	158. AN	PS	199. IM	PC
36. EV	PC	77. AN	PS	118. AS	PC	159. AS	PS	200. AN	PS
37. AN	PC	78. AS	PC	119. AS	PS	160. IM	E	201. IM	PS
38. AS	PC	79. IM	E	120. IM	E	161. IM	PC	202. IM	PC
39. PL	PC	80. IM	E	121. AS	PC	162. IM	E	203. PL	E
40. IM	PS	81. AS	PC	122. AN	PS	163. PL	H	204. IM	PC
41. EV	PC	82. AN	PC	123. AN	PS	164. EV	PS	205. IM	PC

206.	IM	PC	216.	PL	H	226.	IM	PS	236.	AN	PC	246.	IM	H
207.	EV	H	217.	PL	E	227.	AN	PC	237.	IM	PC	247.	AN	PS
208.	AS	PS	218.	IM	PC	228.	IM	PS	238.	IM	PS	248.	AN	PC
209.	IM	PC	219.	IM	PC	229.	AN	PS	239.	IM	PC	249.	AN	PC
210.	AS	PS	220.	IM	PC	230.	AS	PS	240.	IM	PS	250.	IM	PS
211.	IM	PS	221.	AN	PC	231.	IM	PS	241.	IM	E	251.	PL	PC
212.	IM	E	222.	AS	PC	232.	IM	H	242.	IM	PC	252.	IM	PC
213.	IM	PC	223.	PL	E	233.	EV	H	243.	IM	PS	253.	IM	PC
214.	IM	PC	224.	IM	PC	234.	IM	PS	244.	PL	H	254.	AN	PC
215.	IM	E	225.	IM	E	235.	AN	H	245.	IM	PC			

Section 3: Nursing Care of the Adult

1.	IM	PS	47.	AN	PS	93.	AN	E	139.	IM	H	185.	PL	E
2.	IM	PS	48.	AN	PS	94.	AS	PS	140.	AN	PS	186.	IM	H
3.	AN	PS	49.	AS	PS	95.	AN	PS	141.	AN	PS	187.	AS	PS
4.	PL	PS	50.	AS	PS	96.	AN	PS	142.	AN	PS	188.	AN	PS
5.	AS	PS	51.	AS	PS	97.	AS	PS	143.	IM	E	189.	IM	E
6.	AN	PS	52.	AN	PS	98.	AN	PS	144.	AS	PS	190.	AS	PS
7.	AS	PS	53.	IM	E	99.	IM	H	145.	PL	E	191.	AS	PS
8.	AN	PS	54.	AN	PS	100.	AN	PS	146.	AS	PS	192.	AS	PS
9.	AN	PS	55.	AN	PS	101.	AS	PS	147.	AS	H	193.	AN	E
10.	AS	PS	56.	AS	PS	102.	AN	PS	148.	EV	PS	194.	AN	PS
11.	EV	PS	57.	AS	PS	103.	AN	PS	149.	AS	PS	195.	AN	PS
12.	AN	PS	58.	AN	PS	104.	PL	PS	150.	IM	E	196.	AS	PS
13.	AN	PS	59.	AS	PS	105.	AS	PS	151.	AS	PS	197.	PL	E
14.	AS	PS	60.	IM	PS	106.	AN	PS	152.	AN	PS	198.	AN	PS
15.	AN	PS	61.	AN	PS	107.	AN	PS	153.	IM	PS	199.	IM	H
16.	AN	PS	62.	PL	PS	108.	AS	PS	154.	IM	E	200.	AS	PS
17.	AN	PS	63.	AN	PS	109.	PL	PS	155.	IM	PS	201.	IM	E
18.	AN	PS	64.	IM	E	110.	IM	PS	156.	AN	E	202.	AS	PS
19.	AN	PS	65.	IM	H	111.	AN	PS	157.	AS	PS	203.	IM	E
20.	AN	PS	66.	IM	H	112.	AN	PS	158.	AN	PS	204.	AN	PS
21.	AN	PS	67.	AS	PS	113.	IM	E	159.	PL	PS	205.	IM	E
22.	AN	PS	68.	PL	PS	114.	AS	PS	160.	AN	S	206.	AS	E
23.	IM	PS	69.	AN	PS	115.	EV	PS	161.	EV	PS	207.	AN	PS
24.	IM	PS	70.	IM	PS	116.	AS	PS	162.	AS	PS	208.	AN	PS
25.	AN	PS	71.	AS	PS	117.	AS	PS	163.	PL	E	209.	AN	H
26.	AN	PS	72.	AN	PS	118.	PL	H	164.	PL	PS	210.	AN	PS
27.	IM	H	73.	IM	E	119.	AN	PS	165.	AN	PS	211.	AS	PS
28.	AN	PC	74.	AN	PS	120.	IM	H	166.	PL	E	212.	AN	H
29.	IM	PS	75.	AS	PS	121.	IM	PS	167.	IM	E	213.	AS	PS
30.	EV	PS	76.	AS	PS	122.	AN	PS	168.	AS	PS	214.	AS	PS
31.	AS	PS	77.	AN	PS	123.	AS	PS	169.	AS	PS	215.	PL	PS
32.	AN	PS	78.	AN	PS	124.	IM	H	170.	AN	PS	216.	IM	PC
33.	AN	PS	79.	IM	PS	125.	IM	H	171.	AN	PS	217.	AS	PS
34.	AN	PS	80.	AN	PS	126.	AN	E	172.	IM	E	218.	IM	PS
35.	AN	PS	81.	AN	PS	127.	AN	PS	173.	IM	E	219.	IM	PC
36.	AN	PS	82.	AS	PS	128.	AN	PS	174.	IM	E	220.	IM	PS
37.	AN	PS	83.	AN	PS	129.	AN	PS	175.	AN	PS	221.	IM	PS
38.	AN	PS	84.	AS	PS	130.	AN	PS	176.	IM	PS	222.	IM	H
39.	AS	PS	85.	AS	PS	131.	AN	PS	177.	PL	E	223.	IM	H
40.	IM	PS	86.	AS	PS	132.	AN	PS	178.	IM	H	224.	AS	PS
41.	IM	H	87.	AS	PS	133.	AN	PS	179.	AN	PS	225.	PL	E
42.	PL	H	88.	PL	E	134.	AN	PS	180.	AN	PS	226.	PL	E
43.	AN	H	89.	AN	PS	135.	AN	PS	181.	IM	PS	227.	AS	PS
44.	AS	PS	90.	AS	PS	136.	AN	PS	182.	AS	PS	228.	IM	H
45.	IM	H	91.	AN	PS	137.	AS	PS	183.	AN	PS	229.	AS	PS
46.	AN	PS	92.	IM	E	138.	AN	PS	184.	PL	PS	230.	IM	PC

231.	IM	PS	288.	AS	PS	345.	IM	PS	402.	AS	PS	459.	PL	E
232.	AS	PS	289.	AN	PS	346.	AN	PS	403.	AN	PS	460.	PL	E
233.	EV	H	290.	AN	PS	347.	AN	PS	404.	PL	E	461.	AN	PS
234.	EV	H	291.	AN	PS	348.	IM	E	405.	AN	H	462.	AN	PS
235.	IM	H	292.	AS	PS	349.	AS	PS	406.	PL	PS	463.	IM	PS
236.	AS	E	293.	AS	PS	350.	IM	H	407.	AN	E	464.	IM	H
237.	IM	E	294.	AS	PS	351.	PL	PS	408.	IM	E	465.	IM	PC
238.	AN	PS	295.	AS	PS	352.	AS	PS	409.	PL	H	466.	IM	PC
239.	AS	E	296.	AN	PS	353.	PL	PS	410.	PL	H	467.	AS	PS
240.	AS	PS	297.	IM	E	354.	AN	PS	411.	AN	PS	468.	IM	E
241.	IM	PC	298.	IM	E	355.	AN	PS	412.	AS	PS	469.	EV	H
242.	IM	PS	299.	AS	PS	356.	AN	PS	413.	AN	PS	470.	AN	PS
243.	IM	PS	300.	IM	E	357.	AN	PS	414.	AS	PS	471.	PL	E
244.	AN	PS	301.	IM	PS	358.	AN	PS	415.	AN	PS	472.	PL	H
245.	AS	PS	302.	AN	H	359.	AN	PS	416.	PL	E	473.	AN	H
246.	IM	PS	303.	PL	PC	360.	AN	H	417.	AS	PS	474.	EV	H
247.	AS	PS	304.	AN	PS	361.	IM	H	418.	PL	H	475.	AN	H
248.	AN	PS	305.	AN	PS	362.	AS	PS	419.	AN	PS	476.	IM	H
249.	AN	PS	306.	AN	PS	363.	AS	PS	420.	AN	PS	477.	AS	H
250.	IM	E	307.	AN	PS	364.	PL	PS	421.	IM	E	478.	AS	H
251.	AS	PS	308.	AN	E	365.	AN	PS	422.	AN	PS	479.	AN	PS
252.	AN	PS	309.	IM	PS	366.	EV	PS	423.	PL	H	480.	PL	E
253.	IM	H	310.	AN	PS	367.	AS	PS	424.	PL	H	481.	AN	PS
254.	PL	E	311.	AS	PS	368.	PL	PS	425.	IM	E	482.	AN	PS
255.	AS	PS	312.	AN	PS	369.	PL	E	426.	PL	PS	483.	AN	PS
256.	AN	PS	313.	IM	PS	370.	PL	PS	427.	IM	PS	484.	PL	E
257.	AN	PS	314.	EV	H	371.	AN	PS	428.	IM	H	485.	IM	E
258.	AN	PS	315.	IM	PC	372.	AS	PS	429.	AS	PS	486.	IM	PC
259.	AN	PS	316.	PL	PS	373.	AS	PS	430.	AN	PS	487.	PL	PS
260.	AN	PS	317.	PL	PS	374.	AN	PS	431.	PL	E	488.	AN	PS
261.	AN	PS	318.	PL	PS	375.	EV	PS	432.	PL	PS	489.	AN	PS
262.	IM	PS	319.	AN	PS	376.	AS	PS	433.	AN	PS	490.	AS	PS
263.	IM	PS	320.	AS	PS	377.	IM	H	434.	AN	H	491.	AS	PS
264.	PL	PS	321.	AS	PS	378.	IM	PS	435.	IM	PS	492.	IM	PC
265.	IM	E	322.	AN	PS	379.	AN	PS	436.	IM	E	493.	IM	PS
266.	IM	PS	323.	PL	E	380.	AN	H	437.	PL	E	494.	IM	PC
267.	IM	PS	324.	PL	PS	381.	AS	PS	438.	AN	PS	495.	AN	H
268.	AN	PS	325.	IM	PS	382.	AS	PS	439.	AS	H	496.	IM	PC
269.	IM	H	326.	AN	PS	383.	AN	PS	440.	PL	H	497.	IM	E
270.	EV	H	327.	IM	PS	384.	PL	PS	441.	IM	PS	498.	IM	PS
271.	AS	PS	328.	IM	PS	385.	AS	PS	442.	IM	PS	499.	IM	H
272.	AS	E	329.	AN	PS	386.	PL	E	443.	AN	PS	500.	AS	PS
273.	IM	E	330.	IM	PS	387.	AS	PS	444.	AS	E	501.	AN	PC
274.	PL	PS	331.	AN	PS	388.	AN	PS	445.	IM	E	502.	AN	PS
275.	AN	PS	332.	AN	PS	389.	AN	PS	446.	IM	E	503.	AS	PC
276.	AN	PS	333.	AN	PS	390.	EV	PS	447.	IM	PS	504.	AN	E
277.	AS	E	334.	AN	PS	391.	AN	PS	448.	AN	PS	505.	PL	E
278.	IM	E	335.	AS	PS	392.	AS	PS	449.	AS	PS	506.	AN	E
279.	IM	PS	336.	AS	PS	393.	AN	PS	450.	AS	PS	507.	IM	H
280.	IM	E	337.	AN	PS	394.	AN	PS	451.	IM	H	508.	PL	E
281.	PL	E	338.	AN	PS	395.	AN	PS	452.	AS	PS	509.	IM	PS
282.	AN	PS	339.	PL	E	396.	IM	PS	453.	IM	PS	510.	IM	H
283.	PL	H	340.	AS	PS	397.	AN	PS	454.	AN	PS	511.	IM	H
284.	IM	E	341.	AN	PS	398.	PL	E	455.	AS	PS			
285.	IM	E	342.	AS	E	399.	PL	PS	456.	AN	PS			
286.	IM	E	343.	PL	E	400.	AN	PS	457.	AN	PS			
287.	IM	PS	344.	AN	PS	401.	AS	PS	458.	AN	PS			

Section 4: Nursing Care of the Childbearing Family

1.	AS	PS	37.	AN	PS	73.	EV	PS	109.	AS	PS	145.	AN	PS
2.	AN	PS	38.	AS	PS	74.	AS	H	110.	AS	PS	146.	IM	H
3.	AN	PS	39.	AS	PS	75.	IM	PS	111.	AS	PS	147.	PL	E
4.	IM	H	40.	AN	PS	76.	AN	E	112.	IM	E	148.	IM	H
5.	IM	H	41.	AN	PS	77.	AS	PC	113.	IM	PC	149.	AS	PS
6.	IM	PS	42.	IM	PS	78.	IM	PC	114.	AN	PS	150.	AS	H
7.	AS	PS	43.	IM	E	79.	AN	PC	115.	IM	H	151.	AN	PS
8.	AN	PS	44.	IM	E	80.	IM	H	116.	IM	PS	152.	AS	H
9.	IM	PS	45.	IM	PC	81.	EV	PC	117.	AN	PS	153.	IM	H
10.	AS	PS	46.	AS	PS	82.	AS	PS	118.	IM	E	154.	IM	PS
11.	AN	PS	47.	AS	PS	83.	IM	PS	119.	AN	PS	155.	AS	PS
12.	IM	H	48.	IM	E	84.	AS	PS	120.	IM	PC	156.	AS	PS
13.	AS	PS	49.	AN	PS	85.	IM	PS	121.	IM	PC	157.	AS	PS
14.	EV	H	50.	AN	PS	86.	EV	PS	122.	AS	PS	158.	AS	PS
15.	IM	PC	51.	IM	PS	87.	IM	E	123.	IM	PC	159.	AS	PS
16.	AS	E	52.	IM	PS	88.	IM	E	124.	AN	PS	160.	AS	H
17.	IM	E	53.	IM	E	89.	AN	E	125.	IM	E	161.	IM	PS
18.	IM	H	54.	PL	E	90.	AN	PS	126.	IM	E	162.	AN	PS
19.	EV	H	55.	AN	PS	91.	AN	PS	127.	IM	PS	163.	IM	H
20.	AS	PS	56.	IM	PS	92.	AS	PS	128.	AN	PS	164.	IM	H
21.	PL	H	57.	AN	PS	93.	IM	PS	129.	IM	PS	165.	AS	PS
22.	IM	PC	58.	IM	E	94.	AN	PS	130.	IM	H	166.	AS	PS
23.	AS	PS	59.	AS	PS	95.	AS	PS	131.	EV	H	167.	AN	PS
24.	IM	E	60.	PL	E	96.	IM	PS	132.	AS	PS	168.	IM	E
25.	IM	E	61.	PL	E	97.	IM	PS	133.	AN	PS	169.	AN	PS
26.	IM	PC	62.	AN	PS	98.	IM	PS	134.	AS	PS	170.	IM	H
27.	AN	PC	63.	IM	H	99.	IM	PS	135.	IM	PS	171.	IM	E
28.	EV	PS	64.	AS	PS	100.	AN	PS	136.	AS	PS	172.	AS	PS
29.	IM	H	65.	IM	PS	101.	IM	H	137.	IM	H	173.	AS	PS
30.	IM	H	66.	AN	PS	102.	IM	E	138.	AN	PS	174.	IM	PC
31.	EV	E	67.	PL	E	103.	IM	E	139.	AN	PC	175.	IM	PS
32.	IM	PS	68.	AS	PC	104.	IM	PS	140.	IM	PS	176.	AN	PS
33.	AN	PS	69.	IM	PC	105.	IM	E	141.	AN	PS	177.	AN	PS
34.	IM	PS	70.	AN	PS	106.	AS	E	142.	AS	PS	178.	AN	PS
35.	IM	H	71.	AS	PS	107.	AN	E	143.	IM	H	179.	AN	PS
36.	IM	E	72.	AN	PS	108.	IM	PS	144.	IM	E	180.	IM	PC

Section 5: Nursing Care of the Child

1.	AS	H	19.	IM	H	37.	PL	PS	55.	PL	E	73.	AN	PS
2.	AS	PS	20.	PL	H	38.	IM	H	56.	AN	PC	74.	EV	PC
3.	AN	H	21.	PL	H	39.	IM	H	57.	IM	PC	75.	AS	PS
4.	IM	H	22.	AN	H	40.	AS	PS	58.	PL	E	76.	AN	PS
5.	AN	H	23.	AN	PC	41.	IM	H	59.	IM	H	77.	PL	E
6.	PL	H	24.	PL	PC	42.	AN	PS	60.	IM	E	78.	PL	PS
7.	IM	H	25.	PL	E	43.	PL	PS	61.	AS	PS	79.	PL	PS
8.	IM	H	26.	IM	H	44.	IM	H	62.	IM	PS	80.	AS	H
9.	IM	H	27.	IM	E	45.	IM	PS	63.	PL	PS	81.	AS	PS
10.	IM	H	28.	AN	E	46.	IM	PS	64.	IM	PS	82.	PL	PS
11.	IM	PS	29.	PL	PS	47.	PL	H	65.	AN	PS	83.	PL	H
12.	IM	H	30.	AN	E	48.	EV	PS	66.	IM	PS	84.	AS	H
13.	AS	PC	31.	AN	PS	49.	AS	H	67.	AS	PS	85.	PL	PS
14.	IM	PS	32.	IM	E	50.	AS	PS	68.	AN	PS	86.	AN	PS
15.	PL	H	33.	AN	E	51.	IM	H	69.	PL	PS	87.	IM	PS
16.	AS	PS	34.	AS	PC	52.	IM	H	70.	PL	PS	88.	AN	PS
17.	IM	H	35.	AN	PS	53.	IM	H	71.	EV	H	89.	IM	PS
18.	AN	PC	36.	AS	PS	54.	AN	PS	72.	IM	PC	90.	AS	PS

91. IM H	117. AN PS	143. AN PC	169. PL H	195. AN PS
92. AN PS	118. AN PS	144. IM PC	170. AS PS	196. AS PS
93. AS H	119. AN H	145. PL PS	171. PL H	197. IM H
94. IM PS	120. IM H	146. IM E	172. AS PS	198. IM PC
95. IM PC	121. PL PS	147. IM H	173. AN PS	199. IM E
96. AN PC	122. IM PS	148. AN PC	174. AN PC	200. PL PS
97. PL E	123. IM PS	149. AN PC	175. IM E	201. AN H
98. IM H	124. AN PS	150. IM PC	176. IM PS	202. IM PS
99. AS PS	125. AN PS	151. IM PC	177. PL PS	203. IM PS
100. AS PS	126. AN PS	152. AS PS	178. IM PS	204. IM PS
101. IM E	127. IM PS	153. PL PS	179. AN PS	205. AS H
102. IM H	128. IM PS	154. PL PS	180. IM PS	206. AN PS
103. AS PS	129. IM PC	155. IM PS	181. EV PS	207. AN PS
104. PL PC	130. PL H	156. IM PS	182. AS PS	208. PL PS
105. AN PS	131. EV H	157. IM E	183. AS PS	209. AN PS
106. IM PS	132. IM PC	158. IM E	184. PL PS	210. AN PS
107. AN PS	133. AN PC	159. IM E	185. AS PS	211. IM PS
108. EV H	134. AS H	160. IM PS	186. IM E	212. AN PS
109. AS H	135. AN E	161. IM PS	187. EV PS	213. AS PS
110. AS PS	136. PL E	162. PL E	188. IM PS	214. IM H
111. AS PS	137. IM E	163. IM PS	189. IM PS	215. PL PS
112. AS H	138. IM H	164. IM PS	190. AS H	216. PL PS
113. IM PC	139. AN PC	165. AS H	191. AS PS	217. PL H
114. IM PC	140. AS PC	166. AS PS	192. AN PC	218. IM H
115. IM PC	141. EV H	167. IM H	193. AN PC	
116. AS PS	142. AS H	168. IM H	194. IM H	

Section 6: Sample Tests
Test 1, Book I

1. AS E	20. AN PS	39. AN PC	58. IM H	77. AS PC
2. AS PS	21. IM PS	40. IM PC	59. PL E	78. IM E
3. IM E	22. IM PS	41. IM PC	60. IM PS	79. IM PC
4. PL E	23. AN PS	42. IM PC	61. AS PS	80. IM PC
5. AN PC	24. AS PS	43. AN PC	62. AS E	81. PL PC
6. AS PC	25. IM H	44. IM PC	63. IM H	82. EV PC
7. IM E	26. IM PS	45. AS PS	64. IM H	83. PL PC
8. AN PC	27. IM H	46. IM PS	65. IM PS	84. IM PS
9. AN PC	28. IM H	47. AN PS	66. AN PS	85. IM PS
10. EV PC	29. AS PS	48. AS PS	67. AN PS	86. AN PC
11. EV PC	30. AS PS	49. AS PS	68. AN PS	87. AN PS
12. AS PS	31. AN PS	50. AS PS	69. AN PS	88. IM E
13. AN PS	32. IM PS	51. PL E	70. EV H	89. AN PC
14. IM PS	33. IM E	52. AN PS	71. AN PS	90. AS PS
15. AN PS	34. AN PS	53. AN PS	72. IM PS	91. AN PS
16. AN PS	35. AN PS	54. IM H	73. IM PS	92. IM PS
17. PL PS	36. AN PC	55. EV H	74. PL PS	93. PL PS
18. IM E	37. AN PC	56. IM PC	75. AN PC	94. AN PS
19. PL E	38. IM PC	57. AS PS	76. AN PC	95. AN PS

Test 1, Book II

1. IM E	7. AS PS	13. AN PS	19. IM PS	25. IM PS
2. AN PS	8. AN H	14. AN PS	20. AS PS	26. AN PC
3. IM PS	9. PL PC	15. AN PS	21. AN PS	27. IM PC
4. AN PS	10. AN PS	16. AN PS	22. AS PS	28. AN PS
5. AS PS	11. AS PS	17. AN PS	23. IM E	29. AN PS
6. AN PS	12. IM PS	18. AS PS	24. IM H	30. PL E

31.	AS	PS		44.	AN	PC		57.	IM	PC		70.	PL	PS		83.	AN	PS
32.	AN	PS		45.	IM	PC		58.	AS	H		71.	PL	E		84.	PL	E
33.	IM	H		46.	PL	PC		59.	AN	PS		72.	IM	PC		85.	IM	PS
34.	PL	PS		47.	PL	E		60.	AS	PS		73.	IM	PC		86.	EV	PS
35.	EV	H		48.	IM	PC		61.	IM	E		74.	AN	PS		87.	AN	PS
36.	AS	PS		49.	IM	PC		62.	AN	PS		75.	AN	PS		88.	IM	PS
37.	IM	PS		50.	IM	PC		63.	AS	PS		76.	AN	PS		89.	AS	PS
38.	AS	PS		51.	IM	PC		64.	PL	PS		77.	IM	PC		90.	PL	PS
39.	AS	PS		52.	EV	PC		65.	AN	PS		78.	IM	PC		91.	AN	PS
40.	AS	PS		53.	AS	H		66.	EV	PS		79.	IM	PC		92.	IM	H
41.	PL	E		54.	AN	PS		67.	IM	E		80.	EV	PC		93.	IM	PS
42.	PL	PS		55.	PL	E		68.	PL	PS		81.	IM	H		94.	AN	PS
43.	AN	H		56.	PL	H		69.	AS	PS		82.	IM	PC		95.	AN	PS

Test 1, Book III

1.	AN	PS		20.	AS	PS		39.	AN	PS		58.	IM	PC		77.	IM	E
2.	AS	PS		21.	AS	PS		40.	AN	PS		59.	IM	PC		78.	AN	PS
3.	PL	E		22.	PL	E		41.	IM	PS		60.	AN	PS		79.	AS	PS
4.	IM	PC		23.	PL	E		42.	AN	PS		61.	AS	PS		80.	EV	PS
5.	IM	H		24.	PL	PS		43.	AN	PS		62.	AS	PS		81.	IM	PC
6.	AN	PC		25.	AN	PS		44.	AN	PS		63.	AS	PS		82.	IM	PS
7.	AN	PC		26.	AN	PS		45.	AN	PS		64.	PL	E		83.	IM	PS
8.	AS	PC		27.	IM	PC		46.	AS	PS		65.	IM	PS		84.	EV	PS
9.	AN	PC		28.	IM	E		47.	AN	PC		66.	AS	PS		85.	AS	PS
10.	IM	PC		29.	IM	PC		48.	AN	H		67.	EV	H		86.	AN	PS
11.	AN	PS		30.	IM	E		49.	IM	PS		68.	AS	PS		87.	IM	PS
12.	PL	PS		31.	IM	E		50.	PL	E		69.	AN	PS		88.	AS	PS
13.	AS	PS		32.	AS	PS		51.	IM	PS		70.	IM	PS		89.	AS	PS
14.	IM	E		33.	AN	PS		52.	IM	H		71.	AN	PS		90.	AN	PS
15.	PL	PS		34.	AS	PS		53.	AS	PC		72.	AN	PS		91.	AN	PS
16.	IM	E		35.	AN	PS		54.	AS	PC		73.	IM	E		92.	IM	PS
17.	AS	PS		36.	AN	PS		55.	PL	E		74.	AS	PS		93.	PL	PS
18.	IM	PC		37.	IM	PS		56.	IM	PC		75.	AN	PS		94.	AN	PS
19.	AS	H		38.	EV	H		57.	IM	PC		76.	AS	PS		95.	AN	PS

Test 1, Book IV

1.	IM	PC		20.	IM	E		39.	AN	PS		58.	IM	PC		77.	EV	H
2.	AN	PC		21.	PL	PS		40.	IM	PS		59.	IM	PC		78.	AS	PS
3.	AS	PC		22.	PL	PS		41.	AS	PS		60.	AS	PS		79.	AS	PS
4.	AS	PC		23.	AS	PS		42.	IM	H		61.	AS	PS		80.	AS	PS
5.	AS	PC		24.	EV	H		43.	IM	H		62.	AN	PS		81.	PL	PS
6.	AS	PC		25.	IM	PS		44.	AN	PS		63.	PL	E		82.	AN	PC
7.	AN	PC		26.	IM	H		45.	IM	PS		64.	AS	PS		83.	PL	PS
8.	AS	PS		27.	AS	PS		46.	PL	H		65.	AN	PS		84.	IM	PS
9.	AS	PS		28.	PL	PS		47.	AN	PS		66.	IM	PC		85.	EV	PS
10.	AN	PS		29.	IM	H		48.	PL	H		67.	AN	PS		86.	IM	PS
11.	IM	PC		30.	AN	PS		49.	AS	PS		68.	IM	PS		87.	IM	E
12.	AS	PC		31.	AS	H		50.	AS	PS		69.	AS	PS		88.	IM	PS
13.	AN	PC		32.	AS	PS		51.	PL	E		70.	IM	PS		89.	PL	E
14.	AS	PS		33.	AN	PS		52.	IM	PS		71.	PL	PS		90.	IM	PS
15.	AS	PS		34.	IM	PS		53.	PL	PS		72.	AN	PS		91.	IM	PS
16.	AS	PS		35.	AN	PS		54.	IM	E		73.	AN	PS		92.	IM	PS
17.	PL	PS		36.	AN	PS		55.	AS	PC		74.	PL	PS		93.	IM	PS
18.	AN	PS		37.	AN	PS		56.	AN	PC		75.	IM	E		94.	IM	PS
19.	AS	PS		38.	AN	PS		57.	IM	PC		76.	IM	H		95.	IM	H

Test 2, Book I

1. AS H	20. AN PS	39. AS PS	58. AS PS	77. IM PS
2. IM PC	21. AS PS	40. AN PS	59. AN PS	78. AN PS
3. IM H	22. PL E	41. AN PS	60. IM PS	79. AN PS
4. IM H	23. PL E	42. EV PS	61. IM PS	80. AS PS
5. AN PS	24. PL PS	43. AN PS	62. AN PS	81. AS PS
6. AN PS	25. AN PS	44. AS PS	63. AN PS	82. IM PC
7. AS PS	26. AS PS	45. AN PS	64. AN PS	83. IM PS
8. AN PS	27. AN PS	46. AN PS	65. IM PS	84. AS PS
9. PL PS	28. AS PS	47. PL H	66. AS PS	85. AS PS
10. AN PS	29. IM PS	48. IM PC	67. PL PS	86. IM E
11. AS PS	30. EV H	49. IM PC	68. IM PS	87. AN PS
12. AS PS	31. AS PC	50. AN PC	69. PL H	88. IM H
13. IM PC	32. IM H	51. PL PC	70. IM PS	89. AN PS
14. IM PS	33. IM PS	52. AS PC	71. EV H	90. PL E
15. PL PC	34. EV E	53. AN PC	72. IM H	91. EV H
16. IM PS	35. AS E	54. IM PC	73. AS PC	92. PL PS
17. AN PS	36. AN PC	55. AN PC	74. AS PS	93. AN PS
18. IM PS	37. PL PC	56. AN PC	75. EV H	94. IM E
19. IM PS	38. IM PS	57. AN H	76. IM E	95. AN PS

Test 2, Book II

1. AN PS	20. AN PS	39. AN PC	58. AS PC	77. AS PS
2. PL PS	21. PL E	40. IM PC	59. AN PC	78. PL PC
3. PL PS	22. PL E	41. IM PC	60. IM PC	79. IM PC
4. AN PS	23. PL E	42. PL E	61. AN PC	80. IM PS
5. AN PS	24. PL E	43. PL E	62. AN PC	81. AN PS
6. AN PS	25. AS PS	44. AS PS	63. AS PS	82. AS PS
7. AN PS	26. IM PC	45. AN PS	64. AN PS	83. AS H
8. IM PS	27. AS PS	46. AN PS	65. AN PS	84. IM E
9. AS PC	28. IM PS	47. AN PS	66. AN PS	85. IM PS
10. AN PC	29. IM PC	48. IM E	67. PL E	86. PL E
11. IM PC	30. AS H	49. AN PS	68. PL H	87. IM PS
12. AS PS	31. IM H	50. IM H	69. AN PS	88. AN H
13. IM E	32. AN PS	51. IM PC	70. AN PS	89. IM H
14. EV H	33. EV H	52. AS H	71. AS PS	90. IM H
15. AS PC	34. AS PC	53. IM PS	72. AN PS	91. AS PS
16. IM H	35. AS PC	54. IM H	73. AS PS	92. AN PS
17. AS PS	36. IM PC	55. AN H	74. AS PS	93. PL E
18. IM PC	37. IM PC	56. PL H	75. IM PS	94. PL PS
19. AS PS	38. IM H	57. AN E	76. IM PS	95. IM PS

Test 2, Book III

1. AN PS	12. AS PC	23. IM E	34. IM H	45. EV PC
2. IM PS	13. AN PS	24. IM H	35. IM H	46. AN PC
3. IM PS	14. IM E	25. PL E	36. EV H	47. PL PS
4. AN PS	15. PL PS	26. AN PS	37. EV H	48. PL PS
5. AN PS	16. AN PS	27. PL PS	38. PL PS	49. IM PC
6. IM PS	17. AN H	28. AN H	39. AN PC	50. AS PS
7. IM PS	18. AN PS	29. IM PS	40. PL E	51. PL PS
8. AN PC	19. AS PS	30. AS PS	41. AN PC	52. PL PS
9. PL E	20. PL PS	31. PL PS	42. IM PC	53. IM PS
10. IM PC	21. AN PS	32. AN PS	43. AN PC	54. IM PS
11. IM PC	22. AN PS	33. PL PS	44. EV PC	55. AN PS

56.	AS	PS	64.	PL	PS	72.	IM	PS	80.	IM	PC	88.	AS	PS
57.	AN	PS	65.	EV	E	73.	IM	PS	81.	EV	H	89.	PL	E
58.	AN	PS	66.	PL	H	74.	IM	PS	82.	AS	PS	90.	AS	PS
59.	AS	PS	67.	AN	PS	75.	IM	PS	83.	PL	PS	91.	AN	PS
60.	IM	PS	68.	AN	PC	76.	IM	H	84.	IM	PC	92.	IM	PS
61.	AN	PS	69.	AS	PC	77.	IM	H	85.	PL	PS	93.	AN	PS
62.	AN	PS	70.	AS	PC	78.	AS	PC	86.	AN	PS	94.	AS	PS
63.	AS	PS	71.	IM	PC	79.	IM	E	87.	AS	PS	95.	IM	H

Test 2, Book IV

1.	AZ	PS	20.	AS	PS	39.	AS	PS	58.	AN	PC	77.	IM	E
2.	IM	PS	21.	AS	PS	40.	EV	H	59.	IM	PC	78.	AS	H
3.	AZ	PS	22.	PL	E	41.	IM	PS	60.	AN	PS	79.	AN	PS
4.	AZ	PS	23.	EV	E	42.	AN	PC	61.	AN	PC	80.	IM	PS
5.	AZ	H	24.	IM	PS	43.	IM	PS	62.	AN	PC	81.	IM	PS
6.	AZ	PS	25.	EV	H	44.	IM	PS	63.	AS	PC	82.	IM	PS
7.	PL	PS	26.	IM	PS	45.	PL	E	64.	PL	E	83.	AS	PS
8.	PL	PS	27.	AN	PS	46.	EV	PC	65.	IM	PC	84.	AS	PS
9.	IM	E	28.	AS	PS	47.	AS	E	66.	IM	PC	85.	AN	PS
10.	AS	PC	29.	IM	PS	48.	PL	E	67.	EV	H	86.	PL	PS
11.	AZ	PC	30.	AN	PS	49.	IM	PS	68.	AN	PS	87.	AN	PS
12.	AS	PC	31.	AN	PS	50.	PL	E	69.	IM	H	88.	AS	PS
13.	IM	PC	32.	IM	H	51.	AS	PS	70.	AN	PS	89.	AN	PS
14.	IM	PC	33.	IM	PS	52.	AS	PS	71.	IM	E	90.	IM	PS
15.	EV	PC	34.	AS	PS	53.	AS	PS	72.	IM	PS	91.	IM	E
16.	IM	PC	35.	IM	PS	54.	AN	PS	73.	AS	PS	92.	IM	E
17.	IM	PC	36.	EV	PS	55.	PL	E	74.	IM	PS	93.	AS	PS
18.	IM	PC	37.	AN	PS	56.	AS	E	75.	IM	PS	94.	AN	PS
19.	AS	PS	38.	AS	PS	57.	IM	H	76.	EV	PS	95.	IM	H

Index

A = Adult   C = Child   CF = Childbearing Family   P = Psychosocial   T1B1 = Test 1 Book 1   T1B2 = Test 1 Book 2   T1B3 = Test 1 Book 3   T1B4 = Test 1 Book 4   T2B1 = Test 2 Book 1   T2B2 = Test 2 Book 2   T2B3 = Test 2 Book 3   T2B4 = Test 2 Book 4

The letters and numbers that follow each entry refer to the clinical section and the question number. For example: A481 following "Abdominoperineal resection" indicates equation 481 in *Nursing Care of the Adult*.